Case Studies in Emergency Medicine

Colin G. Kaide • Christopher E. San Miguel
Editors

Elena Ko
(Special Pharmacy Editor)

Case Studies in Emergency Medicine

LEARNing Rounds: Learn, Evaluate,
Adopt, Right Now

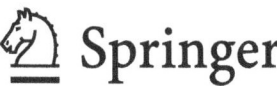 Springer

Editors
Colin G. Kaide
Wexner Medical Center
Ohio State University
Columbus
OH
USA

Christopher E. San Miguel
Wexner Medical Center
Ohio State University
Columbus
OH
USA

ISBN 978-3-030-22444-8   ISBN 978-3-030-22445-5   (eBook)
https://doi.org/10.1007/978-3-030-22445-5

This Springer imprint is published by the registered company Springer Nature Switzerland AG
The registered company address is: Gewerbestrasse 11, 6330 Cham, Switzerland

Foreword

The "holy grail" of medical education rests on three pillars: engaging the learner, providing important clinical information, and ensuring knowledge retention. Colin Kaide's and Christopher San Miguel's *LEARNing Rounds* accomplishes all three and more!

The book starts by engaging the reader with a case, based on an actual patient encounter from the authors' real-life practice, encouraging us to consider how would we have further evaluated and managed the complaint. Clinical information is thoroughly described with priming questions, background on the diagnosis, pathophysiology, and an exploration of how to "work up" the patient and concludes with recommendations for treatment. But none of this matters if the reader does not remember the lessons described—enter the "hook" of *LEARNing Rounds*. To improve knowledge retention, the authors have imbedded throughout each chapter "orienting" boxes with key points, tips on pattern recognition, pictures, and a case discussion by national emergency medicine experts.

It is hard to imagine a more focused and colorful format—in a sea of online education, textbooks, journal articles, and abstract summaries, we now have a resource which will be fun to read and which will not only make bedside care in the emergency department easier but most importantly improve patient care. I can't wait to get my hands on this "holy grail" of medical education!

Michael B. Weinstock, MD
Creator of *Bouncebacks! Emergency Department Cases: ED Returns*
Associate Program Director, Adena Emergency Medicine Residency
Director of Medical Education and Research, Adena Health System
Professor of Emergency Medicine, Adjunct, Department of Emergency Medicine
Wexner Medical Center at The Ohio State University
Associate Editor Clinical Content, *The Journal of Urgent Care Medicine* (JUCM)
Executive Editor, *Urgent Care Reviews and Perspectives* (UC RAP)
Risk Management Section Editor, *Emergency Medicine Reviews and Perspectives* (EM RAP)
Medical Director, Ohio Dominican University Physician Assistant Studies Program
Columbus, OH, USA

Foreword

I wish to acknowledge the expert work of the editors, Colin Kaide, MD and Chris San Miguel, MD and the chapter authors in formulating an informative, instructive text applicable to the general practice of emergency medicine. Much like the specialty of emergency medicine, each chapter is introduced by a real undifferentiated case as they presented to the ED. The case presentation is followed by diagnostic tests, preliminary diagnosis, and initial treatment and disposition in a similar manner to how we typically evaluate, treat, and disposition patients every day in the emergency department. The case presentations in general are more complex and sophisticated than many other case presentation formats and thus lend themselves well to in-depth discussion and teaching. The fact that these are actual case presentations provides a more realistic and interesting approach to the intended emergency medicine provider, be they students, residents, and advanced practice providers or attending. As emergency medicine providers are very comfortable in reading and learning from individual case presentations, this text should be very well received by the emergency medicine community.

Mark Angelos, MD
Professor and Chair
Department of Emergency Medicine at
The Ohio State University
Wexner Medical Center
Columbus, OH, USA

Preface

The initial inspiration for LEARNing Rounds originated in a teaching exercise performed at the bedside with residents and medical students rotating in the emergency department at The Ohio State University Wexner Medical Center Emergency Department. We would find an interesting case and gather around the bedside to discuss the clinical aspects of the case. We would start out with some background about the disease in question and proceed to a discussion of the physiology/pathophysiology involved and then on to making the diagnosis and treating the patient. These were originally called teaching rounds. I would have the resident who was involved in the case write a brief description and some important learning points. I would then edit these, add to them, and send them out to our faculty and residents. Many of our internal medicine rotating residents found these cases to be interesting and a good source of information so we began to distribute them to our IM colleagues. As time went on, the level of complexity used in the writing of one of these documents increased. I thought the name "LEARNing Rounds" would be more fitting as it puts emphasis on the learners' role in understanding, alongside the initiative and innovation of the teacher. LEARNing Rounds was also an acronym for learn, evaluate, adopt, right now. After having spent so much time putting these cases together, I thought it would be a fun and educational endeavor to bring them together in one publication.

The focus of learning rounds is to highlight cases that were not so rare as to reach the status of "Zebra" but at the same time were not bread-and-butter emergency medicine presentations. The goal was to create the right mix of diagnoses that were very clinically important but not regularly seen by emergency physicians. In a Grand Rounds lecture I have given a number of times, I referred to these as "syndromes you can't afford to miss."

In this book, I and my coeditor attempt to create a case-based approach to learning about these selected topics that would be fun and creative and help to cement fundamental concepts in the minds of the readers. We focused on providing enough information on each diagnosis to be practical without creating an exhaustive treatise on the subject. We began by soliciting the attendings and residents in our department and in other programs to find interesting and not-so-common cases that would be best suited to our format. The plan was to pair a resident with an attending to create a chapter using our format. We even have a few medical student-attending and attending-attending chapters. The response was excellent with more cases proposed than we could put together in a single book! As very involved editors (and co-authors of many cases), we provided our writers with images and drawings and any help possible to make their cases fun and memorable.

To put this book together, I chose my coeditor wisely! Dr. Christopher San Miguel was well known to me, having completed his EM residency at OSU, where he was a chief resident and resident lecturer of the year. He also completed an education fellowship in our EM program. His dedication to both the practice of emergency medicine and his passion for education made him the perfect choice. We also engaged one of our former emergency medicine pharmacy fellows extraordinaire, Elena Ko, to assist with editing chapters that were heavy in pharmacology. She brought a very specialized knowledge to the book and helped us immensely to assure the reader of accurate and up-to-date drug information.

We would like to extend a huge thanks to the many very knowledgeable and motivated contributors to this book for their interesting cases, personal experiences, and passion for education. We could never have gotten this done without their contributions!

We sincerely hope you enjoy and learn from this book as much as we did in developing and editing the content.

Colin G. Kaide

I want to be clear and say that the concept for this book and all the legwork for what went into its evolution over the years is the byproduct of Colin Kaide's excellent work as an educator. When he approached me with the offer to join him in bringing his ideas through to publication, I was honored and immediately agreed to coedit this project. As a resident, Colin was one of my favorite attendings. In addition to being an excellent clinician and overall great guy, Colin always asks the question, "Why?" His natural curiosity leads him to develop a deeper level of understanding of clinical medicine than even other excellent clinicians. At the same time, he is remarkably practical and doesn't get bogged down in unnecessary details. This unique combination of traits allows him to bring a deeper level of comprehension to his learners while keeping them actively engaged. It was our goal to bring those same characteristics to print in this book. This is not meant to be an introduction to emergency medicine text. I envision this as the text to read as a second-year resident. The basics have already been learned, and you now need to learn about the uncommon pathologies or unique situations that may encounter in your emergency department. It helps the clinician clinically think through their next patient encounter and ask the question, "Is there anything else I need to be worried about?" I hope you find that this book helps inform your clinical practice and allows you to continue providing excellent emergent care.

Christopher E. San Miguel

Contents

About the Editors

Colin Kaide is an associate professor of emergency medicine at the Wexner Medical Center at The Ohio State University (OSU) in Columbus, Ohio. As a native of Chicago, Illinois, he completed Undergraduate Studies and Medical School at the University of Illinois, Urbana-Champaign. He completed a residency in emergency medicine at the Ohio State University (1993–1996). After residency, he served as the assistant director of the emergency department in Lima, Ohio, for 3 years while serving as part-time faculty at OSU. In 2000 he joined the department at OSU as a full-time faculty member. He is board-certified in emergency medicine and hyperbaric medicine. In addition to emergency medicine and hyperbarics, he completed advanced training in wound care and is certified by the Council for Medical Education and Testing.

His academic interests include medical education, rapid-sequence intubation and the advanced management of the difficult airway, hematological and oncological disorders, anticoagulation and its reversal, procedural sedation, and hyperbaric medicine. He was honored as "Teacher of the Year" for the Department of Emergency Medicine (2008) and has received both the OSU College of Medicine Excellence in Teaching Award (2004) and Outstanding Teaching Award (2008). At the 2017 American College of Emergency Physicians (ACEP) Scientific Assembly, he was presented with the 2016–2017 Outstanding Speaker of the Year Award. This award is designed to recognize a single faculty member who has consistently demonstrated teaching excellence through performance, versatility, and dependability during ACEP educational meetings throughout the year. He is core faculty in the emergency medicine residency program at OSU.

One of his outside interests is martial arts. He has participated in the combative arts since 1978 and holds a 3rd-degree black belt in Goshin Jitsu. He has been a teacher of self-defense since high school and has developed a specialized course for EMS providers and healthcare professionals. He has also been a principal developer and chief medical editor for a medical software company that produces a computer-based electronic medical record product that creates computerized ED and inpatient discharge instructions, prescriptions, and work excuses with over 800 hospitals using the software and instructions. Finally, he is a lifelong Chicago Cubs fan and was ecstatic when his team finally broke a 108-year drought!

Christopher San Miguel is an assistant professor of emergency medicine at the Wexner Medical Center at The Ohio State University in Columbus, Ohio. During Colin's intern year, he completed first grade, but he did manage to attend a couple of emergency medicine conference days with his father, who was also an emergency medicine intern at the time. He grew up in southeastern North Carolina and attended North Carolina State University as a Park Scholar. He received his MD from the University of North Carolina School of Medicine in Chapel Hill before completing his residency in emergency medicine at The Ohio State University, where he served as chief resident. During his chief year, he received the department's "Resident Teacher of the Year" award. He subsequently completed a medical education fellowship at The Ohio State University. As part of his fellowship and continued professional development, he is pursuing a Master of Education in Health Professions through Johns Hopkins University. His professional interests include curriculum development and innovation, simulation, and cognitive errors in medical decision-making.

Elena (You Jung) Ko is an emergency medicine clinical pharmacy specialist at Hurley Medical Center, Flint, Michigan. After graduating from the University of Connecticut School of Pharmacy in 2016, she completed a PGY-1 pharmacy residency at Maine Medical Center and a PGY-2 EM pharmacy residency at The Ohio State University Wexner Medical Center. Currently, she is tasked with establishing a new EM pharmacy practice at an urban community teaching hospital associated with the University of Michigan School of Medicine. Her areas of interest include anticoagulation reversal, trauma, and precepting with a goal to develop a PGY-2 EM pharmacy residency of her own.

Contributors

Joshua K. Aalberg Department of Emergency Medicine, Wexner Medical Center at The Ohio State University, Columbus, OH, USA

Daniel Z. Adams Department of Pulmonology and Critical Care Medicine, Washington University/Barnes-Jewish Hospital, St. Louis, MO, USA

Eric Adkins Department of Emergency Medicine, Wexner Medical Center at The Ohio State University, Columbus, OH, USA

Leslie Adrian Department of Emergency Medicine, Wexner Medical Center at The Ohio State University, Columbus, OH, USA

Michelle Axe Wright State University, Dayton, OH, USA

David Bahner Department of Emergency Medicine, Wexner Medical Center at The Ohio State University, Columbus, OH, USA

Kimberly Bambach Department of Emergency Medicine, Wexner Medical Center at The Ohio State University, Columbus, OH, USA

Michael Barrie Department of Emergency Medicine, Wexner Medical Center at The Ohio State University, Columbus, OH, USA

Jason J. Bischof The University of North Carolina School of Medicine, Department of Emergency Medicine, Columbus, OH, USA

Department of Emergency Medicine, Wexner Medical Center at The Ohio State University, Columbus, OH, USA

Natasha Boydstun Doctors Hospital Emergency Department, Columbus, OH, USA

PGY4, Emergency Medicine Resident, Columbus, OH, USA

Mena Botros Department of Emergency Medicine, Wexner Medical Center at The Ohio State University, Columbus, OH, USA

Department of Pediatrics – Nationwide Children's Hospital, Columbus, OH, USA

Creagh Boulger Department of Emergency Medicine, Wexner Medical Center at The Ohio State University, Columbus, OH, USA

Lauren Branditz Department of Emergency Medicine, Wexner Medical Center at The Ohio State University, Columbus, OH, USA

Colleen J. Bressler Department of Emergency Medicine, Nationwide Children's Hospital, Columbus, OH, USA

Katherine H. Buck Department of Emergency Medicine, Wexner Medical Center at The Ohio State University, Columbus, OH, USA

Zachary E. Cardon The University of North Carolina School of Medicine, Department of Emergency Medicine, Columbus, OH, USA

M. Scott Cardone Department of Emergency Medicine, Wexner Medical Center at The Ohio State University, Columbus, OH, USA

Justin Carroll Department of Emergency Medicine, Wexner Medical Center at The Ohio State University, Columbus, OH, USA

Andrew D. Chou Department of Emergency Medicine, Wexner Medical Center at The Ohio State University, Columbus, OH, USA

Mark J. Conroy Department of Emergency Medicine, Wexner Medical Center at The Ohio State University, Columbus, OH, USA

Jennifer Cotton Division of Emergency Medicine, Department of Surgery, University of Utah Hospital, Salt Lake City, UT, USA

Priyanka Dube Department of Emergency Medicine, Wexner Medical Center at The Ohio State University, Columbus, OH, USA

Greg Eisinger Department of Emergency Medicine, Wexner Medical Center at The Ohio State University, Columbus, OH, USA

Geremiha Emerson Department of Emergency Medicine, Wexner Medical Center at The Ohio State University, Columbus, OH, USA

Bradley M. End Department of Emergency Medicine, Robert C. Byrd Health Sciences Center, West Virginia University, Morgantown, WV, USA

Jessica A. Everett Department of Emergency Medicine, Wexner Medical Center at The Ohio State University, Columbus, OH, USA

Joshua Faucher Rush Oak Park Hospital, Oak Park, Illinois, USA

Nicholas S. Fern The Queen's Medical Center, Honolulu, HI, USA

Natalie Ferretti Department of Emergency Medicine, Wexner Medical Center at The Ohio State University, Columbus, OH, USA

James Flannery Department of Emergency Medicine, Wexner Medical Center at The Ohio State University, Columbus, OH, USA

Caitlin Hackett Department of Emergency Medicine, Wexner Medical Center at The Ohio State University, Columbus, OH, USA

David Hartnett Department of Emergency Medicine, Wexner Medical Center at The Ohio State University, Columbus, OH, USA

Hani Abou Hatab Harlem Hospital Center, New York, NY, USA

Hannah Hays Department of Emergency Medicine, Wexner Medical Center at The Ohio State University, Columbus, OH, USA

Central Ohio Poison Center, Columbus, OH, USA

Nationwide Children's Hospital, Columbus, OH, USA

Elaise Hill Nationwide Children's Hospital, Columbus, OH, USA

Serena Hua Department of Emergency Medicine, Wexner Medical Center at The Ohio State University, Columbus, OH, USA

Christopher Jones Nationwide Children's Hospital, Columbus, OH, USA

Colin G. Kaide Department of Emergency Medicine, Wexner Medical Center at The Ohio State University, Columbus, OH, USA

Kelsey Kauffman Department of Emergency Medicine, Wexner Medical Center at The Ohio State University, Columbus, OH, USA

Sorabh Khandelwal Department of Emergency Medicine, Wexner Medical Center at The Ohio State University, Columbus, OH, USA

Andrew King Department of Emergency Medicine, Wexner Medical Center at The Ohio State University, Columbus, OH, USA

Seth Klein Department of Emergency Medicine, Wexner Medical Center at The Ohio State University, Columbus, OH, USA

Nick Kman Department of Emergency Medicine, Wexner Medical Center at The Ohio State University, Columbus, OH, USA

Alex Koyfman The University of Texas Southwestern Medical Center, Department of Emergency Medicine, Dallas, TX, USA

Ashley Larrimore Department of Emergency Medicine, Wexner Medical Center at The Ohio State University, Columbus, OH, USA

Christopher Lee Department of Emergency Medicine, Wexner Medical Center at The Ohio State University, Columbus, OH, USA

Cynthia G. Leung Department of Emergency Medicine, Wexner Medical Center at The Ohio State University, Columbus, OH, USA

Seth Linakis Department of Emergency Medicine Nationwide Children's Hospital, Columbus, OH, USA

Simiao Li-Sauerwine Department of Emergency Medicine, Wexner Medical Center at The Ohio State University, Columbus, OH, USA

Brit Long Brooke Army Medical Center, Department of Emergency Medicine, Fort Sam Houston, TX, USA

Christine Luo Department of Emergency Medicine, Wexner Medical Center at The Ohio State University, Columbus, OH, USA

Matthew Malone Department of Emergency Medicine, Wexner Medical Center at The Ohio State University, Columbus, OH, USA

Amal Mattu Department of Emergency Medicine, University of Maryland School of Medicine, Baltimore, MD, USA

Ryan McGrath Department of Emergency Medicine, Wexner Medical Center at The Ohio State University, Columbus, OH, USA

Jennifer E. Melvin Nationwide Children's Hospital, Columbus, OH, USA

Matthew Michalik Department of Emergency Medicine, University of North Carolina at Chapel Hill School of Medicine, Chapel Hill, NC, USA

Jennifer Mitzman Nationwide Children's Hospital, Columbus, OH, USA
Department of Emergency Medicine, Wexner Medical Center at The Ohio State University, Columbus, OH, USA

Brooke M. Moungey Department of Emergency Medicine, Wexner Medical Center at The Ohio State University, Columbus, OH, USA

Michelle Nassal Department of Emergency Medicine, Wexner Medical Center at The Ohio State University, Columbus, OH, USA

Kurt Neltner Department of Emergency Medicine, Wexner Medical Center at The Ohio State University, Columbus, OH, USA

Bridget Onders Department of Emergency Medicine, Wexner Medical Center at The Ohio State University, Columbus, OH, USA

Nkeiruka Orajiaka Department of Emergency Medicine, Wexner Medical Center at The Ohio State University, Columbus, OH, USA

Ashish Panchal Department of Emergency Medicine, Wexner Medical Center at The Ohio State University, Columbus, OH, USA

Michael Purcell Department of Emergency Medicine, Wexner Medical Center at The Ohio State University, Columbus, OH, USA

Yuxuan (Tony) Qiu Department of Emergency Medicine, Wexner Medical Center at The Ohio State University, Columbus, OH, USA

Rahul M. Rege Department of Emergency Medicine, Wexner Medical Center at The Ohio State University, Columbus, OH, USA

Maegan Reynolds Department of Emergency Medicine Nationwide Children's Hospital, Columbus, OH, USA

Grace Rodriguez Department of Emergency Medicine, Wexner Medical Center at The Ohio State University, Columbus, OH, USA

Erica Ross Department of Emergency Medicine, Wexner Medical Center at The Ohio State University, Columbus, OH, USA

Caitlin Rublee Department of Emergency Medicine, Wexner Medical Center at The Ohio State University, Columbus, OH, USA

Christopher E. San Miguel Department of Emergency Medicine, Wexner Medical Center at The Ohio State University, Columbus, OH, USA

Matthew Schwab Department of Emergency Medicine, Wexner Medical Center at The Ohio State University, Columbus, OH, USA

Annaliese G. Seidel Department of Emergency Medicine, Wexner Medical Center at The Ohio State University, Columbus, OH, USA

Meenal Sharkey USACS, Canton, OH, USA

Doctors Hospital Emergency Department, Columbus, OH, USA

Travis Sharkey-Toppen Department of Emergency Medicine, Wexner Medical Center at The Ohio State University, Columbus, OH, USA

Benjamin Smith Department of Emergency Medicine, University of North Carolina at Chapel Hill School of Medicine, Chapel Hill, NC, USA

Patrick Sylvester Department of Emergency Medicine, Wexner Medical Center at The Ohio State University, Columbus, OH, USA

Caleb J. Taylor Department of Emergency Medicine, Wexner Medical Center at The Ohio State University, Columbus, OH, USA

Tatiana Thema Department of Emergency Medicine, Wexner Medical Center at The Ohio State University, Columbus, OH, USA

Betty Y. Yang Department of Emergency Medicine, Wexner Medical Center at The Ohio State University, Columbus, OH, USA

Jennifer Yee Department of Emergency Medicine, Wexner Medical Center at The Ohio State University, Columbus, OH, USA

Bleeding on Anti-Xa Drugs: *"Does All Bleeding Really Stop?"*

Colin G. Kaide and Kelsey Kauffman

Case

Pertinent History

A 57-year-old male presents as a trauma alert following a rollover MVC. The patient was pulled from the driver's seat by a good Samaritan who stopped at the crash site. The patient has been disoriented since EMS arrived and throughout transport by the aeromedical crew. On arrival to the Emergency Department (ED), the patient had a Glasgow Coma Score (GCS) of 13 and was repetitive with questions. He admits to being on blood thinners, but does not know the name of the drug or when he took his last dose.

PMH, SH, FH Unknown

Medication Unknown, possibly a blood thinner.

Pertinent Physical Exam

- BP 105/62, HR 112, temperature 98.2 °F, RR 18, SpO2 98% on room air

Except as noted below, the findings of the complete physical exam are within normal limits.

C. G. Kaide (✉) · K. Kauffman
Department of Emergency Medicine, Wexner Medical Center at The Ohio State University, Columbus, OH, USA
e-mail: Colin.kaide@osumc.edu; Kelsey.kauffman@osumc.edu

© Springer Nature Switzerland AG 2020
C. G. Kaide, C. E. San Miguel (eds.), *Case Studies in Emergency Medicine*,
https://doi.org/10.1007/978-3-030-22445-5_1

- Constitutional: Alert, confused male who appears to be in moderate distress.
- Head: Contusions to the face and scalp with a scalp laceration and hematoma. The laceration is actively bleeding.
- Eyes: Pupils are equal and reactive at 4 mm bilaterally.
- Neck/Spine: Midline c-spine tenderness is noted. No thoracic or lumbar spine tenderness was noted.
- Cardiovascular: S1/S2, increased rate with an irregularly irregular rhythm.
- Pulmonary/chest: Clear bilaterally. Bruising was noted on the lower right chest wall.
- Abdomen: Soft, with abdominal tenderness in the right upper quadrant.
- Musculoskeletal: Extremities appear intact with good distal pulses.
- Neurologic: He is alert but confused and repetitive (GCS +4), he opens his eyes to verbal command (GCS +3), and he obeys commands (+6). His total GCS = 13.

ED Management (21:14)

The patient was a level 2 trauma activation. On arrival his GCS was 13. A FAST (focused assessment with sonography for trauma) exam was performed and showed no free fluid. Direct pressure on the scalp laceration was applied, and bleeding was slowed but not completely stopped. The wound was stapled closed to help control immediate bleeding, but oozing continued. Chest and pelvis X-rays were performed. The pelvis was normal, but the chest X-ray revealed right-sided rib fractures in ribs 10, 11, and 12. With concerning exam findings, a head, cervical spine, and abdominal CT were ordered.

Pertinent Results

Lab results			
Test	Results	Units	Normal range
WBC	15.4	K/uL	3.8–11.0 $10^3/mm^3$
Hgb	11.8	g/dL	(Male) 14–18 g/dL
			(Female) 11–16 g/dL
Platelets	162	K/uL	140–450 K/uL
Sodium	143	mEq/L	135–148 mEq/L
Potassium	4.9	mEq/L	3.5–5.5 mEq/L
Chloride	110	mEq/L	96–112 mEq/L
Bicarbonate	22	mEq/L	21–34 mEq/L
BUN	13	mg/dL	6–23 mg/dL
Creatinine	1.3	mg/dL	0.6–1.5 mg/dL
Glucose	140	mg/dL	65–99 mg/dL
Lactate	1.4	mmol/L	<2.0
INR	3.2	–	≤1.1
PTT	28	seconds	21–35 seconds

Bifrontal Cerebral Contusions

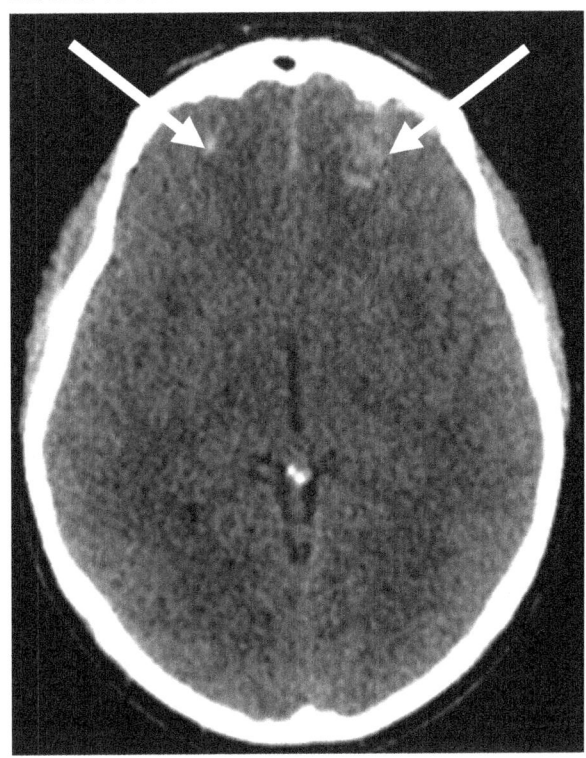

Grade I Liver Laceration

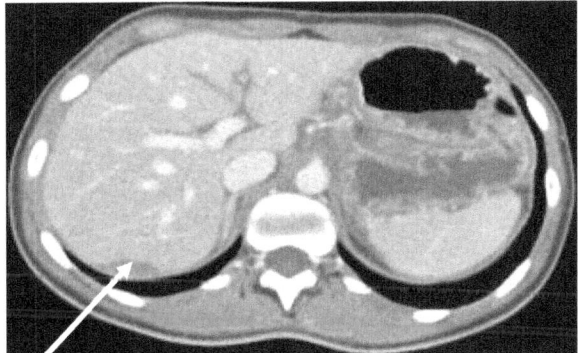

Update 1 on ED Course (21:53)
The patient returned from CT scan, and initial ED physician interpretation of the head CT showed bilateral frontal contusions (left > right). The abdominal CT shows what appeared to be a grade 1 liver laceration (ED attending interpretation). Given the findings in the face of a reported "blood thinner" and elevated INR, anticoagulant therapy was presumed. Initially, the surgery attending wanted to give 4-factor prothrombin complex concentrate (4F-PCC), assuming the patient was on warfarin. The ED attending concurred initially but raised concern for the possibility that the patient could be on a factor Xa inhibitor (FXaI), because the INR was very elevated without a concomitant rise in PTT (which is normally slightly elevated with warfarin due to its effects on the common pathway). Kcentra® (4F-PCC) was ordered.

Update 2 on ED Course (22:05)
While the team was assessing the patient, a social worker obtained contact information for the patient's wife and called to provide an update to her. During the phone call, the patient's wife reported the patient is very good at taking his prescription medications and he took his evening medications with dinner 4 hours ago. She also added the following information:

PMH Atrial fibrillation, HTN

Medications
Lisinopril 20 mg daily
Carvedilol 6.25 mg BID
Aspirin 81 mg daily
Rivaroxaban 20 mg daily with evening meal
Acetaminophen PRN

Because of the new information confirming the patient was on an FXaI, rivaroxaban (Xarelto®), the decision was made to hold the 4F-PCC and start andexanet (Andexxa®), a specific reversal agent for bleeding on that drug.

Update 3 on ED Course (2230)
Just as andexanet was started, the patient began to show signs of deterioration in mental status with his GCS falling to 9. With this change, expansion of the contusion was suspected. The patient was intubated using rapid sequence intubation (etomidate and succinylcholine). He was taken for a repeat head CT, which showed a significant enlargement of the contusion on the left side of the brain. He was admitted to the surgical ICU for monitoring and possible intervention if further expansion was seen.

Contusion CT #2

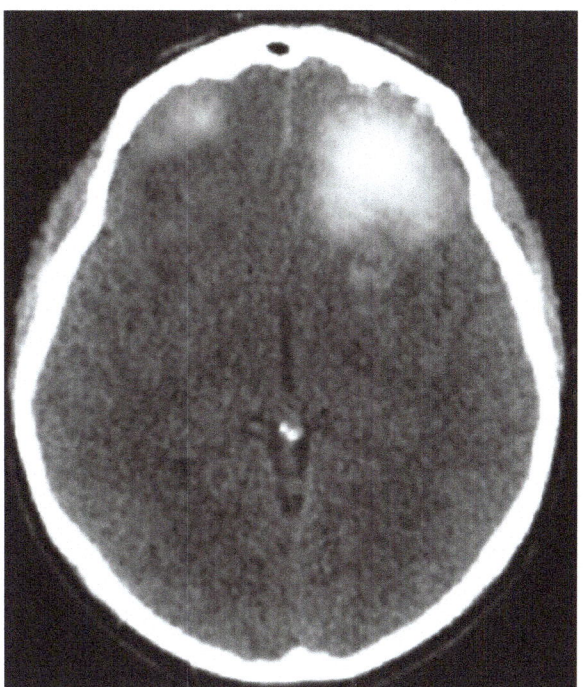

Learning Points

Priming Questions

1. What strategies can you use to determine if the patient is on an anticoagulant when that information is not readily available?
2. What additional information do you need to know to help decide whether to reverse the anticoagulation, or to watch and wait?
3. If the patient is on an FXaI anticoagulant, how should their coagulopathy be managed?
4. Does andexanet work to stop bleeding from FXaI drugs?
5. In the absence of availability of andexanet, what other drugs could be used and do they work?

Introduction/Background

1. Millions of people in the United States are taking an anticoagulant medication for treatment or prevention of venous thromboembolism (VTE) or prevention of thromboembolic complications from diseases such as atrial fibrillation (AF) or a mechanical valve. Of those, a significant proportion are on FXaIs, one type of direct oral anticoagulant (DOAC).
   - Frequency of FXaI use is on a trajectory to increase significantly as there is a desire in the medical community to move away from warfarin. This is further fueled by the FDA approval of a reversal agent that specifically targets FXaIs.
2. Rivaroxaban (Xarelto®) was the first FXaI approved by the FDA in 2011, shortly followed by apixaban (Eliquis®) in 2012. More recently, edoxaban (Savaysa®) and betrixaban (Bevyxxa®) also became available in 2015 and 2017, respectively.
3. As with older anticoagulant medications such as warfarin, DOAC use is associated with an increased risk of bleeding. Clinical trial data indicates annual major bleeding rates range between 2% and 4% with FXaIs [1, 2], and reported mortality rates are as high as 20% [3]. When DOACs first became available, many providers were initially resistant to prescribing them (rather than warfarin) for their patients due to the lack of an FDA approved reversal strategy. Nevertheless, despite this concern, DOAC use has continued to grow. The introduction of idarucizumab (Praxbind®) allayed some of the fears of using the antifactor II agent, dabigatran (Pradaxa®). Availability of a FXaI-specific reversal agent had been an ongoing concern, until recently.

Physiology/Pathophysiology

1. Overview of hemostasis: This overview is purposefully simplified! Non-hematologists only need to have a functional knowledge of this topic as it pertains to management of anticoagulants and their reversal.
   Hemostasis occurs as part of a tightly regulated balance between clot formation and clot breakdown, which develops through an interaction of two independent processes – primary and secondary hemostases.
   - *Primary hemostasis.* When damaged vascular endothelium is exposed, platelets bind via von Willebrand's factor to the endothelium. Bound and activated platelets release various substances, which attract, activate, and facilitate aggregation of other platelets [4]. The efficacy of primary hemostasis depends on both the number of platelets available (platelet count) and the platelet's ability to correctly function during the process. Many medications (aspirin, nonsteroidal anti-inflammatory drugs, and other antiplatelet drugs) can "poison" the ability of platelets to aggregate.
   - *Secondary hemostasis* [5]. The goal of secondary hemostasis (coagulation) is the formation of fibrin. Activation of the clotting cascade can be initiated by two separate pathways – the tissue factor (TF) pathway (a.k.a. the extrinsic pathway) and the contact activation pathway (a.k.a. the intrinsic pathway) *(See* Fig. 1.1).

Fig. 1.1 Simplified coagulation cascade showing parts that are clinically relevant to the emergency practitioner∗. ∗For ease of understanding, Roman Numerals have been replaced with numbers. (Published with kind permission of © Colin G. Kaide 2019. All Rights Reserved)

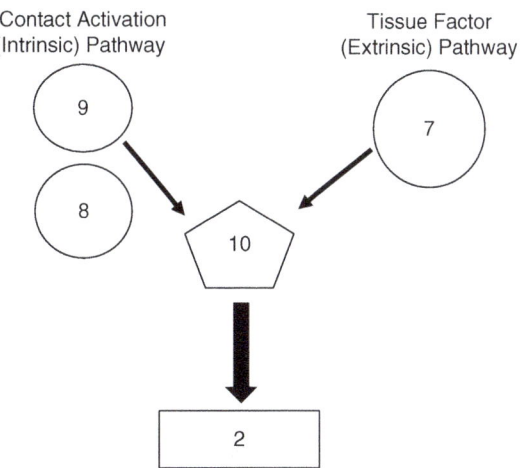

When an injury to the blood vessel allows factor VII (FVII) to come in contact with tissue factor (found on stromal fibroblasts and leukocytes), the FVII–TF complex activates the common pathway, leading to a large thrombin burst. This pathway generates the most fibrin in the shortest time. When collagen in the basement membrane of a blood vessel is exposed, a complex of high-molecular-weight kininogen (HMWK), prekallikrein, and FXII is formed, activating the contact activation pathway. This causes the sequential activation of factors, culminating in the activation of the common pathway. The common pathway leads to the formation of fibrin, which cross-links platelets, strengthening the primary platelet plug. For coagulation to work properly, there has to be an adequate amount of functional clotting factors.

2. Effects of anticoagulants: Using Fig. 1.1, one can explain where all anticoagulants work within the system, making this figure very crucial to know about the otherwise incredibly complicated coagulation system. A more detailed "bigger picture" illustration can be seen in Fig. 1.2.

   - Apixaban (Eliquis®), rivaroxaban (Xarelto®), edoxaban (Savaysa®), and betrixaban (Bevyxxa®) reversibly and competitively inhibit free and clot-bound factor Xa [6].
   - Dabigatran exelate is a reversible competitive direct factor II inhibitor pro-drug, which assumes its active form while in the intestines. Dabigatran prevents the downstream cleavage of fibrinogen to fibrin [7].
   - Warfarin inhibits hepatic synthesis of active forms of vitamin K-dependent coagulation factors, II, VII, IX, and X [8].
   - Unfractionated heparin binds to antithrombin through a high-affinity penta-saccharide. This complex then binds to factors II and X irreversibly [9].
     - Low-molecular-weight heparins (LMWHs) are prepared by depolymerizing heparin. LMWH indirectly inhibits factor Xa activity by activating the antithrombin III complex, similar to heparin. This complex then inactivates factor Xa with some minimal anti-II effect [10].

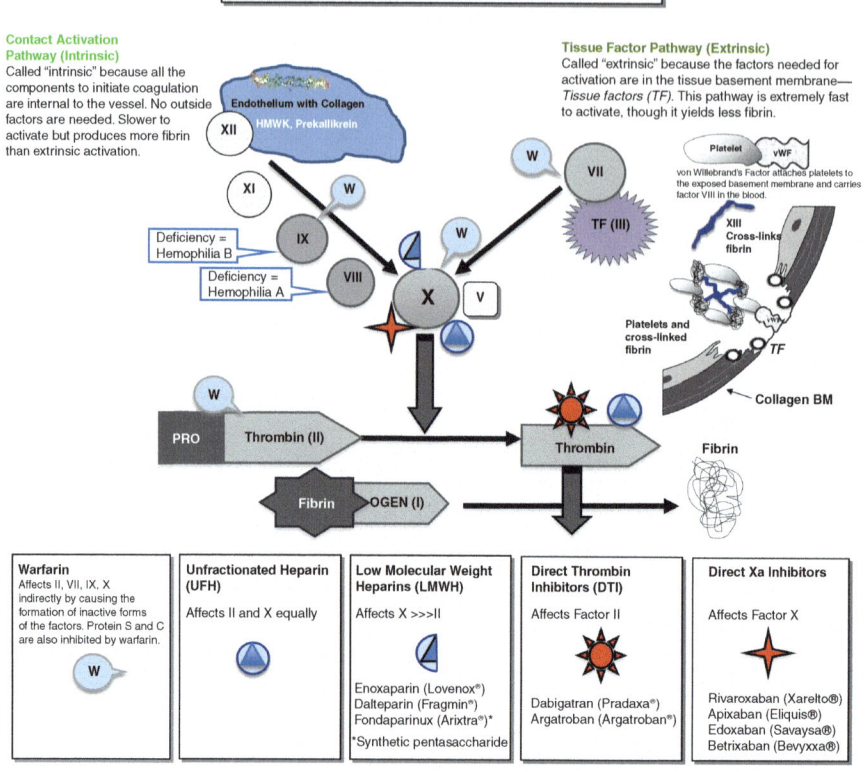

Fig. 1.2 Coagulation and its inhibitors. Published with kind permission of © Colin G. Kaide 2019. All Rights Reserved

– Fondaparinux is a synthetic pentasaccharide that serves as a highly selective factor Xa inhibitor. It selectively binds to antithrombin III to inhibit factor Xa. Unlike heparin or LMWH, it does not inhibit factor II. There is rapid and complete bioavailability, and elimination half-life is 17–21 hours [11].

Making the Diagnosis

Differential Diagnosis[a]
- Anticoagulant therapy with warfarin
- Anticoagulation with a DOAC
- Anticoagulation with LMWH
- Antiplatelet therapy
- Inherited coagulopathy (Hemophilia A or B)
- Inherited coagulopathy (von Willebrand's disease)
- Spontaneous factor inhibitor

[a]Differential diagnosis for inappropriate bleeding in general

1. Consider past medical history, if known. Patients with a history of atrial fibrillation, recent knee or hip replacement surgery, venous thromboembolism, coronary artery disease, and peripheral artery disease will likely be on some form of anticoagulation. FXaIs are approved for all of these indications.
   - Suspicion for anticoagulant use should be high in these patient populations, especially when they present with acute bleeding requiring intervention.
2. Testing the System
   - Activated partial thromboplastin time (aPTT): The aPTT is a measure of the contact activation (intrinsic) coagulation pathway. While the aPTT becomes prolonged in a predictable fashion in patients on heparin, it is not a reliable measurement of anticoagulation in patients on LMWH or synthetic pentasaccharides. The aPTT will however be prolonged in patients who are taking the factor II inhibitor dabigatran (Pradaxa®) in a nonlinear relationship that cannot be used to reliably tell how much anticoagulation is happening with any given level of dabigatran. The aPTT can help to identify a patient who has recently taken dabigatran, in that a completely normal aPTT makes significant anticoagulation very unlikely, especially with a simultaneous normal thrombin time (TT) [12].
   - Prothrombin time (PT): Prothrombin time and INR (international normalized ratio – a way of standardizing PT measurement across labs) measure anticoagulant effect on the tissue factor (extrinsic) pathway. INR is prolonged with the use of warfarin and can reliably predict the degree of warfarin anticoagulation. PT can also be prolonged with the use of rivaroxaban (Xarelto®), an FXaI drug; however, the magnitude of PT/INR elevation is not an effective measure of the degree of anticoagulation. PT/INR may be much less sensitive for detecting the presence of other anti-Xa agents apixaban (Eliquis®) or edoxaban (Savaysa®) [12, 13]. Data has not yet been published on betrixaban.
   - Anti-factor Xa activity assay: Anticoagulation from drugs affecting factor Xa (including the direct agents, LMWH, and fondaparinux) can be measured using anti-Xa activity levels. Newer bedside tests are available that can at least partially quantify anti-Xa activity. These have not yet become commonplace in emergency medicine. Formal, fully quantitative tests usually cannot be obtained in real time, making them less useful in decision making in the ED setting.
   - Thrombin time and ecarin clotting time (ECT): Thrombin time (TT) directly assesses factor II activity by reflecting the conversion of fibrinogen to fibrin. ECT assays test for factor II generation and have a strong linear correlation with the plasma concentrations of dabigatran [14, 15]. Much like anti-Xa levels, these tests are not readily available or used in the clinical setting but mainly utilized in laboratory research (Table 1.1).
   - **Thromboelastography:** Thromboelastography (TEG®) and rotational thromboelastometry (ROTEM®) are functional tests of coagulation, which measure the interaction of clotting factors, fibrinogen, and platelets. The test determines the viscoelasticity of the clot during formation and breakdown.

Table 1.1 Testing the system

Test	Range	Components tested	Medications
Prothrombin time (PT/INR)	12–13 seconds/0.8–1.2	Tissue factor pathway and common pathway (2, 7, 10)	Warfarin, anti-Xa agents (rivaroxaban[a], apixaban[a], edoxaban[a])
Partial thromboplastin time (PTT)	30–60 seconds	Contact activation and common pathways (all factors except factor 7)	Heparin, factor II inhibitors (dabigatran[b])
Anti-Xa assay	0.0	Factor X	LMWH, anti-Xa agents (rivaroxaban[a], apixaban[a], edoxaban), fondaparinux
Thrombin time	12–14 seconds	Factor II activity	Factor II inhibitors (dabigatran)
Ecarin clotting time (ECT)	22.6–29.0 seconds At trough: >3× the upper limit of normal suggests bleeding risk	Factor II activity	Factor II inhibitors (dabigatran)

Published with kind permission of © Colin G. Kaide 2019. All Rights Reserved
[a]PT is frequently elevated with these agents, but a prediction as to the degree of anticoagulation is unreliable with these agents
[b]PTT is useful in determining the presence of an anti-factor II activity; however, it cannot be used to monitor the degree of anticoagulation produced by these medications

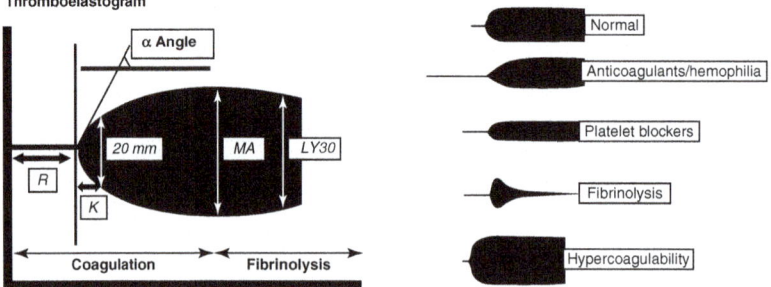

Thromboelastogram

R (Reaction Time) represents the time until initial fibrin formation. R reflects the coagulation factor levels present in the individual.
K (Coagulation Time), from R until the amplitude of the TEG reaches 20 mm.
MA (Maximum Amplitude) describes the maximum strength of the clot and reflects platelet function and fibrinogen activity.
α Angle measures the speed of fibrin accumulation and cross linking and assesses the rate of clot formation.
LY30 is the percentage diminution of the amplitude at 30 minutes after the maximum amplitude has been reached.
It represents a measure of the degree of fibrinolysis.
https://creativecommons.org/licenses/by/2.0/legalcode
By Luis Teodoro da Luz, Bartolomeu Nascimento, and Sandro Rizoli

Fig. 1.3 Thromboelastography and rotational thromboelastometry. Published with kind permission of © Colin G. Kaide 2019. All Rights Reserved

Changes in this parameter are converted into electrical signals, which then form a graphical representation (Fig. 1.3). Measurements of the different phases of clotting and fibrinolysis are shown as changing of the shape of the graphic [16]. Although TEG and ROTEM use slightly different nomenclatures, the results are interchangeable.

- TEG/ROTEM, in addition to the INR and PTT, can improve the understanding of the patient's overall coagulation picture and help guide transfusion of various blood components. Because TEG tracings can identify anomalies in the coagulation process, they can help identify the presence of an anticoagulant and the degree to which it affects clotting.

Treating the Patient

1. Universal measures: Management strategies that should be implemented for all patients with anticoagulant-associated bleeding include discontinuation of the anticoagulant medication, mechanical compression at the bleeding site if possible, and general supportive care to provide hemodynamic support, volume transfusion, and blood transfusion.
2. Determine the need to reverse anticoagulation: To determine if a patient's anticoagulant-associated coagulopathy requires intervention to reverse the medication's effects on the coagulation cascade, consider the following:
   - Is this a major, potentially life-threatening, or uncontrolled bleed?
     - Bleeding at a critical site. Examples include but are not limited to:
       o Intracerebral or any CNS location including intraspinal
       o Intraocular
       o Pericardial
       o Gastrointestinal
       o Retroperitoneal
       o Traumatic bleeding (spleen, liver, pelvis, etc.)
       o Other causes
     - Hemodynamic instability with persistent hypotension
     - Overt bleeding with ≥2 g/dL hemoglobin decrease, or ≥2 units PRBCs administered
   - Is the anticoagulant still present? By establishing time since last anticoagulant dose relative to its expected half-life, as well as considering the presence or absence of renal and hepatic dysfunctions, one can make an educated deduction about whether or not the medication still may be present and exerting an effect in the body. To determine this, ask three additional questions:
     - When did the patient take their last dose?
     - What is the medication's elimination half-life? (See Table 1.2)
     - Does the patient have organ dysfunction that will extend the drug's half-life beyond what is normally expected?

Table 1.2 Duration of FXaI action

Drug	Elimination half-life (hours)[a]	Approximate washout period (hours)[a]
Rivaroxaban	5–9	15–30
Edoxaban	10–14	30–45
Apixaban	12	40
Betrixaban	19–27	60–90

[a]Assumes normal renal/hepatic function, and absence of significant drug–drug interactions

3. Nonspecific reversal: Historically, when the determination was made that a patient on a FXaI required pharmacotherapeutic reversal to manage life-threatening bleeding, nonspecific reversal strategies including 4F-PCC or its activated form, FEIBA® (factor eight inhibitor bypassing activity), have been the only available treatment options [17, 18]. 4F-PCC (Kcentra®) is a concentrated mixture of factors 2, 7, 9, and 10 in their inactivated forms along with protein S and protein C. FEIBA® also contains factors 2, 7, 9, and 10, but a portion of the factors (especially 7) are in the activated form. The theory behind the use of these nonspecific agents such as 4F-PCC, FEIBA, and rFVIIa is that they attempt to overwhelm the effect of a circulating FXaI by supplementing either upstream factors (rVIIa), or factor X along with both upstream and downstream factors. It is important to remember that patients taking FXaIs have normal levels of clotting factors and supplementation (in light of a circulating inhibitor) may not be effective, calling into question the potential efficacy of this strategy.
   - Current evidence from prospective studies examining the ability of 4F-PCCs and aPCCs to reverse FXaI activity in humans is mostly limited to healthy patient populations [19–22]. The one study that looked at 4F-PCC's effect on anti-Xa levels showed measured anti-Xa activity was identical after infusion of saline and 4F-PCC [17].
   - A clinical study (Gemer et al) looking at PCCs given for DOAC-associated intracranial hemorrhage failed to show any decrease in hematoma expansion rate [23].
   - Nevertheless, this approach is recommended by a variety of medical bodies and, thus, is widely employed when FXaI-targeted reversal is unavailable. 4F-PCC is recommended first line for FXaI reversal. Anti-inhibitor coagulant complex, or FEIBA®, is commonly recommended as a second-line reversal option [24, 25]. Although the risk for thromboembolic complications with 4F-PCC and anti-inhibitor coagulant complex use in this clinical scenario likely varies from patient to patient based on many factors such as anticoagulant indication, other comorbidities, and dose of reversal agent used, it should be considered when weighing the risk versus benefit of administering a reversal agent (Table 1.3).
4. Additional nonspecific options:
   - Activated charcoal may be considered if the time of dose ingestion is within 1–2 hours of presentation. Keep in mind this is not an appropriate option for patients with altered mental status, airway compromise, or in patients with

Table 1.3 Nonspecific reversal agent dosing

Factor product	Contents	Dose	Additional information
Four-factor PCC (Kcentra®)	Factors II, VII, IX, and X; proteins C and S; heparin	25–50 Units / kg (maximum recommended dose 5000 units. Repeat dosing not recommended)	First-line treatment option Contraindicated in patients with a history of heparin-induced thrombocytopenia
Anti-inhibitor coagulant complex (FEIBA®)	Factors II, VII, IX, and X	50 Units / kg (may consider redosing for ongoing clinical bleeding after 6 hours)	Second-line treatment option

any other reason for concern of aspiration. The dose is 1 g/kg, rounded to the nearest 25 g.

- Other reversal strategies including antifibrinolytics (tranexamic acid, amino-caproic acid), vitamin K, fresh frozen plasma, and other factor products (recombinant factor VIIa and 3-factor PCC, or Profilnine®) have been attempted in this patient population but have not been shown to be effective and therefore are not routinely recommended.

5. Specific reversal agents: Andexanet alfa (Andexxa®) is now officially known by the FDA-given, new, and approved generic name of "coagulation factor Xa (recombinant), inactivated-zhzo." This is too many words for us, so we will unofficially continue to call it andexanet. Andexanet is the first reversal agent that specifically targets FXaIs to be approved by the FDA [26]. Although it was approved in May of 2018, owing to mass production issues, it only became widely available in February of 2019. It is labeled for the reversal of life-threatening bleeding associated with rivaroxaban and apixaban only. It is a factor X decoy molecule that lacks the ability to participate in the coagulation process and functions to directly bind and inactivate circulating FXaIs [27].

   - In two studies, ANNEXA-R (rivaroxaban) and ANNEXA-A (apixaban), healthy volunteers received andexanet alfa or placebo after being given either rivaroxaban or apixaban. They had a 92% and 94% reduction in anti-Xa activity, respectively, along with almost complete restoration of thrombin generation. There were no thrombotic complications observed [28].
   - The first study to look at the efficacy of andexanet in bleeding patients is ANNEXA-4 (Connolly, et al). Published in the February of 2019, this study looked at 352 patients with primarily intracranial (64%) and gastrointestinal (GI) bleeding (26%). Safety was evaluated in all 352 patients, while efficacy was evaluated in 254 patients. There were two coprimary outcomes – percent change in anti-Xa activity after infusion of andexanet and the percent of patients with excellent or good hemostasis at 12 hours post infusion of andexanet. It came to the following conclusions: [26]
     - The median anti-Xa activity decreased by 92% for patients treated with rivaroxaban or with apixaban.
     - 85% of patients with GI bleeding had excellent or good hemostatic efficacy.
     - 80% of patients with intracranial bleeding had excellent or good hemostatic efficacy.
     - 10% of patients had a thrombotic event within 30 days of receiving andexanet, with 11 patients having the event within 5 days; 11 patients had an event between days 6 and 14, and 12 had the event between 15 and 30 days.
       - Of note, 62% of the patients were restarted on (at least one dose of) their anticoagulation within 30 days. Only 2% of these had a thrombosis after restarting anticoagulation.
   - Andexanet is given as a bolus followed by an infusion that lasts 2 hours. It is believed that during the infusion time, adequate clotting is formed to stop bleeding and, therefore, when the infusion is stopped and anticoagulant effect of the FXaI returns, no further bleeding develops. Exact dosing is based on

Table 1.4 Andexanet dosing [27]

Dose	Last FXaI exposure	IV bolus	IV infusion
Low dose	*Last dose <8 hours or unknown*	400 mg at 30 mg/min	4 mg/min for 120 min
	Rivaroxaban ≤10 mg		
	Apixaban ≤5 mg		
	Last dose ≥8 hours		
	Any FXaI at any dose		
High dose	*Last dose <8 hours or unknown*	800 mg at 30 mg/min	8 mg/min for 120 min
	Rivaroxaban >10 mg or unknown dose		
	Apixaban >5 mg or unknown dose		

the specific FXaI ingested, most recent time of exposure, and the dose taken. Data does not exist to guide the appropriateness or effectiveness of repeat dosing (Table 1.4).

Criteria for Determining Hemostatic Efficacy [26]

- GI bleeding: Hemostasis was considered effective if there was a <10% (excellent) or ≥10% to ≤20% (good) decrease in both corrected hemoglobin/hematocrit at the 12-hour post-andexanet infusion time point, compared with baseline.
- ICH: Criteria for effective hemostasis included serial CT or MRI scans that were reviewed by an independent core laboratory. For intracerebral hematoma, hemostasis was considered excellent if there was ≤20% increase from baseline in hematoma volume, or good if there was >20% to ≤35% increase from baseline in hematoma volume, at 1 or 12 hours post infusion. The assessment of effective hemostasis for subarachnoid and subdural bleeding events was similar, except that the maximal hematoma thickness was used.

Case Conclusion

Shortly after the repeat CT showing hematoma expansion and after infusion of andexanet was started, the decision was made to move to the operating room for evacuation of the frontal hematoma. The patient remained in the SICU post-op for 4 days and was transferred to the floor and subsequently to the rehabilitation hospital for significant cognitive deficits. At 4 weeks post therapy, he had made significant improvements and was discharged for outpatient speech and cognitive therapy.

Discussion

When a patient presents with potentially life-threatening bleeding, determining if an anticoagulant medication is contributing to the patient's coagulopathy is paramount. If the patient is unable to provide any medication history, there are a variety of strategies you or another member of the medical team can utilize to find this information. Be a detective! If you are too young to remember Quincy or Columbo, reruns are available on YouTube! Options include: Interview or call family/friends and ask "what medications does the patient take?" You can ask about which pharmacy the patient uses, as a quick-call to most pharmacies will yield the needed information. You can review refill records available through your local EMR or other similar resource. You can also run a report via your state's online controlled substance reporting system. Though the report will not include anticoagulants, it may tell you location(s) where the patient fills prescriptions. You can then call pharmacies to ask about additional refill history, specifically anticoagulant medications. Results of coagulation parameters such as PT/INR and PTT may provide information. If the next level of testing is available, TEG or rapid anti-Xa levels (or ECT and TT) can be very revealing.

Owing to both financial and more importantly, physiologic costs (inappropriate thrombotic events), it behooves the clinician to decide not only if the patient is anticoagulated, but if their degree of anticoagulation warrants reversal. It is important to understand that patients are on anticoagulants for a reason. They have either a diagnosed thrombotic event (DVT/PE, etc.) or have conditions prone to thrombosis, atrial fibrillation being a classic example. Also remember that even in the face of overt bleeding, sudden reversal of anticoagulation (especially with an underlying prothrombotic state – Factor V Leiden, prothrombin gene mutation, antiphospholipid antibody syndrome, etc.) can lead to thrombotic events. Re-initiation of anticoagulation as soon as it is appropriate is paramount in preventing inappropriate clotting.

Every emergency practitioner should identify reversal strategies available at his or her practice site(s) before they become necessary. Andexanet alfa, the only FDA-approved FXaI-targeted reversal agent, is only beginning to make its way into hospital formularies following its recent FDA approval. Owing to the recent approval and staggering cost (~$25,000/dose), it may not be readily available or approval for its use may lie out of the emergency practitioner's locus of control. Become familiar with alternative reversal strategies. Even then, smaller hospitals do not always have PCC products such as Kcentra® and FEIBA® on hand at all times. If this is the case, starting with blood products may be the only management option available until the patient is transferred to another facility for ongoing care.

Finally, never underestimate the ability of an anticoagulant to make an otherwise simple problem a potential catastrophe!!

Pattern Recognition

- Unexpected bleeding, either spontaneous or after trauma
- An historical reason the patient might be on anticoagulants (DVT/PE, atrial fibrillation, artificial valves, etc.)
- Abnormal tests of coagulation (PT/INR, PTT, TEG, etc.)

Disclosure Statement Kelsey Kauffman has no disclosures to report.

Colin Kaide reports affiliation with Callibra inc. No relevance to this chapter.

Also Colin Kaide provides Lecturing for Portola pharmaceuticals. All possible biases were explored by both authors and every attempt to provide unbiased information was made, including final editing by Kelsey Kauffman who has no Portola connections.

References

1. Patel MR, Mahaffey KW, Garg J, et al; ROCKET AF Investigators. Rivaroxaban versus warfarin in nonvalvular atrial fibrillation. N Engl J Med. 2011;365(10):883–91.
2. Granger CB, Alexander JH, McMurray JJ, et al; ARISTOTLE Committees and Investigators. Apixaban versus warfarin in patients with atrial fibrillation. N Engl J Med. 2011;365(11):981–92.
3. Piccini JP, Garg J, Patel MR, et al; ROCKET AF Investigators. Management of major bleeding events in patients treated with rivaroxaban vs. warfarin: results from the ROCKET AF trial. Eur Heart J. 2014;35(28):1873–80.
4. Sangkuhla K, Shuldinerc AR, Kleina TE, Altmana RB. Platelet aggregation pathway. Pharmacogenet Genomics. 2011;21(8):516–21.
5. Furie B, Furie BC. Thrombus formation in vivo. J Clin Invest. 2005;115(12):3355–62.
6. Roehrig S, Straub A, Pohlmann J, et al. Discovery of the novel antithrombotic agent 5-chloro-N-({(5S)-2-oxo-3-[4-(3-oxomorpholin-4-yl)phenyl]-1,3-oxazolidin-5-yl}methyl)thiophene-2-carboxamide (BAY 59-7939): an oral, direct factor Xa inhibitor. J Med Chem. 2005;48(19):5900–8.
7. Blommel ML, Blommel AL. Dabigatran etexilate: a novel oral direct thrombin inhibitor. Am J Health Syst Pharm. 2011;68(16):1506–19.
8. Frumkin K. Rapid reversal of warfarin-associated hemorrhage in the emergency department by prothrombin complex concentrates. Ann Emerg Med. 2013;62(6):616–26. e8
9. Hirsh J, Raschke R. Heparin and low-molecular-weight heparin: the Seventh ACCP Conference on Antithrombotic and Thrombolytic Therapy. Chest. 2004;126(3. Suppl):188S–203S.
10. Weitz JI. Low-molecular-weight heparins. N Engl J Med. 1997;337(10):688–98.
11. Weitz JI, Hirsh J. New anticoagulant drugs. Chest. 2001;119(1 Suppl):95S–107S.
12. Cuker A, Siegal DM, Crowther MA, Garcia DA. Laboratory measurement of the anticoagulant activity of the nonvitamin K oral anticoagulants. J Am Coll Cardiol. 2014;64(11):1128–39.
13. Cuker A, Husseinzadeh H. Laboratory measurement of the anticoagulant activity of edoxaban: a systemic review. J Thromb Thrombolysis. 2015;39(3):288–94.
14. van Ryn J, Stangier J, Haertter S, et al. Dabigatran etexilate – a novel, reversible, oral direct thrombin inhibitor: interpretation of coagulation assays and reversal of anticoagulant activity. Thromb Haemost. 2010;103(6):1116–27.
15. Nowak G. The ecarin clotting time, a universal method to quantify direct thrombin inhibitors. Pathophysiol Haemost Thromb. 2003;33(4):173–18.
16. da Luz LT, Nascimento B, Rizoli S. Thrombelastography (TEG®): practical considerations on its clinical use in trauma resuscitation. Scand J Trauma Resusc Emerg Med. 2013;21:29.

17. Levi M, Moore KT, Castillejos CF, et al. Comparison of three-factor and four-factor prothrombin complex concentrates regarding reversal of the anticoagulant effects of rivaroxaban in healthy volunteers. J Thromb Haemost. 2014;12(9):1428–36.
18. Mao G, King L, Young S, et al. Factor Eight Inhibitor Bypassing Agent (FEIBA) for reversal of target-specific oral anticoagulants in life-threatening intracranial bleeding. J Emerg Med. 2017;52(5):731–7.
19. Eerenberg ES, Kamphuisen PW, Sijpkens MK, et al. Reversal of rivaroxaban and dabigatran by prothrombin complex concentrate: a randomized, placebo-controlled, crossover study in healthy subjects. Circulation. 2011;124(14):1573–9.
20. Song Y, Wang Z, Perlstein I, et al. Reversal of apixaban anticoagulation by four-factor prothrombin complex concentrates in healthy subjects: a randomized three-period crossover study. J Thromb Haemost. 2017;15(11):2125–37.
21. Brown KS, Wickremasingha P, Parasrampuria DA, et al. The impact of a three-factor prothrombin complex concentrate on the anticoagulatory effects of the factor Xa inhibitor edoxaban. Thromb Res. 2015;136(4):825–31.
22. Zahir H, Brown KS, Vandell AG, et al. Edoxaban effects on bleeding following punch biopsy and reversal by a 4-factor prothrombin complex concentrate. Circulation. 2015;131(1):82–90.
23. Gerner ST, Kuramatsu JB, Sembill JA, et al. Association of prothrombin complex concentrate administration and hematoma enlargement in non-vitamin K antagonist oral anticoagulant-related intracerebral hemorrhage. Ann Neurol. 2018;83(1):186–96.
24. Kaatz S, Kouides PA, Garcia DA, et al. Guidance on the emergent reversal of oral thrombin and factor Xa inhibitors. Am J Hematol. 2012;87(Suppl 1):S141–5.
25. Tomaselli GF, Mahaffey KW, Cuker A, et al. 2017 ACC expert consensus decision pathway on management of bleeding in patients on oral anticoagulants: a report of the American College of Cardiology Task Force on Expert Consensus Decision Pathways. J Am Coll Cardiol. 2017;70(24):3042–67.
26. Connolly SJ, Crowther M, Eikelboom JW, et al; ANNEXA-4 Investigators. Full study report of andexanet alfa for bleeding associated with factor Xa inhibitors. N Engl J Med. 2019. https://doi.org/10.1056/NEJMoa1814051.
27. Andexanet alfa (Andexxa) [package insert]. South San Francisco: Portola Pharmaceuticals, Inc; 2018.
28. Siegal DM, Curnutte JT, Connolly SJ, et al. Andexanet alfa for the reversal of factor Xa inhibitor activity. N Engl J Med. 2015;373(25):2413–24.

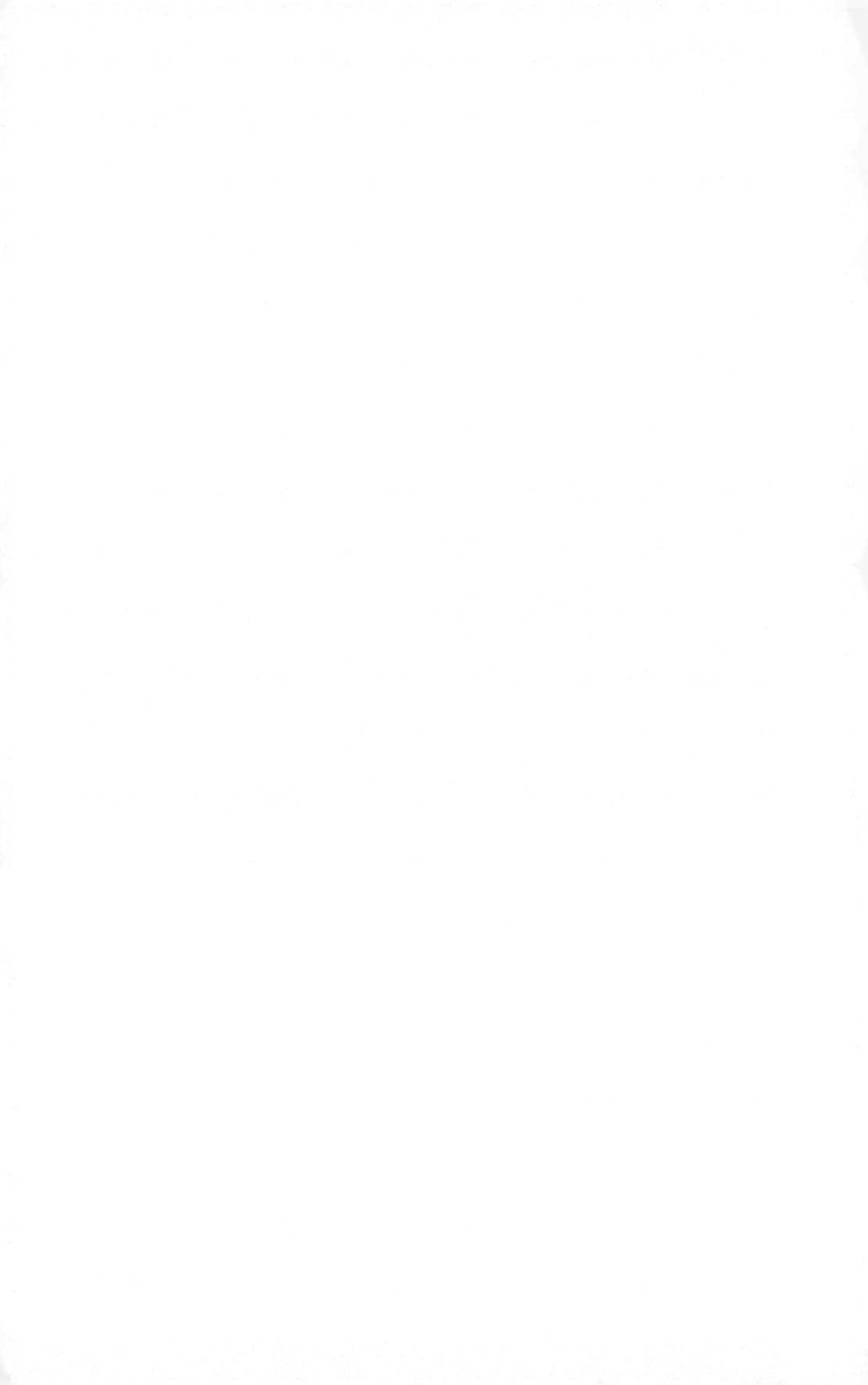

Beta-Blocker Overdose: *"You know, the green pill."*

2

Katherine H. Buck and Colin G. Kaide

Case

Sad, Young, Bradycardic and Hypotensive

Pertinent History A 28-year-old male with no past medical history presented to triage with report of a suicide attempt by ingestion of his grandmother's medications. This was witnessed by his girlfriend approximately 20 minutes prior to arrival. He does not know what medications his grandmother takes, but he reports he took all of the "green ones." Neither he nor his girlfriend knows how many pills were in the bottle. He currently denies chest pain or shortness of breath. He has no known psychiatric history or history of suicide attempts.

His girlfriend shares that he has stopped exercising and meeting with friends, since he was laid off about 3 weeks ago.

Pertinent Physical Exam

- Pulse 45 | Respiratory rate 16 | SpO2 100% on RA | Blood pressure 116/85 | Temperature 98.1F/36.7°C.
- Constitutional: Well-appearing male patient sitting in bed.
- HEENT: Normocephalic, atraumatic. Moist mucous membranes.
- Cardiac: Bradycardic, regular rhythm. No murmurs, rubs or gallops.
- Pulmonary: Clear lung sounds bilaterally.
- Abdomen: Soft, nondistended and nontender.
- Neuro: A&O x3. No CN deficits. No tremors. 5/5 strength of bilateral UE and LEs.
- Skin: No rashes. No wounds.

K. H. Buck (✉) · C. G. Kaide
Department of Emergency Medicine, Wexner Medical Center at The Ohio State University, Columbus, OH, USA
e-mail: Katherine.buck@osumc.edu; Colin.kaide@osumc.edu

© Springer Nature Switzerland AG 2020
C. G. Kaide, C. E. San Miguel (eds.), *Case Studies in Emergency Medicine*,
https://doi.org/10.1007/978-3-030-22445-5_2

No PMH, FH related to presentation.

SH Denies tobacco, alcohol, and drug use.

Pertinent Test Results Within normal limits:

- CBC
- Chem 10
- Hepatic function panel
- Acetaminophen level
- Salicylate level
- Venous blood gas
- UA

Pending labs:

- Urine drug screen
- Chest radiograph

EKG: Sinus bradycardia

ED Management

This patient presented reporting an overdose of a "green pill." Pharmacy was called but without having the pills, it was hard to narrow what he took. As he was well-appearing, our differential remained wide, but with the reported overdose in mind ordered: CBC, chem 10, hepatic function panel, acetaminophen level, salicylate level, urine or blood drug screen, blood gas, EKG. We placed him on the monitor, ordered suicide precautions, and requested that our nurses alert us immediately of any changes.

Update 1

While awaiting the initial workup, the nurse called to report that the patient's pulse was now 30. When we arrived at the bedside, he was newly hypotensive with a blood pressure of 64/palp. As we walked into the room, patient's girlfriend handed us a sheet of paper with the grandmother's medication list on it:

Medication List

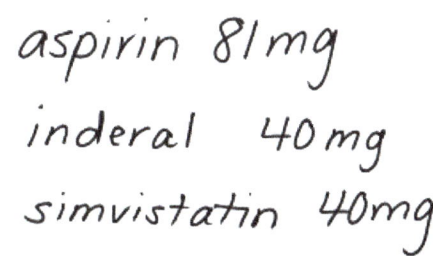

aspirin 81mg

inderal   40mg

simvistatin 40mg

With this medication list and the turn of events, a beta-blocker overdose was at the top of the differential. Our pharmacist was also able to confirm that Inderal (propranolol) 40 mg is a green pill.

Because the overdose was reported to have occurred so recently, the patient was given 50 grams of activated charcoal and 1 mg of atropine. He then received 5 mg of glucagon. Shortly after that, he sat up and vomited a black cloud of charcoal and little green pills. He remained hypotensive and bradycardic and received 5 mg of glucagon and an infusion was started at 5 mg/h along with 3 grams of calcium gluconate. High-dose insulin was ordered as a 1 unit/kg bolus, followed by an infusion of 1 unit/kg/h. After epinephrine was started at 5 mcg/minute, his pressure increased to 100 systolic and his heart rate to 70.

We considered lipid emulsion therapy, since propranolol is lipid soluble but held off initially after the poison center recommended against it.

Update 2

After an initial stabilization of vital signs, the patient again became bradycardic and hypotensive (40 and 60/p). We initiated 1.5 mL/kg of 20% Intralipid followed by an infusion of 0.25 mL/kg/minute. Shortly after starting lipids and titrating the epinephrine drip, the patient stabilized and was admitted to the ICU. After starting lipids and titrating the epinephrine drip, the patient improved and was stabilized. He was subsequently admitted to the ICU.

Learning Points

Priming Questions
1. What is the workup for a suspected beta blocker overdose?
2. How do beta blockers cause toxicity?
3. How do you treat a stable beta blocker overdose?
4. How do you treat an unstable beta blocker overdose?

Introduction/Background

1. The first beta-blocker was synthesized in 1958 (pronethalol). It was never used clinically. Propranolol was introduced in the USA in 1973.[A(1)]
   - Today, there are about 20 beta-blocker agents that are approved for use in the USA.
2. Each year, there are approximately 25,000 overdose cases that include a beta-blocker that are reported to poison centers across the USA.[1(2)]
   - Owing to the wide range of diagnoses for which it is prescribed (including anxiety, stress, and depression), propranolol accounts for a disproportionate number of overdoses and deaths [1].
3. In only about half of the cases (10,500) was beta-blocker was the only drug ingested [2]. Therefore, one must always consider a coingestion, especially if the patient's presentation is atypical for a beta-blocker overdose.

Physiology/Pathophysiology

1. Beta-blockers are class II antiarrhythmic agents commonly prescribed for tachydys-rhythmias, cardiovascular disorders, and elevated blood pressure. They are also used for congestive heart failure, migraine headaches, benign essential tremor, panic attacks, stage fright, hyperthyroidism, and topically for ophthalmic conditions.
   - Therapeutic effects
     - They cause a decrease blood pressure, heart rate, cardiac contractility, and cardiac depolarization through effects on both the SA and AV nodes.
     - They also block the peripheral manifestations of catecholamine stimulation such as tremor, sweating, and anxiety.
   - Overdose effects
     - Hypotension, hypoglycemia, respiratory depression, CNS depression bronchospasm, seizures, and arrhythmias.
2. Sotalol has class III antidysrhythmic properties along with beta-blocking effects. This leads to prolongation of QTc interval, increasing the risk of developing *Torsades de Pointes.* Unlike other beta-blockers, sotalol poisoning can present in a delayed fashion with symptoms developing up to 24 h after overdose.
3. Propranolol has significant membrane-stabilizing effects, acts to block sodium channels, and can cause a prolonged QRS, leading to arrhythmias [3].
   - A "Brugada-like" EKG pattern has been reported in some cases of propranolol overdose [4].
   - Propranolol is concentrated in synaptic vesicles and can interfere with synaptic function by inhibiting membrane ion pumps (sodium, potassium, and magnesium ATPase). This may be the reason propranolol can cause more significant CNS symptoms such as delirium, coma, and seizures than other beta-blockers [5].
   - One study looked at propranolol compared to other beta-blockers in overdose and found 29% of the propranolol overdoses experienced seizures verses none in the nonpropranolol group [6].
   - EKG findings can mimic a tricyclic overdose.

4. In overdose, beta-selectivity is lost and both beta-1 and beta-2 receptors are affected.
5. Lipophilicity can indicate the possible usefulness of lipid therapy in overdose.

Lipid Solubility of Beta-Blockers
- *High Lipophilicity*:
  - Propranolol, labetalol
- *Intermediate Lipophilicity*:
  - Metoprolol, bisoprolol, carvedilol, acebutolol, timolol, pindolol
- *Low Lipophilicity (hydrophilic beta-blockers)*:
  - Atenolol, nadolol, and sotalol

Making the Diagnosis

Differential Diagnosis (Bradycardia)
- Sinus bradycardia
- Primary cardiac events
- Metabolic derangements
- Hypothyroidism
- Ingestion (beta blockers, calcium channel blockers, digoxin, cholinergic medications, clonidine)

---

1. Most importantly, think of beta-blocker overdose as a cause for a a patient presenting with significant bradycardia.
   - This patient presented with a reported ingestion. Not all patients will volunteer this history!
2. Always consider overdose as the cause for presentation in an altered and/or unstable patient.
3. The history provided by potential overdose patients can be is unreliable [7, 8] and you MUST consider beta-blocker overdose in order to treat it.
4. As the situation permits, conduct a thorough history and physical exam and use all resources available to you (family members, police, EMS, etc.) to obtain as much history as possible.
5. Send a laboratory evaluation that will help identify other common patterns of ingestions (e.g., elevated transaminases in acetaminophen overdose or chemistries and a blood gas to uncover an anion gap acidosis which can suggest a differential diagnosis). In some cases, this additional testing can help confirm or refute some suspected diagnoses or indicate a coingestion.
   - CBC
   - Chem 10
   - Hepatic function panel
   - Acetaminophen level

- Salicylate level
- Blood gas
- EKG
- Chest or abdominal plain film
- Urine or blood drug screen

6. The problem with routine toxicology screening is in the interpretation of the results. Even if a qualitative tox screen is positive for a drug, it doesn't tell you if the patient ingested a normal dose or a toxic dose. Further, one needs to know what the particular tox screen in question is capable of detecting. A "negative tox screen" that is not capable of finding the offending drug is useless to you. On the other hand, if a quantitative test tells you the level of the drug in question is above a certain threshold, it can be useful to guide treatment (acetaminophen, valproic acid, phenytoin, lithium, iron, and salicylate levels).

EKG Findings in Beta-Blocker Overdose
- Sinus bradycardia
- Prolonged PR interval
- Widening of the QRS (seen in propranolol overdose)
- A terminal R wave in lead aVR of 3 mm or greater (seen in propranolol overdose—mimics tricyclic antidepressant EKG findings)
- QTc Prolongation, without QRS widening (seen in sotalol overdose)

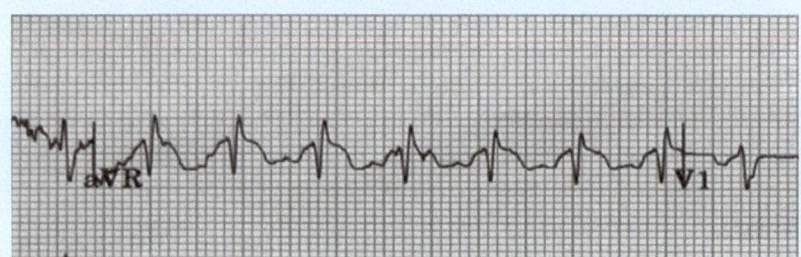

Terminal R wave in aVR—Propranolol OD. Published with kind permission of © Colin G. Kaide 2019. All Rights Reserved

Treating the Patient

1. *Glucagon.* The first line of treatment for a patient with symptomatic beta-blocker overdose is glucagon, which will reverse the effects of the beta-blocker by causing increased myocardial contractility, heart rate and AV nodal conduction.
   - The initial bolus is 3–5 mg intravenously (0.03–0.15 mg/kg × 1 in pediatric patients). The bolus can be repeated. There is no ceiling dose for glucagon, but up to 30 mg (cumulative bolus dose) has been described.
     - Repeat the dose in 10 minutes if the patient is still hypotensive and bradycardic.

- Remember, this bolus will only work temporarily, so start a continuous infusion at the dose the patient responded to. For example, if the patient responded to 10 mg, then start the drip at 10 mg/h. You can escalate this drip to 15 mg/h; however, data on the effectiveness at greater than 10 mg/h is lacking. The pediatric drip rate is 0.07 mg/kg/h.

2. *Insulin*: High-dose insulin has an inotropic effect. The mechanism by which insulin works in these overdoses is not clear. One proposed action is to facilitate glucose entry into the cell. Under normal conditions, the heart uses fatty acid oxidation as an energy source. When stressed, the myocardium shifts to glucose metabolism. This may play a minor role in increasing contractility. Several other intracellular operations involving calcium handling and the phosphinositide 3-kinase pathway are enhanced by high-dose insulin, leading to increased contractility [9].
   - Give 1 unit/kg intravenous bolus of regular insulin followed by continuous infusion of 1 unit/kg/h and titrate to blood pressure goals.
   - As this could cause hypoglycemia, administer concomitant dextrose as a 25 g bolus followed by continuous infusion of 0.5 g/kg/h with frequent blood glucose monitoring.

3. *Calcium*: Increases intracellular calcium and enhances contractility.
   - Calcium can increase blood pressure but does not have an effect on heart rate.
   - Use 1 g (20 mg/kg up to 1 g in pediatric patients) of calcium chloride up to 3 grams in adults OR calcium gluconate 3 g (50–100 mg/kg up to 2 g in pediatric patients) up to 9 grams in adults.

4. *Epinephrine*: Hypotensive patients should be started on epinephrine, chosen for the mixed alpha-1 and beta-1 properties.
   - Start at 1 mcg/minute with MAP goal of 60 and titrate quickly to as higher doses than normal may be required.
   - As higher doses are likely required, this should NOT be the sole pressor used.

Mean Arterial Pressure

$$MAP = \frac{1}{3}\text{Systolic Pressure} + \frac{2}{3}\text{Dialostic Pressure}$$

OR

$$MAP - \frac{\text{Systolic Pressure} + \left(2 \times \text{Diastolic Pressure}\right)}{3}$$

5. *Milrinone*: Consider milrinone as your additional agent.
   - Milrinone (a phosphodiesterase inhibitor) inhibits phosphodiesterasemediated cylcic-AMP breakdown and will improve contractility without affecting heart rate. This works via a different pathway than catecholamines.
   - Give a 50 mcg/kg IV bolus followed by continuous infusion of 0.375–0.75 mcg/kg/minute.

6. *Sodium Bicarbonate*: Patients with QTc greater than 120 ms should receive sodium bicarbonate. Propranolol can have sodium channel–blocking effects in overdose.
   - 1–2 mEq/kg IV bolus every 3–5 minutes until QTc has decreased to less than 120 ms.
   - Consider a bicarb drip if the lipophilic propranolol continues to leech out of the lipid compartment causing persistent or worsening QTc prolongation after the initial bolus wears off.
7. *Atropine*: If the patient has symptomatic bradycardia, consider atropine.
   - 0.5–1 mg IV (0.02 mg/kg in pediatric patients up to 1 mg). Repeat if needed.
   - Be cautioned that patients may have minimal response to atropine.
8. *Cardiac Pacing*: Pacing can also be attempted in symptomatic bradycardia.
   - However, cardiac pacing may be ineffective due to decreased calcium stores and higher than normal voltages may be required.
   - Additionally, if capture is successful, pacing often fails to improve hypotension in beta-blocker overdose.
9. *Activated Charcoal*: This should only be considered if the patient presents within 1–2 h of ingestion; in these patients, it can reduce absorption by 40% [10].
   - When deciding to use charcoal, remember that there is a high risk of aspiration if altered mental status develops.
10. *Intralipid*: Lipid therapy is an emerging treatment for beta-blocker toxicity, but patient selection is paramount.
    - The data in animal studies is unclear, but there are countless clinical case reports that boast success in periarrest patients [11–14].
    - Theoretically, intralipid binds lipophilic beta-blockers, thereby decreasing the blood concentrations. Another theory is that intralipid provides the heart with its preferred substrate of fatty acids. It can also increase calcium in the cell. You can find more information at http://www.lipidrescue.org/.
    - 1.5 mL/kg of 20% intralipid emulsion via IV push followed by infusion of 0.5 mL/kg/minute for 30–60 minutes up to a maximum of 10–12 mL/kg over the first 30–60 minutes.
    - There is no evidence showing adverse events with the administration of intralipid and severe beta-blocker overdose can be fatal.
      - Therefore, lipids should be considered in severe cases of beta-blocker overdose.
11. *Extracorporeal Membrane Oxygenation (ECMO)*: ECMO can be used to provide circulatory support in a patient who is refractory to initial therapy [13]. For it to be effective, it would need to be thought of early in the resuscitation so that if it becomes necessary, the resources can be mobilized to get the patient on the circuit quickly. This modality is usually available at larger medical centers; however, owing to the uncommon nature of ECMO use in poisoned patients, the cardiothoracic team that usually initiates the process may need to be quickly brought up to speed as to the nature of these severe, life-threatening overdoses. It is best to find out what is available at your center or your referral centers BEFORE you encounter a situation where it might be needed.

Mechanisms of Beta-Blocker Overdose Treatments

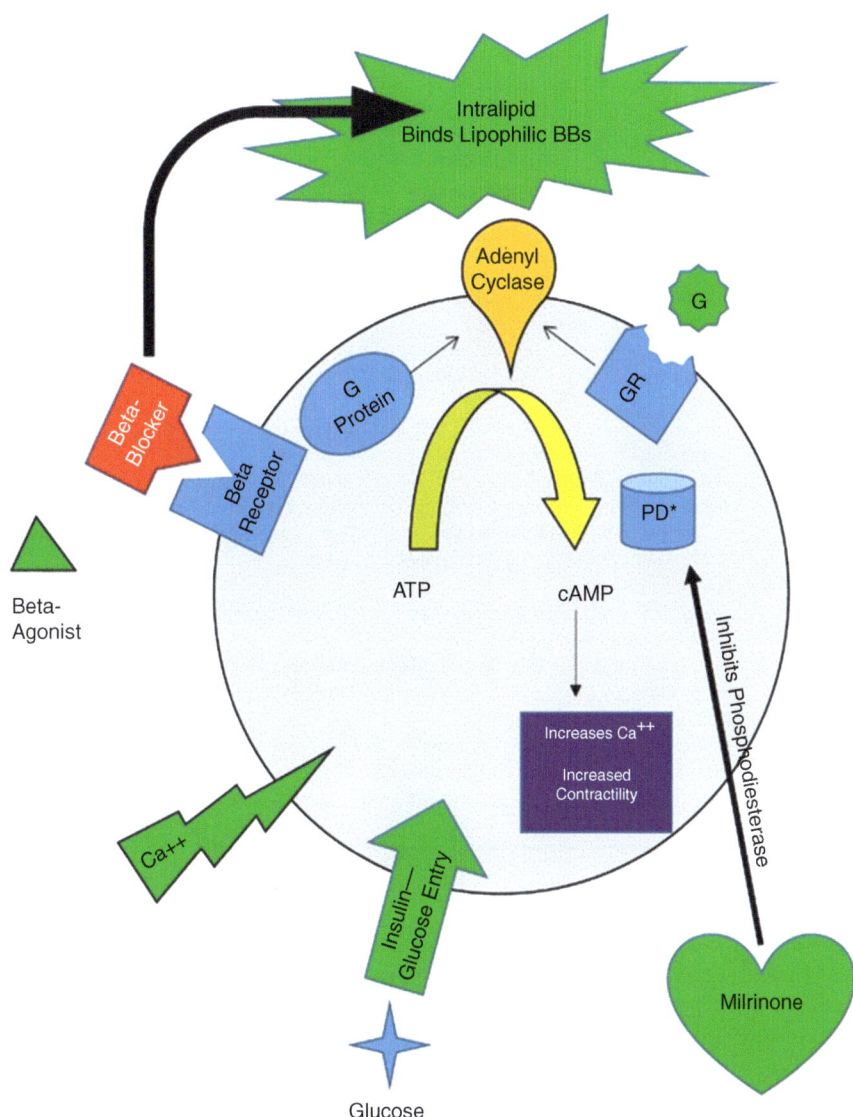

G = Glucagon
Ca^{++} = Calcium
* PD = Phosphodiesterase. PD breaks down cyclic AMP

Drugs for Treatment of Beta-blocker Overdose		
Drug	Dosage	Comment
Glucagon	*Bolus*: 3–5 mg intravenously (0.03– 0.15 mg/kg in pediatric patients). Repeat dose in 10 minutes if needed *Infusion*: 2–5 mg/h (or at bolus dose where it was effective per hour) In pediatric patients 0.07 mg/kg/h	Can escalate the drip to 15 mg/h if needed
Insulin (Regular)	*Bolus*: 1 unit/kg intravenous bolus *Infusion*: 1 unit/kg/h and titrate to blood pressure goals	Dextrose as a 25 g bolus followed by continuous infusion of 0.5 g/kg/h with frequent blood glucose monitoring may be needed
Calcium	*Bolus*: Calcium chloride—1 g (20 mg/kg up to 1 g in pediatric patients) OR Calcium gluconate—3 g (50–100 mg/kg up to 2 g in pediatric patients)	Calcium chloride has more calcium per gram than the gluconate form necessitating a higher dose
Epinephrine	*Infusion*: Start at 1 mcg/minute with and titrate quickly to MAP goal of 60	Higher doses than normal may be required
Milrinone	*Bolus*: 50 mcg/kg IV *Infusion*: 0.375–0.75 mcg/kg/minute	Should be used as an adjunctive to primary catecholamine infusion
Sodium Bicarbonate	*Bolus*: 1–2 mEq/kg IV bolus every 3–5 minutes until QTc has decreased to less than 120 ms	Useful in propranolol and sotalol overdoses
Atropine	*Bolus*: 0.5–1 mg IV (0.02 mg/kg in pediatric patients). Repeat as needed	May not be effective
Lipid Emulsion	*Bolus*: 1.5 mL/kg of 20% lipid emulsion IV push *Infusion*: 0.5 mL/kg/minute for 30–60 minute up to a maximum of 10–12 mL/kg for the first 30–60 minutes	May be effective in lipid soluble beta-blockers

Case Conclusion

The rapid treatment after identification of possible beta-blocker overdose in this case was successful and, after an ICU stay, the patient received psychiatric treatment for his depression which was determined to be related to his recent job loss. After discharge, he found a new job and has been very successful with no return visits or further suicide attempts to date.

Discussion

This patient presented well-appearing and then quickly decompensated. He had a witnessed overdose of "green pills." Most physicians (and pharmacists) will not be able to identify the medication by only this description. However, there are a few clues. The medication belonged to his grandmother, and the patient was bradycardic on presentation. Beta-blocker or calcium channel blocker ingestion should be high on your list of potential diagnoses.

Always be ready for rapid decompensation in beta-blocker overdoses as well as with calcium channel blockers, tricyclic antidepressants, salicylates, organophosphates, and cyanide overdoses. As the physician, when you suspect one of these ingestions, make sure the staff is constantly watching the patient regardless of what else is happening in the emergency department.

Beware of propranolol as it has a membrane-stabilizing effect and can cause significant CNS changes along with QRS widening and subsequent arrhythmias. Sotalol also has Class III antiarrhythmic effects along with beta-blockade and can cause a prolonged QTc, leading to arrhythmias. Moreover, sotalol can have a delayed onset of toxicity.

What if the patient does decompensate? Does that mean you waited too long and should have treated earlier? No. Many of these patients will remain stable and be appropriate for observation. However, when the patient begins to decompensate, you must treat quickly and with all of the modalities available to you.

Dialysis can also be considered in certain beta-blocker overdoses (acebutolol, atenolol, nadolol, and sotalol), but will require time to initiate and take effect. Importantly, dialysis is never effective in calcium channel blocker overdose.

Beta-blocker overdose is associated with PEA arrest [15] and epinephrine may be less effective. If you are treating a suspected beta-blocker overdose and the patient has cardiac arrest, it is important to continue treating the beta-blocker overdose. However, you should also consider what other options may save this patient's life. Sodium bicarbonate may help reverse a long QTc in patients with propranolol overdose. ECMO should be considered early in patients who are refractory to initial treatments [13, 16]. Aortic balloon pumps [17] and prolonged CPR also have reported success.

Pattern Recognition

Beta-Blocker Toxicity
- Bradycardia
- Hypotension
- CNS depression
- Bronchospasm

Disclosure Statement   Katherine Buck: Nothing to disclose
Colin Kaide: Callibra, Inc. Discharge 123 medical software company. Medical Advisory Board Portola Pharmaceuticals. I have no relationship with a commercial company that has a direct financial interest in subject matter or materials discussed in article or with a company making a competing product.

References

1. Brubacher JR. β-Adrenergic antagonists. In: Hoffman RS, Howland MA, Lewin NA, et al., editors. Goldfrank's toxicologic emergencies. 10th ed. Columbus: McGraw-Hill Education; 2015.

2. Mowry JB, Spyker DA, Brooks DE, Zimmerman A, Schauben JL. 2015 Annual Report of the American Association of Poison Control Centers' National Poison Data System (NPDS): 33rd Annual Report. Clin Toxicol (Phila). 2016;54(10):924–1109. https://doi.org/10.1080/1556365 0.2016.1245421.
3. Wang DW, Mistry AM, Kahlig KM, Kearney JA, Xiang J, George AL. Propranolol blocks cardiac and neuronal voltage-gated sodium channels. Front Pharmacol. 2010;1:144. https://doi.org/10.3389/fphar.2010.00144.
4. Rennyson SL, Littmann L. Brugada-pattern electrocardiogram in propranolol intoxication. Am J Emerg Med. 2010;28(2):256.e7–8.
5. Gopalaswamy UV, Satav JG, Katyare SS, et al. Effect of propranolol on rat brain synaptosomal Na(+)-K(+)-ATPase, Mg(2+)-ATPase and Ca(2+)-ATPase. Chem Biol Interact. 1997;103:51–8.
6. Reith DM, Dawson AH, Epid D, Whyte IM, Buckley NA, Sayer GP. Relative toxicity of beta blockers in overdose. J Toxicol Clin Toxicol. 1996;34(3):273–8.
7. Erickson TB, Thompson TM, Lu JJ. The approach to the patient with an unknown overdose. Emerg Med Clin North Am. 2007;25(2):249–81; abstract vii. https://doi.org/10.1016/j.emc.2007.02.004.
8. Perrone J, De Roos F, Jayaraman S, Hollander JE. Drug screening versus history in detection of substance use in ED psychiatric patients. Am J Emerg Med. 2001;19(1):49–51. https://doi.org/10.1053/ajem.2001.20003.
9. Engebretsen KM, Kaczmarek KM, Morgan J, Holger JS. High-dose insulin therapy in betablocker and calcium channel-blocker poisoning. Clin Toxicol. 2011;49(4):277–83.
10. Chyka PA, Seger D, Krenzelok EP, Vale JA, American Academy of Clinical T, European Association of Poisons C, et al. Position paper: single-dose activated charcoal. Clin Toxicol (Phila). 2005;43(2):61–87.
11. Harvey M, Cave G, Lahner D, Desmet J, Prince G, Hopgood G. Insulin versus lipid emulsion in a rabbit model of severe propranolol toxicity: a pilot study. Crit Care Res Pract. 2011;2011:361737. https://doi.org/10.1155/2011/361737.
12. Jovic-Stosic J, Gligic B, Putic V, Brajkovic G, Spasic R. Severe propranolol and ethanol overdose with wide complex tachycardia treated with intravenous lipid emulsion: a case report. Clin Toxicol (Phila). 2011;49(5):426–30. https://doi.org/10.3109/15563650.2011.583251.
13. Escajeda JT, Katz KD, Rittenberger JC. Successful treatment of metoprolol-induced cardiac arrest with high-dose insulin, lipid emulsion, and ECMO. Am J Emerg Med. 2015;33(8):1111 e1–4. https://doi.org/10.1016/j.ajem.2015.01.012.
14. Le Fevre P, Gosling M, Acharya K, Georgiou A. Dramatic resuscitation with Intralipid in an epinephrine unresponsive cardiac arrest following overdose of amitriptyline and propranolol. BMJ Case Rep. 2017;2017 https://doi.org/10.1136/bcr-2016-218281.
15. Youngquist ST, Kaji AH, Niemann JT. Beta-blocker use and the changing epidemiology of out-of-hospital cardiac arrest rhythms. Resuscitation. 2008;76(3):376–80. https://doi.org/10.1016/j.resuscitation.2007.08.022.
16. Maskell KF, Ferguson NM, Bain J, Wills BK. Survival after cardiac arrest: ECMO rescue therapy after amlodipine and metoprolol overdose. Cardiovasc Toxicol. 2017;17(2):223–5. https://doi.org/10.1007/s12012-016-9362-2.
17. Lane AS, Woodward AC, Goldman MR. Massive propranolol overdose poorly responsive to pharmacologic therapy: use of the intra-aortic balloon pump. Ann Emerg Med. 1987;16(12):1381–3.

Acute Blast Crisis/Hyperviscosity Syndrome: *Blasting Off!*

Colin G. Kaide and Geremiha Emerson

3

Case

Pertinent History

This patient is a 74-year-old male who presented to the Emergency Department at 0800 with 5 days of shortness of breath, nonproductive cough, and generalized fatigue. He denied any associated fevers/chills, abdominal pain, nausea, vomiting, dysuria, melena, or hematochezia. He does note a diffuse non-pruritic rash.

PMH
- Hypertension, hyperlipidemia
- Meds: Amlodipine, Simvastatin

SH Smoker (1 PPD × 20 years), denies alcohol or drug use

Pertinent Physical Exam

- BP 135/60, Pulse 102, RR 24, SpO2 90% (RA), Temperature 98.7 °F (37.1 °C)

Except as noted below, the findings of a complete physical exam are within normal limits.

- General: Awake and alert. Appears uncomfortable and frail.
- Cardiovascular: Tachycardic with regular rhythm. No rubs, gallops or murmurs. Sluggish capillary refill. No peripheral edema.

C. G. Kaide · G. Emerson (✉)
Department of Emergency Medicine, Wexner Medical Center at The Ohio State University, Columbus, OH, USA
e-mail: Colin.kaide@osumc.edu; Geremiha.Emerson@osumc.edu

© Springer Nature Switzerland AG 2020
C. G. Kaide, C. E. San Miguel (eds.), *Case Studies in Emergency Medicine*,
https://doi.org/10.1007/978-3-030-22445-5_3

- Pulmonary: Tachypnea with increased work of breathing. Diffuse rhonchi and faint wheezing appreciated in all fields.
- Integument: Diffuse petechial rash.

Petechiae

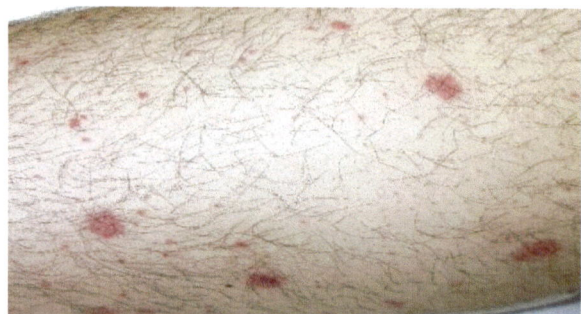

Pertinent Diagnostic Testing

Chest X-ray Interstitial infiltrates suggestive of pulmonary edema. Bilateral peri-bronchovascular infiltrates in the bilateral lower lung zones.

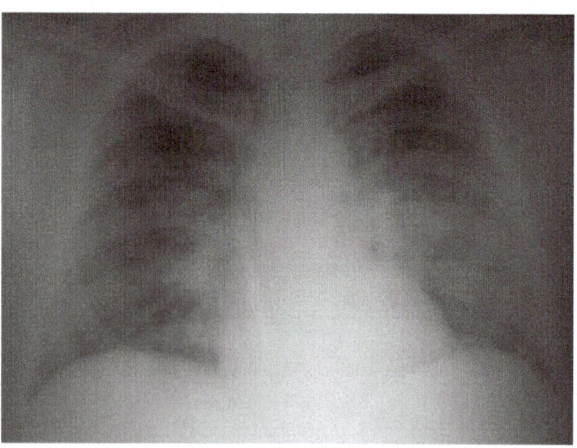

ECG Sinus tachycardia. Normal axis and intervals. No concerning ST segment or T-wave changes.

Plan
Bilevel noninvasive positive pressure ventilation, cardiac workup including troponin and BNP, labs including CBC, basic metabolic panel (BMP), and coagulation studies

- *Update 1 (0900)*: The patient showed some modest improvement in his respiratory status with the noninvasive PPV. He continues to remain tachycardic and afebrile, and as such antimicrobials were held. Laboratory tests were slow to return, which the technicians attributed to multiple abnormal levels.
- *Update 2 (1015)*: The patient remained stable with ongoing shortness of breath and mild tachycardia. Labs returned (see below), and many show marked abnormalities, including marked leukocytosis, thrombocytopenia, critical hyperkalemia, and AKI.
- Cardiac markers returned within normal limits. Concerns were raised for an acute hematologic malignancy, and arrangements are made for transfer to a nearby cancer center. Given concerns for pulmonary edema, IV fluids were withheld, as were antibiotics, given the absence of infectious symptoms. The patient is given insulin + dextrose for the hyperkalemia.

Lab Results

Test	Results	Units	Normal range
WBC	160	K/uL	3.8–11.0 10^3/mm^3
HGb	11.6	g/dL	(Male) 14–18 g/dL
			(Female) 11–16 g/dL
Platelets	62	K/uL	140–450 K/uL
BUN	26	mg/dL	6–23 mg/dL
Creatinine	2.29	mg/dL	0.6–1.5 mg/dL
Potassium	>10	mEq/L	3.5–5.5 mEq/L
Lactate	2.5	mmol/L	<2.0
LDH	1490	U/L	50–150 U/L
Uric Acid	11.6	mg/dL	(3.5–7.7 mg/dL)
Troponin	<0.01	ng/dl	< 0.04
BNP	60	pg/ml	<100
INR	1.6	–	≤ 1.1

- *Update 3 (1230)*: Patient leaves ED as a transfer to the cancer center. Shortly thereafter, a critical alert is called by the lab, reporting that the differential includes >85% blast cells.

Learning Points: Acute Blast Crisis and Leukostasis

Priming Questions
1. What is a blast crisis and in which type of leukemia patients can it develop?
2. What is Leukostasis and how does it manifest clinically?
3. What role do leukapheresis and hydroxyurea play in the management of these patients?

Introduction/Background

1. Acute blast crisis is defined as the presence of abnormal blast cells, either in the peripheral circulation or in the bone marrow.
   - Variably (and somewhat artificially) defined as >20% blast cells [1].
     – Healthy bone marrow contains <5% blasts; peripheral blood should contain no blasts [1].
   - These cells can be lymphoid (lymphocytes) or myeloid (erythrocytes, thrombocytes, monocytes, neutrophils, basophils, eosinophils) [1].

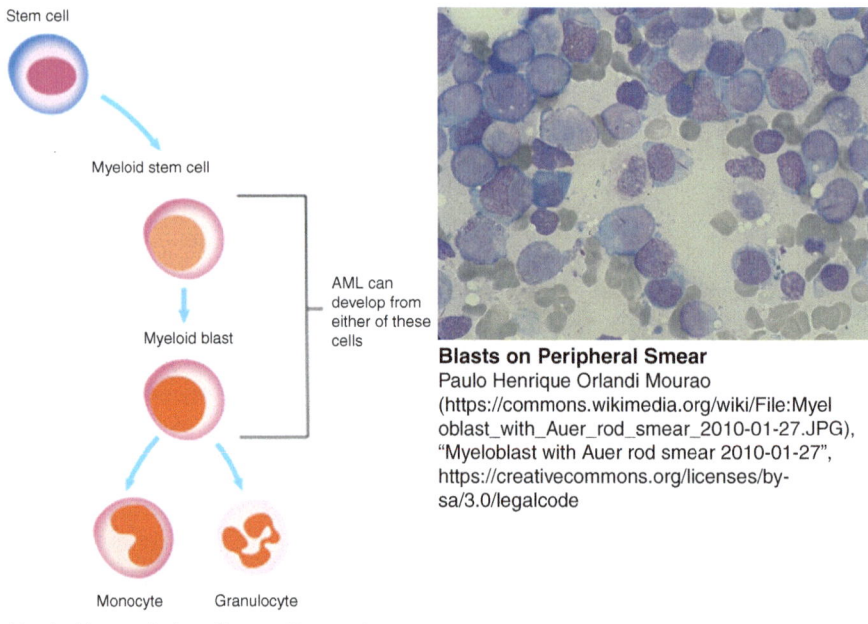

Blasts on Peripheral Smear
Paulo Henrique Orlandi Mourao
(https://commons.wikimedia.org/wiki/File:Myel
oblast_with_Auer_rod_smear_2010-01-27.JPG),
"Myeloblast with Auer rod smear 2010-01-27",
https://creativecommons.org/licenses/by-
sa/3.0/legalcode

Used with permission: Cancer Research
UK / Wikimedia Commons

2. Clinical manifestations of blast crisis can be broadly divided into two categories:
   - Manifestations are related to markedly elevated white blood cell count.
     – Hyperleukocytosis refers to white blood cell counts >50,000/ml.
     – Leukostasis refers to symptomatic hyperleukocytosis and primarily manifests as neurologic and/or pulmonary signs and symptoms.
   - Manifestations related to bone marrow infiltration.
     – Anemia, thrombocytopenia, immunosuppression, and bone pain.

3. Leukostasis is a true hematologic emergency!
   - It is more commonly seen with myeloid malignancies, including acute myeloid leukemia (AML) and chronic myeloid leukemia (CML) with acute conversion to blast crisis.
     - Hyperleukocytosis complicates 10–20% of cases of AML [2].
     - Leukostasis is more common in myeloid malignancies owing to their larger and less deformable morphology, as well as increased likelihood for endothelial adhesion [3].
     - While rare, leukostasis can be seen in patients with CML if there is progression to the blast phase [4].
   - While marked hyperleukocytosis is not uncommon in lymphocytic malignancies (ALL and CLL), leukostasis is a rare complication in these patients.

Physiology/Pathophysiology

1. The pathophysiology of leukostasis is poorly understood and likely multifactorial.
   - Increased blood viscosity results in microvascular accumulation of relatively rigid blast cells leading to vessel occlusion and tissue ischemia [5, 6].
     - Subsequent extravasation of blast cells may produce local tissue damage [7].
   - Liberation of inflammatory cytokines by blast cells leads to endothelial activation and increased cell adhesion [8].
   - High metabolic demand of rapidly dividing blast cells leads to local endothelial hypoxia, resulting in endothelial damage and malfunction [8].
2. The end result of the above processes leads to microvascular obstruction, endothelial dysfunction, and tissue hypoxia with subsequent organ dysfunction. The lungs and the central nervous system (CNS) are most commonly involved [9], though renal dysfunction [10], digit ischemia, retinal damage [11], and priapism [12] are also potential manifestations.
   - CNS manifestations include ischemic and/or hemorrhagic stroke, cerebral edema.
     - Commonly reported signs and symptoms include: confusion/AMS, ataxia, blurred vision, focal numbness/weakness.
   - Pulmonary manifestations include infiltrates (interstitial and alveolar), alveolar hemorrhage.
     - Commonly reported signs and symptoms include dyspnea, tachypnea, hypoxia, rales, and wheezing.
3. Systemic microvascular occlusion and dysfunction may ultimately lead to disseminated intravascular coagulation (DIC).
   - Can been seen in up to 40% of cases of acute leukostasis [9].
4. Spontaneous tumor lysis syndrome (TLS) complicates ~10% of cases of leukostasis [9].

Making the Diagnosis

The Differential: Markedly Elevated White Blood Cell Count
- AML, ALL, CML and CLL
- Leukemoid reaction
- Polycythemia vera
- History of splenectomy
- Recent administration of bone marrow stimulant

1. Leukostasis should be considered in any patient presenting with hyperleukocytosis with signs and symptoms suggestive of CNS and/or pulmonary dysfunction.
2. Laboratory assessment should include a comprehensive blood count with differential and peripheral smear, comprehensive metabolic panel, coagulation studies, as well as LDH and uric acid levels.
   - Most patients with leukostasis are in blast crisis.
   - Anemia and thrombocytopenia are common and related to bone marrow suppression by blast cells.
   - Evidence of hemolysis is common.
3. Evidence of DIC includes coagulopathy, decreased fibrinogen, and an elevated D-Dimer.
4. Evidence of tumor lysis syndrome includes hyperkalemia, hyperphosphatemia, hypocalcemia, and elevated uric acid.
5. Patients with hyperleukocytosis may have markedly elevated serum potassium levels with routine lab testing. This can be the result of in vitro cell lysis after lab draw. This "pseudohyperkalemia" can be corrected by running whole blood samples with blood gas analysis [13].
6. There are no imaging studies that are diagnostic for leukostasis. CNS imaging may demonstrate cerebral edema, infarction, or hemorrhage, while pulmonary imaging modalities may demonstrate interstitial and/or alveolar infiltrates. All findings, however, are nonspecific, and should not be used in isolation to make or refute the diagnosis of leukostasis.

Blast Basics

As a causal viewer of peripheral smears, you will probably not feel confident that you can definitively identify a blast. Further, there are different criteria depending on the type of the blast. You may however identify that some white cells don't look quite right!

No single characteristic identifies a blast. In general, blasts are medium to large cells, which have a large nucleus that takes up most of the cell. They usually have a prominent nucleolus, and much less cytoplasm than you would expect to see in a normal white cell. In promyelocytic leukemia, Auer rods (orange-pink, needle-like cytoplasmic structures) may be seen.

Not all blasts will have all of these features. In the right context (very elevated white cells and symptoms of possible leukostasis), the presence of very abnormal looking cells (purple blobs) can be a big clue that this might be a blast crisis.

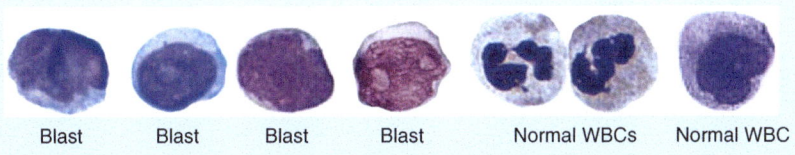

| Blast | Blast | Blast | Blast | Normal WBCs | Normal WBC |

Published with kind permission of © Colin G. Kaide 2019. All Rights Reserved

Treating the Patient

1. The ultimate goal is for rapid reduction of peripheral WBC count, which can be accomplished by leukapheresis and/or emergent induction chemotherapy [2, 9, 14–16].
   - While leukapheresis has been shown to improve short-term outcomes, it has not been shown to improve mortality [17, 18]. Leukapheresis should be viewed as a temporizing modality to provide stabilization until chemotherapy can be safely initiated.
2. Volume expansion with IV fluids can be helpful for reducing viscosity [19, 20].
3. Early administration of broad-spectrum antibiotics should be considered [9].
   - Most patients with leukostasis have some degree of immunosuppression. Remember that blasts are not functional white cells!
   - Fever is common and happens in 80% of patients with blast crisis, though this can be related to cytokine release by blast cells rather than secondary to infection [9].
4. Patients should receive a platelet transfusion to maintain levels of 20–30,000 in order to reduce risk of serious bleeding, including intracranial hemorrhage [20].
5. Red blood cell transfusion should be avoided unless absolutely necessary, as this can increase viscosity and worsen leukostasis [9, 21].
6. If leukapheresis and/or chemotherapy is not immediately available, therapeutic phlebotomy followed by aggressive volume expansion can be considered as a temporizing modality while arrangements are made for transfer for definitive care.
7. In patients with asymptomatic hyperleukocytosis, hydroxyurea is often used to provide the swift reduction in WBC count and prevent complications of hyperleukocytosis, including leukostasis [22].

Case Conclusion

The patient was admitted to the medical intensive care unit for combined emergent leukapheresis and induction chemotherapy. Laboratory tests confirm the diagnosis of acute promyelocytic leukemia, a subtype acute myeloid leukemia. The patient showed initial improvement in his respiratory symptoms. However, within 1 week of diagnosis, the patient experienced a decompensation with fever, altered mental status, and hypotension. He was found to have sepsis without clear source. Despite aggressive measures, the patient subsequently expired on day 8 of his hospitalization. The final diagnosis was acute myeloid leukemia with blast crisis and leukostasis, complicated by sepsis.

Discussion

These observations are made based on these writers' experience with blast crisis and leukostasis:

- Acute blast crisis with leukostasis is a rare complication of hematologic emergencies. Symptoms are often vague and nonspecific, and a high index of suspicion is needed to make the diagnosis. Emergency medicine providers must be familiar with the diagnosis and its potential confounders and complicating factors.
- If the provider works in a setting where the technologists in the hematology lab won't report blasts until confirmed by a pathologist, it becomes important for the emergency physician to do the unthinkable—learn to identify blasts and actually go to the lab and look at the smear under the microscope! Ok, so it is not always easy because of variability of blasts in different types of leukemia, but in general, if you can at least make a good guess in the obvious cases, it might make a big difference in how the hematologist looks at the case, especially in the middle of the night!
- Clinicians must rule out leukostasis in any patient presenting with hyperleukocytosis. Early identification and swift initiation of definitive management is essential to maximize the likelihood of a positive outcome for the patient. Involve consultants and/or transfer to higher levels of care early.
- Expert management of leukostasis in the emergency department includes supporting the ABCs, having a low threshold for the early administration of broad-spectrum antibiotics (when indicated), correction of electrolyte and platelet abnormalities, and volume expansion to reduce blood viscosity.

Pattern Recognition

- Vague and nonspecific symptoms
- Markedly elevated WBC count
- Central nervous system and/or pulmonary manifestations
- Indolent course with rapid decompensation

Disclosure Statement Geremiha Emerson has no disclosures. Colin Kaide: Callibra, Inc.-Discharge 123 medical software company. Medical Advisory Board Portola Pharmaceuticals. I have no relationship with a commercial company that has a direct financial interest in subject matter or materials discussed in article or with a company making a competing product.

References

1. Vardiman JW, Harris NL, Brunning RD. The World Health Organization (WHO) classification of the myeloid neoplasms. Blood. 2002;100(7):2292–302.
2. Dutcher JP, Schiffer CA, Wiernik PH. Hyperleukocytosis in adult acute nonlymphocytic leukemia: impact on remission rate and duration, and survival. J Clin Oncol. 1987;5(9):1364–72.
3. Canaani J, et al. Long term impact of hyperleukocytosis in newly diagnosed acute myeloid leukemia patients undergoing allogeneic stem cell transplantation: an 9analysis from the acute leukemia working party of the EBMT. Am J Hematol. 2017;92(7):653–9.
4. Jabbour E, Kantarjian H. Chronic myeloid leukemia: 2014 update on diagnosis, monitoring, and management. Am J Hematol. 2014;89(5):547–56.
5. Lichtman MA. Rheology of leukocytes, leukocyte suspensions, and blood in leukemia possible relationship to clinical manifestations. J Clin Invest. 1973;52(2):350–8.
6. Lichtman MA, Weed RI. Peripheral cytoplasmic characteristics of leukocytes in monocytic leukemia: relationship to clinical manifestations. Blood. 1972;40(1):52–61.
7. Schiffer CA, Wiernik PH. Functional evaluation of circulating leukemic cells in acute nonlymphocytic leukemia. Leuk Res. 1977;1(4):271–7.
8. Stucki A, Rivier AS, Gikic M, et al. Endothelial cell activation by myeloblasts: molecular mechanisms of leukostasis and leukemic cell dissemination. Blood. 2001;97:2121.
9. Porcu P, et al. Hyperleukocytic leukemias and leukostasis: a review of pathophysiology, clinical presentation and management. Leuk Lymphoma. 2000;39(1–2):1–18.
10. Perazella MA, et al. Renal failure and severe hypokalemia associated with acute myelomonocytic leukemia. Am J Kidney Dis. 1993;22(3):462–7.
11. Awh CC, et al. Leukostasis retinopathy: a new clinical manifestation of chronic myeloid leukemia with severe hyperleukocytosis. Ophthalmic Surg Lasers Imaging Retina. 2015;46(7):768–70.
12. Ali AM, et al. Leukostasis in adult acute hyperleukocytic leukemia: a clinician's digest. Hematol Oncol. 2016;34(2):69–78.
13. Bellevue R, et al. Pseudohyperkalemia and extreme leukocytosis. J Lab Clin Med. 1975;85(4):660–4.
14. Karp DD, Beck JR, Cornell CJ. Chronic granulocytic leukemia with respiratory distress: efficacy of emergency leukapheresis. Arch Intern Med. 1981;141(10):1353–4.
15. Lane TA. Continuous-flow leukapheresis for rapid cytoreduction in leukemia. Transfusion. 1980;20(4):455–7.
16. Eisenstaedt RS, Berkman EM. Rapid cytoreduction in acute leukemia: management of cerebral leukostasis by cell pheresis. Transfusion. 1978;18(1):113–5.
17. Bug G, et al. Impact of leukapheresis on early death rate in adult acute myeloid leukemia presenting with hyperleukocytosis. Transfusion. 2007;47(10):1843–50.
18. Giles FJ, et al. Leukapheresis reduces early mortality in patients with acute myeloid leukemia with high white cell counts but does not improve long term survival. Leuk Lymphoma. 2001;42(1–2):67–73.
19. Ganzel C, et al. Hyperleukocytosis, leukostasis and leukapheresis: practice management. Blood Rev. 2012;26(3):117–22.
20. Ruggiero A, et al. Management of hyperleukocytosis. Curr Treat Options in Oncol. 2016;17(2):7.
21. Harris AL. Leukostasis associated with blood transfusion in acute myeloid leukaemia. Br Med J. 1978;1(6121):1169–71.
22. Grund FM, Armitage JO, Patrick Burns C. Hydroxyurea in the prevention of the effects of leukostasis in acute leukemia. Arch Intern Med. 1977;137(9):1246–7.

Black Widow Spider Bite: *"Can't We Just Get a Divorce?"*

4

Annaliese G. Seidel and Colin G. Kaide

Case

Pertinent History

This patient is a 7-year-old male who presented after falling from a tree. The child was climbing the tree and lost his balance falling approximately 7 feet, landing on a pile of broken branches. He suffered an injury to his left arm, resulting in a deformity. He was initially seen in the emergency department without a trauma activation. He denied loss of consciousness, neck pain, or back pain. His primary concern was the pain in his arm. Over the course of next 20 minutes, patient developed abdominal rigidity, tachycardia, and mild hypertension. He was then converted to a trauma activation.

Pertinent Physical Exam

Except as noted below, the findings of the complete physical exam were within normal limits.

- Vital signs: Blood pressure 160/95, heart rate 120, respiratory rate 18, temperature 99.4 °F
- HEENT: Atraumatic, pupils equal round and reactive to light (7 mm bilaterally), mild ptosis is noted.
- Neck: No cervical spine tenderness or bruising noted.
- Heart: S1-S2, regular rhythm and tachycardia.
- Lungs: Clear bilaterally to auscultation.

A. G. Seidel (✉) · C. G. Kaide
Department of Emergency Medicine, Wexner Medical Center at The Ohio State University, Columbus, OH, USA
e-mail: Annaliese.seidel@osumc.edu; Colin.kaide@osumc.edu

© Springer Nature Switzerland AG 2020
C. G. Kaide, C. E. San Miguel (eds.), *Case Studies in Emergency Medicine*,
https://doi.org/10.1007/978-3-030-22445-5_4

- Chest wall: No significant bruising or deformity.
- Abdomen: Rigid with involuntary guarding and no rebound. Bowel sounds are present.
- Extremities: Left upper extremity has a silver fork deformity with swelling noted around the wrist. All other extremities appear intact.
- Neuro: Patient moves all extremities and appears to have normal sensation and strength bilaterally.
- Skin: Warm and dry.

Pertinent Test Results

Lab Results			
Test	Results	Units	Normal range
WBC	14.9	K/uL	3.8–11.0 10³/mm³
Hgb	14.2	g/dL	(Male) 14–18 g/dL
			(Female) 11–16 g/dL
Platelets	190	K/uL	140–450 K/uL

CT abdomen: Poor-quality study, motion artifact. No evidence of obvious intra-abdominal injury.

ED Management

After the development of abdominal rigidity, he was converted to a level II trauma and was seen by the trauma team. He had an IV established and was given 25 μg of fentanyl for pain. His arm was splinted. A FAST exam was performed, showing no intraperitoneal fluid. The decision was made to send him for an abdominal CT scan.

Updates on ED Course

Update 1
During the CT scan, the technician called back to say that the patient continues to move and appears to be in substantial discomfort. He was given additional 25 μg of fentanyl. A second call was received, and the team went in to examine the patient. He appeared to have fasciculations and muscle spasms in his abdomen, chest, arms, and legs. His blood pressure was 170/100 mmHg with a heart rate of 140 bpm. The patient was diaphoretic and appeared uncomfortable. He received 1 mg of lorazepam IV, which did not help with the muscle spasms. A second 1 mg of lorazepam was given with little effect.

Update 2
The patient had worsening muscle spasms and now developed labored respirations. At this time, ED and trauma teams were perplexed as to what was causing the patient's symptoms. Bedside pulmonary function test was performed showing a negative inspiratory force of negative 15 mmHg. End-tidal CO_2 was measured at 52 mmHg. He was electively intubated using rocuronium and etomidate. Hypersalivation was noted during the procedure. His sedation was maintained with

propofol. His postintubation BP was 200/110 mmHg. He was started on a titratable nicardipine drip with SBP goal of less than 140 mmHg. He was taken for head and cervical spine CT, which were interpreted as normal.

The providers re-examined the patient from head to toe and found a small red patch on his right flank with what appeared to be two small puncture marks. The emergency medicine attending postulated that this might be a black widow envenomation given his symptomatology, including hypertension, muscle rigidity, increased secretions, and respiratory compromise along with the noted wound. The surgery attending was skeptical at first but became more convinced when the emergency physician contacted a toxicology fellow that had a particular interest in envenomation. The fellow confirmed that these findings were in fact indicative of a black widow spider envenomation, although worse than most. The fellow himself admitted to having been bitten by a widow spider on a camping trip when he was in the boy scouts and could attest to the very real nature of the abdominal muscle spasms. Toxicology was formally consulted, and the patient was admitted to the Pediatric ICU after being cleared by the trauma team.

Learning Points

Priming Questions
1. What is the classic presentation of a black widow envenomation?
2. What important features of the history and physical exam point to envenomation?
3. What diagnostic findings may mislead black widow spider bites as a surgical emergency?
4. What is the treatment of black widow spider bites?

Introduction/Background

1. The black widow spider is a member of the genus Latrodectus, which roughly translates into the "bandit biter." There are 31 species of widow spider but only three are found in North America. These are L. mactans (the Southern widow), L. hesperus (Western widow) and L. variolus (the Northern widow). They are all called black widow spiders.
2. Black widow spiders are found across the United States, and are considered the most clinically significant spider envenomation [1]. Building webs in uninhabited dark places such as barns, garages, outhouses, fences, and woodpiles, they only bite when unexpectedly disrupted or their web is disturbed. Both males and females have the typical red hourglass-shaped marking on the underside of these otherwise black or brown spiders. Females are larger, have longer fangs, and are typically more capable of causing systemic toxic responses in humans. Mild black widow spider bites may cause local pain with minimal swelling, but severe bites may present with greater systemic severity such as autonomic dysfunction. Classically seen in the hospital with impressive abdominal rigidity, the pain may

be severe, but the prognosis is good and mortality is rare. Treatment is generally supportive and focuses on pain control, but the clinical presentation warrants ruling out other concerning differential diagnoses (Figs. 4.1, 4.2, 4.3, and 4.4).

Fig. 4.1 *Latrodectus mactans* and egg sac. (Photo WikiCommons image. Mark Chappell of University of California, Riverside) (Published with kind permission of © Colin G. Kaide 2019. All Rights Reserved)

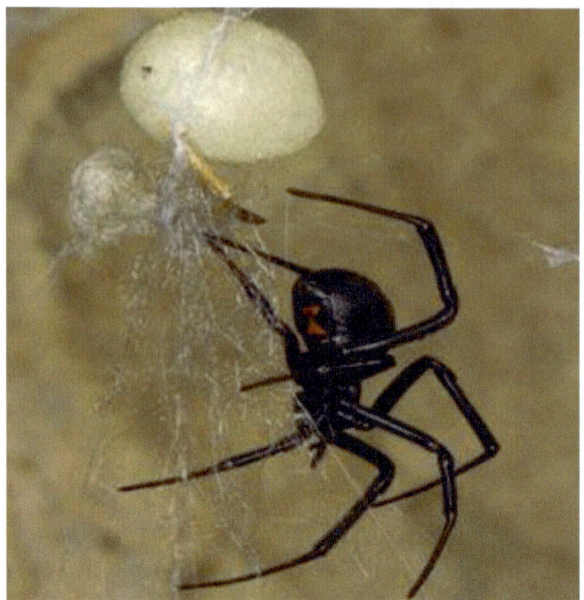

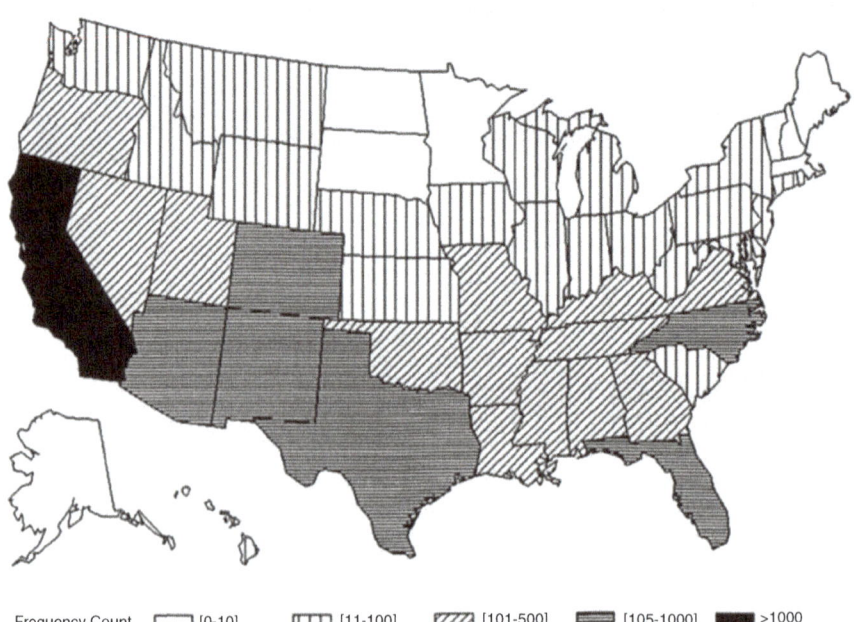

Fig. 4.2 Black widow spider envenomation with at least minor outcomes by state, 2000–2008. (Graphic from AA Monte et al., 2011) [1]) (Published with kind permission of © Colin G. Kaide 2019. All Rights Reserved)

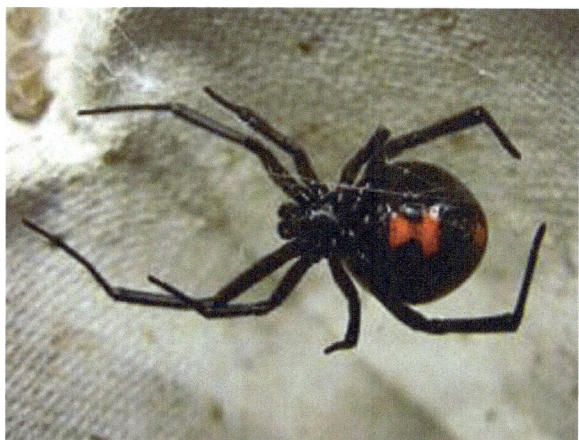

Fig. 4.3 *L. mactans* with characteristic hourglass marking Photo Shenrich91 (https://commons. wikimedia.org/wiki/ File:Adult_Female_Black_ Widow.jpg), https:// creativecommons.org/ licenses/by-sa/3.0/ legalcode (Published with kind permission of © Colin G. Kaide 2019. All Rights Reserved)

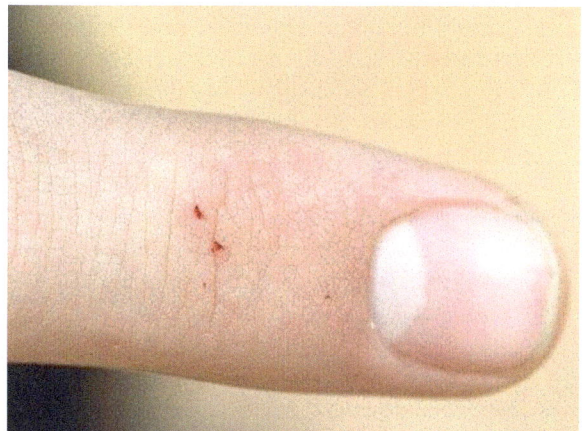

Fig. 4.4 Black widow spider bite. (Photo courtesy of David O'Connor) (Published with kind permission of © Colin G. Kaide 2019. All Rights Reserved)

Physiology/Pathophysiology

1. Black widow spider venom is a neurotoxin called latrotoxin. The venom has a high affinity for neuromuscular junctions and stimulates the release of presynaptic vesicles. The primary neurotransmitter released is acetylcholine, leading to the classic symptom of muscle cramping. Norepinephrine is also released, contributing to further autonomic dysregulation. Toxicity from alpha-latrotoxin in humans is known as *latrodectism*.

2. Pain begins locally within few minutes, and regional or systemic symptoms may follow within few hours. Signs and symptoms can wax and wane and last several days. Despite the severe pain of envenomation, the toxicity rarely causes long-term injury or death.

3. The classic symptoms of black widow toxicity are muscle rigidity and cramping, especially in the abdomen, chest, and back. Cramping causes extreme muscle pain that can be accompanied by weakness, paralysis, muscle fasciculation, or spasms. Patients may present with severe restlessness that can make patient history and physical exam difficult to obtain.

    Other symptoms are detailed below:
    - The bite site typically is painful, but an actual bite or puncture marks may not be seen. Occasionally, a target lesion (erythema with central clearing) may be observed, but is not required to make the diagnosis.
    - Diaphoresis may occur locally or systemically. Additionally, flushing, increased secretions, headache, nausea, and vomiting are common.
    - Respiratory distress can present due to pain and respiratory muscle weakness.
    - Less common symptoms include anxiety, irritability (often in pediatrics), compartment syndrome, or priapism. Pregnant patients may develop severe cramping with a risk of precipitating premature labor [2].
4. Fever, tachycardia, tachypnea, and hypertension regularly occur. Hypertension may result from the venom, pain, or anxiety, and may be an indicative sign of envenomation, especially in pediatric patients [3].
5. Black widow envenomation is classified by 3 severity grades [2, 4]. Most hospitalized patients are of moderate (Grade 2) to severe (Grade 3) and require medical intervention.
    - Grade 1 envenomation may have no symptoms or be limited to local pain at the bite site. No changes in vital signs are seen.
    - Grade 2 envenomation has local pain that spreads to the trunk muscles. They may also have diaphoresis at the bite site only, but vital signs remain normal.
    - Grade 3 envenomation denotes a severe systemic response. All grade 2 symptoms are seen, in addition to widespread muscle pain, diaphoresis far from the bite site, nausea, vomiting, and headache. Alterations in vital signs may include tachycardia and hypertension with potential hypertensive urgency and respiratory distress.

Making the Diagnosis

Differential Diagnosis
- Acute surgical abdomen
- Tetanus
- Other envenomations
- Substance withdrawal
- Organophosphate poisoning

1. History taking may be straightforward when the patient has seen the spider when they were bitten. If the spider has not been identified, inquire about the appearance of the spider or the location where the incident took place as this may be helpful in identifying envenomation by black widow spiders. For example, if the patient recently cleaned out a garage or was retrieving firewood from a woodpile, it might

make an envenomation more likely. In these cases, it is important to know the timing of the bite, symptoms, and any treatments the patient may have already tried (i.e., pain medications or antihistamines). If the patient is symptomatic, but does not know if they were bitten, questions to rule out other diagnoses should be considered:

- Any exposures to chemicals or poisons?
- History of alcohol or substance abuse?
- Any outdoor activity that would expose the patient to other insects or ticks?
- New skin markings or rashes?
- Last tetanus vaccination?
- Recent infection or symptoms of nausea, vomiting, hematemesis, melena, constipation, diarrhea, hematuria, etc.?
- Sexual activity or possibility of being pregnant?
- Other trauma or injuries?

2. The physical exam depends on the timing of presentation and the waxing and waning evolution of the envenomation. Local pain at the bite site can begin within minutes. Extension of pain and spasm of the trunk may be seen soon or develop hours later after local pain. A careful examination of a rigid abdomen must be performed to differentiate an acute surgical abdomen. Extreme pain and restlessness of the patient can make this difficult. When present, the combination of abdominal rigidity and autonomic dysregulation (hypertension, tachycardia, diaphoresis, salivating, or flushing) should put black widow envenomation on the differential. Any change of vital signs is an indication of a severe toxicity.

3. There are no specific labs or imaging for black widow envenomation. A general workup may include complete blood count, chemistry panel, and urinalysis, showing leukocytosis and albuminuria. Muscle spasms can lead to an increase in creatinine kinase (CK).
   - Again, as the differential for an undiagnosed spider bite is broad, the workup may be done to rule out other conditions: EKG, troponins, drug screening, blood or urine organophosphate metabolites, or pregnancy test.
   - Imaging studies, such as abdominal x-ray or CT, are unnecessary, but often done to rule out acute surgical abdomen [2]. Free air and intraperitoneal fluid will not be seen after a widow spider bite. A FAST scan in the ED may be done to assess for these findings before irradiating the patients.

4. It is important to keep black widow spider bites on the differential when the patient's presentation does not fit other diagnoses. Examples are patients with acute abdomen without free air or fluid on imaging and no preceding symptoms (such as melena), or patients with diaphoresis and tremor concerning for withdrawal without alcohol or substance abuse history.

Treating the Patient

1. Treatment of black widow spider bites is primarily supportive. For minor reactions, local cleansing, application of ice, and tetanus prophylaxis as needed are sufficient. Initial pain management can be provided with oral nonsteroidal anti-inflammatory drugs.

2. For more severe cases, pain control is the mainstay of treatment. Patients may require large doses of opioid analgesics, muscle relaxants, and benzodiazepines for muscle spasm and pain. Intravenous fentanyl or morphine, as well as diazepam (or lorazepam/midazolam), are often used for symptom control. The administration of these medications requires close respiratory monitoring. Additionally, antihypertensive drugs, such as nicardipine or, less often, sodium nitroprusside, help to control blood pressure.
   - Dantrolene and calcium gluconate have minimal effectiveness and are no longer recommended [5]. Likewise, prophylactic antibiotics are generally unnecessary.
3. A *Latrodectus* antivenin does exist, but its use is controversial. Clinical trials have never been done to prove its effectiveness, but it is still widely accepted to be safe and useful in severe cases [5, 6]. A recent study showed no evidence for improved outcomes with the antivenom compared to placebo [7], but anecdotal support seems to suggest in favor of its use for relief of intractable pain and shortened duration of symptoms. Its use in refractory cases is encouraged, especially in elderly, pediatric, and pregnant women [8].
   - To administer the antivenin, one vial (2.5 mL) diluted in 50–100 mL normal saline is given intravenously over 15–30 minutes [3, 9]. Unlike other envenomation, such as snakes, one vial is typically enough for complete treatment [2]. No relapse of symptoms has been recorded following antivenin administration [9].
   - The antivenin is an equine IgG derivative and has potentially serious side effects. While rare, anaphylaxis and hypersensitivity reactions, such as serum sickness, have been observed, leading to one death in the United States [9]. As a result, individuals with severe allergies or asthma requiring antivenin should receive diluted antivenin over a longer infusion time [10]. Pretreatment with antihistamines or steroids may be considered, but effectiveness of preventing the side effects is unproven [9]
   - A new antivenin made of a Fab antibody specific for alpha-latrotoxin is in development and undergoing clinical trials [11]. This product would carry a lower risk of hypersensitivity reaction, a distinct safety advantage in the treatment of black widow spider envenomation.
4. Patients with adequate symptom control after observing for several hours can be discharged. This includes patients who received antivenin and had relief of symptoms. Children, pregnant women, and patients with refractory pain or a history of hypertension should be considered for admission [4]. Even when admitted, patients are generally discharged within 1–3 days with no sequelae [5] (Fig. 4.5).

Case Conclusion

With presumptive diagnosis of latrodectism and the severity of the reaction, the toxicologist recommended antivenin. The vital signs stabilized over the next few hours, and the child was moved out of the ICU the next day and discharged 2 days later.

Drug	Dose	Comment
Pain Control		
Morphine	0.1-0.15 mg/kg—Repeat as needed	100 kg patient gets 10-15 mg
Hydromorphone	0.01-0.015 mg/kg—Repeat as needed	100 kg patient gets 1-1.5 mg
Fentanyl	1-1.5 mcg/kg—Repeat as needed	100 kg patient gets 100-150 mcg
Muscle Spasms/Anxiolytics		
Lorazepam	0.05 mg/kg (Peds). 1-2 mg doses in adults	May require multiple doses
Diazepam	5-10 mg in adults	May require multiple doses
Antivenin		
Alpha-Latrotoxin Antivenin	One Vial—2.5 ml diluted in 50-100 mL normal saline	A full antibody. Can cause serum sickness or other allergic response.

Fig. 4.5 Treatment of Black Widow Spider Bites. (Published with kind permission of © Colin G. Kaide 2019. All Rights Reserved)

After the patient's family was informed about the possible spider bite, the parents went to the site of the fall and found a tattered, irregular-shaped web with what appeared to be an egg sac suspended from the web. Dad doused the small woodpile with gasoline, tossed a match into it, and, in a bit of ironic karma, suffered minor flash burns when the gasoline vapor ignited explosively. The spider and her young did not survive.

Discussion

The pediatric patient in this case is a great example of how black widow spider envenomation can mimic other conditions. This patient had a trauma activation, CT scan, and was intubated prior to recognition of envenomation. A thorough history and physical exam is required on every patient, and in this case, a detailed reassessment helped to find the bite site and prompted the toxicology team to be consulted.

For such severe pain, impressive abdominal rigidity, and autonomic dysfunction including hypertension, the lack of sequelae in this patient is remarkable. Fortunately, black widow spider bites have low mortality, both from the toxin response and from the antivenin use. With the development of a new antivenin in process, future treatment of black widow spider bites may change. Until then, take care not to disturb any residents with the red-hourglass warning in outhouses.

Pattern Recognition

Black Widow Spider Envenomation Symptoms
- Environmental situation making a spider bite possible
- Abdominal rigidity and extreme pain
- Autonomic dysregulation
  - Hypertension
  - Fever
  - Diaphoresis
- Respiratory distress

Disclosure Statement   Annaliese Seidel: Nothing to disclose

Colin Kaide: Callibra, Inc-Discharge 123 Medical Software Company. Medical Advisory Board Portola Pharmaceuticals. I have no relationship with a commercial company that has a direct financial interest in subject matter or materials discussed in article or with a company making a competing product.

References

1. Monte AA, Bucher-Bartelson B, Heard KJ. A US perspective of symptomatic Latrodectus spp. envenomation and treatment: a National Poison Data System review. Ann Pharmacother. 2011;45(12):1491–8.
2. Glatstein M, Carbell G, Scolnik D, Rimon A, Hoyte C. Treatment of pediatric black widow spider envenomation: a national poison center's experience. Am J Emerg Med. 2018;36(6):998–1002.
3. Rahmani F, Banan Khojasteh SM, Ebrahimi Bakhtavar H, Shahsavari Nia K, Faridaalaee G. Poisonous spiders: bites, symptoms, and treatment; an educational review. Emerg (Tehran). 2014;2(2):54–8.
4. Camp NE. Black widow spider envenomation. J Emerg Nurs. 2014;40(2):193–4.
5. Auerbach PS, Cushing TA, Harris NS. Auerbach's wilderness medicine. Seventh edition. Philadelphia: Elsevier; 2017. 2 volumes (xxxi, 2631, 76 pages) p.
6. Offerman SR, Daubert GP, Clark RF. The treatment of black widow spider envenomation with antivenin latrodectus mactans: a case series. Perm J. 2011;15(3):76–81.
7. Isbister GK, Page CB, Buckley NA, Fatovich DM, Pascu O, MacDonald SP, et al. Randomized controlled trial of intravenous antivenom versus placebo for latrodectism: the second Redback Antivenom evaluation (RAVE-II) study. Ann Emerg Med. 2014;64(6):620–8. e2.
8. Shackleford R, Veillon D, Maxwell N, LaChance L, Jusino T, Cotelingam J, et al. The black widow spider bite: differential diagnosis, clinical manifestations, and treatment options. J La State Med Soc. 2015;167(2):74–8.
9. Clark RF, Wethern-Kestner S, Vance MV, Gerkin R. Clinical presentation and treatment of black widow spider envenomation: a review of 163 cases. Ann Emerg Med. 1992;21(7):782–7.
10. Clark RF. The safety and efficacy of antivenin Latrodectus mactans. J Toxicol Clin Toxicol. 2001;39(2):125–7.
11. Dart RC, Bogdan G, Heard K, Bucher Bartelson B, Garcia-Ubbelohde W, Bush S, et al. A randomized, double-blind, placebo-controlled trial of a highly purified equine F(ab)2 antibody black widow spider antivenom. Ann Emerg Med. 2013;61(4):458–67.

Radiology Case 1

5

Priyanka Dube and Joshua K. Aalberg

Indication for the Exam A 76-year-old female with a PMH of IBD presents with diffuse abdominal pain.

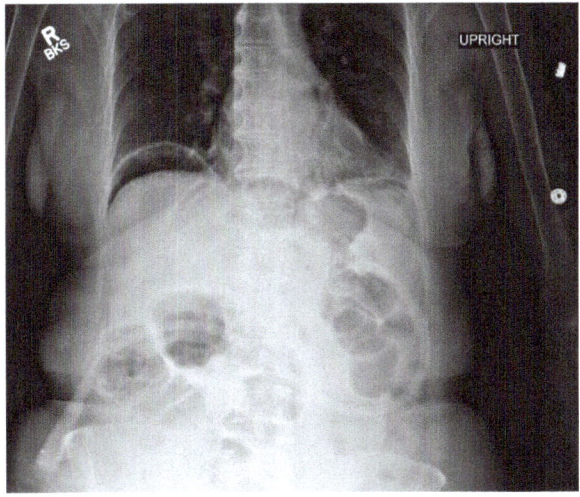

Radiologic Findings Upright abdominal radiograph demonstrating free air under the right hemidiaphragm.

P. Dube · J. K. Aalberg (✉)
Department of Emergency Medicine, Wexner Medical Center at The Ohio State University, Columbus, OH, USA
e-mail: Priyanka.Dube@osumc.edu; joshua.aalberg@osumc.edu

© Springer Nature Switzerland AG 2020   51
C. G. Kaide, C. E. San Miguel (eds.), *Case Studies in Emergency Medicine*,
https://doi.org/10.1007/978-3-030-22445-5_5

Diagnosis Pneumoperitoneum.

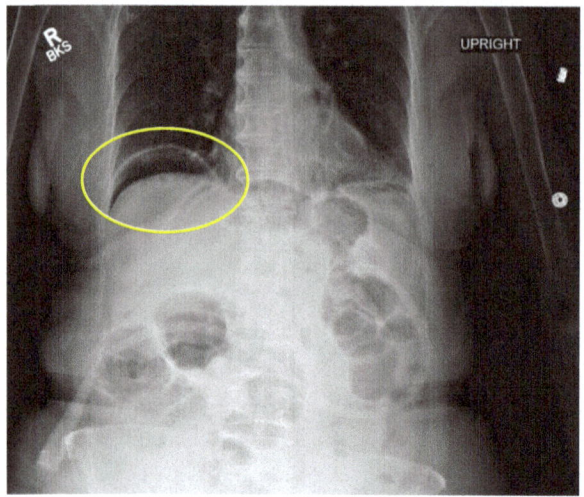

Learning Points

Priming Questions
1. Which radiographic features help to identify pneumoperitoneum?
2. What are some common causes of pneumoperitoneum?
3. In the neonatal population, what might one consider when a patient presents with pneumoperitoneum?

Introduction/Background

Free air/gas within the peritoneum, also known as pneumoperitoneum, can be a sign of a critical pathology, postoperative complication, trauma, or can arise from iatrogenic causes [1, 2]. Prompt and accurate diagnosis is life-saving in this population to reduce enteric contamination. Surgical intervention is often indicated.

Pathophysiology/Mechanism

Pneumoperitoneum occurs when the wall of a hollow viscus organ is disrupted [1]. The differential diagnosis is broad, and hence, combining clinical history with the location of free air is important in determining etiology.

Making the Diagnosis

- *Upright* chest and abdominal radiographs and left lateral decubitus radiographs are sensitive imaging modalities to diagnose pneumoperitoneum [3].
- On an upright chest radiograph, the presence of subdiaphragmatic gas indicates free intraperitoneal air as seen on the above radiograph. On supine chest imaging, free air located midline underneath the central diaphragmatic tendon can also suggest free intraperitoneal air; however, it is less sensitive (free air moves up with gravity) [1–3].
- Radiographs are not as sensitive for small foci of free air/microperforations; hence, in these situations, computerized tomography should be utilized [1].

Common Causes

Adults [1]
- Peptic ulcer disease (most common)
- Perforated appendicitis and diverticulitis
- Inflammatory bowel disease
- Iatrogenic/mechanical (postoperative, colonoscopy, CPR)
- Trauma
- Ischemic bowel

Neonates [1]
- Necrotizing enterocolitis (most common)
- Meconium ileus
- Hirschsprung disease
- Peptic ulcer disease
- Iatrogenic/mechanical

> **Major Mimicker's of Pneumoperitoneum** [2]
> - Gas within skin folds
> - Diaphragmatic contour/eventration
> - Subcutaneous emphysema
> - Interposed Bowel

Treating the Patient

In general, all patients with pneumoperitoneum necessitate a surgical evaluation in the Emergency Department. In many cases, emergent surgical intervention is warranted (e.g., perforated viscus, sepsis, hemodynamic instability). When patients are stable, the amount of free air is minimal, and there is a lack of peritoneal signs, clinicians may elect for conservative management and observation [4].

The emergency physician should initiate antibiotic treatment, covering for Gram-positive, Gram-negative, and anaerobic coverage. Ciprofloxacin/Metronidazole, Piperacillin/Tazobactam, and Ertapenem are all common regimens. Fluid resuscitation is also generally indicated, though should be based on the overall clinical picture.

Discussion

- Pneumoperitoneum can suggest time critical emergencies. In most cases, surgical intervention is required due to peritoneal contamination from a perforated viscus. In clinically stable patients, sometimes, clinicians will elect conservative management and observation especially if the amount of free air is small.
- The most common cause for pneumoperitoneum in the adult population is gastric disruption secondary to peptic ulcer disease. Timely diagnosis helps reduce complications and improve recovery time.
- Upright/semierect radiographs are quick, inexpensive, and sensitive imaging modalities to diagnose pneumoperitoneum to reduce the risk of peritonitis. Right-sided subdiaphragmatic air typically indicates free intraperitoneal air.
- Causes for pneumoperitoneum in adults differ from those in children. While GI tract perforation, including PUD, is a common cause in adults, one should consider necrotizing enterocolitis, meconium ileus, and Hirschsprung disease in the neonatal population.

References

1. Sharma R, Jones J. Pneumomediastinum. Radiopaedia. Accessed 6 Jun 2018. https://radiopaedia.org/articles/pneumomediastinum.
2. Sureka B, Bansal K, Arora A. Pneumoperitoneum: what to look for in a radiograph? J Family Med Prim Care. 2015;4(3):477. https://doi.org/10.4103/2249-4863.161369.
3. Baker SR. Pneumoperitoneum—the radiographic and clinical virtues of the supine abdominal film. Emerg Radiol. 2012;19(6):547–8. https://doi.org/10.1007/s10140-012-1075-7.
4. Tanaka R, Kameyama H, Nagahashi M, Kanda T, Ichikawa H, Hanyu T, Wakai T. Conservative treatment of idiopathic spontaneous pneumoperitoneum in a bedridden patient: a case report. Surg Case Rep. 2015;1(1) https://doi.org/10.1186/s40792-015-0073-x.

Botulism: *"I don't need to talk, but I do need to swallow!"*

Daniel Z. Adams and Colin G. Kaide

6

Case

Diplopia, Dysarthria, and Dysphagia

Pertinent History

A 30-year-old male with a history of type 1 diabetes presents to the Emergency Department with 3 days of worsening blurred and double vision, difficulty speaking, and progressive dysphagia. He states that he initially noted a mild, dull diffuse headache and blurred vision for which he was evaluated at an outside hospital. During that visit, he was treated for a migraine headache with improvement of his symptoms and discharged. However, while the headache had resolved, his blurred vision progressed to double vision, and he noted difficulty in formulating words and swallowing both solids and liquids, with associated hoarseness of his voice. At present, his voice is muffled, his speech is slurred almost like he is intoxicated, and he has pooling secretions in his oropharynx. No others around him have been sick. He did not eat anything unusual. He denies recent travel, wounds, or environmental exposures.

Past Medical History (PMH) Type 1 diabetes

Social History (SH) Former IV drug user, but has "been clean for sometime now"

D. Z. Adams (✉)
Department of Pulmonology and Critical Care Medicine,
Washington University/Barnes-Jewish Hospital, St. Louis, MO, USA

C. G. Kaide
Department of Emergency Medicine, Wexner Medical Center at The Ohio State University,
Columbus, OH, USA
e-mail: Colin.kaide@osumc.edu

© Springer Nature Switzerland AG 2020
C. G. Kaide, C. E. San Miguel (eds.), *Case Studies in Emergency Medicine*,
https://doi.org/10.1007/978-3-030-22445-5_6

Pertinent Physical Exam

- Vital Signs: BP 165/90, HR 90, RR 16, Temperature 99.4 ° F/37.4 C

Except as noted below, the findings of the complete physical exam are within normal limits.

- Head, eyes, ears, nose, throat (HEENT): Bilateral ptosis and ophthalmoplegia including cranial nerves 3 and 6, with a weak gag reflex and pooling secretions in the oropharynx. He has an asymmetrical rise in his palate when trying to say "aah."
- Neurological Exam: Symmetrically decreased 1/4 upper extremity reflexes, and 2/4 lower extremity reflexes. He is notably ataxic on ambulation but with a normal motor and sensory exam otherwise.

Pertinent Diagnostic Testing

- CBC, serum chemistry, liver function testing, urinalysis – within normal limits
- Negative inspiratory force: −40 cm H_2O (normal −80 to −100 cm H_2O)
- Vital capacity: 2.8 liters (3–5 liters)

ED Management

Our differential diagnosis included Guillain–Barre syndrome, specifically the Miller–Fisher syndrome, as well as neuromuscular junction disorders such as myasthenia gravis, infiltrative central nervous system processes (i.e., lymphoma, metastatic cancer, neurosarcoidosis), Lyme disease, botulism, and tick paralysis. Neurology was consulted with continued airway monitoring in the ED. An immediate MRI of his brain was unremarkable, as were the results of a lumbar puncture. He was subsequently admitted to the ICU for monitoring given concerns for impending respiratory failure.

Test results for HIV, Lyme disease, acetylcholine receptor antibody, and ganglioside antibody panel were negative. He was empirically started on IVIG for presumed Miller–Fisher variant Guillain–Barre syndrome while awaiting other studies. Further inpatient questioning revealed that he had, in fact, recently relapsed and started using IV heroin again, sharing needles with multiple persons. He had initially withheld this information to prevent his family from finding out about his addiction. Shortly after admission, he was intubated for inability to handle secretions and impending respiratory failure. Given the new history, concerns were focused on the possibility of wound botulism.

Learning Points

Priming Questions
1. What are the classic presenting features of botulism?
2. What historical clues can help you delineate the diagnosis?
3. What diagnostic workup and treatment should be provided?
4. What are the characteristics of some important members of the differential diagnosis?

Introduction/Background

1. Botulism is a rare, neurotoxin-mediated illness produced by the Gram-positive, anaerobic spore-forming bacilli *Clostridium botulinum* [1, 2]. Four different categories are described for surveillance purposes, including foodborne, wound, infant, and others.
    - Wound Botulism: The bacteria, *C. botulinum,* infects the wound and produces the toxin, which is responsible for the neurological symptoms. This is most often associated with the intramuscular or subcutaneous injection of black tar heroin.
    - Infant Botulism: Accounts for 80% of laboratory-confirmed botulism cases. Infants less than 1 year of age may become infected by ingesting germinated *C. botulinum* spores, which then elicit neurotoxin while in the gastrointestinal tract. The classically described association is with the ingestion of honey; however, the majority of infant botulism cases are actually caused by swallowing dust particles, which contain *C. botulinum spores.*
    - Foodborne Botulism: In contrast, foodborne botulism seen in adults and children greater than 1 year of age is acquired by ingestion of preformed toxin, as the matured gastrointestinal tract does not allow for spore germination. In this type of botulism, there is no actual infection with *C. botulinum.*

Physiology/Pathophysiology

1. Regardless of the means of acquisition, weakness and paralysis result when the toxin irreversibly binds with presynaptic peripheral cholinergic nerve endings (i.e., neuromuscular junction and autonomic ganglia), preventing stimulation-induced acetylcholine release by the presynaptic nerve [2, 3].

Nerve ending at neuromuscular junction. US National Institutes of Health, National Institute on Aging created original. Marked as public domain. (Published with kind permission of © Colin G. Kaide 2019. All Rights Reserved)

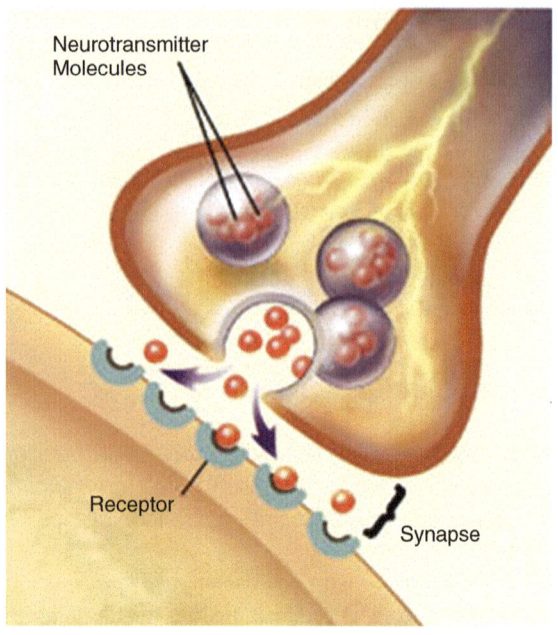

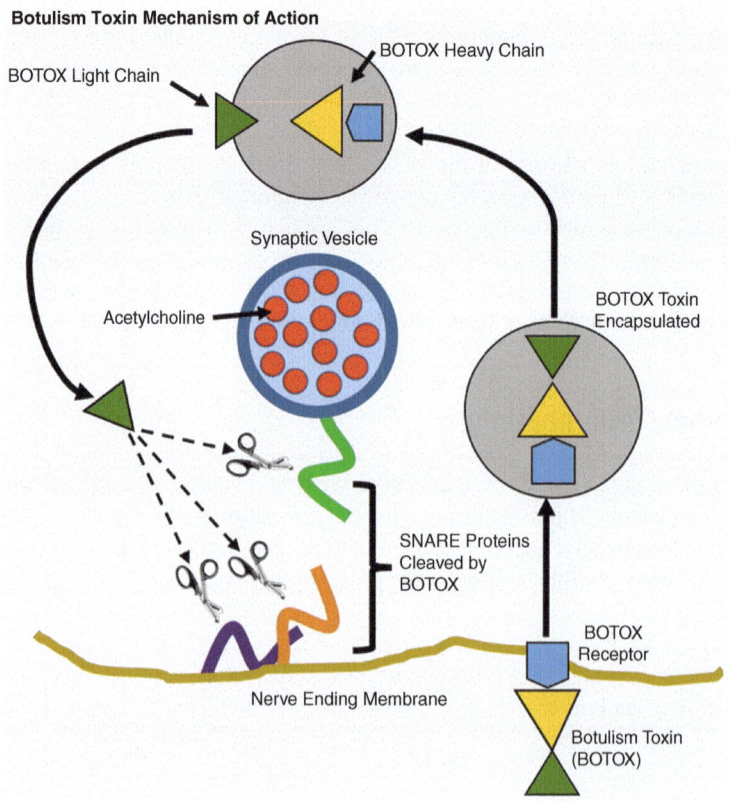

2. Recovery only results when new nerve terminals sprout and form new synaptic contacts in a process that may take months.
3. Outbreaks of botulism have been described with ingestion of contaminated food, usually secondary to poor food preparation including home canning with an associated anaerobic, low acid, and low solute environment [4].
   - Of note, a major outbreak of foodborne botulism was noted in 2015 associated with a church potluck meal in Lancaster, Ohio, causing one of the largest outbreaks in United States (US) history with 21 confirmed cases, resulting in one death. The culprit was potato salad made from home canned potatoes [4].
4. REMEMBER the "four D's" – Diplopia, Dysarthria, Dysphagia, and Dry mouth [5]. However, initial symptoms depend on the source of the infection.
   - GI symptoms including nausea, vomiting, and diarrhea may predominate early on with foodborne botulism.
   - Otherwise, cranial nerves and bulbar muscles are most often affected initially, leading to gaze paralysis, blurred vision from loss of accommodation, ptosis, and other cranial neuropathies.
     – Loss of deep tendon reflexes with associated motor weakness progresses in a *descending* fashion.
     – *Anticipate respiratory muscle paralysis.*
     – Autonomic symptoms include orthostatic hypotension, urinary retention, and constipation.
     – Sensation is spared.

Beware of the "Floppy Baby" – Noticeably weak with a poor suck
Constipation and poor feeding are usually the first manifestation of infant botulism → cranial nerve dysfunction (decreased suck, poor eye movement, ptosis) → hypotonia and autonomic dysfunction (decreased tear production, hemodynamic instability) [6].

Making the Diagnosis

Differential Diagnosis
- Guillain–Barre syndrome
- Miller–Fisher syndrome, a Variant of Guillain–Barre syndrome
- Myasthenia gravis
- Lambert–Eaton syndrome
- Tick paralysis

1. As with every patient, start with a thorough history and physical exam.
   - Have they had recent unusual food exposures?
   - Do they eat home canned goods?
   - Has anyone else been affected?

- Any recent wounds?
- Any history of IV drug abuse?
- In the case of an infant, pay attention to age … Either way, inquire as to a history of constipation, poor feeding, decreased suck reflex, hypotonia, honey ingestion, etc.
  - <1 year, likely to be *infected* by germinated spores producing toxin.
  - >1 year, more likely to have ingested *preformed toxin.*
2. A *presumptive diagnosis* should be made in any of the following situations based on history and physical.
  - Adult
    - Acute onset of descending, symmetric flaccid paralysis with cranial nerve involvement in the absence of fever.
    - Don't forget, it may crop up in clusters (i.e., foodborne outbreaks or bioterrorism)!
  - Infant
    - Constipation with development of a weak suck, ptosis, and hypotonia.
3. The three clinical criteria listed in Table 6.1 have been reported to be sensitive in helping clinicians to consider botulism but lack specificity, and the absence of one criterion does not rule out the possibility of botulism [7].
  - When suspected, contact the state health department immediately for assistance.
  - If infant botulism is suspected, call the California Department of Health Services, Infant Botulism Treatment and Prevention Program (www.infantbotulism.org or 510-231-7600).

Table 6.1 Helpful Screening Criteria For Botulism[a]

Absence of Fever[b] PLUS
One of the following symptoms
Blurred vision
Double vision
Difficulty speaking, including slurred speech
Any change in sound of voice, including hoarseness
Dysphagia/pooling of secretions/drooling
Thick tongue
One of the following signs
Ptosis
Extraocular palsy/decreased tracking of objects
Fatigability manifested by averting light shining in the eye
Facial paresis/loss of facial expression/pooling of secretions or milk
Poor feeding/poor suck using pacifier
Fatigability while eating
Fixed pupils
Descending paralysis beginning with cranial nerves

[a]Reported sensitivity of all three criteria 89%
[b]May be febrile for another reason, such as in wound botulism or complications such as urinary tract infection secondary to urinary retention, aspiration pneumonia, etc

4. Send confirmatory *botulinum toxin assay* from serum, stool/vomit, or food sources +/− cultures from suspected wound sources [8].
   - *Do not await results to administer antitoxin.*
   - Serum assays will be negative in infant botulism but suspected to be positive in stool samples.
   - Serum toxin assays are suspected to be positive in foodborne botulism.
   - A culture from the wound that isolates *C. botulinum* is diagnostic.
     - It is pointless in these cases to send toxin assay from stool/vomit.
   - If bioterrorism is suspected, do not be reassured by lack of toxin in serum or other specimens, because levels may not be high enough (i.e., lack of detection does not rule it out) [9].
5. *EMG* findings can be supportive, with expected results showing decreased compound muscle action potential amplitudes

Treating the Patient

1. Pay special attention to the *ABC's*!
   - Monitor pulse oximetry and respiratory parameters (negative inspiratory force, vital capacity).
     - Respiratory failure is what kills, and early intubation decreases the risk of death.
     - *Consider intubating patients with a vital capacity less of than 30% predicted.*
2. Administer *antitoxin* as soon as possible.
   - Antitoxin binds remaining neurotoxin but cannot reverse paralysis that has already occurred. That only gets better when new nerve terminals and synapses develop.
     - Early administration prevents deterioration.
     - Contact local state health department for help with obtaining and administering the antitoxin.
       ○ Watch for side effects including serum sickness and anaphylaxis when using heptavalent botulinum antitoxin.
     - *Infants < 1 year should receive botulinum immune globulin instead (aka BIG-IV or BabyBIG).*
3. Antibiotic therapy is only indicated for cases of *wound botulism* and *after* antitoxin has been given [10].
   - Treating wound botulism with an antibiotic prior to giving antitoxin can increase toxin release and also rapidly worsen the symptoms.
   - Suggested regimen – penicillin G or metronidazole for penicillin allergy.
   - All wounds regardless of appearance should be debrided – consider surgical consultation.
     - Update tetanus!

Other Considerations
Miller–Fisher Syndrome (MFS)

Our initial impression of this patient's presentation was MFS given the predominant cranial nerve findings and minimal motor weakness. MFS is a GBS variant that classically presents with a triad of limb-ataxia, areflexia, and ophthalmoplegia, with or without pupillary areflexia [11, 12]. Many patients, however, will not have all three classic findings. About half of patients with MFS present with facial nerve involvement, with other cranial nerves variably affected. Mild sensory involvement has been reported as well. Extremity involvement in MFS is rare but can occur in about one-third of cases, as would be seen in GBS [13]. Only a minority of patients with MFS clinically deteriorate to the point of needing mechanical ventilation for respiratory support. In cases that do not progress, clinical improvement is seen in 2–4 weeks, with near-complete resolution by 6 months. Given the similarity in symptoms between MFS and botulism, a thorough history (including recent infection, intravenous drug use, case clustering, etc.) and physical examination are paramount for guiding the appropriate diagnostics and treatment. A strong recommendation can be made to specifically question patients presenting in this fashion about intravenous drug use after they have been separated from family members who may inhibit truthful responses. Further, assurances of confidentiality may go a long way to facilitate open and honest communication.

Bioterrorism

Consider if large numbers of individuals are affected or there are suspicious circumstances surrounding the presentation.

- Mode of transmission – inhalation of aerosolized toxin or possibly gastrointestinal [14].

Case Conclusion

An EMG was performed showing decreased compound muscle action potential amplitudes, strongly suggestive of a diagnosis of botulism. Confirmatory studies for botulism were sent as well as blood cultures. He received penicillin G and botulism antitoxin. He recovered adequately over the next week to be extubated and was transferred to a rehabilitation facility to assist during his prolonged anticipated recovery.

Discussion

In particular, wound botulism has been described as a complication of intravenous drug abuse, and we should consider this diagnosis in patients with a known history of IVDA and suggestive clinical signs and symptoms [15].

The case presented here is interesting in that he presented as a bounce-back to our facility after a visit to an outside hospital. His initial presentation was atypical in that he complained of headache and blurred vision initially. When he was being discharged from the first visit, he told us he said to the discharging nurse, "I don't have to talk right, but I really need to be able to swallow!" His symptoms obviously progressed with increased bulbar muscle dysfunction and the classic "four D's," with blurred vision, double vision, slurred speech, and difficulty handling his secretions. While our initial consideration was Miller–Fisher variant Guillain–Barre, the patient's history of intravenous drug use is what really helped nail down the diagnosis. As with almost all ED diagnoses, the biggest clues were discovered by obtaining a thorough history and physical examination. In the case of botulism, a presumptive diagnosis should be immediately followed by contacting the local state health department and administration of antitoxin or BabyBIG depending on age of the patient.

Pattern Recognition

Botulism
- Adults – the "four D's" (diplopia, dysarthria, dysphagia, dry mouth)
- Pediatrics – constipation and poor feeding ➔ hypotonia
- Descending motor paralysis with normal sensory exam
- Normal mental status
- Possible or impending respiratory failure

Disclosure Statement   Daniel Adams: Nothing to disclose

Colin Kaide: Callibra, Inc.-Discharge 123 medical software company. Medical Advisory Board Portola Pharmaceuticals. I have no relationship with a commercial company that has a direct financial interest in subject matter or materials discussed in article or with a company making a competing product.

References

1. Ganti L, Rastogi V. Acute generalized weakness. Emerg Med Clin North Am. 2016;34(4):795–809.
2. Brook I. Botulism: the challenge with diagnosis and treatment. Rev Neurol Dis. 2006 Fall;3(4):182–9.
3. Sugiyama H. Clostridium botulinum neurotoxin. Microbiol Rev. 1980;44(3):419–48.
4. McCarty CL, Angelo K, Beer KD, et al. Large outbreak of botulism associated with a church potluck meal – Ohio, 2015. MMWR Morb Mortal Wkly Rep. 2015;64(29):802–3.
5. Hughes JM, Blumenthal JR, Merson MH, et al. Clinical features of types A and B food-borne botulism. Ann Intern Med. 1981;95:442–5.
6. Long SS. Infant botulism. Pediatr Infect Dis J. 2001;20(7):707.
7. Rao AK, Lin NH, Griese SE, et al. Clinical criteria to trigger suspicion for botulism: an evidence-based tool to facilitate timely recognition of suspected cases during sporadic events and outbreaks. Clin Infect Dis. 2018;66(suppl_1):S38.
8. Rao AK, Lin NH, Jackson KA, Mody RK, Griffin PM. Clinical characteristics and ancillary test results among patients with botulism – United States, 2002-2015. Clin Infect Dis. 2017;66(suppl_1):S4.

9. Hodowanec A, Bleck TP. Clostridium botulinum (Botulism). In: Bennet JE, Dolin R, Blaser MJ, editors. Mandell, Douglas, and Bennett's principles and practice of infectious diseases. 8th ed. Philidelphia: Elsevier Saunders; 2015. p. 2763.
10. American Academy of Pediatrics. Botulism and infant botulism (Clostridium botulinum). In: Kimberlin DW, Brady MT, Jackson MA, Long SS, editors. Red book: 2015 Report of the Committee on Infectious Diseases. 30th ed. Elk Grove Village: American Academy of Pediatrics; 2015. p. 294.
11. Lo YL. Clinical and immunological spectrum of the Miller-Fisher syndrome. Muscle Nerve. 2007;36(5):615–27.
12. Fisher M. An unusual variant of acute idiopathic polyneuritis (syndrome of ophthalmoplegia, ataxia and areflexia). N Engl J Med. 1956;255:57–65.
13. Ropper AH, Wijdicks EFM, Truax BT. Guillain-Barré syndrome. Contemporary Neurology Series. F.A. Davis Company. 1991.
14. Arnon SS, Schechter R, Inglesby TV, et al. Botulinum toxin as a biological weapon: medical and public health management. JAMA. 2001;285(8):1059–70.
15. Wenham TN, Kensington C, Moor L. Botulism: a rare complication of injection drug use. Emerg Med J. 2008;25:55–6.

Button Battery Ingestion: *The Battery That Is Not as Cute as a Button*

7

Ashley Larrimore and Justin Carroll

Case

Foreign Body Ingestion

Pertinent History

A 5-year-old male presents at 2 pm with throat discomfort, coughing, gagging, and drooling for the past hour. He has a fever and is irritable. He was unable to eat or drink water without difficulty prior to arrival and had two episodes of nonbilious emesis. His mother had found him and his younger sibling playing in the tool drawer. She denies a history of asthma or allergies. The home medicine cabinet is locked, and sibling does not have any symptoms.

Pertinent Physical Exam

- BP 95/46, Pulse 130, Temp 100.4 °F (38 °C) RR 37, SpO_2 96%

Except as noted below, the findings of a complete physical exam are within normal limits.

- Constitutional: anxious appearing child; mild diaphoresis.
- HEENT: Increased secretions, moist mucous membranes, normal oropharynx with no tonsillar edema or erythema, uvula midline, no lymphadenopathy.
- Respiratory: Tachypnea, Equal breath sounds bilaterally. No wheeze or rhonchi.
- Cardiovascular: Tachycardia with regular rhythm, normal heart sounds, and intact distal pulses. Exam reveals no gallop and no friction rub or murmur heard.
- Imaging: X-ray soft tissue neck: unremarkable

A. Larrimore (✉) · J. Carroll
Department of Emergency Medicine, Wexner Medical Center at The Ohio State University, Columbus, OH, USA
e-mail: ashley.larrimore@osumc.edu

© Springer Nature Switzerland AG 2020
C. G. Kaide, C. E. San Miguel (eds.), *Case Studies in Emergency Medicine*,
https://doi.org/10.1007/978-3-030-22445-5_7

- CXR: 15 mm radio-opaque disk-shaped foreign body with 2 step-border within the upper third of the esophagus
- Plan: Stat GI consult. Contact The National Battery Ingestion Hotline (NBIH) (202)-625-3333

Update 1 (1530) Based on the size of the battery, the patient's age, and his symptoms, GI plans to take the patient to the endoscopy suite to remove the battery. The patient has stopped vomiting and is able to control his airway and secretions. He remains slightly tachycardic but is otherwise hemodynamically stable.

Update 2 (1600) The patient is transported to the endoscopy suite.

Learning Points: Button Battery Ingestion

Priming Questions
1. What symptoms should cause you to suspect your patient may have ingested a button battery?
2. How do you distinguish between a button battery and a coin on xray and how does the size of the battery impact patient treatment?
3. What types of complications result from button battery ingestions and how long after ingestion do these complications occur?

Introduction/Background

1. The number of button battery ingestions (BBIs) has remained stable over the past 30 years [1], although the number of ED visits has increased over the past decade [2]. The incidence of morbidity and mortality has also increased 7-fold. This increase is related to a change in battery production using higher-voltage lithium cells and battery sizes [1]
2. More than 90% of serious outcomes are due to ingestions of batteries greater than 20 mm in diameter, which are more likely to become lodged in the esophagus [1]. In fact, 12.6% of children who ingested a 20-mm battery suffered severe or fatal injuries [3].
3. Most ingestions are unwitnessed and are by small children under 6 years old, with 2 years old being the most common age for ingestion. This often leads to a delay in recognition and diagnosis. More than 50% of serious outcomes due to BBI occur after unwitnessed ingestions, in which case, there is likely a delay in recognition and diagnosis [3].

Physiology/Pathophysiology

1. Button batteries lodged in the mucosal tract cause caustic injury, mucosal ulceration, and, if impacted long enough, perforation. The esophagus is the most common site for impaction. The severity of esophageal damage is determined by the length of time that the battery is lodged in place, the amount of electrical charge remaining in the battery, and the size of the battery [4–6].
   - Damage to the esophagus may begin as early as 2 hours after ingestion with more severe damage occurring after 8–12 hours [4, 7].
   - Injury to tissue is worse near the negative pole of batteries. The flow of electrical current from the battery to the surrounding tissues occurs near the negative pole, causing corrosive tissue injury. Even "dead" batteries retain enough voltage and storage capability to generate an external current and mucosal damage [8].
   - Over 90% of fatalities or serious injuries from button batteries involve batteries that are 20 mm or more in diameter [1, 8]. This is likely because most batteries that are 20–25-mm in diameter are lithium batteries. These batteries have higher voltage and capacitance and are more likely to lead to esophageal burns, fistulas, perforations, and deaths.
   - In acidic environments like the stomach, the seal or crimp of the battery may erode and potentially release chemical contents including sodium or potassium hydroxide. As these alkaline solutions react with the mucosal surface of the GI tract, they cause liquefaction necrosis [9–11]. Systemic heavy metal or lithium poisoning is extremely rare.
2. Long-term complications from button batteries are rare but devastating. Severe esophageal burns and perforations occur adjacent to the negative pole of the battery. This can lead to tracheoesophageal fistula, esophageal perforation, vocal cord paralysis, perforation of the aortic arch, gastric hemorrhage, and intestinal perforation. Death can occur and is usually associated with ingestion of large lithium cell batteries [1, 4, 11–14].

Making the Diagnosis

This is a presentation that is easy to misdiagnose! Patients often present with early signs and symptoms that suggest other more common conditions that do not require chest X-ray. A high suspicion should be kept to avoid delay in diagnosis and poor outcomes.

Differential Diagnosis
- Foreign body ingestion
- Pharyngitis
- Esophagitis
- Pneumonia
- Esophageal rupture

1. The majority of coin and button battery ingestions are not witnessed. Have a high suspicion as children can have a benign early presentation. Common clinical findings on presentation include wheezing, coughing, drooling, voice changes, dysphagia, and stridor. More severe presentation can include chest pain, vomiting, fever, and hematemesis. Make sure to also ask about coingestions like magnets that can worsen complications from button battery ingestion [1].

2. Plain radiographs are the recommended modality for suspected ingestion of button battery or other foreign body. An AP and lateral chest X-ray should be obtained. Neck and abdominal imaging should also be considered [1, 15, 16].
   - In the AP view, a "halo sign" or "double-rim effect" on the AP view can be used to delineate a disk battery from coin ingestion, though occasionally, two ingested coins can mimic this finding (Fig. 7.1).
   - In the lateral view, you may see soft tissue thickening between the battery and trachea that can indicate soft tissue swelling. The narrowest end of the battery can be seen on this view and indicates the negative pole. This is significant as this is the end most likely to corrode first and is often the site of the most severe injury. This can be remembered as the 3 N's: Negative, Narrow, Necrotic [17].
   - You can often determine the imprint code (located at the + end) and the diameter of the battery with a radiograph. This can be helpful with identification when contacting the National Battery Ingestion Hotline (800-498-8666) and with risk stratification [16].
   - Other nonspecific findings suggesting severe injury such as esophageal rupture may be seen on radiograph including [18]:
     - Pneumomediastinum
     - Abnormal cardiomediastinal contour
     - Pneumothorax or pleural effusion
   - Think about insertions into other orifices if a foreign body is not visualized on chest or abdominal X-ray. Consider skull X-ray to assess for nasal or ear battery/foreign body insertion.

3. Other testing in the ED is usually not necessary. Labs do not aid in making the diagnosis. Assays for blood or urine mercury or other battery contents are not recommended as mercury toxicity from battery ingestions is extremely rare. Advanced imaging techniques such as CT or MRI may be used to assess the

Fig. 7.1 The bilaminar structure of the button battery gives it a double ring appearance on plain film. (Courtesy of Colin Kaide, MD)

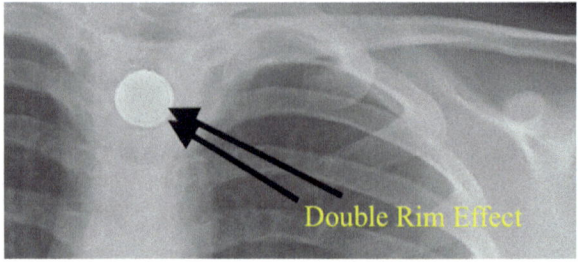

Double Rim Effect

severity of injury after endoscopy but are rarely needed in the emergency department. Fluoroscopy may be helpful if there is suspicion of a button battery masquerading as an ingested coin [18, 19].

Treating the Patient

Treatment of the patient depends on the age of the patient, the size of the battery, the location of the battery, and whether a magnet was coingested.

1. Look for signs of airway obstruction and control the airway if necessary. Aggressively resuscitate patients with signs of shock or hematemesis. Be sure that the patient is kept NPO. Do not attempt to induce vomiting or give medications in an attempt to "move the battery along." These treatments have not been shown to be effective.
2. Patients with esophageal batteries identified on X-ray must undergo immediate endoscopic examination for removal and direct visualization of tissue injury. It is crucial that you do not wait for symptoms to develop – by that point, the patient has already sustained injury from the battery [1, 16]
3. Although not a substitute for endoscopic removal (and should therefore not delay definitive treatment), a single study of cadaveric porcine tissue demonstrated protective effects of both honey and sucralfate in the simulated setting of BBI.
   - Both substances decreased the alkaline effect of the battery and therefore limited the depth of the resultant injury.
   - Do not give if there is concern for esophageal perforation or ingestion occurred >12 hours ago.
   - Honey: 10 mL (2 teaspoons) by mouth every 10 minutes for up to 6 doses.
     - Do not give if the child is less than 12 months of age.
   - Sucralfate: 10 mL (of 1 g/10 mL suspension) by mouth every 10 minutes, up to 3 doses
4. The treatment varies for patients who have a battery that is located in the stomach or beyond [16]:
   - If a magnet was coingested, the patient must have immediate endoscopic removal of the button battery. If the battery is unable to be removed endoscopically, the patient must undergo surgical removal of the battery
   - Patients who are symptomatic, even with minor symptoms, should also undergo immediate endoscopic removal of the battery:
     - If endoscopic removal is not possible, surgical removal is usually reserved for patients with occult or visible bleeding or severe symptoms like vomiting, signs of an acute abdomen, or decreased appetite.
   - If the child is younger than 6 years old or ingested a battery larger than 15 mm, an X-ray should be obtained 4 days after ingestion:
     - If the battery remains in the stomach, it should be removed endoscopically regardless of symptoms.

  – While awaiting the repeat imaging, the patient can be allowed to eat a regular diet at home.
  – If the patient develops symptoms at any time, they should also immediately return for re-evaluation.
- Children who are asymptomatic and over age 6 may be managed at home. Battery passage should be confirmed by inspecting stool:
  – Consider X-ray if passage is not confirmed in 10–14 days
  – If symptoms develop at any time, the patient should be re-evaluated and removal of the button battery should be considered.

Case Conclusion

A rigid esophagoscopy was performed and a 3V lithium button battery with some ulcerated mucosal tissue was identified at the upper esophageal sphincter and was subsequently removed. No other coingestions were found. The patient was provided symptom control and admitted. He had an uneventful inpatient stay. No complications were found at a 2-month follow-up encounter.

Discussion

1. Most button battery ingestions are not witnessed, so you must have a high suspicion in the correct patient population. Consider the possibility of button battery ingestion in any pediatric patient with airway obstruction, difficulty swallowing, wheezing/noisy breathing, drooling, vomiting, and chest or abdominal pain. Also consider ingestion in patients who ingested an unknown object: parents may report a "shiny object" being placed in the mouth or missing batteries from open electronic devices. Remember that early on, many patients may be asymptomatic.

2. Button batteries are everywhere – remote controls, keyless entry fobs, toys, bathroom scales, and hearing aids are just a few places you may find button batteries. Although we don't tend to think a lot about prevention in the emergency department, if you do have a patient who has a button battery ingestion/insertion, this might be a great time to talk about safety and prevention with the family (assuming the child is stable and doesn't need a procedure). Remind parents never to leave button batteries out and to store them out of sight and out of reach of small children. Tell them to check all household devices to ensure the battery compartment is secured tight and to try and only purchase products that require a tool to open the battery compartment or to have a child-resistant locking mechanism.

3. Although we tend to think about children when we talk about button battery ingestion, don't forget that older adults may also swallow button batteries accidentally or purposefully. Typically, adult patients will swallow batteries after putting them in their mouths to "test" them or, due to poor vision, they may mistake them for medication or food. Remember that adults can also have adverse effects from these batteries and to treat accordingly.

Pattern Recognition

- Young child
- "Shiny object in mouth" or missing battery from open device
- Coughing, gagging, drooling or dysphagia
- "Halo" sign on X-ray

Disclosure Statement   The authors of this chapter report no significant disclosures.

References

1. Litovitz T, Whitaker N, Clark L, White NC, Marsolek M. Emerging battery-ingestion hazard: clinical implications. Pediatrics. 2010;125(6):1168–77.
2. Sharpe SJ, Rochette LM, Smith GA. Pediatric battery-related emergency department visits in the United States, 1990-2009. Pediatrics. 2012;129(6):1111–7.
3. Litovitz T, Whitaker N, Clark L. Preventing battery ingestions: an analysis of 8648 cases. Pediatrics. 2010;125(6):1178–83.
4. Sigalet D, Lees G. Tracheosophageal injury secondary to disc battery ingestion. J Pediatr Surg. 1988;23(11):996.
5. Rumack BH, Rumack CM. Disc battery ingestion. JAMA. 1983;249(18):2509.
6. Temple DM, McNeese MC. Hazards of battery ingestion. Pediatrics. 1983;71(1):100.
7. Thompson N, Lowe-Ponsford F, Mant TG, Volans GN. Button battery ingestion: a review. Adverse Drug React Acute Poisoning Rev. 1990;9(3):157.
8. Langkau JF, Noesges RA. Esophageal burns from battery ingestion. Am J Emerg Med. 1985;3(3):265–8.
9. Bass DH, Miller AJ. Mercury absorption following button battery ingestion. J Pedaiatr Surg. 1992;27(12):1541.
10. Rebhandl W, Steffan I, Schramel P, Puid S, Paya K, Schwanzer E, Strobl B, Horcher E. Release of toxic metals from button batteries retained in the stomach: an in vitro study. J Pediatr Surg. 2002;37(1):87–92.
11. Samad L, Ali M, Ramzi H. Button battery ingestion: hazards of esophageal impaction. J Pediatr Surg. 1999;34(10):1527.
12. Wall SJ, Nadel DM, Handler SD. Airway compromise caused by disc battery ingestion. Otolaryngol Head Neck Surg. 1999;121(3):302.
13. Chiang MC, Chen YS. Tracheoesophageal fistula secondary to disc battery ingestion. Am J Otolaryngology. 2000;21(5):333.
14. Krom H, Visser M, Hulst JM, Wolters VM, Van Den Neucker AM, de Meij T, van der Doef HPJ, Norbruis OF, Benninga MA, Smit MJM, Kindermann A. Serious complications after button battery ingestion in children. Eur J Pediatr. 2018;177(7):1063.
15. Pugmire BS, Lin TK, Pentiuk S, de Alarcon A, Hart CK, Trout AT. Imaging button battery ingestions and insertions in children: a 15-year single-center review. Pediatr Radiol. 2016;47(2):178–85.
16. NBIH Button Battery ingestion triage and treatment guideline. National Capital Poison Center. www.poisonorg/battery/guideline.asp (Accessed on 29 June 2018).
17. Maves MD, Lloyd TV, Carithers JS. Radiographic identification of ingested disc batteries. Pediatr Radiol. 1986;16(2):154.
18. Kramer RE, Lerner DG, Lin T, et al. Management of ingested foreign bodies in children: a clinical report of the NASPGHAN Endoscopy Committee. J Pediatr Gastroenterol Nutr. 2015;60(4):562–74.
19. Litovitz T, Schmitz BF. Ingestion of cylindrical and button batteries: an analysis of 2382 cases. Pediatrics. 1992;89(4 Pt 2):747.

Central Retinal Artery Occlusion with Sudden Vision Loss—*"Ay, Ay, My Eye!"*

8

Bradley M. End and Colin G. Kaide

Case

Sudden Monocular Blindness

Pertinent History

This patient is a 62-year-old male with a history of hypertension and hyperlipidemia who presents left-sided vision loss. Patient says that he had sudden onset of painless, unilateral (left-sided), vision loss approximately 24 hours ago. He said his left eye went completely dark over about 25 seconds. He had no headache or any other focal neurologic symptoms. He was seen at an outside hospital within 60 minutes of onset of symptoms and had a CT scan of his brain and a CT angiogram (CTA) of his head and neck. He had a normal intraocular pressure. Ophthalmology was contacted and the decision was made to have the patient follow-up as an outpatient. The patient was not seen by ophthalmology that evening. A retinal and pupillary exam was not documented in the outside hospital (OSH) record. He followed up the next afternoon with ophthalmology and was told that he may have a central retinal artery occlusion (CRAO) and nothing could be done this far after onset. He was sent to the emergency department to have a workup for possible embolic sources.

B. M. End
Department of Emergency Medicine, Robert C. Byrd Health Sciences Center, West Virginia University, Morgantown, WV, USA
e-mail: Bend@hsc.wvu.edu

C. G. Kaide (✉)
Department of Emergency Medicine, Wexner Medical Center at The Ohio State University, Columbus, OH, USA
e-mail: Colin.kaide@osumc.edu

© Springer Nature Switzerland AG 2020
C. G. Kaide, C. E. San Miguel (eds.), *Case Studies in Emergency Medicine*,
https://doi.org/10.1007/978-3-030-22445-5_8

Pertinent Physical Exam

Except as noted below, the findings of the complete physical exam are within normal limits.

- BP 160/95, P 80, RR16, Temp 98.8, SPO2 98%
- *Constitutional*: He is oriented to person, place, and time. He appears well-developed and well-nourished.
- *Head:* Normocephalic and atraumatic.
- *Eyes:* Conjunctivae and extraocular movements are normal. Right eye exhibits no discharge. Left eye exhibits no discharge. *Left eye demonstrates an afferent pupillary defect.* R eye is reactive to light.
- *Fundoscopic Exam*: Right—Normal, *L—Cherry red spot with pale retina.*
- *Neck*: Neck supple.
- *Cardiovascular*: Normal rate, regular rhythm, and normal heart sounds. No murmur.
- *Neurological*: He is alert and oriented to person, place, and time. He has normal strength. No sensory deficit.

Past medical history (PMH)
Hypertension and hyperlipidemia.

Social History (SH)
Daily tobacco use. Occasional alcohol (ETOH) use. No illicit drug use.

Family History (FH)
Coronary artery disease (CAD), Hypertension (HTN), Diabetes

Pertinent Test Results

Outside Hospital Findings: CT/CTA

1. No extracranial carotid or vertebral artery stenosis.
2. Unremarkable intracranial CT angiogram without focal branch occlusion seen.
3. No intracranial mass lesion, acute hemorrhage, or midline shift.
4. No cervical soft tissue mass or pathological lymphadenopathy seen.

Emergency Department Management

The patient was admitted to the hospital for further testing for cardiovascular disease and possible initiation of hyperbaric therapy.

Learning Points

Priming Questions
1. What is the differential and management of painless unilateral vision loss in the ED?
2. What treatment options are available to those presenting with CRAO?
3. Does hyperbaric therapy offer any therapeutic benefit to patients presenting with CRAO?

Introduction/Background

1. Pattern recognition can frequently get you out of potential trouble. Acute ischemia of the retina is a very specific pattern that every EM physician MUST know! Missing a patient with a classic presentation can be financially and emotionally unrewarding. Sudden, rapidly evolving (20–30 seconds) painless, mostly complete, monocular vision loss is central retinal artery occlusion (CRAO), *until proven otherwise.* Similar, vision loss can occur with central retinal vein occlusion (CRVO) and retinal detachment; however, it is usually subacute and incomplete.
2. The incidence of CRAO is estimated to be around 1–10/100,000 persons with at least one study showing that 80% of the patients present with a visual acuity of <20/400.
   - Risk factors include hypertension, carotid artery disease, diabetes mellitus, cardiac disease (especially atrial fibrillation and valvular disease), vasculitis, temporal arteritis, and sickle cell disease.
   - Irreversible vision loss is typically thought to occur within 90 minutes based on primate studies; however, irreversible vision loss has been demonstrated with occlusion times of as little as 15 minutes, while other studies have noted some visual recovery with up to 48 hours of ischemic time [7, 13].

Physiology/Pathophysiology

1. Understanding the blood flow to the retina is useful in helping to understand the presentation and prognosis of CRAO.
   - The central retinal artery (CRA) is a branch of the ophthalmic artery that is a branch of the internal carotid artery. It supplies blood to the optic disk. It then branches into superior and inferior branches, which then divide into the nasal and temporal branches. These all together supply blood to all 4 quadrants of the retina [6].
   - The outer retina is perfused by a branch of the ciliary artery called the choriocapillaris.

2. About 15–25% of the population has an anatomical variation with the presence of an additional artery called the cilioretinal artery. It supplies the macula where the highest number of photoreceptors live. Since this artery is not a branch of the central retinal artery, the macula may remain perfused in these patients who develop CRAO. This might allow for preservation of the most important part of the visual field [8].

Making the Diagnosis

Differential Diagnosis [14]
- CRAO
- CRAO
- CRAO
- CRAO
- CRAO
- CRVO
- Retinal detachment
- Vitreous hemorrhage

1. Fundoscopic findings: Early findings performed within 7 days of CRAO showed the following results:
   - Retinal opacity in the posterior pole (58%).
   - Cherry-red spot (90%) (may also be seen with sphingo- and mucolipidoses) [12].
   - Cattle trucking (19%).
   - Retinal arterial attenuation (32%).
   - Optic disk edema (22%).
   - Pallor (39%).
   - At later stages, fundoscopic findings showed opticatrophy (91%), retinal arterial attenuation (58%), cilioretinal collaterals (18%), and macular retinal pigment epithelial changes (11%).

Funduscopic Findings: Normal, CRAO, CRVO

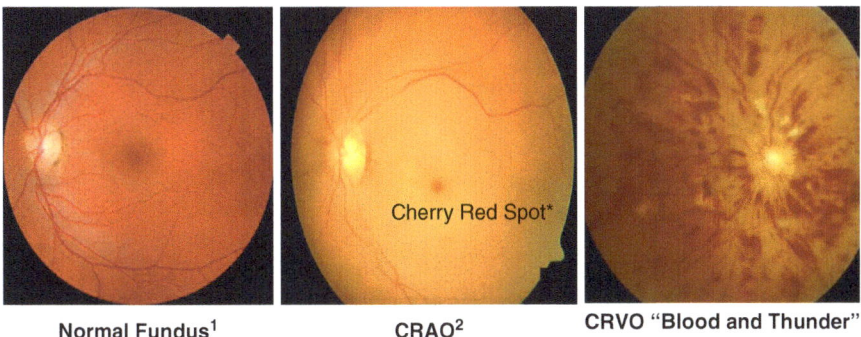

| Normal Fundus[1] | CRAO[2] | CRVO "Blood and Thunder" |

*The cherry red spot develops because the blood supply to the macula is via the choriod (long and short posterior ciliary arteries) and it stays relatively pink while the ischemic retinal tissue becomes pale

[1]Häggström M. Medical gallery of Mikael Häggström 2014. WikiJournal of Medicine. 1(2); 2014. https://doi.org/10.15347/wjm/2014.008. ISSN 2002-4436. Public Domain

[2]Achim F, Ömer C, Stephan K, Sven H, Inez F, Ulrich HS. https://commons.wikimedia.org/wiki/File:Cherry_Red_Spot_Fiess.jpg), *Cherry Red Spot Fiess,* https://creativecommons.org/licenses/by/2.0/legalcode

CRVO: Public domain image. (Published with kind permission of © Colin G. Kaide 2019. All Rights Reserved)

"Cattle-Trucking" or "Box-Car" Appearance of the Blood Column in the Branch Arteries

Public Domain Image. (Published with kind permission of © Colin G. Kaide 2019. All Rights Reserved)

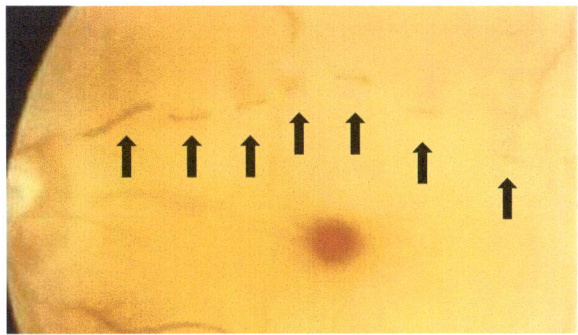

2. An afferent pupillary defect is usually present in CRAO, also known as the Marcus Gunn pupil. This is best assessed using the swinging flashlight test. Using a steady source of light, the light is shined from one eye to another until one of the following observations is made:
   • No Relative Afferent Pupillary Defect: Both pupils constrict equally. Hippus, or non-rhythmic fluctuations in pupillary size with constant illumination, may be noted and is a normal finding.

- Mild Relative Afferent Pupillary Defect: The affected pupil constricts weakly and then dilates to a greater size.
- Moderate Relative Afferent Pupillary Defect: The affected pupil initially does not constrict and then dilates to a greater size.
- Severe Relative Afferent Pupillary Defect: The affected pupil immediately dilates.

Normal and Abnormal Swinging Light Test

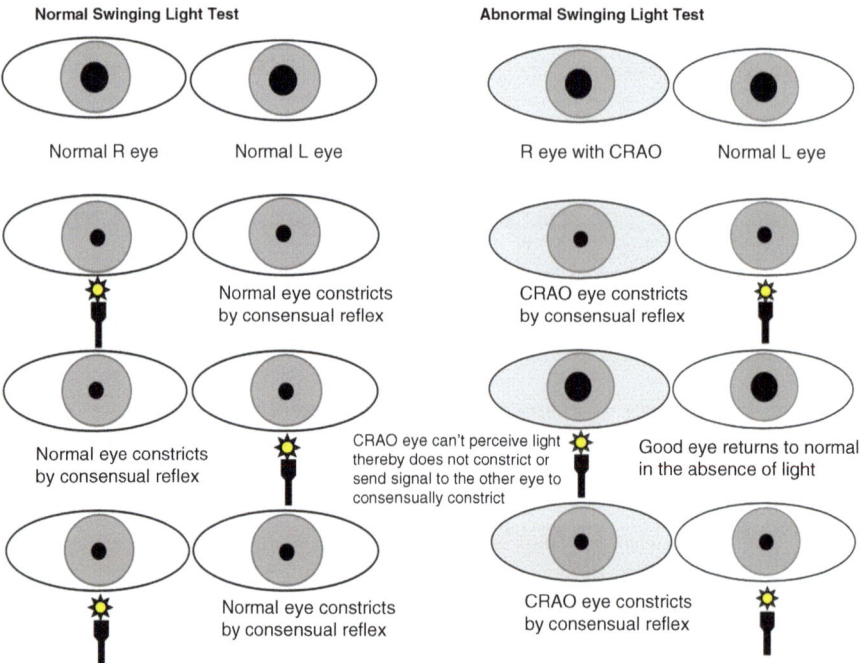

3. A study comparing a cohort of medicare beneficiaries with CRAO to a similar cohort evaluated for hip fracture demonstrated a 28-fold and 33-fold increase in the risk of CVA in the first and second week following CRAO respectively [3].
4. Unlike TIA(s), thromboemboli in CRAO are more likely to originate from carotid disease, while stuttering symptoms may be due to severe carotid stenosis [4].
5. Other things presenting with painless monocular vision loss:
   - Central Retinal Vein Occlusion (CRVO): CRVO usually presents with subacute monocular decrease in vision or acute worsening of gradually deteriorating vision. Complete sudden vision loss *is not* characteristic of CRVO; however, vision loss may be persistent without proper treatment [15]. The risk of CRVO is related to the patient's risk for developing thrombosis.

- Retinal Detachment: Usually presents with acute monocular vision loss but typically has characteristic onset pattern such as a sensation of a curtain drawn over the eye, flashers and floaters, or the description of spider webs or dust in the visual field. The vision loss is usually progressive and incomplete.
6. If vision loss is painful, consider alternative diagnoses such as acute angle closure glaucoma, optic neuritis, and temporal arteritis (which causes CRAO).

Suggested workup for CRAO [11]
- *Exclude Temporal Arteritis*: ESR, CRP
- *Common Vascular Risk Factors*: BP, Cholesterol, Blood Sugar
- *Embolic Sources:* Carotid Doppler, Cardiac Echo
- *Patients with no Risk Factors*:
  - Hypercoagulable screen: Protein C&S, factor V Leiden, prothrombin gene mutation, anti-phospholipid antibody, Methylenetetrahydrofolate reductase Vasculitic screen (ANA, ENA, ANCA, ACE); Myeloproliferative or sickle cell disease screen

Treating the Patient

Treatment from the perspective of the emergency physician is aimed at attempts to restore blood flow to the CRA. Many things have been tried, but few have been shown to be successful in restoring significant vision. It should be noted that some episodes of apparent CRAO may be due to "low-flow" states or partial occlusion and as such even patients presenting hours after symptom onset require immediate treatment and specialist consultation [2]. Treatment modalities include

1. Use of sublingual isosorbide dinitrate or systemic pentoxifylline or inhalation of a carbogen, hyperbaric oxygen to increase blood oxygen content and dilate retinal arteries.
2. Ocular massage to attempt to dislodge emboli.
3. Intravenous acetazolamide and mannitol, plus anterior chamber paracentesis, followed by withdrawal of a small amount of aqueous fluid from the eye to increase retinal artery perfusion pressure by reducing intraocular pressure. This method is preferred in the setting of a visualized embolus on the optic disk [8].
4. Multimodal stepwise conservative approaches involving combinations of: Ocular massage, globe compression, sublingual isosorbide dinitrate, intravenous acetazolamide, followed by intravenous mannitol, methylprednisolone, retrobulbar tolazoline, and different anticoagulants [1, 5, 6].
5. Intra-arterial tPA (IAT) has been studied in a few small studies with mixed results. Several small studies showed to be effective in 60–70% of the study subjects. The European Assessment Group for Lysis in the Eye (EAGLE) was a multicentered prospective randomized controlled trial of 84 patients with CRAO

within 20 hours of symptom onset. The study did not find a statistically significant difference in clinical improvement between the lysis and standard therapy groups (60.0 vs. 57.1%). A recent systematic review/meta-analysis that included 5 retrospective controlled studies and the EAGLE trial demonstrated outcomes favoring IAT [10].

6. Hyperbaric Oxygen Therapy (HBO) can be considered in patients who are diagnosed early in the period before permanent damage can occur.

Rationale for Hyperbaric Oxygen Therapy (HBO) in the Management of Central Retinal Artery Occlusion (CRAO)

Given the dismal outcome with standard therapy and the lack of harm associated with HBO, strong consideration should be given to initiating therapy very early on in the patient's course. For it to be useful, HBO should be started as soon as possible. Consult the HBO physician on call to initiate therapy. Similar to CVA, the visual signs and symptoms of CRAO are dependent on the particular vessel occluded, location and degree of occlusion and the presence or absence of a cilioretinal artery. During periods of occlusion or flow restriction, the inner retinal layers (ganglion cell and inner nuclear layer) that are normally supplied by the retinal circulation may maintain function if the patient is exposed to elevated partial pressures of oxygen through diffusion from the choroidal circulation. This has been demonstrated in animal models during complete restriction of retinal blood flow. Success of therapy is contingent upon preserved choroidal circulation; if choroidal circulation is also occluded, HBO will not be effective. In considering HBO therapy for CRAO, it should be noted that therapy must be initiated before irreversible damage occurs to retinal cells and an adequate partial pressure of O2 must be maintained until circulation through the CRA is restored. In partial occlusions, patients may respond at lower partial pressures of O2 [9].

Case Conclusion

The patient underwent multiple treatments with HBO. After his 10th treatment, he had subjective improvement in his vision in the affected eye. Formal vision testing showed approximately a 25% improvement in his vision from the time of the initial exam.

Discussion

Suspect CRAO when a patient presents with painless, nontraumatic unilateral (though bilateral is possible) vision loss. Unlike CRVO, vitreous hemorrhage, and retinal detachment, visual loss is usually complete. Approximately 20% may present with retained central vision due to the presence of collateral circulation from the cilioretinal artery.

Time is retina! CRAO is an ophthalmologic emergency and, as such, emergent consultation should be obtained. Given the relatively high treatment failure rate, discuss with your consultant the preferred management at your institution before initiating medical therapy. You will not be faulted for attempting ocular massage to attempt to dislodge the clot while waiting for additional recommendations.

In elderly patients, remember that temporal arteritis can lead to CRAO. If your patient reports preceding headaches or jaw claudication, you must exclude temporal arteritis. Remember that nonvasculitic CRAO is a stroke of the eye. Patients will require further evaluation for CVA risk.

HBO therapy may improve outcomes in CRAO. Consult with your local hyperbaric medicine doctor early in the workup and management of CRAO.

Pattern Recognition

CRAO
- Painless, non-traumatic vision loss
- Afferent pupillary defect and cherry red spot on macula

Disclosure Statement
- None for Brad End
- Colin Kaide: Callibra, Inc.-Discharge 123 medical software company. Medical Advisory Board Portola Pharmaceuticals. I have no relationship with a commercial company that has a direct financial interest in subject matter or materials discussed in article or with a company making a competing product.
- Portola Pharmaceuticals: No conflict with this chapter material.

References

1. Ropper AH, Samuels MA, Klein JP, Prasad S, Ropper AH, Samuels MA, Klein JP, Prasad S, editors. Disturbances of vision. In: Adams and victor's principles of neurology. 11th ed. New York: McGraw-Hill. https://accessmedicine.mhmedical.com/content.aspx?bookid=1477&sectionid=119126803. Accessed 08 July 2019.
2. Effron D, Forcier BC, Wyszynski RE. Fundoscopic findings. In: Knoop KJ, Stack LB, Storrow AB, Thurman R, editors. The atlas of emergency medicine. 4th ed. New York: McGraw-Hill. http://accessmedicine.mhmedical.com.proxy.lib.ohio-state.edu/content.aspx?bookid=1763&sectionid=125433189. Accessed 08 May 2018.
3. Fraser SG, Adams W. Interventions for acute non-arteritic central retinal artery occlusion. Cochrane Database Syst Rev. 2009;(1):Art. No: CD001989. https://doi.org/10.1002/14651858.CD001989.pub2.
4. French DD, Margo CE, Greenberg PB. Ischemic stroke risk in medicare beneficiaries with central retinal artery occlusion: a retrospective cohort study. Ophthalmol Ther. 2018;24 https://doi.org/10.1007/s40123-018-0126-x.

5. Givre S, Van Stavern GP. Amaurosis fugax (transient monocular or binocular visual loss). In: Brazis PW, Trobe J, Wilterdink JL, editors. UpToDate; 2017. Retrieved 8 May 2018. from https://www.uptodate.com/contents/amaurosis-fugax-transient-monocular-or-binocular-vision-loss.
6. Greenberg RD, Dippold AL. Eye emergencies. In: Stone C, Humphries RL, editors. CURRENT diagnosis & treatment: emergency medicine. 8th ed. New York: McGraw-Hill. http://accessmedicine.mhmedical.com.proxy.lib.ohio-state.edu/content.aspx?bookid=2172&sectionid=165063265. Accessed 08 May 2018.
7. Hedges TR III. Central and branch retinal artery occlusion. In: Brazis PW, Trobe J, Wilterdink JL, editors. UpToDate; 2015. Retrieved 8 May 2018. from https://www.uptodate.com/contents/central-and-branch-retinal-artery-occlusion.
8. Leveque T. Approach to the adult with acute persistent visual loss. In: Trobe J, Sullivan DJ, editors. UpToDate; 2017. Retrieved 8 May 2018. from https://www.uptodate.com/contents/approach-to-the-adult-with-acute-persistent-visual-loss.
9. Mathew R, Sivaprasad S, Augsburger JJ, Corrêa ZM. Retina. In: Riordan-Eva P, Augsburger JJ, editors. Vaughan & Asbury's general ophthalmology. 19th ed. New York: McGraw-Hill. http://accessmedicine.mhmedical.com.proxy.lib.ohio-state.edu/content.aspx?bookid=2186&sectionid=165517649. Accessed 08 May 2018.
10. Murphy-Lavoie H, Butler F, Hogan C. Arterial insufficiencies: central retinal artery occlusion. In: Weaver LK, editor. Hyperbaric oxygen therapy indications. 13th ed. Best Publishing Company, North Palm Beach, FL, USA p. 11–25.
11. Page PS, et al. Intra-arterial thrombolysis for acute central Retinal artery Occlusion: a systematic review and meta-analysis. Front Neurol. 2018;9(76) https://doi.org/10.3389/fneur.2018.00076.
12. Riordan-Eva P. Disorders of the eyes & lids. In: Papadakis MA, McPhee SJ, Rabow MW, editors. Current medical diagnosis & treatment. New York: McGraw-Hill; 2017. http://accessmedicine.mhmedical.com.proxy.lib.ohio-state.edu/content.aspx?bookid=1843&sectionid=135699961. Accessed 08 May 2018.
13. Tabandeh H, Goldberg MF. Use of the hand-held ophthalmoscope. In: Kasper D, Fauci A, Hauser S, Longo D, Jameson J, Loscalzo J, editors. Harrison's principles of internal medicine. 19th ed. New York: McGraw-Hill; 2014. http://accessmedicine.mhmedical.com.proxy.lib.ohio-state.edu/content.aspx?bookid=1130&sectionid=79725409. Accessed 08 May 2018.
14. Tobalem S, Schutz JS, Chronopoulos A. Centeral retinal artery occlusion – rethinking retinal survival time. BMC Ophthalmol. 2018;18:101. https://doi.org/10.1186/s12886-018-0768-4.
15. Vision loss, acute, painless. In: Ferri FF, editors. Ferri's clinical advisor 2018. Philadelphia: Elsevier. p. 1539–1543.

Cervical Fractures: *Who Did Jefferson Bite?*

9

David Hartnett and Michael Barrie

Case

Neck Pain After Trauma

Pertinent History A 42-year-old female presents to the emergency department after a fall with neck pain. She reports that she was drinking alcohol the night prior, fell down from standing in the bathroom, and woke up with a throbbing headache and pain in the neck. Her pain is worsened with movement and has made it difficult to move around her house or complete her normal activities of daily living today.

Pertinent Physical Exam

Except as noted below, the findings of the complete physical exam are within normal limits.

- Blood pressure 161/99 mm Hg, pulse 105 beats per minute, temperature 97 °F (36.1 °C), temperature source Oral, resp. rate 20 breathes per minute, height, SpO_2 99%.
- Head: Normocephalic, atraumatic
- Eyes: Conjunctivae normal, extraocular muscles intact with full range of motion without pain
- Neck: Tenderness in the superior midline cervical spine. Increased pain with range of motion
- Neuro: Cranial nerves 2–12 intact, strength normal in bilateral upper and lower extremities, sensation intact to light touch throughout.

D. Hartnett (✉) · M. Barrie
Department of Emergency Medicine, Wexner Medical Center at The Ohio State University, Columbus, OH, USA
e-mail: David.Hartnett@osumc.edu; Michael.Barrie@osumc.edu

© Springer Nature Switzerland AG 2020
C. G. Kaide, C. E. San Miguel (eds.), *Case Studies in Emergency Medicine*,
https://doi.org/10.1007/978-3-030-22445-5_9

PMH No pertinent past medical history.

SH Current every-day smoker, drinks vodka approximately 3 times a week until she is "drunk," has thought about stopping alcohol consumption before and would like to quit.

FH No pertinent past family history.

Pertinent Test Results

4 view cervical radiographs

1. 3 mm anterior subluxation of C2 on C3 with 15 degrees of forward tilt of C2
2. Asymmetric widening of the atlanto-axial junction
3. No visualized fracture, CT imaging recommended

   Cervical spine Computed Tomography (CT)

1. Mildly displaced fracture involving the right lateral mass and bilateral transverse processes/pars interarticularis of C2 with grade 1 anterolisthesis of C2 on C3. These findings are consistent with hangman's type fracture.
2. Comminuted fracture of the transverse process, articular process, and lamina of C3. There is perched facet on the left contributing to a rotatory component.
3. Small fracture involving the anterior aspect of the transverse process and the superior aspect of the left articular process of C4. Vascular injury not excluded.

   Magnetic Resonance Imaging (MRI)/ Magnetic Resonance Angiogram (MRA) of the neck and cervical spine:

1. Cervical fractures as described in CT
2. No evidence of cord compression, contusion, or hemorrhage
3. Disruption of the anterior longitudinal ligament at C2–C3 with 3 mm of antero-listhesis of C2 on C3. Posterior ligamentous injury at C1–C2.
4. Left vertebral artery occlusion

ED Management

On initial physical exam, the patient was identified to have midline cervical pain, approximately 12 hours after what was believed to be a fall from standing in her bathroom. She did not completely remember the event as she was significantly intoxicated at the time. As she had been ambulatory, was thought to have a low-risk mechanism, and had no neuro-deficits; plain films of her neck were obtained. On plain radiographs, no fractures were identified, but there was anterior subluxation of C2 on C3 with anterior tilt of C2, which is concerning for a nonvisualized hangman's fracture.

The patient was then placed in a cervical collar. As there was no spinal surgery available at the hospital, she was transferred to a tertiary care center while maintaining cervical spine immobilization.

Updates on ED Course

At the tertiary care center, a CT scan of the cervical spine was obtained, which confirmed a type 2 hangman's fracture and also identified multiple high cervical transverse process fractures. Neurosurgery was consulted, recommending an MRI and MRA. The patient was admitted to the neurosurgical service for considerations of internal immobilization versus halo immobilization.

Learning Points

Priming Questions
1. What is the appropriate screening tool for traumatic neck pain?
2. When should you obtain plain films vs CT for traumatic neck pain?

Introduction/Background

1. Cervical spinal fractures and dislocations rarely present to the emergency department. However, providers must remain always vigilant for cervical spine injuries as misdiagnosis can have grave consequences of progressive neurologic deficit and death. Of the millions of patients who present with potential cervical spine trauma, in stable alert patients, less than 1% will have sustained a cervical spine injury [1, 2]. Rates are likely higher in patients with associated head trauma and in unconscious patients.
2. As with most traumatic injuries, there is a bimodal age distribution, with a peak in young adults between ages 15 and 29 when individuals are more likely to engage in riskier behaviors, and then again in adults over the age of 65 when they have other risk factors for cervical injury [3].
3. Blunt cervical spine injury generally requires a high-force mechanism, such as a motor vehicle accident or fall from a great height. However, patients can certainly sustain these injuries from more benign mechanisms such as a fall from standing [4].

Physiology/Pathophysiology

1. The cervical spine consists of seven vertebrae. C1 (atlas) is the most superior, and with C2 (axis) forms the joint connecting the spine to the skull base. C1

lacks a full vertebral body, and instead this piece is fused to C2 to form the odontoid process. This allows for the rotation of the atlas on the axis. Also of importance, the vertebral artery travels through the transverse foramen of the cervical vertebrae.

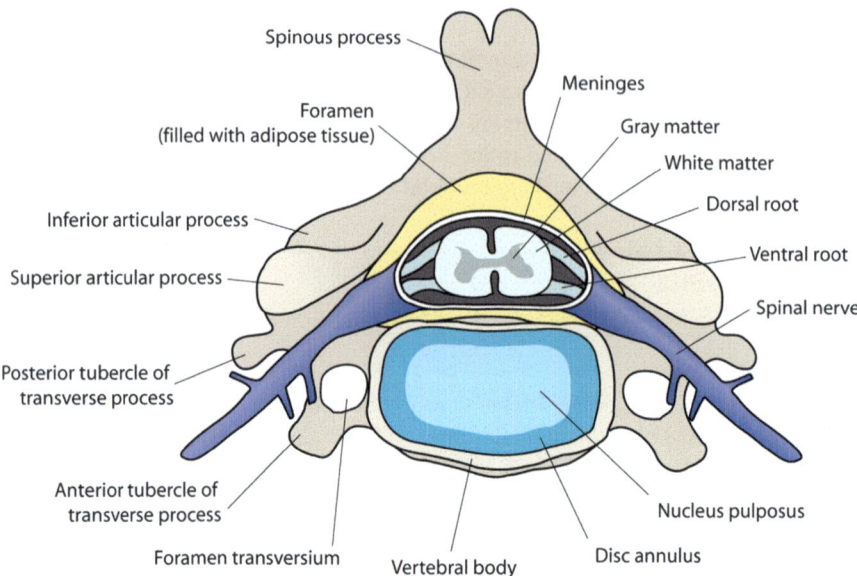

Image courtesy of wiki commons - user:debivort (https://commons.wikimedia.org/wiki/File:Cervical_vertebra_english.png), "Cervical vertebra english", https://creativecommons.org/licenses/by-sa/3.0/legalcode

2. Most commonly, a cervical spine fracture occurs following blunt trauma. In rare cases, patients could experience a pathologic fracture such as with malignant bony metastasis [5]. The most common mechanism of injury is motor vehicle collision.
3. The stability of cervical fractures is perhaps best understood by dividing the cervical vertebrae into two columns. The anterior column includes the vertebral body, the intervertebral disk space, the anterior and posterior longitudinal ligaments, and the disk annulus. The posterior column includes the spinal canal, pedicles, and articulating facets, and the posterior ligament complex, among other structures. In general, if both of these columns are affected, the injury is considered unstable and at high risk for spinal injury. Below are some of the classically described cervical spine fractures that should be recognized. While these are generally considered unstable, there are some exceptions such as Type 1 Jefferson and Odontoid fractures.

- C1 – Atlas fracture, also known as a Jefferson's Fracture. These fractures are more common in the elderly population. Rates and cost of care for atlas fractures are increasing [6].
  - Type I is isolated to the anterior or posterior arch.
  - Type II is a burst fracture with bilateral fractures of anterior and posterior arches.
  - Type III is a unilateral lateral mass fracture.
- C2 – Odontoid fracture. Most frequent fracture location in older adults.
  - Type I odontoid fractures involve avulsion of the tip of the odontoid. There may be associated atlanto-occipital instability.
  - Type II fractures occur through the waist of the odontoid. This is the most common fracture pattern in older adults.
  - Type III fractures extend into the body of C2.
- A Hangman's fracture is a traumatic anterior spondylolisthesis with a fracture dislocation of C2 on C3. These fractures are associated with a high-energy mechanism, making them more common in a younger population. They occur from a forceful extension of the neck with rapid deceleration. The name comes from the association with judicial hangings when the knot was placed under the chin in order to cause forceful extension. This is a helpful mechanism to remember as the same mechanics can occur when a patient falls and strikes their chin on a stationary surface or when an unrestrained driver hits their chin on the steering wheel.
  - Type I – axial loading and hyperextension – minimally displaced. Typically nonoperative.
  - Type II – Hyperextension with rebound flexion, disruption of C2–C3 disk.
  - Type IIA – Severe flexion of body fragment with minimal fracture displacement.
  - Type III – flexion/rebound extension with facet joint dislocations. Least common.
- Other unstable cervical fractures include
  - Atlanto-Occipital Dislocation
  - Bilateral Cervical Facet Dislocation
  - Flexion Teardrop
  - Any cervical fracture/dislocation
  - Wedge fracture with >50% height loss or if present in adjacent vertebrae
- Treatment is discussed below; however, in reality the stability of the injury may be difficult to determine in the emergent setting and often requires advanced imaging such as MRI. Because of this, the nuance in treatment for various injuries, and the high-risk pathology, it is generally recommended that all cervical fractures be immobilized and undergo specialist evaluation. An exemption to this may be an isolated spinous process fracture of the lower

Fig. 9.1 A Common
Mnemonic for Unstable
Cervical Fractures

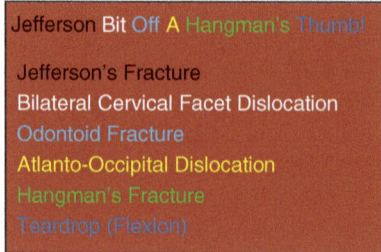

cervical spine, a "clay shoveler's fracture." This is typically treated conservatively with a collar and outpatient follow-up with a spinal surgeon to monitor
healing (Fig. 9.1).
4. While the high cervical fractures are most common in the elderly population,
   fractures involving C6–C7 are the most common pattern in younger patients.
   This is due to the mobility of the lower cervical spine compared to the fixed
   thoracic spine, with fractures occurring near this transition [7].

Making the Diagnosis

Differential Diagnosis
- Contusion
- Sprain
- Strain
- Spinal Shock
- Fracture
- Dislocation
- Subluxation

1. Clinical Exam
   - A careful clinical exam is important in any patient with suspected cervical
     spine injury. This will include palpation of the cervical spine and a neuro-
     logic assessment of cervical spinal levels. This includes strength assessment
     of the upper extremity, along with sensation in the upper extremity.
     Remember the dermatomal map to guide localization of a concerning neuro-
     logical findings – C6 involves the thumb, C7 middle finger, C8 pinky, T1
     lower arm.

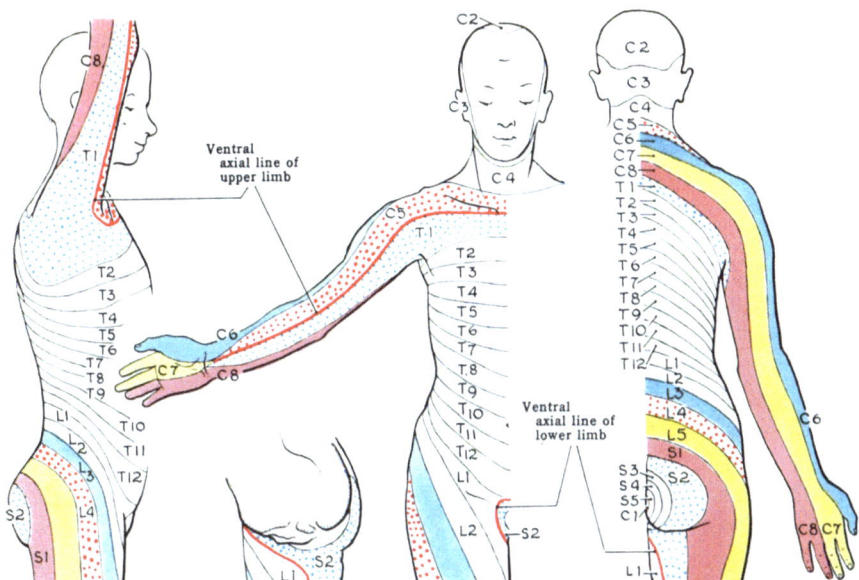

https://en.wikipedia.org/wiki/Dermatome_(anatomy)#/media/File:Grant_1962_663.png
Grant, John Charles Boileau (https://commons.wikimedia.org/wiki/File:Grant_1962_663.png), "Grant 1962 663", marked as public domain, more details on Wikimedia Commons: https://commons.wikimedia.org/wiki/Template:PD-US

- In those without tenderness and without high-risk mechanism, it is also important to perform range-of-motion testing to ensure the patient has normal active range of motion. However, in high-risk patients or those with a concerning neurologic exam, forgo range-of-motion testing to avoid further aggravating a spinal cord injury.
- If the physical exam is considered unreliable in a patient, such as in an unconscious patient, an intoxicated patient, or a patient with severe distracting injuries, imaging is required to exclude potential cervical injury. Alternatively, if overall suspicion is low, the patient can be immobilized and clinically reassessed when they are more reliable, for example, after they are no longer intoxicated.

2. There are well-validated clinical decision rules to support clinicians in the assessment of potential cervical spine injury. These rules are designed to help decrease rates of unnecessary imaging in patients with low risk for clinically significant injuries. The two main clinical decision rules that are utilized are the NEXUS criteria and the Canadian C- spine rules. When applied to an appropriate population, cervical imaging can be deferred if the patient meets either of the following criteria.

- The National Emergency X-Radiography Utilization Study Criteria (NEXUS criteria). [8] Patients do not need imaging so long as they do not have
  - Focal neurologic deficit
  - Midline spinal tenderness
    - This is the most common reason patients fail the nexus criteria. In low-risk patients, it may be appropriate to carefully differentiate paraspinal muscle tenderness from true midline tenderness.
  - Unreliable clinical exam:
    - Altered level of consciousness.
    - Intoxication.
    - Distracting injury – generally, a long bone fracture is considered reliably distracting. The clinician must be able to get an adequate exam despite other injuries. One approach is to ask the patient if they feel any pain, and to gently pinch the skin at the neck and ask if they can appreciate that discomfort.
- The Canadian c-spine rule. [9] Patients do not need imaging so long as they:
  - Do not have
    - Age greater than 65
    - Extremity paresthesias
    - Dangerous mechanism – fall >3 feet/5 stairs, axial load injury, high-speed MVC/rollover/ejection, bicycle collision, motorized recreational vehicle accident
  - Present with at least one low-risk factor:
    - Sitting position in ED
    - Ambulatory at any time
    - Delayed (not immediate) onset of neck pain
    - Simple rear-end MVC (not pushed into traffic, not hit by large truck/ bus, not rollover, not hit by high-speed vehicle)
  - Are able to rotate their neck 45 degrees left and right
3. Special populations:
   - Pediatric patients greater than 1 year of age were included in the initial NEXUS cohort, and the standard clinical decision rules can be applied to the pediatric patient population to avoid imaging [10]. In children less than 8 years old, the most common injury pattern is at or above C3 due to the relatively large head causing high fulcrum. Head injury should also be evaluated using the PECARN clinical decision rule to evaluate need for concurrent head imaging [11]. The Canadian C-Spine rule study excluded patients under 16 years of age, and therefore cannot be applied to most pediatric patients.
   - Geriatric patients were also included in the initial NEXUS cohort; however, there have been reports of decreased sensitivity of the NEXUS criteria in patients older than 65 [12]. One recommendation is to add a change in mental status from baseline, which improved sensitivity [13]. Clearly, all patients over 65 necessitate imaging by the Canadian C-Spine rule as this is considered a high-risk feature, as listed above.

4. Imaging
   - For most patients that fail a clinical decision rule, there is debate as to the imaging modality of choice. Plain film imaging of the cervical spine has the benefit of delivering less radiation and being cheaper than a cervical CT. However, X-ray imaging must be *adequate* to exclude fracture. This means that the entire cervical spine and T1 must be visualized, and there are no baseline bony changes to obscure interpretation. Furthermore, recent studies have demonstrated varying ranges of sensitivity for plain film evaluation, and the Eastern Association for the Surgery of Trauma guidelines recommend against the use of plain films in evaluating for traumatic injuries [14]. Therefore, many clinicians now utilize CT imaging even in low-risk patients who necessitate imaging.
   - It is generally recommended to evaluate geriatric patients with CT cervical spine imaging to rule out fractures [15]. This is because the older patient population is at higher risk for cervical spine injury with lower mechanism injuries, and they more frequently have baseline bony changes.
   - Plain films have been shown to be highly sensitive in pediatric patient population [16].
   - CT imaging is recommended in patients suffering from multiple trauma. They are at the highest risk of cervical spine injury, and many times it is impossible to get an adequate physical exam or X-ray in these patients.
   - Indications for MRI are limited but would include those patients with neurologic deficits but normal CT imaging. MRI may also be needed to assess for ligamentous and spinal injuries in those patients who are shown to have bony abnormalities on CT.
5. Because the vertebral artery travels through the transverse foramen of the cervical spine, arteriogram imaging may need to be considered in patients with traumatic spinal injuries. Multiple screening criteria have been developed, and the Eastern Association for the Surgery of Trauma recommends arterial imaging in the following patients [14]:
   - Any patient with a neurologic abnormality on exam that is unexplained by the diagnosed injuries
   - A blunt trauma patient who develops epistaxis from a suspected arterial source following a trauma
   - Arterial imaging may be considered in patients with
     - GCS less than 8
     - Petrous bone fractures
     - Diffuse axonal injury
     - Cervical spine fractures of C1 through C3 or fractures that extend through the transverse foramen
     - Cervical spine fractures with subluxation or a rotational component
     - Le Fort II (mobile mid face) or Le Fort III (mobile face) fractures

Treating the Patient

1. For the initial management of patients with potential cervical fractures, always consider the ABCs (airway, breathing, circulation). Patients with extensive trauma may have other life-threatening conditions that first require stabilization before fully assessing or managing the cervical spine.
2. Standard practice currently recommends placement of ridged cervical collar in all patients with blunt head or cervical trauma who cannot be initially cleared by clinical decision rules. However, recent evidence is growing to suggest ridged cervical collars may cause harm without measurable benefits [17, 18]. This is certainly an active controversy. A common-sense recommendation is to use a cervical collar when the patient can tolerate it. However, if contraindications are present and the patient is co-operative, it is reasonable to defer the cervical collar while obtaining definitive cervical spine imaging. In these patients, it is still important to limit mobility of the cervical spine with patient cooperation.
3. Patients with injuries limited to penetrating neck trauma are very unlikely to sustain c-spine fracture or dislocation, and immobilization in these patients has been shown to have worse outcomes [19]. It is NOT recommended to immobilize the spine for patients with isolated penetrating neck injury unless there is a focal neurological deficit.
4. Clearing the cervical spine
   - In those that do not have injury on imaging, the cervical spine should be cleared. This involves removing the cervical collar and repeating the physical exam to determine if there is ongoing concern for cervical spine injury.
   - Current guidelines recommend removing the cervical collar in obtunded patients with normal CT imaging [17]. This recommendation can be extrapolated to alert patients with a reassuring clinical exam.
   - Patients should be considered for cervical spine MRI to evaluate for blunt spinal cord injuries or unstable ligamentous injury if there are neurologic deficits or other exam features concerning for spine instability despite normal CT imaging. Fortunately, these sorts of injuries are exceedingly rare in patients with normal CT imaging and a reassuring physical exam.
5. Definitive management of the cervical spine depends on the specific type of fracture. It is always recommended to consult a spinal surgeon in the setting of any spinal injury. Many patients will require surgical fixation.

Case Conclusion

The patient underwent halo external fixation. During her hospitalization, she developed a persistent supraventricular tachycardia that was difficult to control with medical management. She underwent an electrophysiology study with ablation of the secondary pathway. She presented again to the emergency department a few months later and was found to have an intracranial abscess deep to the halo fixation device attachment point and underwent craniotomy and wash out. During her second hospitalization, she developed a Deep Vein Thrombosis (DVT) and Pulmonary Embolus (PE). Eventually, she recovered with neurologic function fully intact.

Discussion

Cervical spine fractures are an uncommon diagnosis but an entity that the provider should always consider in patients with blunt head and neck trauma. There are well-validated clinical decision tools to help guide workup and identify individuals who require imaging. There is significant debate over the best initial imaging study. It is the clinical practice of the authors, to use plain film X-rays to rule out fractures in patients, they consider low-risk by clinical gestalt. However, CT imaging can be the initial modality if there is a high likelihood of an inadequate plain film, such as in the geriatric population, or a higher pretest probability of cervical spine injury, such as in the polytraumatized patient. Placement of rigid cervical collars to "protect" the uncleared cervical spine is somewhat controversial, and we may see practice patterns change in the future to rely less on rigid cervical collars. Patients with normal CT imaging of the spine can be "cleared" even in obtunded trauma patients, unless there is neurologic deficit or concerns for blunt spinal cord injury.

Pattern Recognition

Cervical Fractures
- Mid-line cervical pain and limited range of motion
- Neurological deficit (though this should prompt investigation, most patients with spinal fractures are neurologically intact)
- Geriatric patients with a fall from standing (or more significant trauma)

Disclosure Statement The authors of this chapter report no significant disclosures

References

1. National Center for Health Statistics. National Hospital Ambulatory Medical Care Survey: 2010, 2014.
2. Greenbaum J, Walters N, Levy PD. An evidenced-based approach to radiographic assessment of cervical spine injuries in the emergency department. J Emerg Med. 2009;36(1):64–71.
3. National Spinal Cord Injury Association Resource Center. Available from: www.sci-info-pages.com/factsheets.html.
4. Wang H, Coppola M, Robinson RD, Scribner JT, Vithalani V, de Moor CE, et al. Geriatric trauma patients with cervical spine fractures due to ground level fall: five years experience in a level one trauma center. J Clin Med Res. 2013;5(2):75–83.

5. Davis MA, Taylor JA. A case of vertebral metastasis with pathologic c2 fracture. J Manip Physiol Ther. 2007;30(6):466–71.
6. Daniels AH, Arthur M, Esmende SM, Vigneswaran H, Palumbo MA. Incidence and cost of treating axis fractures in the United States from 2000 to 2010. Spine (Phila Pa 1976). 2014;39(18):1498–505.
7. Morrison J, Jeanmonod R. Imaging in the NEXUS-negative patient: when we break the rule. Am J Emerg Med. 2014;32(1):67–70.
8. Matteucci MJ, Moszyk D, Migliore SA. Agreement between resident and faculty emergency physicians in the application of NEXUS criteria for suspected cervical spine injuries. J Emerg Med. 2015;48(4):445–9.
9. Stiell IG, Clement CM, Lowe M, Sheehan C, Miller J, Armstrong S, et al. A multicenter program to implement the Canadian C-Spine rule by Emergency Department Triage Nurses. Ann Emerg Med. 2018;72:333.
10. Schoneberg C, Schweiger B, Hussmann B, Kauther MD, Lendemans S, Waydhas C. Diagnosis of cervical spine injuries in children: a systematic review. Eur J Trauma Emerg Surg. 2013;39(6):653–65.
11. Runde D, Beiner J. Calculated decisions: PECARN pediatric head injury/trauma algorithm. Pediatr Emerg Med Pract. 2018;15(Suppl 6):Cd3–cd4.
12. Goode T, Young A, Wilson SP, Katzen J, Wolfe LG, Duane TM. Evaluation of cervical spine fracture in the elderly: can we trust our physical examination? Am Surg. 2014;80(2):182–4.
13. Tran J, Jeanmonod D, Agresti D, Hamden K, Jeanmonod RK. Prospective validation of modified NEXUS cervical spine injury criteria in low-risk elderly fall patients. West J Emerg Med. 2016;17(3):252–7.
14. Bromberg WJ, Collier BC, Diebel LN, Dwyer KM, Holevar MR, Jacobs DG, et al. Blunt cerebrovascular injury practice management guidelines: the Eastern Association for the Surgery of Trauma. J Trauma. 2010;68(2):471–7.
15. Paykin G, O'Reilly G, Ackland HM, Mitra B. The NEXUS criteria are insufficient to exclude cervical spine fractures in older blunt trauma patients. Injury. 2017;48(5):1020–4.
16. Cui LW, Probst MA, Hoffman JR, Mower WR. Sensitivity of plain radiography for pediatric cervical spine injury. Emerg Radiol. 2016;23(5):443–8.
17. Patel MB, Humble SS, Cullinane DC, Day MA, Jawa RS, Devin CJ, et al. Cervical spine collar clearance in the obtunded adult blunt trauma patient: a systematic review and practice management guideline from the Eastern Association for the Surgery of Trauma. J Trauma Acute Care Surg. 2015;78(2):430–41.
18. Hauswald M, Braude D. Spinal immobilization in trauma patients: is it really necessary? Curr Opin Crit Care. 2002;8(6):566–70.
19. Vanderlan WB, Tew BE, McSwain NE Jr. Increased risk of death with cervical spine immobilisation in penetrating cervical trauma. Injury. 2009;40(8):880–3.

Radiology Case 2

10

Priyanka Dube and Joshua K. Aalberg

Indication for the Exam 27 y/o m with left knee swelling, lateral tenderness, and pain with rotational movements after a motor vehicle accident.

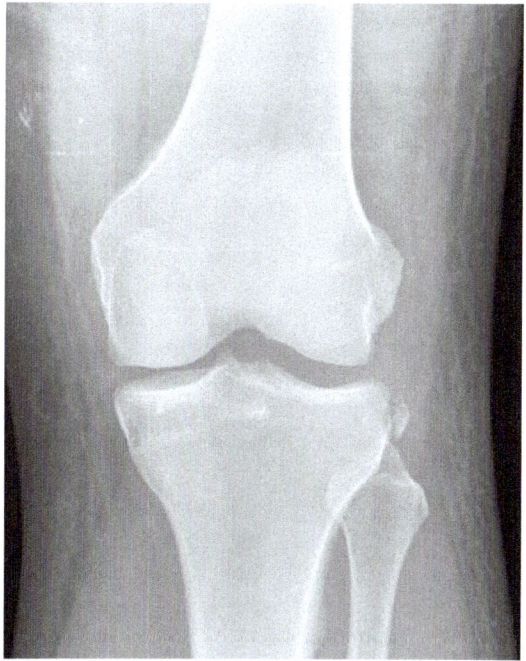

P. Dube · J. K. Aalberg (✉)
Department of Emergency Medicine, Wexner Medical Center at The Ohio State University, Columbus, OH, USA
e-mail: Priyanka.Dube@osumc.edu; joshua.aalberg@osumc.edu

© Springer Nature Switzerland AG 2020
C. G. Kaide, C. E. San Miguel (eds.), *Case Studies in Emergency Medicine*,
https://doi.org/10.1007/978-3-030-22445-5_10

Radiographic Findings AP view of the left knee demonstrating an avulsion fracture of the lateral tibia.

Diagnosis Segond fracture.

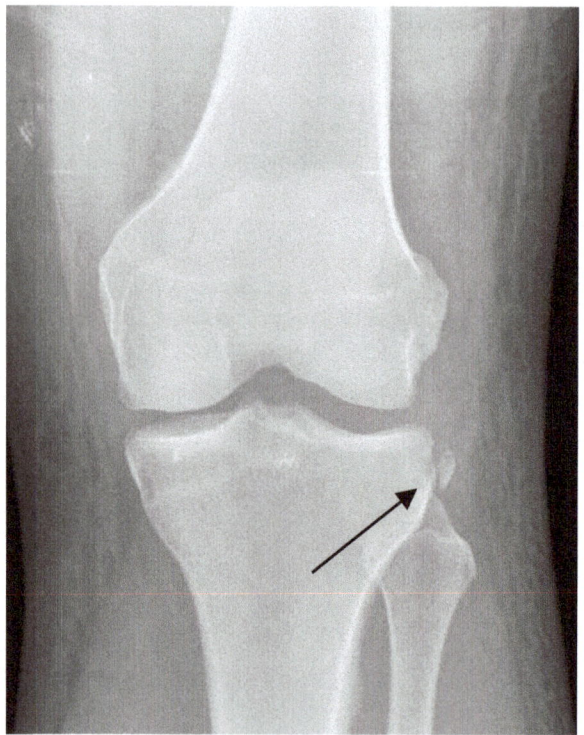

Learning Points

Priming Questions
- What is the mechanism of injury?
- What are additional injuries associated with this fracture?
- What is the Reverse Segond fracture?
- What is the arcuate sign?

Introduction/Background

Named after French surgeon Paul Segond in 1879, a Segond fracture is an avulsion fracture of the tibia at the insertion site of the lateral capsular ligament [1].

Pathophysiology/Mechanism

The Segond fracture occurs from internal rotation of the knee with an external varus stress. This motion increases tension upon the lateral capsular ligament, which then causes a cortical break at its insertion on the tibia. There is a high association of lateral capsular disruption with ACL and meniscal tears. Patients will complain of pain along the lateral aspect of the tibia with lateral rotational instability [1]. Other injuries associated with a Segond fracture can include trauma to the iliotibial band and anterior oblique band of the fibular collateral ligament [2].

Making the Diagnosis

- On AP knee radiographs, an elliptical-shaped bone fragment is seen along the lateral aspect of the tibia just below/adjacent to the lateral tibial plateau. Radiologists will often refer to this as the *lateral capsular* sign [1].
- Conspicuity of the small avulsed bone fragment is best appreciated on cross-sectional imaging; however, AP radiographs of the knee are the initial test of choice.
- It is important to note that nonemergent MRI is indicated for all patients with a Segond fracture given the strong association with anterior cruciate ligament (>70%) (2–3) and meniscal tears [1, 3].
- The *Reverse Segond Fracture* is described as an avulsion injury to the deep capsular medial collateral ligament. An elliptical bone fragment is located adjacent to the medial tibial plateau. This injury occurs with external rotation and valgus stress: the reverse mechanism of a Segond fracture [1].

Other Injuries Associated with Segond Fractures

- ACL injury
- Meniscal Tear
- Avulsion injury of the long head of the biceps femoris ligament
- Avulsion injury of the fibular collateral ligament
- Tibial Plateau Fracture [3]

Major Mimicker of Segond Fractures: The Arcuate Sign

- An avulsion fracture of the styloid process of the fibula where the arcuate ligament complex attaches is known to radiologists as *the arcuate sign* [4].
- This fracture is also commonly associated with cruciate ligament injury. On conventional radiograph, the osseous fragment *is displaced superiorly and medially* to the fibular donor site [4].

- Distinguishing between these two pathologies is difficult but can be accomplished by identification of the donor site (tibia for Segond Fracture and fibula for the arcuate sign), orientation of the bone fragment (generally vertical for Segond Fracture and horizontal for the acuate sign), or via advanced imaging.

Segond Fracture vs. Arcuate Sign		
	Segond Fracture	Arcuate Sign
Donor Site	Lateral Tibia	Styloid process of the Fibula
Orientation of the bone fragment	Vertical	Horizontal
Displacement Direction	Anterior and Lateral to the Lateral Tibia	Superior and Medial to the Fibula

Treating the Patient

In many cases, surgical intervention is eventually warranted due to the extensive ligamentous injury that may occur [2]. Due to the high instance of ligamentous injury, these patients should be treated as though they have a presumed ligamentous tear. Depending on local practice patterns, this may result in an orthopedic consultation and advanced imaging in the Emergency Department or non-weight-bearing status with urgent orthopedic specialist follow-up.

Discussion

- Traumatic injuries to the knee can result in avulsion fractures due to the number of tendons and ligaments that attach. While radiography is typically the initial exam of choice to diagnose fracture, MRI is used to diagnose any associated soft tissue injuries.
- Understanding the appearance of imaging can help the clinician identify mechanism of injury and raise suspicion for any associated injuries. Due to the high instance of associated ligamentous injury with both Segond Fractures and The Arcuate Sign, these patients should be treated as though they have a presumed ligamentous tear.

Disclosure Statement The authors of this chapter report no significant disclosures.

References

1. Gottsegen CJ, Eyer BA, White EA, Learch TJ, Forrester D. Avulsion fractures of the knee: imaging findings and clinical significance. Radiographics. 2008;28(6):1755–70. https://doi.org/10.1148/rg.286085503.
2. Gaillard F. et al. Segond Fracture. Radiopaedia. Accessed 17 Jun 2018. https://radiopaedia.org/articles/segond-fracture.

3. Peltola EK, Mustonen AO, Lindahl J, Koskinen SK. Segond fracture combined with Tibial Plateau fracture. Am J Roentgenol. 2011;197(6) https://doi.org/10.2214/ajr.10.6095.
4. Gaillard F. et al. Arcuate Sign. Radiopaedia. Accessed 17 Jun 2018. https://radiopaedia.org/articles/arcuate-sign-knee.

Cyanide Poisoning—"I'm Mr. Blue..."

11

Jessica A. Everett, Colin G. Kaide, and Hannah Hays

Case 1

Pertinent History

This patient is a 27-year-old female who presents by medic to the emergency department after a syncopal episode in class. She went up to her professor and said she didn't feel well, then collapsed. The medics found her unconscious and apneic at the scene and began bag valve mask ventilation. She arrived in the emergency department unconscious being bagged at a rate of 12 times per minute. Her heart rate initially was 40, and her blood pressure was 40 systolic. No further information was available at the time.

Pertinent Physical Exam

- *Vitals: BP 40/Palp, HR 40, RR 12 (per BVM), Temp 98.9 °F/37.2 °C*

Except as noted below, the findings of the complete physical exam are within normal limits.

J. A. Everett (✉) · C. G. Kaide
Department of Emergency Medicine, Wexner Medical Center at The Ohio State University, Columbus, OH, USA
e-mail: Jessica.Everett@osumc.edu; Colin.kaide@osumc.edu

H. Hays
Department of Emergency Medicine, Wexner Medical Center at The Ohio State University, Columbus, OH, USA

Central Ohio Poison Center, Columbus, OH, USA

Nationwide Children's Hospital, Columbus, OH, USA
e-mail: Hannah.Hays@nationwidechildrens.org

© Springer Nature Switzerland AG 2020
C. G. Kaide, C. E. San Miguel (eds.), *Case Studies in Emergency Medicine*,
https://doi.org/10.1007/978-3-030-22445-5_11

- *General:* Unconscious and apneic female with no signs of external trauma
- *Eyes:* Pupils dilated and nonreactive
- *Lungs:* Clear bilaterally
- *Heart:* S1, S2 Bradycardic rate, regular rhythm
- *Abdomen:* Soft
- *Skin:* No rash. Cool and dry
- *Neuro:* GCS 3. No spontaneous movement noted

PMH
Unknown.

SH/FH
Unknown.

Pertinent Test Results

Pertinent Lab Results						
Test	Result 0923	Result 0945	Result 1026	Result 1142	Units	Normal Range
WBC	19				K/uL	3.8–11.0 10^3/mm^3
Hgb	12.3				g/dL	(Male) 14–18 g/dL (Female) 11–16 g/dL
Platelets	203				K/uL	140–450 K/uL
Sodium	137				mEq/L	135–148 mEq/L
Potassium	4.6				mEq/L	3.5–5.5 mEq/L
Chloride	105				mEq/L	96–112 mEq/L
Bicarbonate	<5				mEq/L	21–34 mEq/L
BUN	12				mg/dL	6–23 mg/dL
Glucose	156				mg/dL	65–99 mg/dL
Serum HCG	Negative				–	Negative
Creatinine	0.9				mg/dL	0.6–1.5 mg/dL
Lactate	20		24		mmol/L	<2.0
pH	6.92	7.02	6.84	6.92	–	7.35–7.45
PaCO2	35	30			mmHg	35–45
PaO2	550	529			mmHg	Depends on FiO$_2$
Carboxyhemoglobin			3		%	<5%
Drugs of Abuse				None	–	None

Pertinent Lab Results

Test	Result 0923	Result 0945	Result 1026	Result 1142	Units	Normal Range
CSF WBC				3	leukocyte/ mcL	0–5
CSF RBC				16	erythrocytes/ mcL	0–10
CSF Gram Stain				No org seen	–	None
Volatile Alcohols				None	–	None
Ethylene Glycol				None		
Serum Measured Osmoles				298	mOsm/kg	285–295
Comprehensive Toxicology				Sertraline, diphenhydramine	–	Negative

ED Management

She was immediately intubated using rapid sequence induction and taken for head CT with the first thought being that this could be an intracranial hemorrhage. Simultaneous to the CT scan, an IV was established with fluids wide open. The CT scan showed no evidence of intracranial hemorrhage. The patient's blood pressure and pulse were unchanged. She received 4 sequential, 1 mg doses of atropine with no change in her heart rate. A norepinephrine drip was started and titrated rapidly with her blood pressure rising to 45 systolic at maximum norepinephrine dosing.

Laboratory work showed a pH of 6.92 with a pO_2 of 550 a pCO_2 of 35 and a bicarbonate of zero. Her lactate was 20. The patient was given 4 Amps of sodium bicarbonate, and her pH on subsequent blood gas was 7.0. She was given 2 additional doses of atropine with no response in her heart rate. An epinephrine drip was substituted for norepinephrine and titrated. Her blood pressure was now around 50 systolic.

A central line was attempted in the right internal jugular, and the resident reported that she thought the blood was arterial, though it was not pulsatile. She then moved to a femoral central line and had a similar report when attempting to place the line. While the needle was in place, a second needle was placed more laterally and blood was obtained, which was pulsatile. The arterial stick was converted to an arterial line, and the initial presumably venous stick was converted to a central line.

Update 1

A repeat blood gas showed a pH at 6.8. She was given 4 more amps of sodium bicarbonate. Additional laboratory testing was performed that included a carbon monoxide level, which was 3, and a repeat lactate, which was now 23. A lumbar puncture was performed showing 2 white cells per high-power field and 10 red cells. No organisms were seen on Gram stain. Her white count came back at 19,000 with a hemoglobin of 12. Broad-spectrum antibiotics were initiated, and toxicologic screening was performed. A FAST scan was performed showing no evidence of intraperitoneal blood. Her heart did not show pericardial effusion; however, contractility was poor. Despite max dosing of epinephrine, her heart rate remained in the mid-40s and her blood pressure did not exceed 50 systolic. She remained unconscious. She was admitted to the ICU with cardiovascular collapse of unknown etiology.

Update 2

Two of her friends arrived in the emergency department and stated that she had been sick for a couple of days prior to this event. She is a Pharmacy Doctorate (PharmD) student and, except for cold symptoms, was otherwise healthy as far as her friends knew. The patient was going to graduate in the next week. After the patient arrived in the ICU, the comprehensive toxicology screen resulted, showing no detected no illicit drugs or medications other than sertraline and diphenhydramine.

Case 2: House Fire

Pertinent History

This patient is a 37-year-old male who was brought to the emergency department by EMS after being rescued from a house fire. He had suffered significant smoke inhalation. EMS said the patient was unresponsive and CPR was initiated, followed by return of spontaneous circulation. Post arrest, he was reported to be hypotensive and bradycardic at the scene. He was intubated at the scene without complication. The fire was reported to have started in a bedroom where it is possible that a family member had been smoking in bed. There were 2 fatalities at the scene.

Pertinent Physical Exam

Vitals: BP 50/P HR 35 RR 14 per BVM Temp 97.2 degrees F.
    Except as noted below, the findings of the complete physical exam are within normal limits.

- *General:* Unresponsive male
- *Eyes:* Pupils dilated and reactive
- *Mouth:* Soot noted in airway
- *Lungs:* Rhonci bilaterally
- *Heart:* S1, S2 Bradycardic rate, regular rhythm
- *Abdomen:* Soft
- *Skin:* No rash. Cool and dry. No burns noted
- *Neuro:* GCS 3. With minimal spontaneous movement

PMH
Unknown

SH/FH
Unknown

Pertinent Test Results

Test	Result 0230	Result 0350	Units	Normal
WBC	12		K/uL	3.8–11.0 10³/mm³
HgB	14.4		g/dL	(Male) 14–18 g/dL
				(Female) 11–16 g/dL
Platelets	187		K/uL	140–450 K/uL
Sodium	139		mEq/L	135–148 mEq/L
Potassium	3.9		mEq/L	3.5–5.5 mEq/L
Chloride	105		mEq/L	96–112 mEq/L
Bicarbonate	9		mEq/L	21–34 mEq/L
BUN	9		mg/dL	6–23 mg/dL
Creatinine	0.6		mg/dL	0.6–1.5 mg/dL
Glucose	190		mg/dL	65–99 mg/dL
Lactate	14		mmol/L	<2.0
pH	7.01	7.29	–	7.35–7.45
PaCO₂	24	30	mmHg	35–45
PaO₂	550	529	mmHg	Depends on FiO₂
Carboxyhemoglobin	16		%	<5

Emergency Department Management

The patient was given 2 mg of atropine with no response in heart rate. He was started on a norepinephrine drip. The critical care laboratory results showed a profound metabolic acidosis with an anion gap and a significantly elevated lactate. The lab abnormalities in conjunction with the clinical findings of altered level of consciousness, persistent hypotension, and bradycardia lead to the diagnosis of cyanide toxicity. The patient was given 5 grams of hydroxocobalamin IV over 15 min. He was also given 12.5 grams of sodium thiosulfate IV (50 ml).

Update 1

Within 20 minutes of receiving the antidotes, the patient had significant improvement in vital signs with his heart rate increasing to 80 and his BP to 120/70. He started to move around. The hyperbaric physician on-call felt the carboxyhemoglobin was likely not the significant contributor to the patient's clinical condition and recommended to continue normobaric oxygen at an FiO₂ of 100% while on the ventilator.

Learning Points

Priming Questions
1. What clinical presentation would lead you to suspect cyanide poisoning?
2. What "natural" sources of cyanide exist?
3. What lab abnormalities do you expect in acute cyanide poisoning?
4. Can you confirm cyanide poisoning prior to initiating treatment?
5. What are the treatment options for acute cyanide poisoning?

Introduction/Background

1. Cyanide exposure can occur from inhalation, skin absorption, ingestion, or metabolism of medications/compounds (e.g., nitroprusside, cyanogenic food sources).
2. They occur in various forms.
   - Inorganic cyanides (cyanide salts) contain anionic form CN^-. Common forms are sodium cyanide and potassium cyanide (NaCN & KCN).
     - Industrial use: Metallurgy, photographic developing, fumigation, plastics manufacturing, mining, electroplating, ore extraction, pharmaceutical manufacturing, chemistry labs where cyanide salts are common reagents [1–3].
     - Cyanide salts + water → hydrogen cyanide [2].
       o Hydrogen cyanide (HCN) is a volatile and highly flammable liquid with boiling point at approximately room temperature. It is produced industrially on a large scale with multiple applications, for example, nylon manufacturing [2, 4].
   - Organic compounds that involve the cyano group and an alkyl residue are called "nitriles" ($R–C\equiv N$). Organic molecules including multiple nitrile groups are called "cyanocarbons." Examples of these include
     - Latex-free medical gloves, nitrile rubber in automotive seals, compounds in superglue (cyanoacrylate), to list a few examples [1, 2, 4, 5].
     - Plants, such as bitter almonds, apricot pits, apple seeds, cassava, and certain lima beans, contain cyanogenic glycosides [2, 6].
     - By the way, there are bitter and sweet almonds. Sweet almonds are what you typically eat as a snack or use in cooking. Bitter almonds (found in the Middle East and Asia) are used in food flavorings and oils. Bitter almonds are not just bitter, but they also contain prussic or hydrocyanic acid in the raw form. They can be significantly toxic to humans and animals, with ingestion of as few as 10 bitter almonds being potentially lethal! [11] Heating and/or processing them can inactivate the toxin.
   - There are several forms of cyanide gas:
     - HCN – hydrogen cyanide is a gas at room temperature with a reported bitter odor.
     - Cyanogen chloride (CNCl) is considered a chemical weapon, since it is easily condensed and colorless [2, 5].
     - Cyanogen gas ($N\equiv C–C\equiv N$) reacts with water to release CN^- [2].

- Nitroprusside, an IV medication used to treat hypertension, can become toxic in 5–10 hours at a rate of 4 mcg/kg/min, and even faster in malnourished or postoperative patients. Each molecule of nitroprusside contains *five* CN molecules [2].
- *Combustion of polyurethane, silk, wool, synthetic rubber, and other common household items can release cyanide gas accounting for potential poisoning in smoke inhalation [2, 4, 5].*

3. The dose required to produce toxicity depends on the form, duration of exposure, route of exposure, and underlying comorbidities [2, 5].
   - The adult oral lethal dose of potassium cyanide is about 200 mg [2].
   - Hydrogen cyanide (HCN) is immediately fatal at a concentration of only 270 ppm.
   - HCN has a low molecular weight and is nonionized, so it readily crosses biologic membranes rapidly crossing alveolar membranes and is therefore quickly distributed to target organs [2].

Physiology/Pathophysiology

1. Cyanide inhibits multiple enzymes including cytochrome oxidase in the electron transport chain ("ETC") of the mitochondria.
   - Hydrogen ions normally combine with oxygen at the end of the ETC. Cyanide inhibits this process – even with sufficient oxygen available, the electron transport chain cannot be utilized, halting production of ATP. This shifts the body to anaerobic respiration and leaves unincorporated hydrogen ions to accumulate, contributing to profound acidemia [7]. *See* Fig. 11.1.
   - Elevated lactic acid follows CN poisoning due to anaerobic metabolism. Pyruvate is converted to lactate [7]. *See* Fig. 11.2.

2. Amount, route of poisoning, duration of exposure, and comorbid conditions affect toxicity including time to onset and ultimate severity of illness [2].
   - Onset of toxicity occurs in seconds with inhalation HCN or IV injection of a water-soluble salt.
   - Onset of toxicity occurs in minutes following ingestion of inorganic salt (usually sodium or potassium cyanide).
   - Onset of toxicity occurs in hours to days for cyanogenic chemicals, which require biotransformation prior to toxicity. An example of this is nitroprusside infusion without coadministration of thiosulfate.

3. Toxicity is nonspecific causing rapid dysfunction of oxygen-sensitive, highly metabolic organs – notably CNS and cardiovascular system [2, 5].
   - CNS: Cyanide acts as a neurotoxin, significantly affecting highly metabolic brain tissue.
     - The most oxygen-sensitive areas of the brain (e.g., basal ganglia, cerebellum, sensorimotor cortex) are particularly susceptible, demonstrating injury on cranial imaging of cyanide-poisoning survivors.
     - Other routes of toxicity involve generation of reactive oxygen species, which interfere with multiple pathways leading to apoptosis, necrosis, and neurodegeneration.

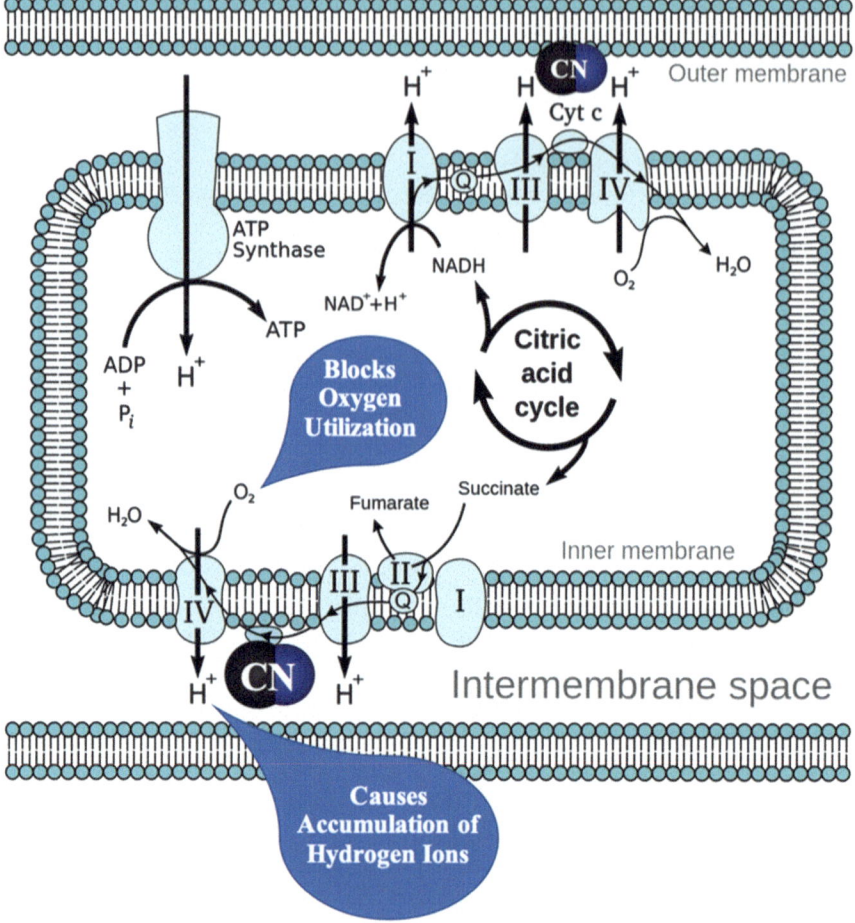

Fig. 11.1 Inhibition of Cytochrome C by CN. CN blocks oxygen utilization and ATP formation and causes accumulation of hydrogen ions. (Published with kind permission of © Colin G. Kaide 2019. All Rights Reserved)

- The chain of events leads to
  - Progressive hypoxia ➔ headache, agitation, anxiety, confusion, lethargy, coma
  - Nonreactive, dilated pupils
  - Centrally mediated tachypnea ➔ bradypnea ➔ apnea
- Cardiovascular: The cardiovascular system has a complex response to cyanide exposure [8].
  - Reflex mechanisms may temporarily prevent obvious dysfunction – initially one may see hypertension, tachycardia, and increased inotropy.
  - This is followed by hypotension often with initial reflex tachycardia.
  - As ATP depletion and acidosis develop, bradycardia and hypotension become inevitable.
  - Ventricular arrhythmias are *not* a predominant feature.

Fig. 11.2 Accumulation of Lactate in the Presence of CN. (Published with kind permission of © Colin G. Kaide 2019. All Rights Reserved)

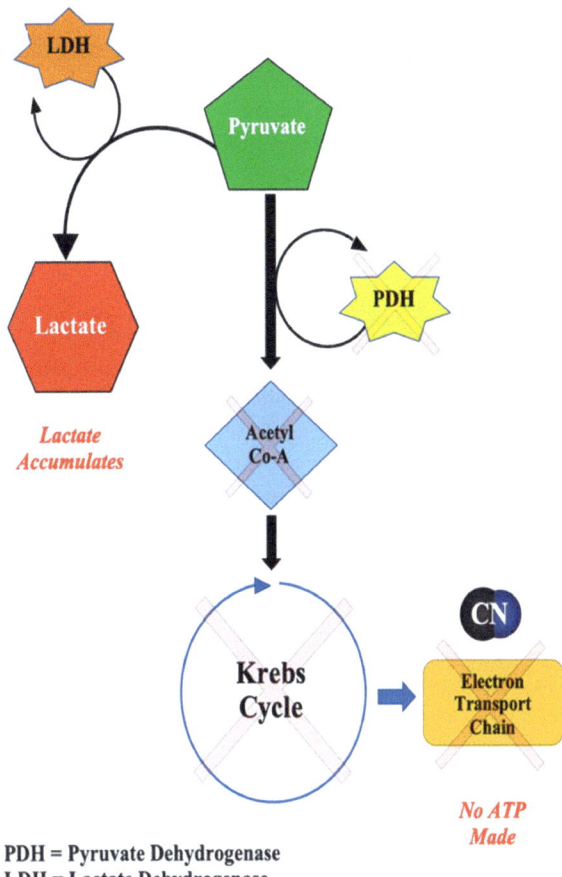

PDH = Pyruvate Dehydrogenase
LDH = Lactate Dehydrogenase

- Pulmonary:
  - Mild corrosive injury to mucosa may be seen.
  - Pulmonary edema has been seen at autopsy.
  - Exhaled air from patient with cyanide toxicity is classically described as having "bitter almond" smell, but this is not sensitive or specific and should not be relied upon for diagnosis.
- Cutaneous: This has variable manifestations.
  - It is historically taught that "cherry red skin" can be seen due to hyperoxia from decreased tissue utilization of oxygen. This may best be seen on funduscopic examination where veins and arteries can appear similar in color.
  - Cyanide does not directly cause cyanosis, despite the name similarity. Cyanosis in toxicity is favored to be from cardiovascular collapse and poor perfusion.
- GI: Symptoms may be seen after ingestion of inorganic cyanide and cyanogens. These include abdominal pain, nausea, and vomiting.
  - Hemorrhagic gastritis can develop over time, due to corrosive effects; however, if the patient suffers rapid deterioration/death, this may not have time to develop.

4. Delayed manifestations [2, 3].
   - May be insidious and nonspecific involving multiple organ systems.
   - Neurologic sequelae, including parkinsonian symptoms, dysarthria, bradykinesia, and rigidity, are the most common and develop over weeks to months as the result of direct cellular toxicity and tissue hypoxia.
   - These are generally poorly responsive to antiparkinsonian medication.
5. Toxicity manifestations in cyanogenic food exposure (e.g., cassava) [6].
   - Sublethal concentrations (≤80 μmol/L) associated with signs/symptoms of acute toxicity can be seen in blood of populations dependent on cyanogenic cassava as a main food source.
   - Ingestion of improperly processed cassava is associated with a syndrome of permanent neurologic deficits, known as "Konzo" (roughly translated from the Yaka language to mean, "tied legs"). Symptoms of Konzo include symmetric spastic paresis (lower extremities more severely affected), gait abnormalities, and hyperreflexia of the lower extremities.
   - Within populations affected, children and women of childbearing age tend to be more affected – members of the population with poor dietary intake of proteins – which is the major source of sulfur necessary for the detoxification process of cyanide.

Making the Diagnosis

Differential Diagnosis
- Shock – choose your favorite flavor
- Carbon monoxide or hydrogen sulfide exposure (cellular toxins)
- Causes of anion gap metabolic acidosis CAT MUDPILES
  - Cyanide
  - Alcoholic Ketoacidosis
  - Toluene (Halogenated Hydrocarbons)
  - Methanol, Metformin
  - Uremia
  - Diabetic Ketoacidosis
  - Paracetamol
  - Isoniazid, Iron, Ibuprofen
  - Lactate
  - Ethylene Glycol
  - Salicylates

1. When to suspect cyanide poisoning [1–3, 5, 6, 9].
   - *Caveat:* many deaths from acute cyanide toxicity/poisoning likely occur "in the field" without presentation to hospital [3].
   - *Caveat 2:* If patients make it to the hospital, ***there is no clear toxidrome. The clinician must have "could this be cyanide?" on the differential diagnosis or he/she will miss it!*** Suspicious scenarios include

- Victims of house fires, the sudden collapse of laboratory or factory/industry workers (as seen in the first case)
- A patient returning from a foreign country who was seeking alternative cancer therapy or purchased a homeopathic "cancer cure" sold online, derived from amygdalin (Laetrile)
- Possible suicide/homicide attempt in a patient with an unexplained acidemia and coma
- Ingestion of cassava that is improperly processed [2, 6]
- Ingestion of pits/seeds of fruits from the genus *Prunus* (apricot, peach, plum, apple, etc.)
- High suspicion in smoke inhalation patients with two or more of the following: [5, 10]
  - Neurologic dysfunction – change in mental status, loss of consciousness, seizure activity
  - Carbonaceous material in oropharynx or sputum
  - Metabolic acidosis
  - Lactate >8

The Laetrile Lie

Amygdalin is a naturally occurring chemical compound found in many plants, but most commonly in the seeds/pits of apricots, bitter almonds, apples, peaches, and plums [1].

Amygdalin is called a cyanogenic glycoside because after ingestion, owing to the action of beta-glucosidase, it releases cyanide and can cause cyanide toxicity. A modified form of amygdalin called "Laetrile," and also misrepresented as a vitamin ("Vitamin B_{17}") was touted as an "alternative cancer treatment" as early as the 1950s. Not only have numerous studies found Laetrile to be ineffective as an antineoplastic agent, they have clearly demonstrated it to be potentially toxic or lethal, inducing cyanide toxicity [12].

An article by Lerner (1981) [13] described this drug and its promotion as a cancer therapy as "the slickest, most sophisticated, and certainly the most remunerative cancer quack promotion in medical history."

2. Workup
   - History
   - Lactate!
     - Lactate >8 mmol/L is commonly found in patients with acute CN poisoning.
     - Lactate >10 mmol/L is sensitive and specific indicator of acute CN poisoning [5].
   - Blood gas [2, 5].
     - Metabolic acidosis, acidemia, elevated lactate, increased anion gap.
     - Elevated venous O_2 saturation due to decreased tissue extraction.

- o Venous O_2 sat >90% from SVC indicates decreased O_2 utilization. *This is not specific to cyanide!*
    - A narrow difference between arterial O_2 and venous O_2 saturations is suggestive of cyanide poisoning in the correct clinical scenario, but it is *not* specific to cyanide!
- Glucose – don't miss hypoglycemia!
- CN levels. Whole blood and serum CN concentrations are generally *unavailable* in timeframe needed and there are many flaws with test [2, 5].
    - Coma, bradypnea seen at concentrations >2.5 mcg/mL in whole blood.
    - Death >3 mcg/mL in whole blood.
    - Urinary thiocyanate (more useful than urinary cyanide) – This is a marker of CN exposure. *The concentration does not correlate with symptoms but can confirm exposure.*
    - Calorimetric paper test strips – used in water treatment facilities can detect CN concentrations >1 mcg/mL.
- Consult regional Poison Control Center (would have expedited diagnosis in Case 1; learners should be encouraged that they do not need to have a definitive diagnosis of poisoning to do so).

Treating the Patient

1. First and foremost – YOU MUST CONSIDER THE DIAGNOSIS OR YOU WILL MISS IT!
2. Initial therapy
   - *Personal protective equipment* – avoid personal exposure!
   - Remove the patient from any possible source and perform decontamination.
       - This is particularly important with inhalational and dermal exposure – remove the victim from the scene, remove clothing, flush skin with water, and irrigate open wounds [7].
   - ABCs – Airway patency, ventilator support, administer 100% O_2, establish IV access, and begin general resuscitation measures/supportive care.
   - Activated charcoal does not significantly adsorb cyanide and is therefore generally not recommended unless the possibility of coingestants exists and the patient's airway is protected.
3. Antidotes.
   - There are four antidote regimens available across the globe for cyanide poisoning [14]:
       - Hydroxocobalamin (Cyanokit)
       - Cyanide Antidote Kit (amyl nitrite, sodium nitrite, sodium thiosulfate)
       - Dicobalt-EDTA (dicobalt-ethylenediamine tetra-acetic acid) (Kelocyanor)
       - DMAP (4-dimethylaminophenol).
   - Hydroxocobalamin (a form of vitamin B12) appears to be best tolerated and has the fewest contraindications, and many consider it to be first-line treatment for suspected cyanide toxicity [5, 14–16], even being called an "...antidote of first resort" [17]. It works by binding the cyanide in a 1:1 fashion, to the cobalt

ion in hydroxocobalamin forming the nontoxic vitamin B12, cyanocobalamin. This removes cyanide from the mitochondrial electron transport chain, thus allowing oxidative metabolism to resume. By also binding nitric oxide (a potent vasodilator), hydroxocobalamin may also improve hemodynamics in a cyanide-poisoned patient by causing transient hypertension [18].

- It is category C in pregnancy; however, the benefits likely outweigh the risks in a truly poisoned patient.
- It is safe for use in smoke-inhalation exposure.
- Adverse effects include allergic reaction, transient reddish discoloration of skin, and urine, interference with colorimetric assays (including hemoglobin, coagulation tests, urinalysis, pH, AST, creatinine, and others), and mild, transient increase in blood pressure [2, 9] (which may be beneficial considering patients may present in shock-like state).
- Dose:
  o 5 g IV over 15 minutes.
  o Additional 2.5–5 g doses can be given if no initial improvement is seen [2, 5].
  o Cited max total dose is 10 g [2].
  o Algorithms for prehospital and hospital-based treatment of suspected cyanide toxicity have been proposed, and rely on hydroxocobalamin as first-line therapy [15].

- Sodium nitrite, dicobalt-EDTA, and DMAP have serious adverse effects including hypotension and formation of methemoglobin, which can exacerbate carbon monoxide–induced functional anemia [5, 14].
  - Nitrites have associated risks of precipitation of hypoxia and hypotension. Though some early and limited studies conclude they *may* be safe if very slowly infused in patients with concomitant CO poisoning/smoke inhalation exposure [19], their use in the age of safer antidotes with more rapid onset of action (hydroxocobalamin) could be considered relatively contraindicated in burn victims already suffering from potentially both cyanide and carbon monoxide (CO) poisoning [5].
    o One way to think about this is if you have carboxyhemoglobin (CO poisoning) and methemoglobin (from nitrite) and carbaminohemoglobin (carries CO_2)...there is not a lot of room to have oxyhemoglobin!

- Sodium thiosulfate (a component of the Cyanide Antidote Kit) potentiates the action of rhodanese (a mitochondrial enzyme): 80% of cyanide elimination occurs by the enzyme rhodanese, which in the presence of thiosulfate converts cyanide to thiocyanate. This is excreted by the kidney. The rate-limiting step in this pathway is the presence of adequate thiosulfate. It is safe to give empirically without fear of hypotension or exacerbation of CO poisoning. Although it has been shown to be effective as a solo-treating agent in cyanide poisoning, this type of use is reserved for cases in which sodium nitrite is contraindicated or hydroxocobalamin is unavailable [20].
  - 50 ml of the 25% solution (12.5 g) is given IV at the rate of 3–5 ml/minute. Pediatric dose is 1.65 ml/kg up to 50 ml.
  - Thiosulfate can be readministered in 1 hour if symptoms persist or recur.

- Dicobalt-EDTA has been associated with anaphylactic reactions, severe hypertension, and cardiac arrhythmias if a patient is not suffering from CN poisoning.
  - ("Kelocyanor" is not available in the USA) [14].
- Hyperbaric oxygen therapy is common for CO poisoning, which can coexist in smoke inhalation patients, but its use for CN toxicity alone is controversial [5]. It is not recommended by most hyperbaric medicine physicians.
- Caution should be taken particularly with burn patients [5, 16] – assume lactic acidosis is underresuscitation until proven otherwise. Burn victims that are volume-depleted and underresuscitated can develop profound hypotension and worsening clinical condition if underresuscitated.

Case Conclusion

Case 1

The attending physician of record in the Emergency Department consulted with a few other ED attendings, with no new ideas uncovered. Just prior to leaving at the end of the shift, the ED attending physician discussed the case with one of the more experienced veteran emergency physicians. The "seasoned doc" was told the same story but in summary form. He was told a grad student suffered a sudden cardiovascular collapse with intractable bradycardia and hypotension despite atropine and vasopressors and that she had a bicarb of zero and a pH of around 6.8, unresponsive to a total of 8 amps of bicarb and 6 of atropine. The "seasoned doc" asked, to the shock and awe of the "green attending," if the patient happened to work in the lab. He was told that the patient is a PharmD student. He wisely looked up and said, "This is cyanide poisoning." The attending of record immediately slapped himself on the forehead and grabbed the Lillie Cyanide Antidote Kit (now discontinued, since this case occurred in the late 1990s) containing sodium thiosulfate and sodium nitrite and amyl nitrate (in the days prior to hydroxocobalamin). He went to the ICU and immediately approached the treating team. The working diagnosis at the time was that this patient had some sort of intra-abdominal abscess and Gram-negative sepsis. The ED attending relayed the other information to the team and despite multiple attempts to convince them that this case was almost certainly cyanide poisoning, the attending emergency physician was told that his help was no longer needed in the ICU and that he should go back downstairs!

The ED attending confronted the 3rd year internal medicine resident and told him that this is the picture-perfect case of cyanide poisoning including the presentation, her place of work and all of the lab findings and that if he didn't act on this and treat for cyanide, that the emergency physician was going to "take him and his ICU attending to the medical director of the hospital and hold them responsible for not acting in the face of overwhelming evidence." He further said he would be happy to testify against them if the case went to medical–legal action. Bodily harm of the resident and ICU attending may have been mentioned in passing!

The emergency physician then went back downstairs with the expectation of receiving a phone call after he had instructed the medicine resident that he needed to give the sodium thiosulfate immediately (because it was relatively harmless) and if the patient had any response, he needed to start the sodium nitrite. The emergency physician received a phone call approximately 20 minutes later with a report that the patient's blood pressure responded "rapidly to the sodium thiosulfate" and that she was actually moving a little bit. The medicine resident was instructed that he needed to start the sodium nitrite. Subsequently, the patient completely recovered cardiovascular function.

The patient regained consciousness and was transferred from the ICU following day and after brief hospitalization was transferred to rehab. She had some memory loss but otherwise regained 90% of her cognitive functioning after 4 weeks of therapy.

The Back Story The patient was a pharmacy graduate student ready to graduate; however, she was from a foreign country and was currently dating an American boyfriend. She was in severe conflict with her family after they told her she must break up with him, because she was promised in marriage to another man in her country of origin. They were coming to pick her up and bring her back home shortly. She had access to sodium cyanide at her workstation and subsequently was found to have put a tablespoon of sodium cyanide into her coffee and drank it: 15 minutes later, she had the sudden collapse and cardiovascular collapse in front of her professor. She was picked up by her family after 2–1/2 weeks of rehab and taken back to her native country.

Case 2

The patient was extubated in the ICU the next day. He had some cognitive deficits that appeared to represent mild anoxic brain injury. He was transferred to a rehab hospital for cognitive therapy and at 3 weeks after treatment, he was manifesting minimal cognitive deficits.

Case Discussion

Cyanide can cause a dramatic and devastating toxicity to individuals who are acutely exposed to its effects. Cyanide poisoning can be ridiculously easy to diagnose if the patient presents hypotensive, altered, and acidotic after a house fire or known industrial exposure to cyanide or cyanide-like compounds. The emergency physician really earns his or her money by being able to diagnose toxicity without historical clues. This can be unfortunately very difficult when a patient appears at the ED with little history and in cardiovascular (CV) collapse. The differential diagnosis for this is unfortunately broad. In the first case discussed, I was the attending of record in my first year after graduating residency (Kaide). Our team included myself and a 3rd year EM resident. We were so caught up in the details of resuscitating this tragically moribund young woman, we stumbled upon so many clues to the diagnosis, but were not able to put them together into a meaningful pattern. We did not have much context to work with nor did either of us have any experience with a pure cyanide ingestion. Using the retrospect-o-scope (which is always so much more accurate), there were some clues we should have put together. First, she had a sudden, unexplained CV collapse with no evidence of persistent arrhythmia, intracranial hemorrhage, or hypoxia (to suggest a PE). These three items were at the top of our differential…after all, what else besides trauma kills a young, otherwise healthy person this suddenly? What we didn't synthesize is that she was profoundly acidotic despite multiple attempts to buffer her pH. She had a lactate that was crazy high for no here-to-for explainable reason. Her PaO_2 was extremely high, and her arterial blood and venous blood were indistinguishable by color. She did not respond meaningfully to any attempts to treat her bradycardia and hypotension, despite large doses of atropine and epinephrine. *Who does that?? Well, for starters, no other patient I have ever treated in my vast experience of 3.5 years of practice.* Oh, and she worked in a LAB!

The reason the more seasoned attending was able to put this case together so quickly was because he saw the forest and not just the individual trees! When presented with the facts minus the drama, the diagnosis was much less mystifying…A young healthy patient who works in a lab presents comatose with cardiovascular collapse and profound acidosis, hypotension, bradycardia, unresponsive to therapy—with no other good explanation! That makes the diagnosis seem a bit more straightforward. I also think had we called the poison center earlier (maybe out of desperation, since we were not really thinking tox), they would have sorted it out!

Looking back in time to 1997 (and now as a PGY-25.5), I still regard this case as at least in the top 2–3 strangest and most dramatic of my career. I will likely never miss this diagnosis again; however, ironically, I will not likely come across this unusual situation in my remaining years as an emergency physician. I guess the best take-home here is to look at the patterns outside of the immediate resuscitation efforts and look for what makes sense and what doesn't!

Pattern Recognition

Cyanide Poisoning
- Metabolic acidosis with an anion gap and elevated lactate >10
- Persistent altered mental status
- Intractable hypotension
- Intractable bradycardia
- Closed-space fire with smoke inhalation
- Exposure risk (works in a lab or in in the jewelry, photography, metallurgy, or textile industries)
- A symptomatic patient who was seeking alternative cancer therapy, possibly after returning from a foreign country

Disclosure Statement
- Jessica A. Everett. Clarius. Not relevant to this publication
- Colin Kaide. Callibra, Inc.-Discharge 123 medical software company. Medical Advisory Board Portola Pharmaceuticals. I have no relationship with a commercial company that has a direct financial interest in subject matter or materials discussed in article or with a company making a competing product.
- Hannah Hays No conflicts

References

1. Hamel J. A review of acute cyanide poisoning with a treatment update. Crit Care Nurse. 2011;31(1):72–81; quiz 2
2. Holstege CP, Kirk MA. Cyanide and hydrogen sulfide. In: Weitz M, Naglieri C, editors. Goldfrank's toxicologic emergencies. 10th ed: McGraw-Hill Education, Columbus, OH, USA; 2015.
3. Reade MC, Davies SR, Morley PT, Dennett J, Jacobs IC, Council AR. Review article: management of cyanide poisoning. Emerg Med Australas. 2012;24(3):225–38.
4. McKenna ST, Hull TR. The fire toxicity of polyurethane foams. Fire Sci Rev. 2016;5(3):1.
5. Huzar TF, George T, Cross JM. Carbon monoxide and cyanide toxicity: etiology, pathophysiology and treatment in inhalation injury. Expert Rev Respir Med. 2013;7(2):159–70.
6. Tshala-Katumbay DD, Ngombe NN, Okitundu D, David L, Westaway SK, Boivin MJ, et al. Cyanide and the human brain: perspectives from a model of food (cassava) poisoning. Ann N Y Acad Sci. 2016;1378(1):50–7.
7. Hydrogen Cyanide - Emergency Department/Hospital Management. CHEMM. 14 January 2015.
8. Fortin JL, Desmettre T, Manzon C, Judic-Peureux V, Peugeot-Mortier C, Giocanti JP, et al. Cyanide poisoning and cardiac disorders: 161 cases. J Emerg Med. 2010;38(4): 467–76.
9. Hays H, McGrath J. Cyanide. In: Dr Carol Rivers' preparing for the written board exam in emergency medicine, vol. 2. 8th ed. Ohio: ACEP; 2017. p. 579.
10. Lawson-Smith P, Jansen EC, Hyldegaard O. Cyanide intoxication as part of smoke inhalation—a review on diagnosis and treatment from the emergency perspective. Scand J Trauma Resusc Emerg Med. 2011;19:14.
11. Bolarinwa IF, Orfila C, Morgan MR. "Amygdalin content of seeds, kernels and food products commercially-available in the UK" (PDF). Food Chem. 2014;152:133–9.
12. Milazzo S, Horneber M. Laetrile treatment for cancer. Cochrane Database Syst Rev. 2015;4:CD005476.
13. Lerner IJ. Laetrile: a lesson in cancer quackery. CA Cancer J Clin. 1981;31(2):91–5.
14. Hall AH, Dart R, Bogdan G. Sodium thiosulfate or hydroxocobalamin for the empiric treatment of cyanide poisoning? Ann Emerg Med. 2007;49(6):806–13.
15. Anseeuw K, Delvau N, Burillo-Putze G, De Iaco F, Geldner G, Holmström P, et al. Cyanide poisoning by fire smoke inhalation: a European expert consensus. Eur J Emerg Med. 2013;20(1):2–9.
16. MacLennan L, Moiemen N. Management of cyanide toxicity in patients with burns. Burns. 2015;41(1):18–24.
17. Hall AH, Saiers J, Baud F. Which cyanide antidote? Crit Rev Toxicol. 2009;39(7):541–52.
18. Thompson JP, Marrs TC. Hydroxocobalamin in cyanide poisoning. Clin Toxicol (Phila). 2012;50(10):875–85.
19. Kirk MA, Gerace R, Kulig KW. Cyanide and methemoglobin kinetics in smoke inhalation victims treated with the cyanide antidote kit. Ann Emerg Med. 1993;22(9):1413–8.
20. Kerns W 2nd, et al. Hydroxocobalamin versus thiosulfate for cyanide poisoning. Ann Emerg Med. 2008;51:338.

ECG Surprise Attack!: *de Winter Aches and Pains*

12

Nicholas S. Fern and Amal Mattu

Case 1

Pertinent History

A 42-year-old African-American male presents to the ED at 0415. He reports that 3 hours ago, he was awakened from sleep by worsening central chest pain radiating to his left arm. He feels significantly short of breath at rest and has been profusely diaphoretic. He denies nausea, vomiting, or recent illness. The patient specifically denies a history of heart attack or venous thromboembolism. He reports that yesterday he was shovelling snow in the driveway and was forced to stop multiple times because of chest pain and extreme fatigue. The patient reports his only medical history is hypertension and hypercholesterolemia but admits that he has not seen a doctor in many years.

PMH
- Hypertension
- Hypercholesterolemia
- Meds: Hydrochlorothiazide, amlodipine, atorvastatin

SH
- Never-smoker, no drug use
- Drinks 8–12 oz beer several times per week

N. S. Fern
The Queen's Medical Center, Honolulu, HI, USA

A. Mattu (✉)
Department of Emergency Medicine, University of Maryland School of Medicine, Baltimore, MD, USA
e-mail: amalmattu@comcast.net

© Springer Nature Switzerland AG 2020
C. G. Kaide, C. E. San Miguel (eds.), *Case Studies in Emergency Medicine*,
https://doi.org/10.1007/978-3-030-22445-5_12

FH

- Extensive family history of Diabetes Type II.
- Father had myocardial infarction at age 50; older brother had myocardial infarction at age 48.

Pertinent Physical Exam

- BP 164/94, Pulse 82, Temp 98.9 °F (37.2 °C), RR 22, SpO2 94% on RA
- BMI 32

Except as noted below, the findings of the complete physical exam are within normal limits.

- *General:* AAM sitting up in bed clutching his chest, distressed, and profusely diaphoretic.
- *Cardiovascular:* Nontachycardic with regular rhythm, normal heart sounds without murmur. No JVD present. No costochondral tenderness. Pulses 2+ all extremities.
- *Respiratory:* Moderate respiratory distress. Increased respiratory rate. Speaking in sentences. Clear breath sounds bilaterally.
- *Extremity:* Distal pulses intact to DP/PT 2+ bilaterally. No pitting edema.

Pertinent Diagnostic Testing

- CBC, CMP, PT/INR, PTT – All unremarkable
- Troponin I: 7.56 ng/mL (Reference Range <=0.06 ng/mL)
- Portable Chest X-Ray (CXR): Lungs are clear. No atelectasis. Costophrenic angles sharp. Widened mediastinum. Mildly tortuous aorta with moderate calcifications.
- 12 Lead Electrocardiogram (ECG):

DeWinter EKG

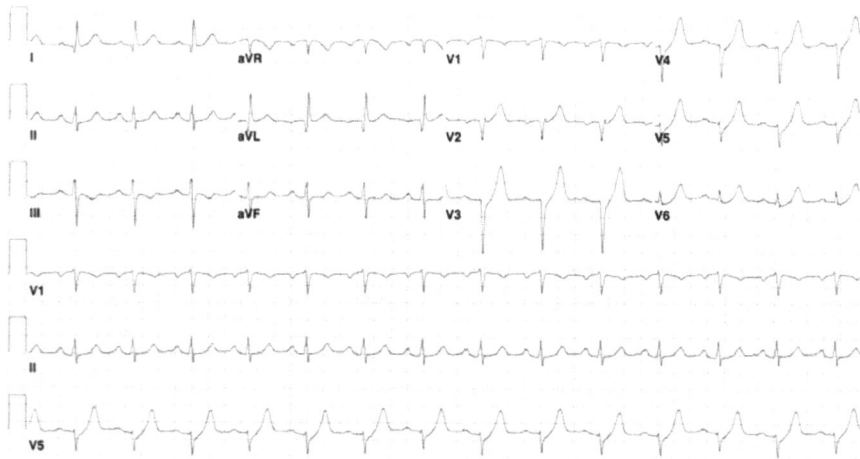

Sinus rhythm, rate 82, poor R-wave progression, slight ST-segment elevation in aVR, upsloping ST-segment depressions with hyperacute T-waves in the anterior precordial leads, consistent with the de Winter T-wave pattern.
ECG Used with Permission, courtesy of Dr. Ammar Ismail.

ED Management

Plan The patient is placed on cardiac monitoring, and a second large bore IV is placed. The patient is administered 324 mg chewable aspirin and 400 mcg sublingual nitroglycerin (NTG) every 5 minutes for 3 doses with minimal improvement in his chest pain. His blood pressure is 124/82 after the third NTG. In consideration of his presentation and ECG, cardiology is paged for emergent cardiac catheterization.

Updates on ED Course

(0435) The cardiology fellow returns the page: She is initially hesitant to activate the cath lab team without clear ST-segment elevation (STE). You explain that the patient's ECG findings and presentation are consistent with the de Winter ECG pattern, and although diagnostic STE may or may not develop, you are concerned for an acutely unstable proximal left anterior descending coronary artery (LAD) occlusion. The patient has not responded to multiple rounds of NTG, despite a reduction in blood pressure and still has severe pain and appears acutely unwell. After a brief discussion with her attending, cardiology then agrees to emergent catheterization.

Learning Points

Priming Questions
1. What coronary lesion(s) are typical culprits in patients presenting with the de Winter pattern?
2. Do patients with the de Winter pattern progress to having overt ST-segment elevation myocardial infarction (STEMI) on serial ECGs?
3. Who is the patient population that generally presents with the de Winter complex and how do these patients differ from our common MI presentations?
4. If you truly believe that a patient needs emergent or urgent cardiac catheterization, how can the cath lab be activated without the patient meeting the traditional "STEMI criteria" (i.e., STE in contiguous leads)?

Introduction/Background

1. The de Winter ECG pattern is an electrocardiographic pattern found in some patients presenting with ischemic chest pain [1]. The pattern is associated with acute proximal LAD occlusion lacking anterior STE on ECG and places the patient at considerable risk for progression to an extensive anterior wall myocardial infarction (MI) [1–3].
   - Many authors contend that the obstructing plaque is often acutely unstable, and therefore, the pattern should be considered a STEMI equivalent and managed emergently [3–9].
   - The de Winter pattern is yet to be included as an indication for emergent reperfusion therapy (i.e., emergent catheterization or administration of fibrinolytics) in the current management guidelines of major cardiovascular societies [10–12] despite increasing literature affirming its association with significant acute coronary disease.
2. The ECG pattern was originally described by de Winter and colleagues in 2008 as: "…1- to 3-mm upsloping ST-segment depression at the J point in leads V1 to V6 that continued into tall, positive symmetrical T waves. The QRS complexes were usually not widened or were only slightly widened, and in some there was a loss of precordial R-wave progression. In most patients there was a 1- to 2-mm ST-elevation in lead aVR" [13]. This pattern has since been refined to the following [2]:

The de Winter EKG Pattern
- Upsloping ST-segment depression (STD) >1 mm at the J point in the precordial leads
- Continuation of the STD into tall, prominent, symmetric T waves in the precordial leads
- STE (0.5–2 mm) in lead aVR
- The absence of other, anatomically oriented, STE

3. There is some debate over the dynamic versus static nature of the de Winter pattern.
   - In the original two articles, the pattern was defined as "static," persisting from initial presentation until the preprocedural ECG and angiography (30–60 minutes). In all cases, the pattern resolved after reperfusion [1, 13].
   - Other authors [4, 14–17] have proposed a dynamic pattern with conversion between traditional de Winter findings and overt STE resulting from ebb and flow between complete coronary occlusion and spontaneous reperfusion.
   - Zhao and colleagues [14] proposed a 2-category division of both static and dynamic, reflecting the possibility that the underlying plaque can be unstable.
4. In the original 2008 series, de Winter and colleagues drew from their primary database of percutaneous coronary interventions identifying 30 patients (2.0%) showing the de Winter pattern among 1532 patients with anterior wall MI [13].
   - In a 2009, a larger cohort from the same database showed identical incidence of the de Winter pattern, 2% (35 patients) of 1890 patients who had undergone primary percutaneous intervention (PCI) of the LAD. Meanwhile, the remaining 1855 LAD patients (98%) all exhibited precordial STE [1].

Physiology/Pathophysiology

1. The de Winter pattern has proven association with LAD occlusion on coronary angiography, specifically the proximal LAD [1].
   - Despite being pathognomonic of LAD occlusion, no cases involve occlusion of its supplying left main coronary artery (LMCA). Most cases (67%) exhibit isolated LAD disease [1].
   - Roughly half of patients were found to have a wraparound LAD, which is associated with a greater region of ischemia [1].

Coronary Anatomy

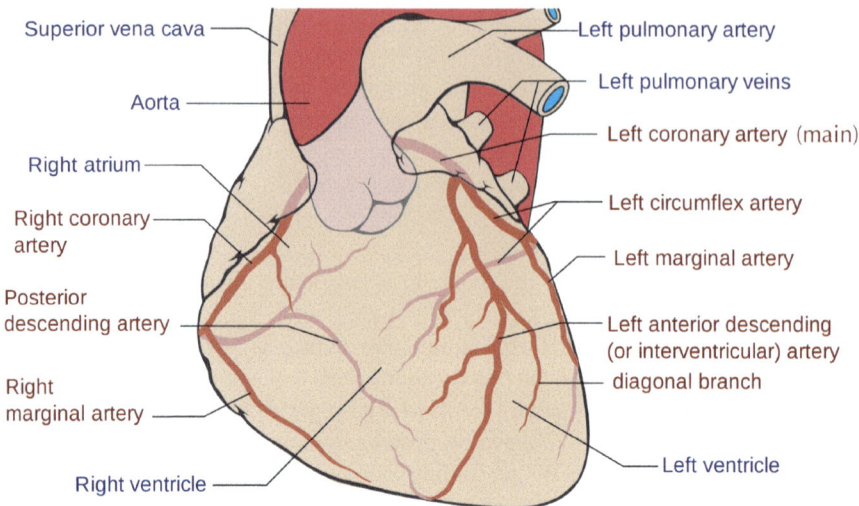

Superior vena cava — Left pulmonary artery

Left pulmonary veins

Aorta — Left coronary artery (main)

Right atrium —

Right coronary artery — Left circumflex artery

Left marginal artery

Posterior descending artery —

Right marginal artery — Left anterior descending (or interventricular) artery

diagonal branch

Right ventricle —

Left ventricle

By Coronary.pdf: Patrick J. Lynch, medical illustratorderivative work: [CC BY-SA 3.0 (https://creativecommons.org/licenses/by-sa/3.0)], via Wikimedia Commons

2. The question arises as to why an anterior infarction may present with this unconventional pattern in 2% of cases while the remaining 98% present with the more typical precordial STE.
   - The electrophysiological explanation for J-point depression and prominent T-waves initially proposed by de Winter et al. [13] suggested the presence of endocardial conduction delay resulting from one of two mechanisms:
     – An anatomical variant of the Purkinje fibers.
     – Ischemia diminishing cardiomyocyte ATP resulting in failure of activation of sarcolemmal ATP-sensitive potassium (K_{ATP}) channels [13], supported by work with K_{ATP} knockout mice in which ligation of the LAD fails to produce STE [18].
   - Sala et al. theorize that the de Winter ST–T complex is created by a delay in subendocardial repolarization with a change in transmembrane action potential shape [16].
   - Verouden et al. suggest that "the area of transmural ischemia (is) very large, such that no injury currents (are) generated towards the precordial leads but only directed upwards to standard lead aVR" [1].
   - Montero-Cabezas propose the absence of STE is secondary to an incomplete occlusion of the LAD [15].

Making the Diagnosis

Differential Diagnosis of Prominent Precordial T Waves in the Patient with Chest Pain
- ACS
  - The de Winter pattern
  - Hyperacute T-waves
- Other Causes of Prominent T Waves
  - Hyperkalemia
  - Early repolarization
  - Left ventricular hypertrophy/high left ventricular voltage
  - Left bundle branch block

1. History and Physical

   The first step in diagnosis of acute coronary syndrome in the initial presentation of the undifferentiated patient with chest pain is through history and physical examination:
   - A thorough history of the event including preceding events: nature, intensity, location, duration, and radiation of the pain; associated symptoms such as nausea, vomiting, diaphoresis, lightheadedness or syncope; and response to treatment.
   - The joint American Heart Association (AHA) and American College of Cardiology (ACC) Guideline for the Management of Patients With Non-ST-Elevation Acute Coronary Syndromes (NSTE-ACS) [11] lists factors that increase the probability of NSTE-ACS: older age, male sex, positive family history of early-onset CAD, the presence of peripheral arterial disease, diabetes mellitus, renal insufficiency, prior MI, and prior coronary revascularization.
     - Patients with the de Winter pattern tend to more often be male, and have hypercholesterolemia, but differ in that they tend to be younger [1].
   - The physical exam may be normal in ACS; however, any signs of heart failure should raise alarm as a possible indication of acute decompensation.
     - The patient with the de Winter pattern will often be extremely ill-appearing and may rapidly progress to STEMI [2].
2. Imaging: Various modes of imaging may be valuable in the chest pain workup. Often the first choice is a quick portable CXR, which may aid in investigation for pulmonary causes of the presentation or may exhibit a widened mediastinum suggesting aortic dissection [11].
3. Lab Testing

   Common laboratory testing when ACS is the provisional diagnosis includes [19]

- Complete blood count – to rule out anemia as the cause of decreased oxygen supply.
- Comprehensive metabolic panel – to investigate for electrolyte disturbances or hyper-/hypoglycemia.
- Cardiac biomarkers – such as Troponin I or T as indicators of myocardial damage. Troponins are the preferred cardiac biomarker in the AHA/ACC guidelines [11, 12, 20]

4. The ECG

The 12-lead ECG is the defining feature of the de Winter pattern of acute proximal LAD occlusion.

- The pattern, as mentioned above, includes upsloping STD >1 mm at the J point continuing into tall, prominent, symmetric T-waves in the precordial leads with concurrent isolated STE (0.5–2 mm) in lead aVR.
- In a systematic review, the de Winter pattern demonstrated diagnostic benefit with a positive predictive value of 95.2–100% (95% CIs of 76.2–99.9%, 69.2–100%, 51.7–100%) for acute coronary occlusion [21].
- The hyperacute T-waves (HATWs) of anterior transmural ischemia are another STEMI equivalent and bear similarities to the de Winter T-waves in their prominence, broad base, and symmetric configuration.
  - However, HATWs are considered a transient and dynamic feature with inevitable progression to overt precordial STE [1, 4].
  - HATWs appear within minutes of acute coronary occlusion and progress quickly to STEMI [5, 13, 22].
  - HATWs are generally not associated with concurrent STD.
  - Wellens syndrome is another important condition with a characteristic ECG pattern of distinct T-wave changes that may be confused with the de Winter ST–T complex [5, 23].
- Wellens syndrome involves biphasic (Type A) or inverted T-waves (Type B) in leads V_2–V_3.
  - These changes are normally caused by chronic or subacute high-grade LAD stenosis as opposed to the acute occlusion of the de Winter pattern.
  - As a result of the chronic or subacute nature of disease, patients with an ECG consistent with Wellens syndrome may instead be evaluated with nonemergent angiography [5], as opposed to the emergent nature of a patient with the de Winter pattern.

The EKG in Type A Wellens Syndrome

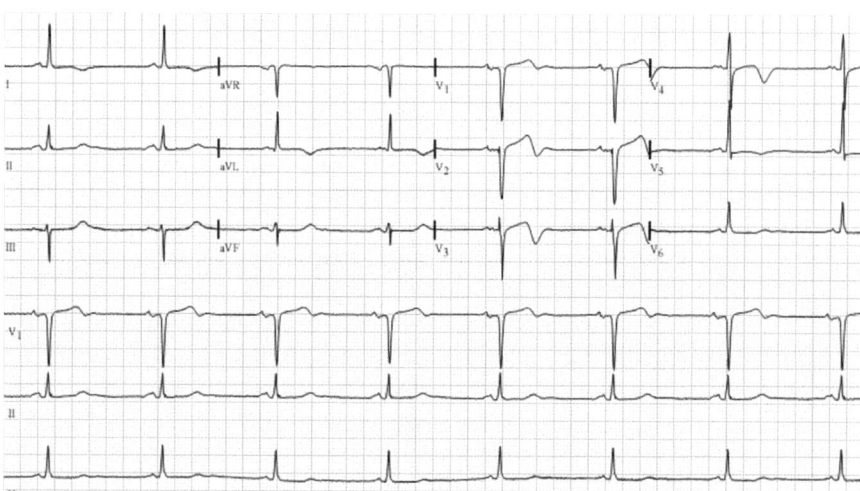

Jer5150 (https://commons.wikimedia.org/wiki/File:Wellens'_Syndrome.png), "Wellens' Syndrome", https://creativecommons.org/licenses/by-sa/3.0/legalcode

5. Coronary Angiography/Cardiac Catheterization

Invasive Coronary Angiography is considered the goldstandard for definitive diagnosis of coronary lesions [24]; however, strictly speaking, the de Winter pattern does not fit the criteria outlined by the AHA and ACC as an indication for emergent coronary angiography [11, 12].

- The accepted definition of STEMI is new STE at the J point in two contiguous leads: ≥1 mm in all leads other than V_2–V_3, and STE in V_2–V_3 ≥ 2 mm in men ≥40 years, ≥2.5 mm in men <40 years, or ≥1.5 mm in women [12, 25].
- These criteria are expanding as evidence emerges, as of the 2013 ACC/AHA guideline [12], patterns concerning for STEMI include
  - STD in ≥2 precordial leads (V_1–V_4) – suggestive of transmural posterior injury.
  - Multilead STD with coexistent STE in aVR – suggestive of LMCA or proximal LAD occlusion. (One could argue that the de Winter pattern is included here.)
  - Hyperacute T Waves – indicative of early STEMI.
- Although the de Winter pattern is not yet expressly included, the guidelines state, "If doubt persists, immediate referral for invasive angiography may be necessary to guide therapy in the appropriate clinical context" [12, 13].
  - This invites the reasonable argument for emergent cath lab activation when the ED physician is concerned for ACS in a patient with an ECG exhibiting the de Winter pattern.

- Per the AHA/ACC Guideline for the Management of Patients With Non-ST-Elevation Acute Coronary Syndromes [11]: NSTE-ACS patients are managed in one of the two treatment pathways: The early invasive and ischemia-guided strategies. Both of these pathways conceivably permit the de Winter patient (if considered as NSTE-ACS due to lack of diagnostic STE in the presence of positive cardiac biomarkers) to advance to cardiac catheterization; however, this may occur with a variable extent of delay.
  - The early invasive strategy advises coronary angiography within 24 hours. This may allow the de Winter patient to progress to catheterization, but they will likely be too acutely unwell to remain stable up to 24 hours, especially with ongoing chest pain.
  - Coronary angiography occurs in the ischemia-guided strategy for patients who
    - Fail medical therapy (refractory chest pain despite vigorous medical therapy) – the de Winter patient will likely fail medical therapy, but this may cause significant delay.
    - Have objective evidence of ischemia.
    - Have clinical indicators of high prognostic risk.
- The NSTE-ACS guideline also allows for urgent coronary angiography in patients with hemodynamic or rhythmic instability [11], which has a reasonable probability of occurring in the de Winter patient.

Treating the Patient

1. ED Management
   The ED management of the patient with chest pain and concern for ACS with or without diagnostic STE includes [11, 12]
   - Obtaining IV access and placing the patient on cardiac monitoring.
   - Administration of supplemental oxygen if arterial oxygen saturation is less than 90%, and the patient is in respiratory distress or has other high-risk features of hypoxemia.
   - Antiplatelet therapy: Administration of 162–325 mg of chewable aspirin.
   - Antianginal therapy: Administration of sublingual or IV NTG (unless contraindicated).
   - Analgesic: Administration of morphine sulfate for continuing chest pain is reasonable.
   - Beta-adrenergic or calcium channel blockers: Administration of oral beta-blockers or calcium channel blockers may be considered.
   - Parenteral anticoagulant therapy: Administration of unfractionated heparin (UFH) or enoxaparin prior to PCI is supported in both NSTEMI and STEMI patients.

- GP IIb/IIIa inhibitors: Administration of GP IIb/IIa inhibitors can be added if the patient is likely to be treated with an early invasive strategy.
- Acute reperfusion therapy (cath lab activation or administration of fibrinolytics) for patients that meet criteria discussed previously.

Case Conclusion

Several hours later, you are called in the ED by the interventional cardiologist to update you on the outcome of the patient. The patient had a 100% proximal LAD occlusion that was successfully stented. The patient has been admitted in stable condition to the coronary care unit with complete resolution of his chest pain and the STEs. The cardiology attending thanks you for advocating for the patient to the fellow, allowing the patient to proceed to cath lab.

Discussion

1. Almost half of AMI patients may have a nondiagnostic ECG [26]. The standard ECG criteria for diagnosis of ACS miss a large proportion of cases of acute coronary occlusion. To improve our sensitivity for selecting patients that would benefit from acute reperfusion therapy we should consider other ECG patterns of acute coronary occlusion that do not meet the traditional STEMI criteria.
   - Posterior myocardial infarction has recently been included as an indication for emergent angiography.
   - The presence of STE in aVR with concurrent STD in multiple leads has gained increased support as a potential STEMI equivalent [2, 5].
   - The de Winter T-wave pattern, as discussed, should warrant strong consideration as a STEMI equivalent and cases should be discussed with the interventional cardiologist based on the patient's presentation.
2. In the event that the interventional cardiologist declines to accept the patient for emergent cardiac catheterization, the patient should be monitored closely and serial ECGs should be obtained until the time of admission because of the possibility that the patient will evolve to develop STE on the ECG. At that point, the cardiologist should be recontacted to reconsider emergent catheterization.
   - If the patient continues to have ischemic chest pain and evidence of ischemia on the ECG despite maximal ED-based therapies, even in the absence of STE, emergent catheterization should be reconsidered.
   - If the patient remains stable without evolution of the ECG to STEMI, he or she should be admitted to a telemetry-monitored bed and the admitting team should be made aware of the significance of the concerning ECG pattern.

Pattern Recognition

Chest pain with the de Winter pattern
- Patients presenting with chest pain – tending to be [1]:
  - Male
  - Younger in age
  - Hypercholesterolemic
- Frequently ill in appearance and rapidly progress to STEMI [2]
- ECG with the following pattern [1, 2]:
  - Upsloping ST-segment depression >1 mm at the J point in the precordial leads.
  - Continuation of the ST-segment depression into tall, prominent, symmetric T waves in the precordial leads.
  - ST-segment elevation (0.5–2 mm) in lead aVR.
  - The absence of other, anatomically oriented, ST-segment elevation.

Disclosure Statement   The authors of this chapter report no significant disclosures.

References

1. Verouden NJ, Koch KT, Peters RJ, et al. Persistent precordial "hyperacute" T-waves signify proximal left anterior descending artery occlusion. Heart. 2009;95(20):1701–6. https://doi.org/10.1136/hrt.2009.174557.
2. Lipinski MJ, Mattu A, Brady WJ. Evolving electrocardiographic indications for emergent reperfusion. Cardiol Clin. 2018;36(1):13–26. https://doi.org/10.1016/j.ccl.2017.08.002.
3. de Winter RW, Adams R, Verouden NJW, de Winter RJ. Precordial junctional ST-segment depression with tall symmetric T-waves signifying proximal LAD occlusion, case reports of STEMI equivalents. J Electrocardiol. 2016;49(1):76–80. https://doi.org/10.1016/j.jelectrocard.2015.10.005.
4. Goebel M, Bledsoe J, Orford JL, Mattu A, Brady WJ. A new ST-segment elevation myocardial infarction equivalent pattern? Prominent T wave and J-point depression in the precordial leads associated with ST-segment elevation in lead aVR. Am J Emerg Med. 2014;32(3):287.e5–8. https://doi.org/10.1016/j.ajem.2013.09.037.
5. Rokos IC, French WJ, Mattu A, et al. Appropriate cardiac cath lab activation: optimizing electrocardiogram interpretation and clinical decision-making for acute ST-elevation myocardial infarction. Am Heart J. 2010;160(6):995–1003.e8. https://doi.org/10.1016/j.ahj.2010.08.011.
6. Hennings JR, Fesmire FM. A new electrocardiographic criteria for emergent reperfusion therapy. Am J Emerg Med. 2012;30(6):994–1000. https://doi.org/10.1016/j.ajem.2011.04.025.
7. Birnbaum Y, Bayés De Luna A, Fiol M, et al. Common pitfalls in the interpretation of electrocardiograms from patients with acute coronary syndromes with narrow QRS: a consensus report. J Electrocardiol. 2012;45(5):463–75. https://doi.org/10.1016/j.jelectrocard.2012.06.011.
8. Lawner BJ, Nable JV, Mattu A. Novel patterns of ischemia and STEMI equivalents. Cardiol Clin. 2012;30(4):591–9. https://doi.org/10.1016/j.ccl.2012.07.002.
9. Gorgels APM. ST-elevation and non-ST-elevation acute coronary syndromes: should the guidelines be changed? J Electrocardiol. 2013;46(4):318–23. https://doi.org/10.1016/j.jelectrocard.2013.04.005.

10. Ibanez B, James S, Agewall S, et al. 2017 ESC guidelines for the management of acute myocardial infarction in patients presenting with ST-segment elevation. Eur Heart J. 2018;39(2):119–77. https://doi.org/10.1093/eurheartj/ehx393.

11. Amsterdam EA, Wenger NK, Brindis RG, et al. 2014 AHA/ACC guideline for the management of patients with non–ST-elevation acute coronary syndromes: a report of the American College of Cardiology/American Heart Association Task Force on Practice Guidelines. J Am Coll Cardiol. 2014;64(24):e139–228. https://doi.org/10.1016/j.jacc.2014.09.017.

12. O'Gara PT, Kushner FG, Ascheim DD, et al. 2013 ACCF/AHA guideline for the management of st-elevation myocardial infarction: a report of the American College of Cardiology Foundation/American Heart Association Task Force on Practice Guidelines. J Am Coll Cardiol. 2013;61(4):78–140. https://doi.org/10.1016/j.jacc.2012.11.019.

13. de Winter RJ, Verouden NJW, Wellens HJJ, Wilde AAM. A new ECG sign of Ppoximal LAD occlusion. N Engl J Med. 2008;359(19):2071–3. https://doi.org/10.1056/NEJMc0804737.

14. Zhao YT, Wang L, Yi Z. Evolvement to the de Winter electrocardiographic pattern. Am J Emerg Med. 2016;34(2):330–2. https://doi.org/10.1016/j.ajem.2015.11.057.

15. Montero-Cabezas JM, van der Kley F, Karalis I, Schalij MJ. The "De Winter Pattern" can progress to ST-segment elevation acute coronary syndrome. Response. Rev Esp Cardiol (Engl Ed). 2015;68(11):1043. http://www.revespcardiol.org/en/el-patron-de-winter-puede/articulo/S1885585715003291/ ER.

16. Fiol Sala M, Bayés de Luna A, Carrillo López A, García-Niebla J. The "De Winter Pattern" can progress to ST-segment elevation acute coronary syndrome. Rev Española Cardiol (English Ed). 2015;68(11):1042–3. https://doi.org/10.1016/j.rec.2015.07.006.

17. Ayer A, Terkelsen CJ. Difficult ECGs in STEMI. J Electrocardiol. 2014;47(4):448–58. https://doi.org/10.1016/j.jelectrocard.2014.03.010.

18. Li RA, Leppo M, Miki T, Seino S, Marbán E. Molecular basis of electrocardiographic ST-segment elevation. Circ Res. 2000;87(10):837–9.

19. Zafari AM. Myocardial infarction: practice essentials, background, definitions. Emedicine. medscape.com. https://emedicine.medscape.com/article/155919-overview. Published 2018. Accessed 24 June 2018.

20. Hillis LD, Smith PK, Anderson JL, et al. 2011 ACCF/AHA guideline for coronary artery bypass graft surgery: a report of the American College of Cardiology Foundation/American Heart Association Task Force on Practice Guidelines. 124; 2011. https://doi.org/10.1161/CIR.0b013e31823c074e.

21. Morris NP, Body R. The de Winter ECG pattern: morphology and accuracy for diagnosing acute coronary occlusion: systematic review. Eur J Emerg Med. 2017;24(4):236–42. https://doi.org/10.1097/MEJ.0000000000000463.

22. Nikus K, Pahlm O, Wagner G, et al. Electrocardiographic classification of acute coronary syndromes: a review by a committee of the International Society for Holter and Non-Invasive Electrocardiology. J Electrocardiol. 2010;43(2):91–103. https://doi.org/10.1016/j.jelectrocard.2009.07.009.

23. de Zwaan C, Bär FWHM, Wellens HJJ. Characteristic electrocardiographic pattern indicating a critical stenosis high in left anterior descending coronary artery in patients admitted because of impending myocardial infarction. Am Heart J. 1982;103(4 PART 2):730–6. https://doi.org/10.1016/0002-8703(82)90480-X.

24. Scirica BM. Acute coronary syndrome. Emerging tools for diagnosis and risk assessment. J Am Coll Cardiol. 2010;55(14):1403–15. https://doi.org/10.1016/j.jacc.2009.09.071.

25. Thygesen K, Alpert JS, Jaffe AS, et al. Third universal definition of myocardial infarction. Eur Heart J. 2012;33(20):2551–67. https://doi.org/10.1093/eurheartj/ehs184.

26. Macias M, Peachey J, Mattu A, Brady WJ. The electrocardiogram in the ACS patient: high-risk electrocardiographic presentations lacking anatomically oriented ST-segment elevation. Am J Emerg Med. 2016;34(3):611–7. https://doi.org/10.1016/j.ajem.2015.11.047.

ECG Surprise Attack!: *Chest Pain and the "Forgotten Lead"*

13

Nicholas S. Fern and Amal Mattu

Case 2

Pertinent History

An 84-year-old Caucasian male presents to the emergency department at 2100 by ambulance. He reports that roughly 45 minutes ago he developed an episode of central chest pressure while walking up the basement stairs after moving some boxes. This was associated with some shortness of breath. His wife then witnessed him have a syncopal episode at the top of the stairs. He regained consciousness quickly without confusion or drowsiness. The patient reports that since that time he has had persistent pressure-like chest pain. He reports he has had occasional chest pain while doing gardening and ascending stairs for several years but has never lost consciousness or experienced persistent pain.

PMH
- Diabetes, Type II
- Hypertension
- Hypercholesterolemia/hyperlipidemia
- Meds: Aspirin, atorvastatin, metoprolol, lisinopril, insulin glargine, insulin Aspart

N. S. Fern
The Queen's Medical Center, Honolulu, HI, USA

A. Mattu (✉)
Department of Emergency Medicine, University of Maryland School of Medicine, Baltimore, MD, USA
e-mail: amalmattu@comcast.net

© Springer Nature Switzerland AG 2020
C. G. Kaide, C. E. San Miguel (eds.), *Case Studies in Emergency Medicine*,
https://doi.org/10.1007/978-3-030-22445-5_13

SH

- Former smoker, 40 pack years (quit 20 years ago)
- Denies drug or alcohol use

FH

- Father – myocardial infarction, age 66
- Mother + father: diabetes, type II

Pertinent Physical Exam

- BP 97/62, Pulse 105, Temp 98.6 °F (37.0 °C), RR20, SpO2 96% on RA.

Except as noted below, the findings of the complete physical exam are within normal limits.

- Cardiovascular: Tachycardia with regular rhythm, normal heart sounds without murmur. JVD to the angle of the jaw. No costochondral tenderness. Pulses 2+ to all extremities. No pitting edema.
- Respiratory: Tachypnea. Speaking 4 words or less at a time. No wheeze. Mild crackles to the bases bilaterally.

Pertinent Test Results

CBC, CMP, PT/INR, PTT – All unremarkable.

Troponin I: 5.31 ng/mL (Reference range < =0.06 ng/mL).

Portable CXR: Mild blunting of the costophrenic angles. Increased pulmonary vasculature. Fluid in the horizontal fissure. Diffuse fluffy opacities present.

12 Lead ECG: (See attached image) Sinus rhythm, rate 98, left axis deviation, STD in leads II, III, aVF, V_3-V_6, STE in lead aVR of 2 mm, T-wave inversions I, aVL, V_3-V_6.

ST Elevations in aVR

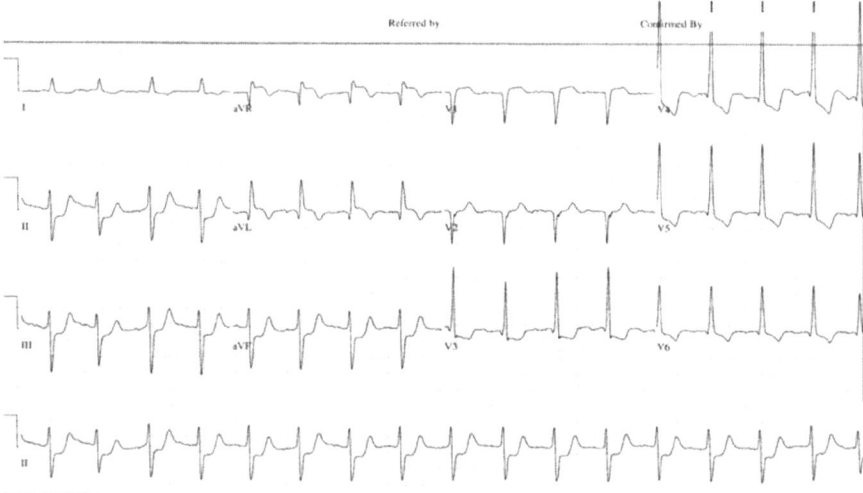

Sinus rhythm, rate 98, left axis deviation, STD in leads II, III, aVF, V_3-V_6, STE in lead aVR of 2 mm, T-wave inversions I, aVL, V_3-V_6
Image used with permission courtesy of Amal Mattu

ED Management

2100 The patient is roomed immediately, seen by the provider, and all investigations are ordered. He is administered 324 mg of chewable aspirin. As the patient is dyspneic, he is immediately placed on non-rebreather mask at 10 LPM with an increase in SpO2 to 100% and mild improvement in respiratory distress. However, his chest pain and hypotension remain.

Updates on ED Course

(2120) Upon examining the patient's ECG and CXR, we elected to immediately call the interventionalist. They agree that the patient should be expeditiously transferred to the cardiac catheterization laboratory (cath lab) for emergent coronary angiography. The cath lab is activated, and the patient is administered a heparin bolus followed by infusion. Though listed in the hospital's pre-cath lab bundle, clopidogrel is withheld.

Learning Points

Priming Questions

1. What specific diagnosis or diagnoses does the ECG with ST-segment elevation (STE) in lead aVR suggest?
2. Is STE in lead aVR indicative of a true STEMI?
3. Should I always be concerned about STE in lead aVR?
4. If sending a patient to cardiac catheterization for STE in aVR, why might you omit some of your hospital's standard precatheterization medications?

Introduction/Background

1. Lead aVR is an augmented unipolar limb lead placed on the right upper extremity providing fundamental information about:
   - The superior right region of the heart including the basal septum.
   - The right ventricular outflow tract.
   - The endocardial surface of the entire left ventricle and apex.
2. Practitioners frequently overlook aVR for several reasons, including [1–3]:
   - Lack of contiguous leads.
   - The presumption that aVR only provides reciprocal information about the left lateral heart (leads aVL, I, II, V_5-V_6) as it is oriented opposite the depolarization vector of these leads [4].
3. ST-segment-elevation (STE) in aVR has proven association to multivessel coronary disease (MVD), and occlusions of the left main coronary artery (LMCA) and proximal left anterior descending (LAD) coronary artery [2, 5–7].
4. Though not recognized by many practitioners as an example of ST-Segment Elevation Myocardial Infarction (STEMI), the diagnostic utility of STE in aVR has been recognized by various guiding international organizations.
   - In 2009, the American Heart Association (AHA), American College of Cardiology (ACC), and the Heart Rhythm Society released a scientific statement advising programming computerized ECG interpretation to suggest MVD or Left Main Coronary Artery (LMCA) ischemia when STE in aVR and/or V_1 is accompanied by ST-segment-depression (STD) ≥ 1 mm in ≥ 8 leads [8].
   - In 2010, an international consensus document recommended prioritizing Acute Coronary Syndrome (ACS) patients for urgent invasive angiography due to high probability of severe angiographic coronary artery disease (CAD) with similar criteria [9]:
     - STD in ≥ 6 leads (maximal in V_4-V_6) **AND** STE in aVR.
5. The importance of recognizing STE in aVR lies in the major coronary artery distributions it displays, its ability to localize coronary lesions, as well as its independent prognostic and diagnostic value:

- Culprit Lesion:
  - Widespread STD and symptoms of ischemia may be indicative of LMCA occlusion regardless of presence of STE in aVR. However, likelihood of LMCA occlusion is increased with concomitant STE in aVR [10].
  - If STE in V_1 is also present, this may indicate either LMCA or proximal LAD occlusion; however, if the STE in aVR $\geq V_1$, this is indicative of a LMCA occlusion as opposed to isolated LAD occlusion [6].
  - Magnitude of STE in aVR is the strongest diagnostic indicator of LMCA and/or MVD [11, 12]:
    - STE ≥ 0.5 mm, OR 19.7, $p < 0.001$.
    - STE ≥ 1 mm, OR 29.1, $p < 0.001$.
    - This supersedes the value of a positive Troponin T (OR 1.27, $p = 0.044$ to OR 3.08, $p = 0.048$).
  - Kosuge et al. found that STE in aVR ≥ 1 mm predicts LMCA and/or MVD with 80% sensitivity and 93% specificity [11].
  - In non-ST-Elevation ACS (NSTE-ACS), STE in aVR is more predictive of LMCA disease or MVD than STD in other leads [11].
  - The prognostic value STE in aVR extends beyond active ACS to include provocative testing as precipitation of STE in aVR via treadmill stress testing denotes stenosis LMCA or proximal LAD [6].

Coronary Anatomy

Coronary Artery Anatomy

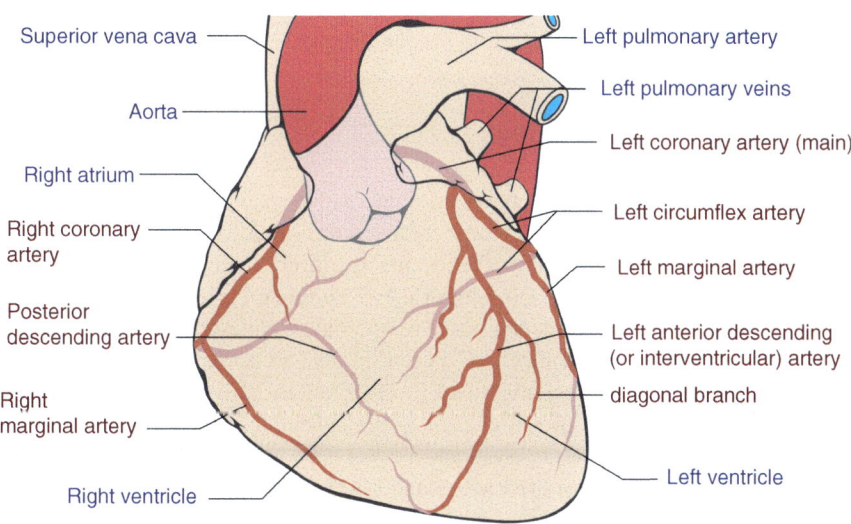

By Coronary.pdf: Patrick J. Lynch, medical illustratorderivative work: Mikael Häggström (Coronary.pdf) [CC BY-SA 3.0 (https://creativecommons.org/licenses/by-sa/3.0)], via Wikimedia Commons

- Mortality – In acute LMCA occlusions, the degree of STE in aVR independently prognosticates increased 30 day mortality [3, 4, 6].
  - STE ≥0.5 mm: mortality increased four times.
  - STE ≥1.0 mm: mortality increased 6–7 times [7].
- Therapy – STE in aVR ≥1.0 mm predicts likely progression to CABG [7, 11].

6. Prompt recognition of STE in aVR and therefore its implicated lesions is crucial as investigation and treatments typically indicated in other cases of ACS may be precluded:
- Stress testing: The culprit high-risk coronary lesions of aVR are *contraindications to exercise stress tests* as they may trigger fatal ischemia or arrhythmias. These patients should be directed to primary coronary angiography [3, 13].
- Coronary artery bypass grafting (CABG): ACS Patients with LMCA and/or MVD are more likely to require CABG than other patterns of occlusion [12].
  - This is vital, as administration of dual antiplatelet therapy (aspirin + clopidogrel) comes with a class I recommendation from the ACC & AHA in NSTEMI patients planned for percutaneous coronary intervention (PCI) [14].
  - The 2011 ACCF/AHA Guideline for Coronary Artery Bypass Graft Surgery advises against administration of clopidogrel, ticagrelor, prasugrel, glycoprotein IIb/IIIa inhibitors, and abciximab for several hours to days preoperatively as they have been associated with increased risk of post-CABG bleeding, transfusion requirement, and major bleeding complications [15].
  - Parenteral anticoagulant therapy such as unfractionated heparin (UFH), enoxaparin, or bivalirudin prior to PCI is supported in both NSTEMI and STEMI patients [14, 16]. However, perioperative enoxaparin has been shown to increase postoperative bleeding and need for re-exploration over UFH [15, 17] and is therefore prudent to avoid.

Physiology/Pathophysiology

1. There are two predominant pathophysiologic pathways that lead to STE in aVR:
- Infarction of the basilar interventricular septum – STEMI via LMCA or proximal LAD occlusion. STE in aVR occurs as a direct change from the transmural infarction of the LVOT or basilar interventricular septum.
- Diffuse endocardial ischemia – as a reciprocal of widespread STD as caused by severe MVD, or mismatch of oxygen supply and demand (e.g., post-ROSC following cardiac arrest, massive PE, or severe tachydysrhythmias). STE in aVR occurs as a reciprocal change to the subendocardial STD in the leads electrically opposite (I, II, aVL, and V_4-V_6).
2. While acute occlusions of the LMCA and LAD typically produce anterior wall ischemia with subsequent precordial STE, due to its perfusion of the posterior myocardium, the LMCA may conversely result in posterior wall ischemia and reciprocal ischemic changes in the precordial leads [6].

3. Occlusive patterns consistent with STE in aVR:
   - LMCA occlusion via massive ischemia.
   - Proximal LAD occlusion via transmural ischemia of the basal septum [15].
   - MVD via diffuse ischemia.
   - Right coronary artery (RCA) occlusion – Due to its role in perfusion of the ventricular septum via septal perforator branches.
4. LMCA occlusion typically results in massive ischemia and is therefore expeditiously fatal. As a result, a large proportion of these patients do not survive to emergency department arrival. This may explain why STE in aVR is a lesser-known sign of ACS.
   - A small subset of patients receives sufficient perfusion via RCA collaterals to survive to ED presentation [18].

Making the Diagnosis

Differential Diagnosis for ST-Segment Elevation in aVR with Multilead ST-Depression [10, 19] – Any Cause of Global Cardiac Ischemia
- ACS
  - LMCA insufficiency
  - Proximal LAD insufficiency
  - Triple vessel disease

Differential diagnoses that will not benefit from the cath lab:

- Other causes of global cardiac ischemia
  - Coronary vasospasm (consider cocaine abuse)
  - Thoracic aortic dissection (potentially involving the coronary arteries or coronary cusps)
  - Massive pulmonary embolism
  - Severe anemia (e.g., massive GI bleed)
  - Post-arrest (within 15 minutes of epinephrine or defibrillation)
- Miscellaneous causes
  - Atrial dysrhythmias with rapid ventricular response (especially AVRT)
  - LBBB & paced rhythms
  - LVH with strain (from severe hypertension)
  - Severe hypokalemia
  - Na + channelopathy (TCA toxicity, hyperkalemia, Brugada syndrome, etc.)
  - Myocarditis

1. History and Physical
   The first step in diagnosis of ACS in the initial presentation of the undifferentiated chest pain patient is thorough history and physical exam:
   - A thorough history of event including preceding events; nature, intensity, location, duration, and radiation of the pain; associated symptoms such as nausea, vomiting, diaphoresis, abdominal pain or syncope; and response to treatment.
   - The joint AHA/ACC Guideline for the Management of Patients With Non-ST-Elevation Acute Coronary Syndromes lists factors that increase the probability of NSTE-ACS as older age, male sex, positive family history of CAD, and the presence of peripheral arterial disease, diabetes mellitus, renal insufficiency, prior MI, and prior coronary revascularization [14].
   - The physical exam may be normal in ACS; however, any signs of heart failure should raise alarm as a possible indication of acute decompensation.
2. Imaging: Various modes of imaging may be valuable in the chest pain workup. Often the first choice is a quick portable CXR, which may aid in investigation for pulmonary causes of the presentation or exhibit the widened mediastinum of aortic dissection [14].
3. Lab Testing: Common laboratory testing when ACS is the provisional diagnosis includes [20]:
   - Complete blood count – to rule out anemia as the cause of decreased oxygen supply.
   - Comprehensive metabolic panel – to investigate for electrolyte disturbances or hyper–/hypoglycemia.
   - Cardiac biomarkers – such Troponin I or T as indicators of myocardial damage. Troponins are preferred in the AHA/ACC guidelines [14–16].
4. The ECG: The 12-lead electrocardiogram is a staple in the patient with chest pain. Its benefit lies not only in its visualization of myocardial perfusion at any given time but in the ease of creating a dynamic image thought serial repetition. *The importance of the ECG in patients with LMCA cannot be understated as STE in aVR > 1 mm is more telling than even the positive troponin.*
   - Electrocardiographic criteria for the diagnosis of STEMI (in the absence of LVH and LBBB) are defined by new STE at the J point in two contiguous leads [16, 21]:
     - ≥ 1 mm – for all leads other than V_2 and V_3.
     - ≥ 2 mm in men ≥ 40 years, ≥ 2.5 mm in men <40 years, or ≥ 1.5 mm in women – for leads V_2–V_3.
   - Contiguous Leads are defined as [21]:
     - Anterior (V1–V6)
     - Inferior (II, III, aVF)
     - Lateral/Apical (I and aVL)
     - Supplemental leads:
   - Free wall of the right ventricle (V_3R and V_4R)

- Inferobasal wall (V_7–V_9)
  - N.B. aVR is the only lead not listed as having a contiguous partner.
5. Coronary Angiography/Cardiac Catheterization.
   Invasive coronary angiography is considered the gold standard for definitive diagnosis of coronary lesions [22].
   - The diagnostic STE criteria above have long been the main indication for emergent invasive coronary angiography. Now, a new group of ECG patterns that do not fit the traditional criteria are gaining recognition: the so-called STEMI equivalents. As evidence emerges, the traditional criteria are expanding to include these STEMI equivalents – as of the 2013 ACC/AHA guideline, patterns concerning for STEMI include [16].
     - STD in ≥2 precordial leads (V_1–V_4) – suggestive of transmural posterior injury
     - Multilead STD with coexistent STE in aVR – suggestive of LMCA or proximal LAD occlusion
     - Hyperacute T waves – indicative of early STEMI
   - STEMI equivalents not yet inducted into the formal criteria are the de Winter pattern and LBBB with Sgarbossa criteria.

Left Main Coronary Artery Occlusion (ST-Elevation in Lead aVR ≥ V_1)

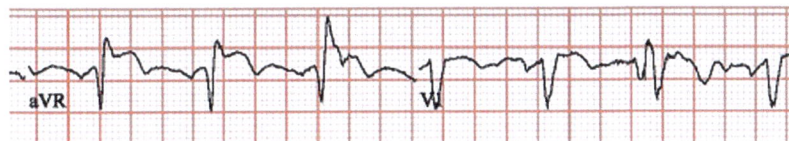

Image courtesy of Amal Mattu

Treating the Patient

1. ED Management: The ED management of the patient with chest pain with concern for ACS includes [14, 16]:
   - Obtaining IV access and placing the patient on cardiac monitoring.
   - Administration of supplemental oxygen if the arterial oxygen saturation is less than 90% or the patient is dyspneic.
   - Antiplatelet Therapy: Administration of 162–325 mg of chewable aspirin.
     - Clopidogrel is advised if the patient has an aspirin allergy, or is planned for PCI. However, as explained above, when STE in aVR is present it is prudent to avoid.
   - Antianginal therapy: Administration of NTG sublingual or IV (unless contraindicated).

- Analgesic: Administration of morphine sulfate (or fentanyl) for continuing chest pain is reasonable.
- Beta-adrenergic or calcium channel blockers: Administration of oral beta-blockers or calcium channel blockers may be considered.
- Parenteral anticoagulant therapy: Administration of unfractionated heparin (UFH) or enoxaparin prior to PCI is supported in both NSTEMI and STEMI patients.
  - As stated earlier, when STE in aVR is present, it is prudent to favor UFH over enoxaparin.
- GP IIb/IIIa inhibitors: Administration of GP IIb/IIa inhibitors is reasonable if the patient is likely to be treated with an early invasive strategy; however, as explained above, when STE in aVR is present, it is prudent to withhold the medication.
2. Invasive Coronary Procedures: The definitive treatments of PCI and coronary artery bypass grafting (CABG) lie beyond the scope of the emergency physician. These procedures are only considered after the patient has first progressed to coronary angiography [23].
- As both PCI and CABG require the patient to first undergo coronary angiography, the emergency physician's goal remains to get the patient to the cath lab expeditiously.

Case Conclusion

(0600) The patient is admitted to the Cardiac ICU. Findings of the catheterization revealed 95% occlusion of the Left Main Coronary Artery, and the patient underwent emergency coronary artery bypass grafting. The patient is recovering well.

Discussion

The clinical significance of STE in aVR has previously been discounted; however, it has recently been gaining increased attention due to its proven diagnostic and prognostic values. We must keep in mind that like almost any sign in medicine, STE in aVR is not flawless. When should we be suspicious of STE in aVR? When a patient presents with alarming (cardiopulmonary) symptoms AND STD in multiple leads (note that isolated STE in aVR is poorly specific for LMCA) [10].

Although some studies suggest that STE in aVR ≤0.5 mm is cause for alarm, our experience and review of the literature indicates that alarm bells should mainly be set off when STE ≥1.0 mm as this is more specific for significant cardiac disease.

Patients presenting with acute LMCA occlusion, MVD, or proximal LAD occlusion will look "sick." Remember, these patients presumably have global cardiac ischemia, and so they are likely to appear ill. Focus your selection of patients for emergent cath lab activation with this point in mind.

Always consider the other causes of STE in aVR that won't benefit from cath lab: thoracic aortic dissection, massive PE, massive GIB, LBBB, LVH with strain pattern, and atrial tachydysrhythmias. The patient's history and physical exam are key in making the distinction between these entities versus those that need emergent catheterization.

PTSD is a useful mnemonic when examining an ECG for STEMI equivalents.

P – **P**osterior MI (isolated): STD + prominent R wave in V_1–V_2.
T – **T** wave abnormalities: de Winter pattern, hyperacute T waves.
S – **S**garbossa criteria.
D – **D**iffuse STD w/ STE in aVR.

All of the STEMI equivalents listed above benefit from emergent coronary angiography with the following caveats:

- Posterior MI (isolated): Data shows that the majority of posterior MIs are presently evaluated with urgent (as opposed to emergent) angiography and this delay correlates with worsened clinical outcomes [24].
- New or presumed new LBBB was previously listed in the ACC/AHA guidelines as an indication for emergent angiography; however, as of the 2013 guidelines, this indication was removed [16, 25].

You may receive pushback from your cardiology consultant regarding STE in aVR. The best approach is to first explain that you are worried because the patient looks "sick." Next, describe the ECG and specifically how these findings are concerning for LMCA occlusion, proximal LAD occlusion, or MVD. Your consultant may agree to immediate activation while others may advise to first attempt medical therapy alone because the patient does not meet "criteria." If the presentation is secondary to one of these severe lesions, then the patient will not become pain-free despite your best medical efforts. At this point, reconsult for activation as the patient "continues to have clinical and electrocardiographic ischemia despite maximal medical therapy."

Pattern Recognition

LMCA Occlusion, Proximal LAD Occlusion, or Severe MVD
- ST elevation in lead aVR ≥1 mm
- Widespread ST depression ≥1 mm (i.e., ≥6 leads).

LMCA Occlusion or Proximal LAD Occlusion
- ST elevation in lead aVR $\geq$1 mm
- Widespread ST depression $\geq$1 mm
- **AND**
- ST elevation in lead V1.

LMCA Occlusion
- ST elevation in lead aVR $\geq$1 mm
- Widespread ST depression $\geq$1 mm
- **AND**
- ST elevation in lead aVR $\geq V_1$ **OR** ST elevation in aVL.

Disclosure Statement The authors of this chapter report no significant disclosures.

References

1. Gorgels APM, Engelen DJM, Wellens HJJ. Lead aVR, a mostly ignored but very valuable lead in clinical electrocardiography. J Am Coll Cardiol. 2001;38(5):1355–6. https://doi.org/10.1016/S0735-1097(01)01564-9.
2. Williamson K, Mattu A, Plautz CU, Binder A, Brady WJ. Electrocardiographic applications of lead aVR. Am J Emerg Med. 2006;24(7):864–74. https://doi.org/10.1016/j.ajem.2006.05.013.
3. Nakamura K. Significance of st-segment elevation in lead avr—diagnosis. Arch Intern Med. 2012;172(5):390–1. https://doi.org/10.1001/archinte.172.5.390.
4. Wong CK, Gao W, Stewart RAH, et al. AVR ST elevation: an important but neglected sign in ST elevation acute myocardial infarction. Eur Heart J. 2010;31(15):1845–53. https://doi.org/10.1093/eurheartj/ehq161.
5. Engelen DJ, Gorgels AP, Cheriex EC, et al. Value of the electrocardiogram in localizing the occlusion site in the left anterior descending coronary artery in acute anterior myocardial infarction. J Am Coll Cardiol. 1999;34(2):389–95. https://doi.org/10.1016/S0735-1097(99)00197-7.
6. Yamaji H, Iwasaki K, Kusachi S, et al. Prediction of acute left main coronary artery obstruction by 12-lead electrocardiography: ST segment elevation in lead aVR with less ST segment elevation in lead V1. J Am Coll Cardiol. 2001;38(5):1348–54. https://doi.org/10.1016/S0735-1097(01)01563-7.
7. Barrabés JA, Figueras J, Moure C, Cortadellas J, Soler-Soler J. Prognostic value of lead aVR in patients with a first non-ST-segment elevation acute myocardial infarction. Circulation. 2003;108(7):814–9. https://doi.org/10.1161/01.CIR.0000084553.92734.83.
8. Wagner GS, Macfarlane P, Wellens H, et al. AHA/ACCF/HRS recommendations for the standardization and interpretation of the electrocardiogram: part VI: acute ischemia/infarction: a scientific statement from the American Heart Association Electrocardiography and Arrhythmias Committee, Council on Clinical Cardiology; the American College of Cardiology Foundation; and the Heart Rhythm Society: endorsed by the International Society for Computerized Electrocardiology. Circulation. 2009;119(10):e262–70. https://doi.org/10.1161/CIRCULATIONAHA.108.191098.

9. Nikus K, Pahlm O, Wagner G, et al. Electrocardiographic classification of acute coronary syndromes: a review by a committee of the International Society for Holter and Non-Invasive Electrocardiology. J Electrocardiol. 2010;43(2):91–103. https://doi.org/10.1016/j.jelectrocard.2009.07.009.
10. Lipinski MJ, Mattu A, Brady WJ. Evolving electrocardiographic indications for emergent reperfusion. Cardiol Clin. 2018;36(1):13–26. https://doi.org/10.1016/j.ccl.2017.08.002.
11. Kosuge M, Ebina T, Hibi K, et al. An early and simple predictor of severe left main and/or three-vessel disease in patients with non-ST-segment elevation acute coronary syndrome. Am J Cardiol. 2011;107(4):495–500. https://doi.org/10.1016/j.amjcard.2010.10.005.
12. Kosuge M, Kimura K, Ishikawa T, et al. Predictors of left main or three-vessel disease in patients who have acute coronary syndromes with non-ST-segment elevation. Am J Cardiol. 2005;95(11):1366–9. https://doi.org/10.1016/j.amjcard.2005.01.085.
13. Gibbons RJ, Balady GJ, Bricker JT, et al. ACC/AHA 2002 guideline update for exercise testing: summary article. A report of the American College of Cardiology/American Heart Association task force on practice guidelines (committee to update the 1997 exercise testing guidelines). Circulation. 2002;106(14):1883–92. https://doi.org/10.1161/01.CIR.0000034670.06526.15.
14. Amsterdam EA, Wenger NK, Brindis RG, et al. 2014 AHA/ACC guideline for the management of patients with non–ST-elevation acute coronary syndromes: a report of the American College of Cardiology/American Heart Association task force on practice guidelines. J Am Coll Cardiol. 2014;64(24):e139–228. https://doi.org/10.1016/j.jacc.2014.09.017
15. Hillis LD, Smith PK, Anderson JL, et al. 2011 ACCF/AHA guideline for coronary artery bypass graft surgery: a report of the American College of Cardiology Foundation/American Heart Association task force on practice guidelines. Circulation. 2011;124:e652–735. https://doi.org/10.1161/CIR.0b013e31823c074e.
16. O'Gara PT, Kushner FG, Ascheim DD, et al. 2013 ACCF/AHA guideline for the management of st-elevation myocardial infarction: a report of the American college of cardiology foundation/american heart association task force on practice guidelines. J Am Coll Cardiol. 2013;61(4):78–140. https://doi.org/10.1016/j.jacc.2012.11.019.
17. Jones HU, Muhlestein JB, Jones KW, et al. Preoperative use of enoxaparin compared with unfractionated heparin increases the incidence of re-exploration for postoperative bleeding after open-heart surgery in patients who present with an acute coronary syndrome: clinical investigation and reports. Circulation. 2002;106(12 Suppl 1):I19–22. https://doi.org/10.1161/01.cir.0000032917.33237.e0.
18. Rokos IC, French WJ, Mattu A, et al. Appropriate Cardiac Cath Lab activation: optimizing electrocardiogram interpretation and clinical decision-making for acute ST-elevation myocardial infarction. Am Heart J. 2010;160(6):995–1003.e8. https://doi.org/10.1016/j.ahj.2010.08.011.
19. Rezaie S, Mattu A. Is ST-segment elevation in lead aVR getting too much respect? with Amal Mattu. R.E.B.E.L. EM. http://rebelem.com/is-st-segment-elevation-in-lead-avr-getting-too-much-respect-with-amal-mattu/. Published 2016.
20. Zafari AM. Myocardial infarction: practice essentials, background, definitions. Emedicine. medscape.com. https://emedicine.medscape.com/article/155919-overview. Published 2018. Accessed June 24, 2018.
21. Thygesen K, Alpert JS, Jaffe AS, et al. Third universal definition of myocardial infarction. Eur Heart J. 2012;33(20):2551–67. https://doi.org/10.1093/eurheartj/ehs184.
22. Scirica BM. Acute coronary syndrome: emerging tools for diagnosis and risk assessment. J Am Coll Cardiol. 2010;55(14):1403–15. https://doi.org/10.1016/j.jacc.2009.09.071.
23. Patel MR, Calhoon JH, Dehmer GJ, et al. ACC/AATS/AHA/ASE/ASNC/SCAI/SCCT/STS 2016 appropriate use criteria for coronary revascularization in patients with acute coronary syndromes: a report of the American College of Cardiology Appropriate Use Criteria Task Force, American Association for Thoracic Surgery, American Heart Association, American Society of Echocardiography, American Society of Nuclear Cardiology, Society for Cardiovascular Angiography and Interventions, Society of Cardiovascular Computed

Tomography, and the Society of Thoracic Surgeons. J Am Coll Cardiol. 2017;69(5):570–91. https://doi.org/10.1016/j.jacc.2016.10.034.

24. Pride YB, Tung P, Mohanavelu S, et al. Angiographic and clinical outcomes among patients with acute coronary syndromes presenting with isolated anterior ST-segment depression: a TRITON-TIMI 38 (trial to assess improvement in therapeutic outcomes by optimizing platelet inhibition with prasugrel-thrombolysis in myocardial infarction 38) substudy. JACC Cardiovasc Interv. 2010;3(8):806–11. https://doi.org/10.1016/j.jcin.2010.05.012.

25. Wilner B, de Lemos JA, Neeland I. LBBB in patients with suspected MI: an evolving paradigm. Am Coll Cardiol. 2017;(Mi). http://www.acc.org/latest-in-cardiology/articles/2017/02/28/14/10/lbbb-in-patients-with-suspected-mi.

Defibrillator Malfunction: *It's Electric! Boogie, Woogie, Woogie!*

14

Matthew Malone and Ashish Panchal

Case

Pertinent History

This patient is a 73-year-old male who presented to the ED approximately 3 hours after a perceived firing of his AICD. He states he was walking to the bathroom when he developed palpitations. He had no chest pain, dyspnea, lightheadedness, or other symptoms. Several seconds later, he felt as though he was "kicked in the chest by a mule." Subsequently, the palpitations he experienced resolved. His only symptom after the event is mild chest discomfort, which is slowly resolving. Patient reports that he forgot to take his metoprolol this morning.

Past Medical History
Hypertension, Type II Diabetes, Coronary Artery Disease, and remote STEMI resulting in ischemic cardiomyopathy with EF 20%.

Medications
Metoprolol, Lisinopril, Lasix, Metformin, Atorvastatin.

Social History
Forty pack-year smoking history, no drug or alcohol use.

M. Malone (✉) · A. Panchal
Department of Emergency Medicine, Wexner Medical Center at The Ohio State University, Columbus, OH, USA
e-mail: Matthew.malone@osumc.edu

© Springer Nature Switzerland AG 2020
C. G. Kaide, C. E. San Miguel (eds.), *Case Studies in Emergency Medicine*,
https://doi.org/10.1007/978-3-030-22445-5_14

Pertinent Physical Exam

- BP 142/90, Pulse 102, Temp 98.1 °F (36.7 °C), RR 14, SpO2 96%.
- Cardiovascular: Borderline tachycardia, regular rhythm, no gallop, friction rub or murmur heard.
- Chest Wall: Left upper chest AICD device without overlying erythema or tenderness to palpation of site.
- Lung: Clear to auscultation bilaterally.

Except as noted above, the findings of a complete physical exam are within normal limits.

Pertinent Test Results

EKG Normal sinus rhythm with old LBBB pattern otherwise unchanged from previous.

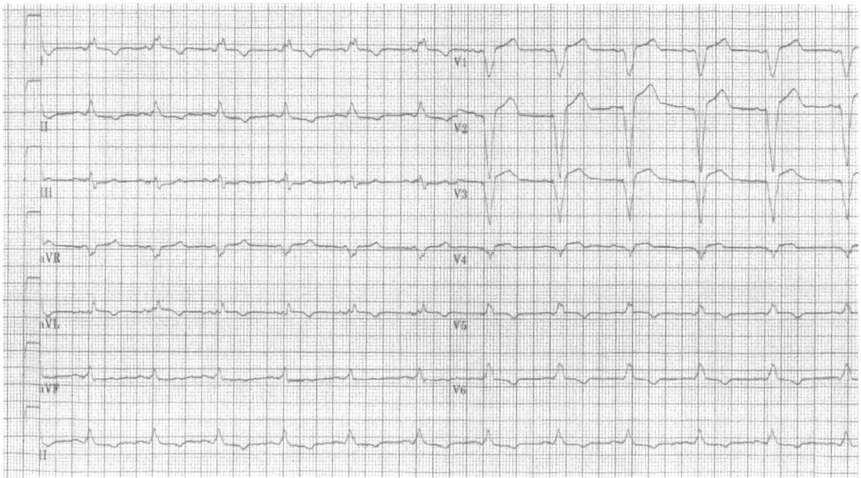

https://en.ecgpedia.org/index.php?title=File:MI_in_LBBB_02.jpg

Laboratory Analysis

Test	Result	Units	Normal Range
WBC	4.55	K/uL	3.8–11.0 10³/mm³
Hgb	14.8	g/dL	(Male) 14–18 g/dL
			(Female) 11–16 g/dL
Platelets	222	K/uL	140–450 K /uL
Sodium	136	mEq/L	135–148 mEq/L
Potassium	2.9 ↓	mEq/L	3.5–5.5 mEq/L
Chloride	106	mEq/L	96–112 mEq/L
Bicarbonate	25	mEq/L	21–34 mEq/L
BUN	13	mg/dL	6–23 mg/dL
Creatinine	1.01	mg/dL	0.6–1.5 mg/dL
Glucose	177 ↑	mg/dL	65–99 mg/dL
Magnesium	1.4 ↓	mg/dL	1.6–2.6 mg/dL
Troponin	<0.13 ↑	ng/dl	<0.11 ng/dl
BNP	350 ↑ (baseline for this patient is 350)	pg/ml	<100 pg/ml

CXR Single chamber AICD in place without evidence of lead fracture or displacement, no other acute cardiopulmonary process.

Device Interrogation Single episode of irregular wide complex tachycardia with rate approximately 177 bpm, successfully aborted by AICD discharge. No other events on device interrogation.

Updates on ED Course

Update 1: The patient's nurse informs you that the patient had four additional AICD firings in the last 10 minutes. You review the cardiac monitor alarms, revealing four episodes of irregular wide complex tachycardia successfully aborted by AICD discharge. You suspect new-onset atrial fibrillation with rapid ventricular response. You place a magnet over the AICD and ask the nurse to notify you if the patient's heart rate increases. Potassium and magnesium were also supplemented.

Update 2: Five minutes later, the nurse notifies you that the patient has had a rhythm change with a heart rate of 175. You enter the room and ask for a 12-lead ECG, which shows recurrence of the irregular wide complex tachycardia. The patient has a BP of 120/70. You administer 15 mg of diltiazem and begin an infusion. The patient's heart rate improves to 130 and BP increases to 120/68.

Update 3: Cardiology was consulted and reviewed the device interrogation report. The consultant believes that this event represents new-onset atrial fibrillation with rapid ventricular response and the shock was inappropriate. She recommends correction of electrolytes, rate control, anticoagulation, and admission for further monitoring and trending of cardiac enzymes. During the admission, the AICD will be adjusted. No recommendation for addition of an antiarrhythmic medication was made at this time. Admission orders were placed and the patient admitted to a monitored unit.

Learning Points: AICD Firing

Priming Questions
1. How can one distinguish between an appropriate and inappropriate AICD discharge?
2. What are the types of inappropriate AICD discharges and how are they treated?
3. Which patients with AICD discharge can be safely discharged home and which require admission?

Introduction/Background

1. Indications for AICD implantation include previous history of monomorphic or polymorphic ventricular tachycardia (VT) or ventricular fibrillation (VF) resulting in cardiac arrest or syncope, sustained VT with structural heart disease, and cardiomyopathy with low ejection fraction, as this is a significant risk factor for developing VT [1, 2].
2. Approximately 50–75% of AICD discharges result from an appropriate device response to a malignant ventricular arrhythmia, either VT of VF. More than 30% of patients with a history of VT or VF experience an appropriate AICD discharge for a malignant ventricular dysrhythmia within the initial 2 years of AICD implantation [3–6].
3. Approximately 20–30% of AICD discharges are considered inappropriate, meaning the device delivered a shock in the absence of a malignant ventricular dysrhythmia [7].
4. Multiple mechanisms for inappropriate electrical discharges exist. Most commonly, inappropriate electrical discharges occur due to false identification of supraventricular tachycardias (e.g., atrial fibrillation, sinus tachycardia) as VT or VF. Devices may also misinterpret large T waves, PVCs, and prominent QRS complexes as dysrhythmias, leading to AICD discharge. Inappropriate discharge may also occur due to device hardware malfunction (e.g., lead fracture, displacement) [1, 2, 8].
5. However, all events need to be evaluated for the underlying dysrhythmia leading to the AICD discharge.

Physiology/Pathophysiology

1. The primary purpose of an AICD is to sense cardiac electrical activity, recognize malignant rhythms such as VT and VF, and terminate these dysrhythmias via defibrillation [1, 2].

2. Malignant arrhythmias (and therefore appropriate shocks) can have many causes, including myocardial ischemia, decompensated CHF, electrolytes imbalances, and acute systemic illnesses [7].
3. Each AICD is programmed for detection of dysrhythmias and will deliver a shock based on ventricular rate and the total time at an accelerated rate. The threshold parameters for rate and duration can be adjusted by a representative of the device manufacturer or a cardiologist.
4. The typical AICD discharge is 40–42 J of electricity and causes most patients significant discomfort [9].
5. Preventing future shocks, both appropriate and inappropriate, is the overall goal in patient management. The effects of AICD defibrillation are not well understood but may include increased mortality as well as increased psychological stress impacting quality of life [7].

Differential Diagnosis

- Appropriate electrical defibrillation of ventricular tachycardia or ventricular fibrillation
- Defibrillation of supraventricular tachycardias including atrial flutter, atrial fibrillation, atrioventricular nodal reentrant tachycardia, atrioventricular reentrant tachycardia, or rapid sinus tachycardia
- Lead fracture or displacement
- Oversensing (e.g., Double counting peaked T waves as QRS)
- External electromagnetic interference
- Phantom shock

Making the Diagnosis

1. The first goal for any patient is to evaluate the patient to determine hemodynamic stability. Place the patient on continuous cardiac monitoring, obtain a full set of vitals, and get a 12-lead ECG to identify the patient's current rhythm.
2. If the patient is able to provide a history, they should be asked about the indication for ICD placement, history of prior shocks, any current cardiac medications (especially antiarrhythmics), and whether they have been able to take them as prescribed. In addition, ask if the AICD has been making "noises" or vibrating, since various models have different methods of notifying the patient of a possible malfunction in the device or the leads.
3. Symptoms preceding the shock and the circumstances surrounding the AICD discharge may also assist in identification of appropriate and inappropriate shocks.

- Chest pain may suggest acute ischemia and prompt an acute coronary syndrome evaluation.
- Shortness of breath, orthopnea, and LE edema may suggest decompensated CHF.
- Palpitations, confusion, lightheadedness, syncope, and anxiety may suggest a arrhythmia with hemodynamically instability.
- AICD discharge while resting, exercising, arm movement, exposure to electromagnetic radiation, or following trauma may help also to identify the cause.

4. Once history has been obtained and the patient has been stabilized, a few additional tests may help to narrow the differential.
   - Electrolyte abnormalities can contribute to both ventricular and supraventricular arrhythmias and should be checked and corrected.
   - Cardiac biomarkers would help exclude acute ischemia
   - Chest radiography can identify lead fracture or displacement
   - Device interrogation is key to confirming that the AICD did discharge and also allows for identification of the underlying cardiac rhythm when it is fired. Device interrogation can also identify device hardware issues, such as an increase in the lead resistance caused by lead displacement or fracture versus a decrease in lead resistance due to lead insulation failure. Further, battery depletion can lead to multiple ineffective shocks for VT and VF.

5. The most common causes of inappropriate shocks are nonventricular tachydysrhythmias, most commonly atrial fibrillation with a rapid ventricular response. Atrial flutter, atrioventricular nodal reentrant tachycardia, and atrioventricular re-entrant tachycardia will also result in the AICD firing if the rate and duration are above the threshold set on the device. Though rare, rapid sinus tachycardia from any cause may also result in shock delivery [1, 2, 8].
   - Dual-chamber ICDs are much more sophisticated and can differentiate between supraventricular and ventricular dysrhythmias. These dual chamber devices have an atrial lead to compare the atrial and ventricular rates and will only fire if the ventricular rate exceeds the atrial rate, as in VT and VF [1, 2].

6. Device interrogation can also identify oversensing, which occurs when the QRS complex and the following T wave (often peaked) are counted as two QRS complexes by the device, resulting in a perceived ventricular rate that is double the actual rate. In addition, oversensing can result from repetitive, rhythmic pectoral muscle movements, which are interpreted by the device as QRS complexes. Oversensing can usually be corrected by device reprogramming [7].

7. In addition to rhythm identification during AICD discharge, device interrogation can also identify AICD hardware issues. High lead impedance usually results from lead fracture and low lead impedance usually results from insulation failure [7].

8. Although far less common in newer devices, older AICDs were subject to interference by external electromagnetic radiation. Metal detectors, magnetic resonance imaging (MRI), external beam radiotherapy, electrical transformers, high-voltage power lines, and transcutaneous electrical nerve stimulation (TENS) units have all been reported to cause inappropriate AICD discharges [10].

9. A phantom shock is a perceived AICD discharge in the absence of shock on device interrogation. Often, these patients have suffered a painful shock in the past and may experience depression, posttraumatic stress disorder, or anxiety about shock recurrence. This is a diagnosis of exclusion.

Treating the Patient

1. If the patient is hemodynamically unstable and has a shockable rhythm, but the AICD is firing without aborting the arrhythmia, the AICD can be disabled by placing a magnet over the device site. External defibrillator pads can be placed on the patient and the patient can be managed according to ACLS algorithms.
2. The underlying etiology of appropriate and inappropriate shocks should be evaluated as above and abnormal findings should be addressed. Electrolytes and volume status should be optimized. If cardiac ischemia or nonventricular tachydysrhythmias are suspected and found, they should be addressed appropriately as well.
3. If device malfunction is confirmed or suspected, defibrillator pads should be placed on the patient and continuous cardiac monitoring should continue. Cardiology should be consulted to determine how best to repair or replace the device.
4. A single AICD discharge, either appropriate or inappropriate, does not necessarily always require hospital admission. Discharge is an option if the patient presents and remains hemodynamically stable during their ED visit, 12-lead EKG demonstrates sinus rhythm without acute changes, the diagnostic workup shows normal electrolytes and no cardiac ischemia, and the patient is comfortable with discharge and has reliable expedited follow-up. After all, if the patient did have a run of VT followed by a shock, then the AICD is doing its job!
5. The use of AICDs makes advanced imaging with MRI more complicated. Many older AICDs are not compatible with MRI, while modern MRI-compatible AICD models require reprogramming before the MRI along with a device check after the MRI. A patient with an AICD should only undergo MRI in close proximity to external defibrillation equipment, after disabling the electrical shock function of the AICD.

Case Conclusion

The patient was admitted to a monitored bed and spontaneously cardioverted to normal sinus rhythm. He had no additional arrhythmias or AICD discharges during his hospitalization. The electrophysiologists recommended rate control, anticoagulation for new-onset atrial fibrillation, and adjusted the parameters on the AICD for sustained tachycardia greater than 180 BPM to lessen the likelihood of any future inappropriate shocks for nonventricular arrhythmias.

Discussion

1. Device interrogation may not be possible in all clinical settings and scenarios but may be necessary to make the diagnosis. Transfer to another facility may be clinically warranted.
2. After initial stabilization, the main task lies in determining if this was an appropriate or inappropriate shock and treating the patient accordingly.
3. In cases of multiple ineffective shocks in the setting of a malignant arrhythmia, the AICD should be inactivated with a magnet and an external defibrillator should be used. The ideal placement of electrodes is anterior–posterior to avoid AICD component damage. If posterior pad positioning is impractical, the pads should be placed at least 10 cm from the AICD device to reduce component damage [7].

Pattern Recognition

- Presence of an AICD
- Patient reported sensation of being kicked or hit in the chest
- Syncope
- +/− palpitations, lightheadedness, chest pain, or dyspnea

Disclosure Statement The authors of this chapter report no significant disclosures.

References

1. Epstein AE, DiMarco JP, Ellenbogen KA, Estes NA 3rd, Freedman RA, Gettes LS, et al. ACC/AHA/HRS 2008 guidelines for device-based therapy of cardiac rhythm abnormalities: a report of the American College of Cardiology/American Heart Association task force on practice guidelines (Writing Committee to revise the ACC/AHA/NASPE 2002 guideline update for implantation of cardiac pacemakers and antiarrhythmia devices): developed in collaboration with the American Association for Thoracic Surgery and Society of Thoracic Surgeons. Circulation. 2008;117(21):e350–408. https://doi.org/10.1161/CIRCUALTIONAHA.108.189742.
2. Epstein AE, DiMarco JP, Ellenbogen KA, Estes NA 3rd, Freedman RA, Gettes LS, et al. 2012 ACCF/AHA/HRS focused update incorporated into the ACCF/AHA/HRS 2008 guidelines for device-based therapy of cardiac rhythm abnormalities: a report of the American College of Cardiology Foundation/American Heart Association task force on practice guidelines and the Heart Rhythm Society. J Am Coll Cardiol. 2013;61(3):e6–75. https://doi.org/10.1016/j.jacc.2012.11.007.
3. Liu CP, Ho YL, Lin YH, Liu YB, Chang WT, Huang CH, et al. Management of patients with implantable cardioverter defibrillators at emergency departments. Emerg Med J. 2007;24(2):106–9. https://doi.org/10.1136/emj.2006.037788.
4. Wathen MS, DeGroot PJ, Sweeney MO, Stark AJ, Otterness MF, Adkisson WO, et al. Prospective randomized multicenter trial of empirical antitachycardia pacing versus shocks for spontaneous rapid ventricular tachycardia in patients with implantable cardioverter-defibrillators: pacing fast ventricular tachycardia reduces shock therapies (PainFREE Rx II) trial results. Circulation. 2004;110(17):2591–6. https://doi.org/10.1161/01.CIR.0000145610.64014.E4.

5. Klein RC, Raitt MH, Wilkoff BL, Beckman KJ, Coromilas J, Wyse DG, et al. Analysis of implantable cardioverter defibrillator therapy in the Antiarrhythmics Versus Implantable Defibrillators (AVID) Trial. J Cardiovasc Electrophysiol. 2003;14(9):940–8.
6. Dichtl W, Wolber T, Paoli U, Brullmann S, Stuhlinger M, Berger T, et al. Appropriate therapy but not inappropriate shocks predict survival in implantable cardioverter defibrillator patients. Clin Cardiol. 2011;34(7):433–6. https://doi.org/10.1002/clc.20910.
7. Iftikhar S, Mattu A, Brady W. ED evaluation and management of implantable cardiac defibrillator electrical shocks. Am J Emerg Med. 2016;34(6):1140–7. https://doi.org/10.1016/j.ajem.2016.02.060.
8. Epstein AE, Miles WM, Benditt DG, Camm AJ, Darling EJ, Friedman PL, et al. Personal and public safety issues related to arrhythmias that may affect consciousness: implications for regulation and physician recommendations. A medical/scientific statement from the American Heart Association and the North American Society of Pacing and Electrophysiology. Circulation. 1996;94(5):1147–66.
9. Stevenson WG, Chaitman BR, Ellenbogen KA, Epstein AE, Gross WL, Hayes DL, et al. Clinical assessment and management of patients with implanted cardioverter-defibrillators presenting to nonelectrophysiologists. Circulation. 2004;110(25):3866–9. https://doi.org/10.1161/01.CIR.0000149716.03295.7C.
10. Akhtar M, Bhat T, Tantray M, Lafferty C, Faisal S, Teli S, et al. Electromagnetic interference with implantable cardioverter defibrillators causing inadvertent shock: case report and review of current literature. Clin Med Insights Cardiol. 2014;8:63–6. https://doi.org/10.4137/CMC.S10990.

Radiology Case 3

15

Priyanka Dube and Joshua K. Aalberg

Indications for the Exam A 71 y/o m presents with sudden-onset abdominal pain, diffusely tender without peritoneal signs.

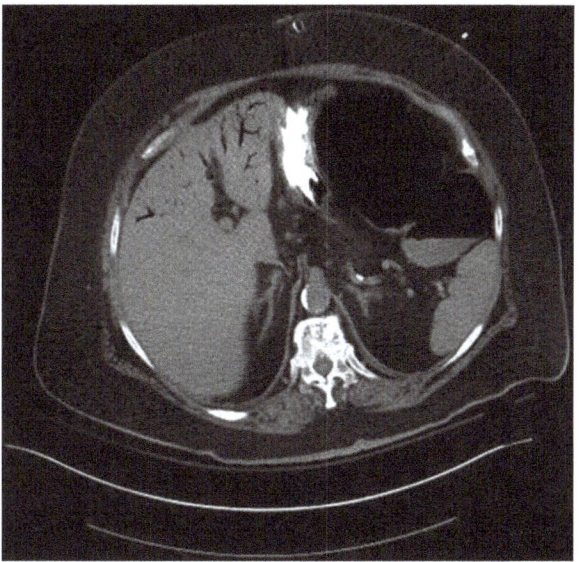

Radiographic Findings Computed tomography (CT) axial image of the abdomen demonstrating portal venous gas.

P. Dube · J. K. Aalberg (✉)
Department of Emergency Medicine, Wexner Medical Center at The Ohio State University, Columbus, OH, USA
e-mail: Priyanka.Dube@osumc.edu; joshua.aalberg@osumc.edu

© Springer Nature Switzerland AG 2020   157
C. G. Kaide, C. E. San Miguel (eds.), *Case Studies in Emergency Medicine*,
https://doi.org/10.1007/978-3-030-22445-5_15

Diagnosis Mesenteric Ischemia.

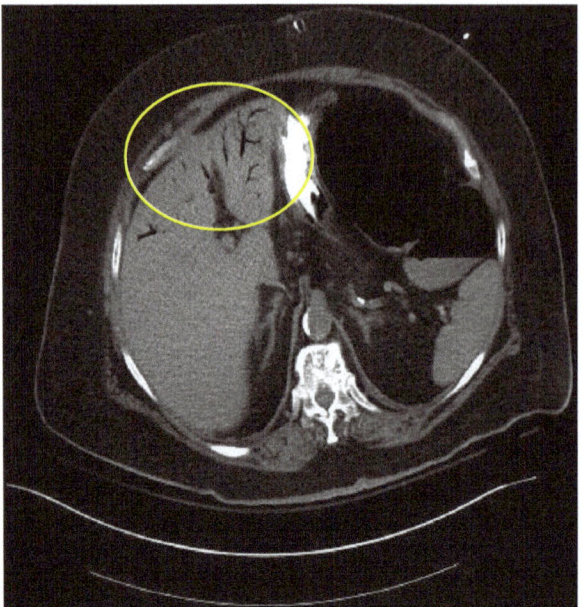

Learning Points

Priming Questions
- What is the pathophysiology that causes portal venous gas and pneumobilia?
- How do you differentiate these on imaging?
- What pathologies are associated with each?

Introduction/Background

The above case is concerning for acute bowel ischemia. On this CT, one can identify gas (dark on CT) within the periphery of the intrahepatic portal veins, indicating *portal venous gas* [1].

A common pitfall is understanding the differences between portal venous gas and pneumobilia. Understanding these diagnostic clues is necessary as they indicate different and serious pathologies. The goal of this section is to educate the reader on these differences to aid in prompt recognition and diagnosis.

Pathophysiology/Mechanism

Sign	Description	Pathophysiology
Portal venous gas	Gas within the portal veins that typically extends to the periphery just beneath the liver capsule	Gas (formed from iatrogenic, gas-forming organisms, and/or increased intraluminal pressure) enters the portal veins through venous/lymphatic drainage of the intestinal wall
Pneumatosis	Gas within the bowel wall [2]	Gas buildup within the bowel wall secondary to ischemia, increased intraluminal pressure, or bowel infarction. May also be from gas-forming organisms
Pneumobilia	Gas in the hepatobiliary tree that is located more centrally	Most commonly, this finding indicates a connection between the biliary tract and the gastrointestinal tract, either iatrogenically or pathologically via a fistula formation. Less commonly, infection of the biliary system with a gas-forming organism can cause pneumobilia

Making the Diagnosis

- *Portal venous gas*
  - Diagnosed from CT, conventional radiography, or ultrasound.
  - CT and ultrasound are the most sensitive imaging modalities to diagnose portal venous gas, especially in small amounts. Findings are subtle on a plain film and fail to demonstrate portal venous gas in 80% of cases [3].
  - Contrast-enhanced (arterial and venous phase) CT will help differentiate acute mesenteric ischemia from other etiologies of causes.
  - Portal venous gas tends to track *peripherally/subcapsular*, while pneumobilia is more *central*.
- *Pneumatosis*
  - The most sensitive imaging modality is CT. On conventional radiographs, there may be a small amount of gas within the bowel wall [4].
  - Pneumatosis can be a benign process; however, bowel wall thickening, dilation, ascites, and portal venous gas may indicate a much more serious etiology with high morbidity/mortality, such as bowel ischemia or infection [4]. Pneumatosis can often coexist with portal venous gas, as the gas tracks from the intestinal wall to the portal system.
  - Cystic fibrosis, COPD, and lung transplant patients are associated with benign etiologies of pneumatosis. The pathophysiology is not completely understood, but it is theorized that pulmonary obstructive disease allows for tracking of some air along vascular inferior to the diaphragm.
  - A thorough history and physical exam is crucial to distinguish between dangerous and benign causes of pneumatosis.
- *Pneumobilia*
  - Diagnosis of pneumobilia can be made from plain radiographs or CT.

- Supine radiographs often demonstrate sword-shaped air pattern in the right upper quadrant, indicating gas within the common duct and the left hepatic duct [5]. Known to radiologists as the *sabre sign*, this may be present in 50% of cases.
- CT will show tubular gas accumulation within the more central portions in the hepatobiliary tree. This is important to distinguish from portal venous gas (gas within the portal veins that extends to the periphery or subcapsular regions of the liver) [5].
- On ultrasound, portal venous gas demonstrates high echogenicity with significant shadowing. This can resemble intrahepatic calcifications.

CT axial image of the abdomen demonstrating pneumobilia

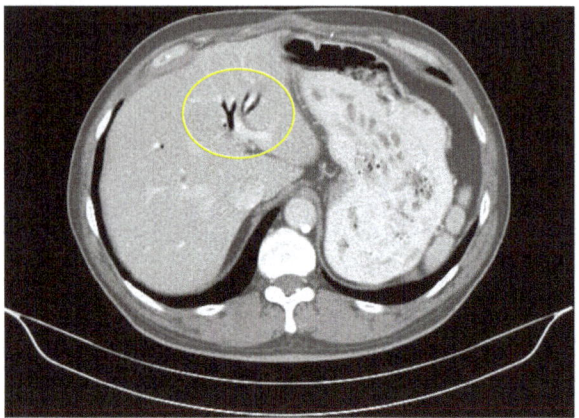

Abdominal X-ray demonstrating pneumatosis

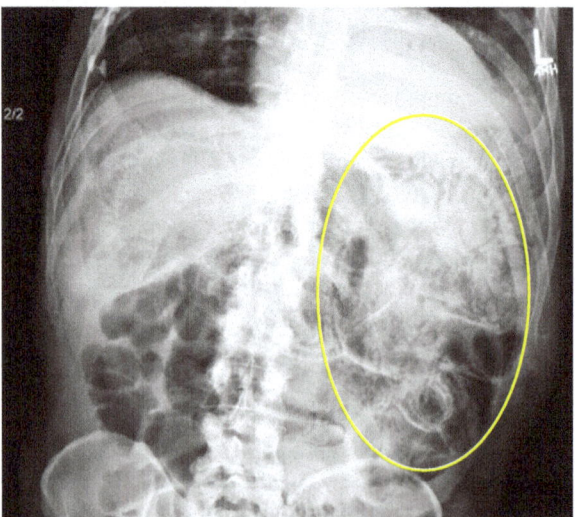

CT axial image of the abdomen demonstrating pneumatosis

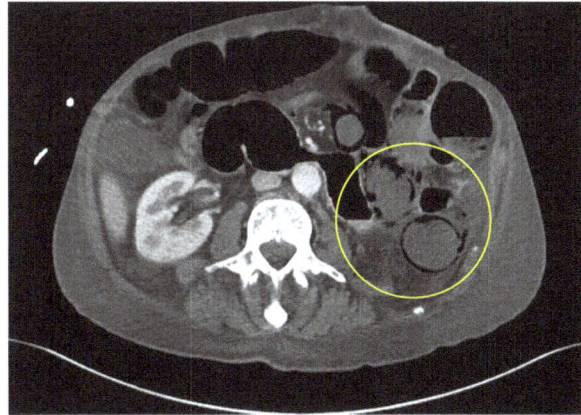

Common associations and causes	
Sign	Associations and causes
Portal venous gas	Ischemic bowel, pneumatosis intestinalis, inflammatory bowel disease, perforated peptic ulcer, necrotizing enterocolitis (pediatric), ileus, bowel obstruction sepsis, diverticulitis, iatrogenic (mechanical), and trauma
Pneumatosis	Bowel ischemia/infarction, necrotizing enterocolitis (pediatric), mechanical, iatrogenic, sepsis, autoimmune, collagen vascular disorders, pulmonary disease, corticosteroid use, and chemotherapy agents [4]
Pneumobilia	Biliary instrumentation, sphincter of Oddi dysfunction, postsurgical anastomoses, trauma, biliary enteric fistulas, and infection [5]

Treating the Patient

The proper treatment will depend on the underlying pathology causing the radiographic findings. Given the extensive list of possible causes, a thorough history and physical exam are needed to determine the proper treatment. For instance, pneumobilia in a patient who has had previous sphincterotomy of the sphincter of Oddi is likely incidental. However, in a patient without instrumentation, who presents with fever and severe right upper quadrant pain, the pneumobilia may be caused by emphysematous cholecystitis, necessitating antibiotics, fluids, and emergent surgery consolation. In general, portal venous gas and pneumatosis are more ominous findings than pneumobilia; however, there are benign and life-threatening causes for all three findings.

Discussion

- Knowing the benign and life-threatening etiologies as well as the differences between portal venous gas and pneumobilia is important to determine management.

- While plain film radiography may assist in making a diagnosis, often times it can be falsely negative when only small amounts of gas are present. Hence, CT will aid in making a diagnosis as well as suggesting possible etiologies.
- Combining imaging findings, physical exam, historical factors, and laboratory findings will aid in making accurate diagnoses.

Disclosure Statement The authors of this chapter report no significant disclosures.

References

1. Hussain A, Mahmood H, El-Hasani S. Portal vein gas in emergency surgery. World J Emerg Surg. 2008;3(1):21. https://doi.org/10.1186/1749-7922-3-21.
2. Jones J, et al. "Intramural Bowel Gas." Radiopaedia. Accessed 17 June 2018. https://radiopaedia.org/articles/intramural-bowel-gas.
3. Abboud B, Hachem JE, Yazbeck T, Doumit C. Hepatic portal venous gas: physiopathology, etiology, prognosis and treatment. World J Gastroenterol. 2009;15(29):3585. https://doi.org/10.3748/wjg.15.3585.
4. Ho LM, Paulson EK, Thompson WM. Pneumatosis intestinalis in the adult: benign to life-threatening causes. Am J Roentgenol. 2007;188(6):1604–13. https://doi.org/10.2214/ajr.06.1309.
5. Gaillard F, et al. "Pneumobilia." Radiopaedia. Accessed 17 June 2018. https://radiopaedia.org/articles/pneumobilia.

Difficult Airway and OMG, There's Blood Everywhere: *Navigating the Difficult Airway*

Caitlin Rublee and Michael Barrie

Case

A 42-year-old male presents to the emergency department with vomiting. The patient's family comes to the front desk and explains that the patient cannot get out of the car and has been vomiting blood. Security and nursing staff extricate the patient to a wheelchair and deliver him to a critical care bay while calling for physician help. You arrive to see the patient slumped in the wheelchair, dark blood pooling in his mouth and covering his shirt. The family tells you that he was just admitted for rectal bleeding, and he had left the hospital against medical advice earlier that morning. His baseline mental status is normal, but he is currently only responsive to painful stimulation. The patient is moved to the critical care bed and initial assessment is started.

Pertinent Physical Exam

Except as noted below, the findings of the complete physical exam are within normal limits.

- Blood pressure 99/40, pulse 143, temperature 97 °F (36.1 °C), temperature source Oral, respiratory rate 28, height 1.803 m (5′ 11″), SpO2 84%.
- Head, Eyes, Ears, Nose Throat: Atraumatic. The patient is actively vomiting. Trachea is midline. There is no appreciated oral edema.

C. Rublee · M. Barrie (✉)
Department of Emergency Medicine, Wexner Medical Center at The Ohio State University, Columbus, OH, USA
e-mail: Caitlin.Rublee@osumc.edu; Michael.Barrie@osumc.edu

© Springer Nature Switzerland AG 2020
C. G. Kaide, C. E. San Miguel (eds.), *Case Studies in Emergency Medicine*,
https://doi.org/10.1007/978-3-030-22445-5_16

- Cardiovascular: Normal S1, S2. Tachycardic. Cool extremities, capillary refill 4 seconds.
- Abdomen: Distended, +fluid wave.
- Skin: Slightly jaundice, spider hemangiomas present on chest, and palmer erythema.
- Neuro: The patient is not following commands, GCS 9 (E2V2M5). Does move all extremities spontaneously. On initial presentation, the patient is more responsive, but during the evaluation, his mental status decreases to GCS 6 (E1V1M4).

Past Medical History Alcoholic cirrhosis with prior variceal bleeding.

Social History Current every day smoker, continues to drink alcohol.

Family History No pertinent past family history.

Pertinent Test Results

Labs were unavailable on initial evaluation. Follow up testing revealed:

Lab Results			
Test	Results	Units	Normal Range
WBC	14.1	K/μL	3.8–11.0 10^3 / mm^3
HGb	5.5	g/dL	(Male) 14–18 g/dL
			(Female) 11–16 g/dL
Platelets	135	K/μL	140–450 K/μL
Creatinine	1.4	mg/dL	0.6–1.5 mg/dL
Potassium	>10	mEq/L	3.5–5.5 mEq/L
Lactate	6.1	mmol/L	<2.0
INR	1.4	–	≤1.1
Glucose	110	mg/dL	65–99 mg/dL
pH	7.11	–	7.35–7.45

Emergency Department Management

The patient was critically ill requiring immediate intervention. He was placed on a monitor, two large-bore peripheral IVs were established, and blood pressure recycled frequently. A definitive airway, given his altered mental status and copious hematemesis (vomiting blood), was an initial priority. He was identified to have a difficult airway given the amount of blood in his oropharynx, high risk of aspiration, and risk for decompensation during intubation given his profound presumed hemorrhagic shock. The patient was immediately placed on a non-rebreather face mask, oxygen turned to "flush," and had a nasal cannula placed with oxygen turned to 15 liters per minute. Team members attempted to suction the airway while others prepared for intubation. The team elected for low-dose etomidate sedation without paralysis given the predicted difficult airway. After induction, the first attempt was performed with direct laryngoscopy with a Macintosh blade. The resident was unable to visualize the vocal cords due to the amount of blood in the airway. A large-bore suction catheter was placed in the posterior oropharynx and left there during the attending physician's second attempt. With the assistance of a bougie device, the patient was successfully intubated with a 7.0 endotracheal tube. The balloon was inflated, and end tidal CO_2 was confirmed with a color-change device. The team continued resuscitation efforts initially with O negative trauma blood and subsequent massive transfusion protocol with O positive blood.

Updates on Emergency Department Course

The patient continued to have profound blood from oral gastric tube. A Blakemore tube was inserted in attempt to tamponade the presumed bleeding esophageal varices. The gastroenterology team was consulted, which recommended against immediate upper endoscopy because the patient was critically unstable. Gastroenterology instead recommended ongoing aggressive resuscitation in the intensive care unit. Interventional radiology was not available to discuss transjugular intrahepatic portosystemic shunt (TIPS) placement.

Learning Points

Priming Questions
1. How do you identify the potentially difficult airway?
2. What special preparations are necessary for the anticipated difficult airway?
3. What techniques will improve chances of success during intubation?

Introduction/Background

1. While managing a patient's airway is a routine aspect of emergency medicine, the anticipated difficult airway often unnerves even the most seasoned emergency physician. Fortunately, these events are rare [1, 2], but the provider must always be prepared for the myriad of airway challenges about to roll in the front door.
2. Applying a step-wise checklist to every airway approached, including the crashing patient with a difficult airway, will provide a sense of security.
3. Even an anticipated "easy" airway can have surprise difficulties. It is best to always prepare for the worst and have a stepwise approach to various backup options, including surgical airway options for the "can't intubate, can't oxygenate" scenario.
4. Brown and Walls have developed approaches for evaluating difficult airways [3]. The first question is whether the patient is crashing—cardiopulmonary arrest, respiratory arrest, and agonal respirations. If not, as the patient in the case was initially, the difficult airway algorithm can be followed using the "P's

of rapid-sequence intubation (RSI)" to maximize first-pass success: This is a slightly modified version of the P's of RSI: Plan B, predict a difficult intubation or bag-valve mask, preparation, "preintubation" optimization, preoxygenation, positioning, paralysis, put to sleep, placement with proof, and postintubation management.

5. Mortality from variceal bleeding has decreased threefold in the last 20 years yet remains a major cause of morbidity and mortality [4]. Avoiding hypoxia, allowing for restrictive transfusion with balanced resuscitation [5], and considering Sengstaken–Blakemore placement for a maximum of 24 hours to tamponade massive bleeding are recommended [6]. Recognizing and managing the factors leading to a difficult airway in the first place are imperative with continued resuscitation.

Physiology/Pathophysiology

1. Airway is placed first on the algorithm for evaluating the critical patient (airway, breathing, circulation) for good reason. Obstruction or failure of the patient's airway will rapidly lead to cardiopulmonary collapse and death.
2. There are many indications for placing a definitive airway.
   - *Respiratory failure*—when the patient is unable to oxygenate or ventilate to adequately meet physiologic needs. This is a clinical decision, but blood gas analysis showing pH < 7.3, $PaCO_2$ > 55 mmHg (or rise of $PaCO_2$ by 10 mmHg acutely in chronic CO_2-retaining patients like COPD), or PaO_2 of less than 60 mmHg on FiO2 > 40% could be suggestive of respiratory failure.
   - *Respiratory muscle fatigue.*
   - *Aspiration protection* if patient is too obtunded to protect their airway.
   - *Mechanical obstruction*—distortion of airway structures could block the airway. Potential etiologies include traumatic disruption, space-occupying lesions (Ludwig's angina, retropharyngeal abscess, malignancy), angioedema, neck hematomas, and foreign bodies.
   - *Other*—less common indications for intubation include intentional hyperventilation for cerebral edema (but rarely used), and core rewarming if patient is profoundly hypothermic.
3. The airway consists of the nose, mouth, posterior oropharynx, epiglottis, larynx, vocal cords, and trachea.

Sphenoid sinus

Internal nares

Entrance to auditory tube

Nasopharynx

Oropharynx

Laryngopharynx

Trachea

Frontal sinus

Nasal conchae
Superior
Middle
Inferior

Nasal cavity

External nares

Hard palate

Soft palate

Oral cavity

Epiglottis

Glottis

Vocal fold

The Upper Respiratory System

By BruceBlaus [7]: Blausen.com staff. ISSN 2002-4436. Own work, CC BY 3.0, https://commons. wikimedia.org/w/index.php?curid=27924400

4. To successfully intubate the patient, the operator must be able to align the airway structures to visualize the vocal cords. Especially when performing direct laryngoscopy, this is best performed by placing the patient in sniffing position [8]. Instead of simply hyperextending the neck, the provider should align the head and neck so the face is looking perpendicular to the bed with the ear lobe aligned with the sternal notch.

Proper Ear-to-Sternal Notch Positioning

Proper positioning with earlobe in line with sternal notch and face parallel to the floor using multiple blankets. (Used with permission courtesy of Colin Kaide)

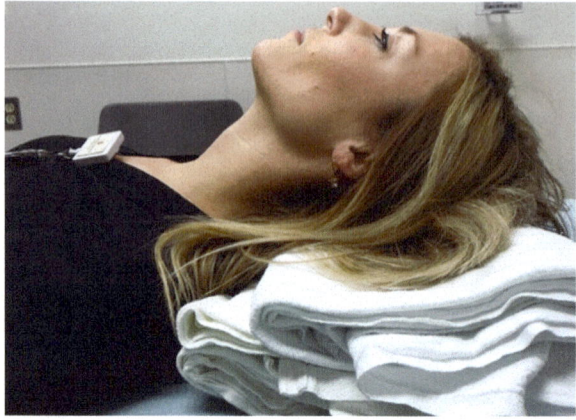

Making the Diagnosis

Differential Diagnosis in this Patient Presentation
- Upper GI bleed
  - Variceal bleeding
  - Peptic ulcer disease
  - Mallory-Weiss tear
  - Dieulafoy's lesions
  - Malignancy
  - Mimics: epistaxis, tonsillar bleeding
- Elevated ammonia leading to altered mental status and aspiration
- Gastroenteritis with vomiting and aspiration
- Coagulopathy

1. The first step in realizing the anticipated difficult airway is to take the time to assess every patient requiring intubation for anticipated difficulties. Generally, taking the time to assess the airway completely will avoid potential pitfalls. It is when the provider rushes to intubate and is not appropriately prepared when disaster can ensue.
   - Consider preexisting difficult airway
   - Special considerations in trauma immobilization
   - Mechanical distortion of the airway
2. A validated tool called the "LEMONS law" can help predict a difficult intubation [3].
   - Look externally—short muscular neck, full dentition, protruding upper incisors, high-arched palate, receding mandible, severe facial trauma, and clinician gestalt

- Evaluate internally—3-3-2 rule
  - The rule describes the ideal external dimensions of the airway.
  - 3- the opening of the jaw should be far enough to accommodate three fingers (3–4 cm)
  - 3- the distance from the tip of the chin to the hyoid bone should be at least 3 fingerbreadths
  - 2- the distance from the floor of the mouth to the thyroid cartilage should be at least 2 fingerbreadths.
- Mallampati- Class I–II have low intubation failure rates while Class IV has failure rates reported over 10% of the time. While difficult to predict, the Mallampati has the highest sensitivity for diagnosing difficult intubation [9].
  - Mallampati Class I: No difficulty: Soft palate, uvula, fauces, and pillars visible
  - Mallampati Class II: No difficulty: Soft palate, uvula, and fauces visible
  - Mallampati Class III: Moderate difficulty: Soft palate and base of uvula visible
  - Mallampati Class IV: Major difficulty: Hard palate only visible

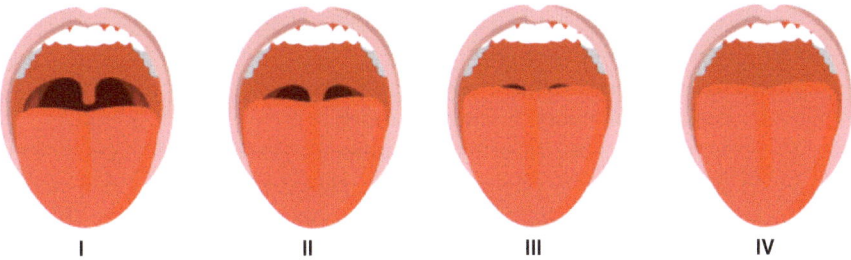

I   II   III   IV

By Jmarchn (Own work) [CC BY-SA 3.0 (https://creativecommons.org/licenses/by-sa/3.0) or GFDL (http://www.gnu.org/copyleft/fdl.html)], via Wikimedia Commons

- Obstruction—Signs include muffled voice, stridor, sense of dyspnea, and difficulty tolerating secretions.
- Neck mobility—Poor neck mobility from cervical spine immobilization or a history of ankylosing spondylitis or rheumatoid arthritis, for examples, restrict optimal sniffing positioning for intubation.
- Saturation—A saturation less than 90% in and of itself can create a difficult intubation as the time before desaturation is significantly less. A saturation this low on maximum oxygenation predicts a rapid desaturation.

3. It is also important to consider if the patient is a potentially difficult cricothyrotomy. Use the SMART mnemonic [10].
   - S—surgery
   - M—mass
   - A—access/anatomy
   - R—radiation (or other scarring)
   - T—trauma

4. It is rare to have a truly "crash" airway, one that must be secured immediately or the patient may rapidly deteriorate. In these rare cases, always assume that the patient will have a difficult airway and have immediate backup plans in mind for failed first attempts.

Treating the Patient

1. With any intubation, the key is using a step-wise approach. One standard approach is to go through the "P's of RSI [3]." Some argue that every approach begins with Plan B as well to assist with anticipating difficulties. Below is a modified version of the "Ps of RSI."

The P's of Rapid-Sequence Intubation
- *Plan B.* Advance planning for multiple contingencies gives the intubator many pre-thought-out options to deal with unanticipated difficulties. Having a strategy that goes beyond A and B can help to set oneself up for success in a potential failure situation. Further, the plan should be verbalized to the team prior to intubation.
- *Predict a difficult intubation.* Use the "LEMONS Law" as described earlier to determine a potentially difficult intubation.
- *Preparation.* Wear personal protection equipment, establish IV access with blood pressure cuff on opposite extremity. Have medications labeled and drawn up. Have equipment (direct and video laryngoscopes, varying sizes of endotracheal tubes, bougie) including Plan B equipment such as scalpel, Laryngeal Mask Airway (LMA) at bedside ready to use.
- *Preintubation optimization.* Resuscitate before you intubate! Optimize blood pressure with fluids or blood products and pressor support anticipating a reduction in blood pressure during RSI.
- *Preoxygenation.* Provide oxygen via non-rebreather turned to wide open. This is also called "flush," and it can provide up to 50 liters per minute (LPM). Begin at least 3 minutes prior to intubation. Place a nasal cannula at 15 LPM and maintain nasal cannula throughout intubation [11]. This combination and flow rate can provide an FIO_2 greater than 90%.
- *Positioning.* Position patient with ear to sternal notch.
- *Paralyze.* Deliver paralytic medications via rapid IV push in rapid succession with induction agents.
- *Put to sleep.* Deliver induction medications via rapid IV push in rapid succession with paralytic agents.
- *Placement with proof.* Pass the tube through the cords. Consider using bougie in setting of difficult airway, some evidence demonstrates increased first-pass success in setting of difficult airway [12]. Confirm placement with end-tidal carbon dioxide detection and pulmonary auscultation.
- *Post intubation management.* Obtain chest X-ray, treat hypotension, and order sedation and analgesia if indicated.

2. Additional tips for success in the difficult airway
   - Endotracheal tube (ET) introducer—bougie
     - Also called the gum elastic bougie, the ET introducer is made of plastic with an angled distal tip. The 30-degree-angled coude tip allows the device to more easily navigate anteriorly around the epiglottis and through the vocal cords. When successfully placed in the trachea, the provider can feel the bougie bumping the anterior tracheal rings, and the angled tip should lodge at the carina or smaller airways. After placement, the provider can slide the ET tube over the introducer into the airway. A few tips and tricks for ET introducer success:
       ○ Do not use an introducer with a hyperangulated blade such as with a glidescope. The bougie introducer is too flexible to follow the hyperangulated course.
       ○ Do not remove the laryngoscope blade when passing the ET tube. This will move the tongue and potentially allow direct visualization of the ET tube entering the airway.
       ○ Consider preloading the ET tube on the introducer. One technique described as the "kiwi grip" or d-loop technique places the distal end of the bougie into the ET tube vent ("Murphy's eye").

Kiwi Grip

Photos courtesy of Michael
Barrie, MD

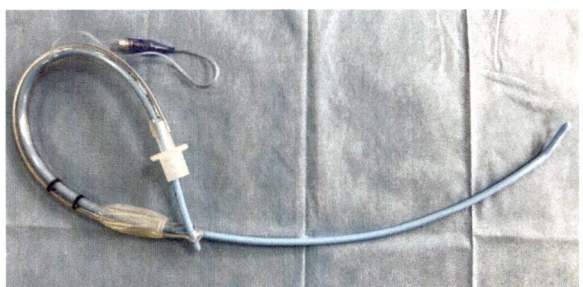

- Suction-assisted laryngoscopy and airway decontamination (SALAD). Coined by anesthesiologist Dr. Jim Ducanto, this process explains how to decontaminate the airway that is full of vomitus or blood [13, 14]. In this description, the endotracheal tube can be attached to a meconium aspirator, and then attached to suction. This converts the ET tube into a large bore suction catheter. The patient then can be intubated using this same ET tube, which will then allow for suctioning of aspirated contents in the airway. Alternatively, this ET tube can be intentionally directed into the esophagus and left on to suction to help clear the airway, and then the patient is intubated with another ET tube.
- Video-assisted laryngoscopy can be useful in the difficult airway, but in this case with a bloody airway, they generally do not work. The camera is easily obscured, and also the hemoglobin in the blood will absorb light, making it even more difficult to see.

3. It is important to always consider surgical airway options in any difficult airway. Generally, the hardest part of a surgical airway is deciding to do one. It is important to realize when other approaches to managing the airway have failed and quickly convert to a surgical approach. Here are three descriptions of common emergency surgical airways.

- Open cricothyrotomy—the cricothyroid membrane is located just below the thyroid cartilage. In an open cricothyrotomy, the only tools the operator needs are a scalpel and a bougie. Perform a vertical incision in the skin over the cricoid cartilage, and then a horizontal incision through the cricoid cartilage. Then, with the blade in the airway, rotate the blade 90° to open up the hole. Slide the bougie into the airway, and then use this in a Seldinger technique to insert the 6–0 ETT.

- Needle cricothyrotomy—this approach uses a Seldinger technique, inserting a needle through the cricoid cartilage until aspirating air, then insert a quide wire into the airway. The needle is removed, and then a device with dilator is inserted over the guidewire. Then the wire is removed.

- Retrograde intubation—similar to the needle cric, enter the airway with a needle until aspirating bubbles, but then guide the wire superiorly out the mouth. The ETT can be delivered over the guidewire through the mouth to orotracheally intubate. This will only be successfully if the upper airway anatomy will cooperate with passing a small endotracheal tube.

Case Conclusion

The patient was admitted to the intensive care unit. However, over the course of hours, the patient became progressively acidotic, with ongoing bleeding despite appropriate Blakemore tube placement, blood product administration, cephalosporin antibiotics, somatostatin analogue, and pressor support. The patient expired from presumed upper gastrointestinal hemorrhage from bleeding varices and decompensated cirrhosis.

Discussion

Fortunately, the difficult airway is a rare event but one that providers should always be prepared for. The first step in managing the difficult airway is recognizing the potential for a difficult intubation. As time allows, prepare for each step of the intubation with multiple back up strategies if initial attempts fail. Be prepared to move to advanced techniques including surgical airway, especially if unable to oxygenate or ventilate the patient. The provider that clearly states their plan to the team and confidently works through their checklist will make management of the difficult airway look routine.

Pattern Recognition

Anticipated Difficult Airway
- Abnormal findings in the LEMONS law
- Abnormal vital signs that could portend peri-intubation arrest
- Vomit or blood in the airway

Disclosure Statement   The authors of this chapter report no significant disclosures.

References

1. Tayal VS, Riggs RW, Marx JA, Tomaszewski CA, Schneider RE. Rapid-sequence intubation at an emergency medicine residency: success rate and adverse events during a two-year period. Acad Emerg Med. 1999;6(1):31–7.
2. Sakles JC, Laurin EG, Rantapaa AA, Panacek EA. Airway management in the emergency department: a one-year study of 610 tracheal intubations. Ann Emerg Med. 1998;31(3):325–32.
3. The walls manual of emergency airway management. 5th ed. 2017.
4. Carbonell N, Pauwels A, Serfaty L, Fourdan O, Levy VG, Poupon R. Improved survival after variceal bleeding in patients with cirrhosis over the past two decades. Hepatology. 2004;40(3):652–9.
5. Wang J, Bao YX, Bai M, Zhang YG, Xu WD, Qi XS. Restrictive vs liberal transfusion for upper gastrointestinal bleeding: a meta-analysis of randomized controlled trials. World J Gastroenterol. 2013;19(40):6919–27.
6. Augustin S, Gonzalez A, Genesca J. Acute esophageal variceal bleeding: current strategies and new perspectives. World J Hepatol. 2010;2(7):261–74.
7. Blaus B. Medical gallery of Blausen Medical 2014. Wiki J Med. 2014;1(2):10.
8. Akihisa Y, Hoshijima H, Maruyama K, Koyama Y, Andoh T. Effects of sniffing position for tracheal intubation: a meta-analysis of randomized controlled trials. Am J Emerg Med. 2015;33(11):1606–11.
9. Roth D, Pace NL, Lee A, Hovhannisyan K, Warenits AM, Arrich J, et al. Airway physical examination tests for detection of difficult airway management in apparently normal adult patients. Cochrane Database Syst Rev. 2018;5:Cd008874.
10. De Regge M, Vogels C, Monsieurs KG, Calle PA. Retention of ventilation skills of emergency nurses after training with the SMART BAG compared to a standard bag-valve-mask. Resuscitation. 2006;68(3):379–84.
11. Weingart SD, Levitan RM. Preoxygenation and prevention of desaturation during emergency airway management. Ann Emerg Med. 2012;59(3):165–75.e1.
12. Driver BE, Prekker ME, Klein LR, Reardon RF, Miner JR, Fagerstrom ET, et al. Effect of use of a bougie vs endotracheal tube and stylet on first-attempt intubation success among patients with difficult airways undergoing emergency intubation: a randomized clinical trial. JAMA. 2018;319(21):2179–89.
13. Kei J, Mebust DP. Comparing the effectiveness of a novel suction set-up using an adult endotracheal tube connected to a meconium aspirator vs. a traditional Yankauer suction instrument. J Emerg Med. 2017;52(4):433–7.
14. Weingart SD, Bhagwan SD. A novel set-up to allow suctioning during direct endotracheal and fiberoptic intubation. J Clin Anesth. 2011;23(6):518–9.

Disseminated Neonatal Herpes Simplex Virus: *Simplex Can Be Very Complex!*

Seth Linakis and Maegan Reynolds

Case

Poorly feeding infant

Pertinent History A 7-day-old patient presented to the emergency department (ED) for decreased feeding and fussiness. The parents reported that the patient previously had been taking about 20–40 mL of formula every 2–3 hours, but over the past 2 days, this had been gradually decreasing, and the patient had to be awakened for the past 2 feeds. The infant was also fussy when awake today, although she would briefly improve when held by parents. She had developed a rash on her chest earlier today, and it had subsequently spread to the whole body. She has had no fevers and no cough. She has had congestion since birth, regular stools, and regular wet diapers.

Past Medical History Full-term healthy neonate born at 39 weeks 3 days via normal spontaneous vaginal delivery. There were no preterm complications. She left the hospital with mother after about 36 hours.

Social History Lives with parents, mother is 20 years old, G2P1, did receive prenatal care, does have a history of chlamydia as a teenager which was treated, mother denies smoking or drug usage during pregnancy.

Pertinent Physical Exam
Temperature 35.1 °C (95.2 °F), heart rate 110 beats per minute, blood pressure 76/48 mmHg, respiratory rate 40 breaths per minute, SpO_2 95% on room air.

S. Linakis (✉) · M. Reynolds
Department of Emergency Medicine Nationwide Children's Hospital, Columbus, OH, USA
e-mail: Seth.Linakis@nationwidechildrens.org; Maegan.Reynolds@nationwidechildrens.org

© Springer Nature Switzerland AG 2020
C. G. Kaide, C. E. San Miguel (eds.), *Case Studies in Emergency Medicine*,
https://doi.org/10.1007/978-3-030-22445-5_17

Except as noted below, the findings of a complete physical exam are within normal limits.

- General: Pale infant with grayish tint to the skin, minimally responsive to painful stimuli.
- Head/Eyes/Ears/Nose/Throat: Anterior fontanelle soft and flat. Moist mucous membranes, and no oral lesions appreciable.
- Cardiovascular: Regular rate and rhythm, normal heart sounds, no appreciable murmurs, faint femoral pulses bilaterally, capillary refill is 4–5 seconds.
- Chest: Mild subcostal and suprasternal retractions, clear breath sounds throughout, and no wheezing.
- Abdomen: Soft, no distension, no appreciable tenderness throughout, no guarding, and no appreciable hepatosplenomegaly.
- Skin: Pale, grayish tint to skin, appears to have jaundice to the mid torso, and diffuse erythematous maculopapular rash to the torso and extremities. Skin poke to the right heel still oozing, pressure applied.
- Plan: Intravenous (IV) line placement, IV dextrose bolus, IV fluid bolus, full septic work up including urine catheterization and lumbar puncture, start empiric antibiotics and acyclovir, and admit.

Triage Evaluation The patient was taken to an intake room for vitals and triage by the nurse. The patient was noted to be minimally responsive and hypothermic. Glucose was obtained and was 40 mg/dL. The patient was immediately brought back to a resuscitation room.

Emergency Department Course The patient was taken to a resuscitation room. An IV was placed with some difficulty and the patient was given a D10 5 mL/Kg IV bolus and IV NS 10 ml/kg bolus. The highest concern was for sepsis, but a cardiac anomaly was also considered so the patient was reassessed following fluid administration. Additionally, a chest x-ray was obtained and did not show pulmonary edema or cardiomegaly. The patient was noted to have continued oozing from any venipuncture attempts.

Pertinent Diagnostic Testing

Test	Results	Units	Normal Range
WBC	16.7	K/µL	3.8–11.0 10^3/mm^3
Hgb	11.7	g/dL	(Male) 14–18 g/dL
			(Female) 11–16 g/dL
Platelets	83	K/µL	140–450 K/µL
Na	132	mEq/L	135–148 mEq/L
Cr	0.4	mg/dL	0.6–1.5 mg/dL
Glucose	40	mg/dL	65–99 mg/dL
pH	7.26	–	7.35–7.45

Test	Results	Units	Normal Range
pCO$_2$	52	mmHg	36.1–52.1 mmHg
ALT	3400	IU/L	8–32 IU/L
AST	7800	IU/L	6–21 IU/L

Urinalysis: Completely negative.

Chest X-ray (CXR): no pulmonary infiltrates, normal cardiac silhouette.

Update An additional IV was placed, and the patient remained minimally responsive despite IV dextrose with a repeat glucose of 126 mg/dL and an additional 20 mL/kg bolus. The patient's respiratory rate decreased, and she was noted to have a brief period of apnea lasting about 15 seconds. She was intubated on the second attempt with a 3.0 cuffed endotracheal tube (ETT). Repeat CXR showed appropriate ETT position and no pulmonary infiltrates. She was given an additional 30 mL/kg for a total of 60 mL/kg, with some improvement in peripheral pulses and a capillary refill of 3 seconds on reassessment. She was given ampicillin and gentamicin and was started on acyclovir given her age. She was admitted to the pediatric ICU.

Update The patient continued to have oozing from IV sites and had pink-tinged sputum suctioned from the ETT. Additional labs showed an international normalized ratio (INR) of 2.1 and an elevated partial thromboplastin time (PTT). Given the concern for coagulopathy, the decision was made to defer performing the lumbar puncture in the ED but to continue resuscitation and empiric antibiotics while awaiting an inpatient bed.

Learning Points: Disseminated Neonatal Herpes Simplex Virus

Priming Questions
1. What is the incidence and pathophysiology of disseminated HSV? What is the morbidity and mortality of this disease?
2. How is the diagnosis of disseminated HSV made? What are key exam and laboratory findings?
3. What is the treatment for disseminated HSV?

Introduction/Background

1. Neonatal herpes simplex virus (HSV) infection is an uncommon but highly morbid condition with substantial short- and long-term implications. In the literature, estimates range from 8 to 60 cases per 100,000 births in the United States, with 13.4/100,000 being a recent estimate [1–5]. If left untreated, neonatal HSV results

in a mortality rate of about 60%, and a high proportion of survivors (up to 50%) experience long-term sequelae, including neurologic impairment and developmental delay as well as recurrent cutaneous manifestations [1, 4].

Physiology/Pathophysiology

1. HSV initially infects skin or mucosal epithelial cells but has a particular affinity for neurons. It is propagated via neuronal tissue and can remain latent in the neuronal nuclei throughout a patient's lifetime. Treatment will not eradicate latent virus.
2. A substantial majority (85%) of neonatal HSV infections occur from exposure during delivery, and most of these cases (50–80%) result from initial maternal HSV infection near term [1, 4]. Infection may also be acquired in utero (5%) or postnatally (10%). Transmission as the result of reactivation of a preexisting maternal infection is rare, occurring in <1% of cases. Overall, HSV-2 is a more common infection in neonates (64–73%) than HSV-1 [1–4, 6–8]. It is important to note that HSV is *not* transmitted via breast milk; mothers may be encouraged to breastfeed if desired [5].
3. Neonatal HSV is distinct from congenital HSV. The latter requires in utero transmission of the disease and results in clinical features which are typically evident at birth such as microcephaly, hydrocephalus, and chorioretinitis [1].

Making the Diagnosis

Differential for the lethargic neonate:
- Sepsis
- Sepsis
- Sepsis
- Hypoglycemia
- Hyperbilirubinemia
- Uncompensated congenital cardiac anomaly
- Intracranial bleed (especially if parental refusal of vitamin K or complicated delivery, i.e., vacuum assisted)
- Congenital metabolic disease (electrolyte abnormalities)
- Seizures

1. There are three primary presentations of neonatal HSV infection. The most common (approximately 45% of cases) is skin-eye-mucous membrane (SEM) disease. SEM disease is typically characterized by vesicular lesions of the skin,

eyes, or mucosa, although this may be absent in up to 20% of cases [1, 4]. Patients with SEM disease are at high risk of progression to disseminated disease if left untreated, but patients appropriately covered with IV acyclovir experience minimal morbidity and mortality [1, 2, 4]. SEM disease typically presents between 10 and 12 days of life [4].

2. The second major form, accounting for approximately 30% of cases, is central nervous system (CNS) disease. CNS disease classically presents between 16–19 days of life with lethargy, poor feeding, and seizures, although presentations can also be nonspecific. Vesicular lesions may be seen but are often not present. Cerebrospinal fluid (CSF) pleocytosis is common, but the preferred diagnostic test is HSV DNA polymerase chain reaction (PCR) from the CSF. If left untreated, mortality from CNS disease is approximately 50%; appropriate acyclovir treatment reduces the mortality to 4–6% [1, 4, 9]. However, approximately 70% of infants who survive CNS HSV infection will experience developmental delay or other long-term neurologic sequelae [1, 4, 6].

3. The third and most severe form of neonatal HSV is disseminated disease. This represents approximately 25% of cases (~3.4/100,000 live births). It typically presents in the first 1–2 weeks of life. In addition to CNS disease (60–75% of patients with disseminated HSV) and cutaneous manifestations (50–80% of patients), infants with disseminated disease may present with respiratory failure, hepatitis or liver failure, pneumonitis, and/or disseminated intravascular coagulopathy (DIC). The overall clinical picture is generally that of sepsis or septic shock. However, neonates with disseminated HSV disease may experience delayed or missed diagnosis, as the presentation is nonspecific. As a result, it has become standard to include evaluation for HSV infection in neonates undergoing a work up for sepsis in the ED. As with CNS disease, HSV DNA PCR is the preferred test for diagnosis [1, 4, 5, 7]. Testing of cutaneous lesions, serum, and CSF is recommended [1, 4].

4. All neonates with suspected HSV infection should undergo cutaneous swabs, swabs of their mucous membranes, blood testing, and cerebrospinal fluid (CSF) testing for HSV.

5. Regardless of type, over half of patients with neonatal HSV are normothermic [2]. The absence of temperature abnormality should not be reassuring to the clinician in an ill-appearing infant or an infant with a concerning history. Similarly, absence of the classic vesicular rash should not decrease suspicion, as it is only present in approximately 50% of infants with HSV [1].

6. There is considerable debate about which nonclassic presentations in ill neonates should be tested and treated. It is our practice to give an empiric dose of acyclovir to all neonates less than 29 days undergoing a serious bacterial illness evaluation. We also give an empiric dose of acyclovir to all ill neonates (≤60 days old) if they are showing signs of severe sepsis, septic shock, DIC, vesicular rash, or have a maternal history of HSV.

Treating the Patient

1. Disseminated disease has an extremely high mortality rate. Left untreated, some 85% of infants will die of disseminated HSV disease. Among survivors, nearly all will have long-term neurologic sequelae without treatment. However, use of appropriate antiviral therapy has demonstrated marked improvement in clinical outcomes. While both vidarabine and acyclovir have shown efficacy in treating neonatal HSV disease, acyclovir has been demonstrated to be superior [1]. Multiple regimens of acyclovir have been tested, and high-dose intravenous acyclovir (20 mg/kg every 8 hours) has been demonstrated to outperform moderate-dose (15 mg/kg every 8 hours) and standard-dose (10 mg/kg every 8 hours) acyclovir in patients with neonatal HSV [10]. CNS and disseminated disease are treated with a 21-day course; for patients with SEM disease only, a 14-day course is recommended [1, 4, 10].
2. If appropriately treated, the impact of neonatal HSV disease may be significantly mitigated. Mortality in disseminated disease decreases from 85% to about 31% in the context of appropriate antiviral therapy, while long-term morbidity drops from nearly 100% to about 17% [1, 4]. As a result, if HSV is included in the differential diagnosis for an ill newborn in the emergency department, treatment with high-dose acyclovir should be strongly considered in addition to standard antimicrobial therapy.
3. Similar to antibiotics in this population, treatment should be started as soon as possible. While reasonable attempts should be made to obtain all the necessary samples for testing prior to initiating therapy, delays in these processes should not cause delays in administration of acyclovir.

Case Conclusion

The patient was taken to the pediatric intensive care unit (PICU) and was continued on mechanical ventilation. Over the next several hours, the patient became hypotensive with poor perfusion and was started on an epinephrine drip. The rash developed some areas that were more pustular or vesicular. Repeat labs showed declining kidney function, increasing liver transaminases, and worsening coagulopathy concerning for DIC. A bedside head ultrasound showed severe intraventricular hemorrhage, and the patient appeared to have some seizure-like activity. The patient coded twice and was resuscitated but continued to show signs of rapidly progressive multi-organ system failure. In discussion with parents, the decision was made to move toward comfort care, and the patient expired approximately 18 hours after initial presentation to the emergency department. Postmortem testing revealed herpes simplex meningitis.

Discussion

Neonatal HSV, while relatively rare, remains an important cause of illness, morbidity, and mortality among infants in the United States. However, early recognition and treatment with acyclovir substantially improves outcomes, including survival and rate of neurologic sequelae. As a result, medical providers should always consider HSV disease when evaluating an ill neonate in the emergency department, particularly in the first 29 days of life. Unfortunately, even with appropriate care, a high proportion of patients with disseminated disease will still die from their illness, as was the case in the patient presented in this chapter.

Pattern Recognition

Neonatal Herpes Simplex Virus
- Lethargic neonate less than 29 days old
- 50% are normothermic and 50% don't have vesicles
- Vesicular lesions of the skin, eyes, or mucosa
- CNS involvement with seizures, poor feeding, and lethargy
- Sepsis with liver failure, multiorgan failure, or DIC
- Febrile or ill neonate with known exposure or maternal history of HSV

Disclosure Statement The authors of this chapter report no significant disclosures.

References

1. Corey L, Wald A. Maternal and neonatal herpes simplex virus infections. N Engl J Med. 2009;361:1376–85.
2. Cruz AT, Freedman SB, Kulik DM, Okada PJ, Fleming AH, Mistry RD, et al. Herpes simplex virus infection in infants undergoing meningitis evaluation. Pediatrics. 2018;141(2):e1–9.
3. Flagg EW, Weinstock H. Incidence of neonatal herpes simplex virus infections in the United States, 2006. Pediatrics. 2010;127(1):e1–8.
4. Kimberlin DW. Herpes simplex virus infections of the newborn. Semin Perinatol. 2007;31:19–25.
5. Krehbiel K, Singh V. Disseminated neonatal herpes simplex virus infection with *Escherichia coli* coinfection. J Forensic Sci. 2018;63(3):935–8.
6. Kimberlin DW, Lin C, Jacobs RF, Powell DA, Frenkel LM, Gruber WC, et al. Natural history of neonatal herpes simplex virus infections in the acyclovir era. Pediatrics. 2001;108(2):223–9.
7. Knezevic A, Martic J, Stanojevic M, Jankovic S, Nedeljkovic J, Nikolic L, Pasic S, Jankovic B, Jovanovic T. Disseminated neonatal herpes caused by herpes simplex virus types 1 and 2. Emerg Infect Dis. 2007;13(2):302–4.
8. Marquez L, Levy ML, Munoz FM, Palazzi DL. A report of three cases and review of intrauterine herpes simplex virus infection. Pediatr Infect Dis J. 2011;30(2):153–7.
9. Caviness AC, Demmler GJ, Selwyn BJ. Clinical and laboratory features of neonatal herpes simplex virus infection: a case-control study. Pediatr Infect Dis J. 2008;27:425–30.
10. Kimberlin DW, Lin C, Jacobs RF, et al. Safety and efficacy of high-dose acyclovir in the management of neonatal herpes simplex virus infection. Pediatrics. 2001;108:230–8.

Dural Venous Sinus Thrombosis: *"Not My Usual Migraine"*

Rahul M. Rege and Brooke M. Moungey

Case

Pertinent History

A 29-year-old woman with a history of Crohn's disease and migraine with aura presented to the emergency department (ED) with a headache. She is 4 weeks post-partum following a term pregnancy and uncomplicated vaginal delivery. She noted that the headache started approximately 5 hours ago with no appreciable trigger, but it "does not feel like my typical migraines." She is usually able to treat her head-aches with 400 mg of ibuprofen and a nap. Today, however, this did not improve her symptoms and instead the pain was slowly worsening. Initially her only symptom was the headache, but now she noticed that "my vision seems a little blurry." This is not like her usual visual aura, which typically includes flashes of color.

She denied sick contacts, had no recent history of travel, ingestions, or environ-mental exposures. She denied numbness, tingling or focal weakness. She has had no fever or chills at home and no neck pain or rashes. She does endorse nausea but no vomiting. Of note, she recently restarted her oral contraceptive pill (OCP). She has a carbon monoxide detector at home.

Past medical history (PMH) Crohn's Disease, migraine with aura.

Social history (SH) Former smoker with 15 pack-year history but quit when she became pregnant, obese with a BMI of 37.

R. M. Rege (✉) · B. M. Moungey
Department of Emergency Medicine, Wexner Medical Center at The Ohio State University, Columbus, OH, USA
e-mail: rahul.rege2@osumc.edu; brooke.moungey@osumc.edu

© Springer Nature Switzerland AG 2020
C. G. Kaide, C. E. San Miguel (eds.), *Case Studies in Emergency Medicine*,
https://doi.org/10.1007/978-3-030-22445-5_18

Family history (FH) Mother and sister with history of deep venous thromboses (DVTs).

Physical Exam

Except as noted below, the findings of the complete physical exam are within normal limits.

- Vital Signs: Blood Pressure 165/90, HR 58, RR 18, oxygen saturation 98% on room air, Temperature 100.3 °F/37.9 °C.
- Neurologic: CNs II–XII intact, no clonus or pronator drift, negative Babinski bilaterally. Normal gait.
- Ocular: Visual Acuity: OD: 20/100 OS: 20/80. She does not use glasses.
  - Pupils equally round and reactive to light, extraocular muscles intact.
  - Peripheral visual fields intact to confrontation.
  - Intraocular pressure normal.
  - Fundoscopic exam completed by ophthalmology shows raised optic disc margins bilaterally, but no retinal tears or detachments, and no vitreal hemorrhage.
- Cardiovascular: Mildly bradycardic rate, regular rhythm, and no murmurs.
- Pulmonary: Lungs clear bilaterally.
- Abdominal: Bowel sounds present and no abdominal pain to palpation.
- Extremities: No lower extremity edema and radial and dorsalis pedis pulses 2+ bilaterally.

Emergency Department Management

Our differential diagnosis included the following: Headache such as migraine, tension, or cluster type as well as atypical migraine, idiopathic intracranial hypertension, subarachnoid hemorrhage, stroke, intracranial mass, preeclampsia, and trigeminal neuralgia and carbon monoxide poisoning.

The patient was treated symptomatically for her headache with Toradol 15 mg IV, Benadryl 25 mg PO, and Compazine 10 mg IV with minimal improvement. About 30 minutes later, the patient had one episode of non-bloody, non-bilious emesis. Lab results and chest x-ray were unremarkable (listed later), showing no evidence of proteinuria to suggest postpartum preeclampsia. A CT head noncontrast was negative for any acute intracranial hemorrhage, large mass, or stroke.

Further attempts at pain control continued to have minimal effect. Given her history regarding being 4 weeks postpartum and recently restarting her estrogen-containing OCP, she was identified to be in a hypercoagulable state. Further history then revealed a family history of DVTs and that the patient had recently resumed smoking cigarettes to cope with the stresses of motherhood. At that time, the patient reported that her headache was worsening and that her vision was becoming blurrier. Visual acuity testing showed diminished acuity bilaterally. Ophthalmology was then consulted, and dilated fundoscopic exam revealed bilateral papilledema. Given these findings, neurology was consulted for increasing suspicion of increased intracranial pressure and recommended lumbar puncture. This revealed an elevated opening pressure but was negative for meningitis and subacute subarachnoid hemorrhage.

Pertinent Diagnostic Testing

Complete blood count, electrolytes, liver function tests, uric acid, lactate dehydrogenase, and urinalysis were within normal limits.

Urine pregnancy: Negative.

Carboxy hemoglobin was 5% (normal is <3% in nonsmokers and up to 10–12% in smokers).

Chest X-ray: No acute cardiopulmonary findings.

CT head (non-contrast): No acute intracranial abnormality.

Lumbar Puncture: Opening pressure 29 mmHg (normal <20 mmHg), RBC: 0–5 (normal =0), WBC: 0–5 (normal <5).

Learning Points

Priming Questions
1. What are the classic presenting features of dural venous sinus thrombosis?
2. What historical clues can help you delineate the diagnosis?
3. What diagnostic work up and treatment should be provided?
4. What are the characteristics of some important members of the differential diagnosis?
5. What are the priorities of acute and chronic management of the disease?

Introduction/Background

1. Dural venous sinus thrombosis is a rare phenomenon which affects <1.5 people per 100,000 annually. In addition to the paucity of cases, clinically, this is a difficult diagnosis to make given its large range of clinical sequalae.

2. Severity of cases can range from a mild headache to profound neurologic impairment with altered mental status and abnormal posturing. While the clinical picture can be varied, headache is the most common presenting symptom [7].
3. The mean age of patients is 39 years, and females are affected with 3× greater frequency than males. The diverse nature of symptoms comes from the variability in clot burden, and accumulation of vasogenic edema and hemorrhage.

Physiology/Pathophysiology

Dural Sinuses

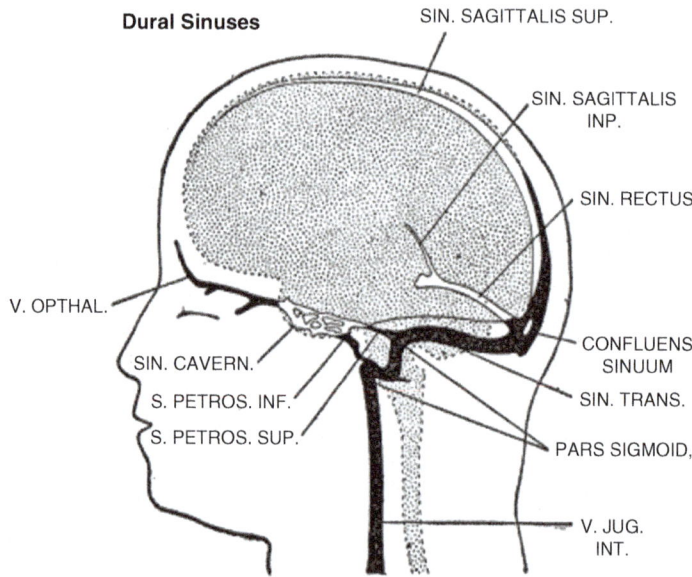

Henry Vandyke Carter creator QS:P170,Q955620 Henry Gray creator QS:P170,Q40319 (https://commons.wikimedia.org/wiki/File:Gray488.png), "Gray488", marked as public domain, more details on Wikimedia Commons: https://commons.wikimedia.org/wiki/Template:PD-1923

Virchow's Triad

(https://commons.wikimedia.org/wiki/File:Virchow's_Triad.svg), "Virchow's Triad", https://creativecommons.org/licenses/by-sa/3.0/legalcode

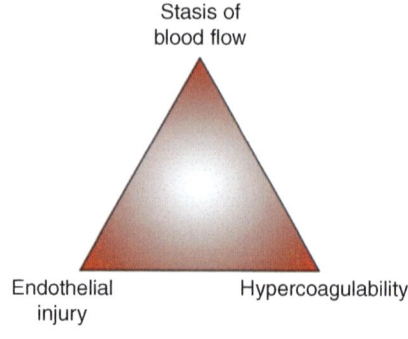

1. Like all deep vein thromboses, a DVST results from some perturbation of Virchow's Triad: Venous stasis, endothelial injury, and hypercoagulability.
2. Risk factors are generally divided into acquired risk factors and genetic risk factors:
   - Common acquired risk factors:
     - Infection (common precipitant in pediatric population) [8].
     - Mechanical (surgery vs. trauma) [1].
     - Pregnancy/Post-partum period [10].
     - Malignancy [13].
     - Exogenous estrogen use.
   - Common genetic prothrombotic risk factors [3].
     - Antithrombin III deficiency
     - Protein S and C deficiency
     - Factor V Leiden
     - Antiphospholipid antibody syndromes
     - Prothrombin gene mutation
     - Protein S and C deficiency
     - Methylenetetrahydrofolate reductase
3. Clot burden leads to two phenomena that cause clinical symptoms: Increased venous pressure and impairment of CSF absorption.
   - Increased venous pressure leads to hemorrhagic infarction of parenchyma leading to focal neurologic deficits. These deficits are dependent on the location of the clot.
     - Decrease in cerebral perfusion: Failure of cellular function leading to cytotoxic edema.
     - Venous and capillary rupture: Parenchymal Hemorrhage
     - Blood-Brain barrier disruption: Vasogenic Edema
   - Impaired CSF absorption leads to increased intracranial pressure which contributes to global headache, papilledema, and visual changes.
4. In the initial phases of pathogenesis, dilation of cerebral venous circulation and formation of collaterals may reduce intracranial pressure [9].

Making the Diagnosis

Differential Diagnosis
- Migraine
- Subarachnoid/intracranial hemorrhage
- Cerebrovascular accident
- Idiopathic intracranial hypertension
- Cerebral neoplasm
- Seizure disorder
- Meningitis
- Trigeminal neuralgia
- Toxic ingestion
- Pre-eclampsia
- Carbon Monoxide Poisoning.

1. As with every patient, start with a thorough history and physical exam.
   - Personal or family history of blood clots?
   - Estrogen hormonal supplements or contraceptives? (Also remember that male to female transgender patients may be using estrogen).
   - Known malignancy?
   - History of recent trauma or surgery?
   - Current or recent smoking history?
   - Is the patient currently pregnant or postpartum?
   - Ask about clear details about timing of symptoms. Acute (<48 hours) sub-acute (48 hours to 30 days) chronic (>30 days).
2. There are two components of making the diagnosis: clinical and imaging-based. Since this diagnosis can present with a wide array of clinical findings, it is a difficult diagnosis to make.
   - Clinical Diagnosis:
     - Headache
       o Often described as a diffuse headache that progresses in severity over days to weeks.
       o May also present as a "thunder clap" or migrainous headache as well [5].
       o Headache without any other neurologic sequalae presents in approximately 25% of patients [5].
     - Physical Exam
       o Papilledema
         - May accompany the headache as a sign of increased intracranial pressure
       o Can be accompanied by a sixth nerve palsy
       o Scalp edema and dilated scalp veins
     - Laboratory Testing
       o Consider testing that will highlight underlying hypercoagulable state, inflammatory state, or infectious process.
       o Complete blood count
       o Chemistry panel
       o Coagulation studies (PT, PTT, INR)
       o Consider early screening for prothrombotic conditions
       o Lumbar Puncture
         - Has no diagnostic utility but can be used to rule out meningitis and subarachnoid hemorrhage.
         - Has shown inconsistent benefits as a therapeutic intervention in patients with intracranial hypertension as a result of DVST.

Localizing the Clot
- Most common location is superior sagittal sinus [2].
- If patient has concomitant ear infection, consider lateral sinus thrombosis.
- Consider cortical involvement with focal neurologic findings.
- With thalamic or basal ganglia infarcts consider deep cerebral venous clot (internal cerebral vein, vein of Galen, and straight sinus) present in 16% of patients [7].

- Imaging Diagnosis (see Radiology Case 9 for a more detailed discussion on imaging)
  - MR Venogram
    - No radiation exposure
    - Good parenchymal definition
    - Studies ongoing to determine sensitivity and specificity
  - CT Venogram
    - Sensitivity of 95% and specificity of 91% for filling defects [11]
    - Able to be used in the emergent setting for acute onset of symptoms

CT Venogram

Heather (https://en.wikipedia.org/wiki/File:Sagital_sinus_thrombus.JPG), "Sagital sinus thrombus", marked as public domain, more details on Wikimedia Commons: https://commons.wikimedia.org/wiki/Template:PD-because

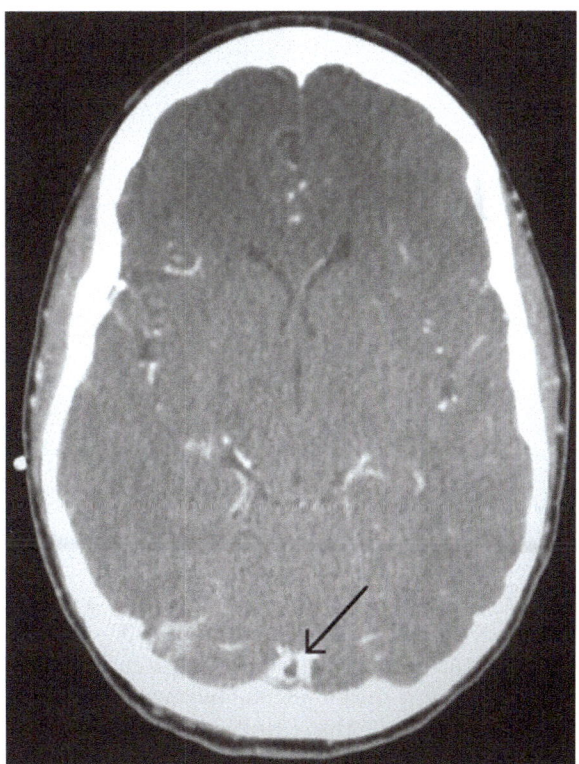

MR Venogram (MRV)

Public Domain Image

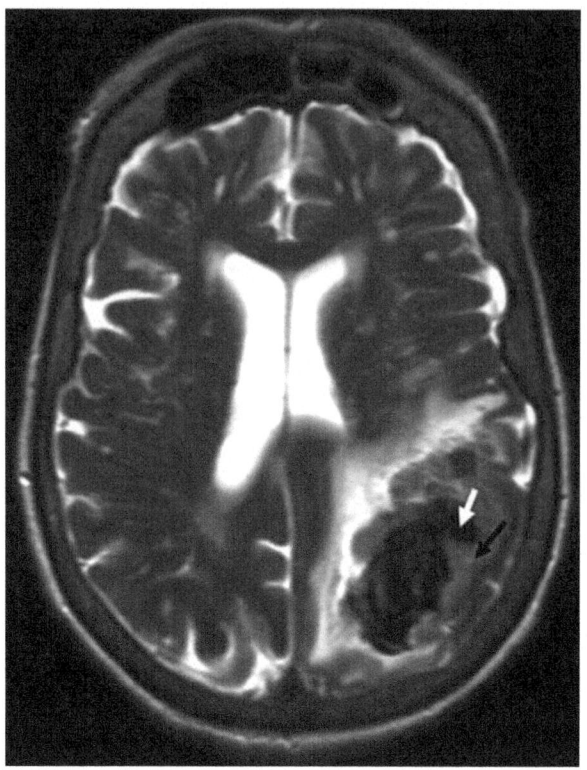

Treating the Patient

1. Pay Attention to the ABCs!
   - The highest cause of mortality for these patients remains symptomatic intracranial hypertension and subsequent herniation.
   - Consider intubating patients early if they show signs of altered mental status.
   - Cushing's reflex is a compensatory mechanism involving hypertension, bradycardia, and irregular respirations suggesting impending herniation.
   - Consider early subspecialty consultation with neurology and neurosurgery, or transfer to a tertiary care facility where these services are available.
2. Anticoagulation
   - Low molecular weight heparin (LMWH) is more effective than unfractionated heparin (UFH) for these patients and equally safe.
   - Hemorrhagic venous infarction is NOT an absolute contraindication to anticoagulation as early anticoagulation shows an all-cause mortality benefit, however, it should be used with care and in combination with subspecialty consultation. LMWH should be followed by ongoing anticoagulation for a period of 3–6 months.

- Endovascular therapy has NOT been shown to be superior to aggressive anti-coagulation (limited studies) [4].
3. Additional Management
   - Elevate head of bed to at least 30°.
   - Consider early administration of mannitol or 3% hypertonic saline.
   - Target therapeutic hyperventilation to a $PaCO_2$ goal of 30–35 mmHg [12].
   - Acetazolamide 500 mg BID versus lasix can be therapeutic alternatives for those who cannot tolerate mannitol.
   - Therapeutic lumbar puncture is not widely recommended due to limited data and no clear improvement in patient morbidity or mortality.
   - Seizures—ongoing seizure activity is treated similar to other epileptic disorders and benzodiazepines remain first-line therapy.
   - Studies have also shown benefit with antiepileptic prophylaxis in patients with supratentorial lesions on imaging and seizure on initial presentation.
   - In DVST with no supratentorial changes on imaging, recurrent seizures have not been shown to occur, and prophylaxis is not recommended.
   - Depakote or Levetiracetam is recommended for prophylaxis in these cases due to limited interaction with anticoagulants.

Case Conclusion

Neurology examined the patient and recommended repeat imaging with a CT Venogram. This showed a clot in the patient's superior sagittal sinus. The patient was immediately started on Enoxaparin and admitted. The patient received a 1.5 g/kg dose of mannitol in the ED, and the angle of the bed was elevated. While inpatient, the patient received a work up for hypercoagulability and was found to have a positive factor V Leiden mutation. The patient made a full recovery, with visual acuity returning to baseline and resolution of headache and nausea prior to discharge.

Discussion

Dural venous sinus thrombosis is a particularly difficult diagnosis to make. While the risk factors associated are similar to those associated with more commonly seen peripheral deep venous thromboses, what makes the diagnosis particularly complex is the variability in presentation and range of clinical severity. Patients can appear asymptomatic, present solely with headache, have seizures, manifest focal neurologic deficits, or present with altered mental status and signs concerning for increased intracranial pressure. Given that it is also an uncommon diagnosis, it requires a high index of suspicion in order to proceed with the necessary diagnostic studies for proper identification and treatment.

The case presented here is particularly interesting because it highlights some of the key risk factors for this disorder. The patient is a smoker, is recently postpartum, and was found to have a previously unknown clotting disorder during the course of her work up. Despite the varying severity of clinical presentation, this patient initially presented with an isolated headache, and we were able to witness the development of focal neurologic sequalae due to increased intracranial pressure. While initial imaging was obtained, it was not completed with contrast or with venogram protocol, and the thrombus was therefore not initially identified.

When other etiologies had been ruled out and the patient exhibited new visual changes along with an abnormal ophthalmoscopic exam, increased intracranial pressure was suspected. However, it is important to note that idiopathic intracranial hypertension is a diagnosis of exclusion, and other intracranial pathology must be ruled out before this diagnosis can be made. Given the patient's young age and risk factors for a hypercoagulopathic state, our index of suspicion for a DVST became higher. Only then did repeat imaging with the appropriate study allow us to visualize the thrombus and tailor the patient's treatment more appropriately.

Pattern Recognition

- Unusual headache
- Evidence of elevated intracranial pressure
- Hypercoagulable state
- Vision changes
- Neurologic findings

Disclosure Statement The authors of this chapter report no significant disclosures.

References

1. Afshari FT, et al. Traumatic dural venous sinus thrombosis; a challenge in management of head injury patients. J Clin Neurosci. 2018;57:169–73.
2. Biousse V, et al. Isolated intracranial hypertension as the only sign of cerebral venous thrombosis. Neurology. 1999;53(7):1537–42.
3. Bombeli T, et al. Prevalence of hereditary thrombophilia in patients with thrombosis in different venous systems. Am J Hematol. 2002;70(2):126–32.
4. Coutinho JM, et al. Thrombolysis or anticoagulation for cerebral venous thrombosis: rationale and design of the TO-ACT trial. Int J Stroke. 2013;8(2):135–40.
5. Cumurciuc R, et al. Headache as the only neurological sign of cerebral venous thrombosis: a series of 17 cases. J Neurol Neurosurg Psychiatry. 2005;76(8):1084–7.
6. Einhaupl K, et al. EFNS guideline on the treatment of cerebral venous and sinus thrombosis in adult patients. Eur J Neurol. 2010;17(10):1229–35.
7. Ferro JM, et al. European stroke organization guideline for the diagnosis and treatment of cerebral venous thrombosis - endorsed by the European Academy of Neurology. Eur J Neurol. 2017;24(10):1203–13.
8. Ferro JM, et al. Prognosis of cerebral vein and dural sinus thrombosis: results of the International Study on Cerebral Vein and Dural Sinus Thrombosis (ISCVT). Stroke. 2004;35(3):664–70.
9. Ferro JM, Pinto F. Poststroke epilepsy: epidemiology, pathophysiology and management. Drugs Aging. 2004;21(10):639–53.

10. Lanska DJ, Kryscio RJ. Risk factors for peripartum and postpartum stroke and intracranial venous thrombosis. Stroke. 2000;31(6):1274–82.
11. Rodallec MH, et al. Cerebral venous thrombosis and multidetector CT angiography: tips and tricks. Radiographics. 2006;26(Suppl 1):S5–18; discussion S42-13.
12. Saposnik G, et al. Diagnosis and management of cerebral venous thrombosis: a statement for healthcare professionals from the American Heart Association/American Stroke Association. Stroke. 2011;42(4):1158–92.
13. Silvis SM, et al. Cancer and risk of cerebral venous thrombosis: a case-control study. J Thromb Haemost. 2018;16(1):90–5.

Endocarditis: *Osler's Challenge*

19

Brit Long and Alex Koyfman

Case

Weakness, fever at home, myalgias, cough, headache

Pertinent History

This patient presented to the emergency department (ED) at 9 pm with several complaints, including weakness, fever to 102 °F, cough, and headache. He is concerned about the flu, as his girlfriend is sick at home and was recently diagnosed with flu by an urgent care physician. His symptoms have been going on for 5 days, and he is able to eat and drink. He denies carbon monoxide exposure or trauma. He has not noticed chest pain, shortness of breath, or neck stiffness, and he has no focal neurologic deficits. However, he has noted generalized weakness and myalgias.

Past Medical History (PMH) Hypertension.

Meds Hydrochlorothiazide.

Surgical History (SH) Smoker, 20 pack year history. Regular alcohol use. Remote IV drug use, but the patient has not used for over 2 years.

Pertinent Physical Exam

- Blood Pressure 150/89 mm Hg, Heart Rate 105 beats/minute, Temperature 99.9°F, RR 18 breaths/minute, SpO2 98% RA.

B. Long (✉)
Brooke Army Medical Center, Department of Emergency Medicine,
Fort Sam Houston, TX, USA

A. Koyfman
The University of Texas Southwestern Medical Center, Department of Emergency Medicine,
Dallas, TX, USA

© Springer Nature Switzerland AG 2020
C. G. Kaide, C. E. San Miguel (eds.), *Case Studies in Emergency Medicine*,
https://doi.org/10.1007/978-3-030-22445-5_19

Except as noted below, the findings of the physical exam are within normal limits.

- Cardiovascular: Tachycardia with regular rhythm, normal heart sounds, and normal distal pulses. No murmur is heard on initial examination.

Pertinent Diagnostic Testing

Test	Results 21:33	Units	Normal Range
WBC	13.3	$10^3/mm^3$	3.8–11.0 $10^3/mm^3$
Hgb	14.2	g/dL	(Male) 14–18 g/dL
			(Female) 11–16 g/dL
Na	132	mEq/L	135–148 mEq/L
K	4.2	mEq/L	3.5–5.5 mEq/L
BUN	40	mg/dL	6–23 mg/dL
Cr	1.5	mg/dL	0.6–1.5 mg/dL
Glucose	168	mg/dL	65–99 mg/dL
pH	7.34	–	7.35–7.45
Lactate	1.9	mmol/L	<2.0

Chest X-Ray (CXR) Multiple consolidations are present. The heart border is normal, and there are no pleural effusions present.

Plan Antibiotics including ceftriaxone IV and azithromycin PO for community-acquired pneumonia, along with IV fluids, followed by reevaluation.

Update 1: (2215) The patient's hemodynamic status has not improved. HR is now 108 beats/minute, and temperature is 100.4 °F. He has received antibiotics and one liter of normal saline. With concern for sepsis from pneumonia, a second liter of normal saline is provided, along with acetaminophen 1 g PO. The patient does not appear to be in distress.

Update 2: (2302) The HR has improved to 95 beats/minute, and the temperature has decreased to 99.5 °F. A reexamination reveals a grade II/VI murmur. Reevaluation of chest X-ray showing multilobar findings is concerning, along with remote history of IV drug use. A bedside ultrasound (US) reveals findings concerning for a tricuspid valve lesion (vegetation) on the periapical four-chamber view.

Tricuspid Valve Vegetation on Apical 4 Chamber View

Image courtesy
of Sambita Basu, MD

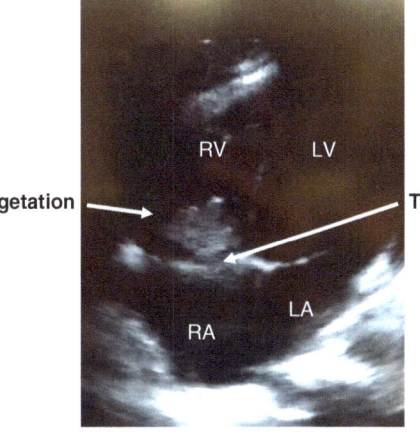

Tricuspid Valve Vegetation on Apical 4 Chamber View

Update 3: (2312)

Three sets of blood cultures are ordered from separate sites due to concern for endocarditis. Cardiology and Infectious Disease consultants recommend obtaining comprehensive echocardiogram with admission. Internal medicine is consulted for admission.

Update 4: (2338)

Patient to internal medicine floor.

Learning Points: Endocarditis

Priming Questions
1. When should endocarditis be considered?
2. How is the diagnosis made, and what roles do laboratory and imaging studies play?
3. How should the Duke Criteria be used in the ED?
4. What is the treatment for endocarditis, and what is required in the ED?

Introduction/Background

1. Infectious endocarditis (IE) is a disease associated with infection of the endocardial surface (heart valves, mural endocardium, or septum). Cardiac effects include valvular insufficiency, myocardial abscess, and congestive heart failure. Infective endocarditis can cause a wide number of systemic findings and symptoms, which makes diagnosis difficult. There is no standard diagnostic test beyond echocardiogram and blood cultures in the ED, and the diagnosis truly

depends on consideration of the disease [1–10]. Duke's Criteria are the standard diagnostic criteria [3, 4, 11]. William Osler put it best in an 1885 lecture: "Few diseases present greater difficulties in the way of diagnosis than malignant endocarditis, difficulties which in many cases are practically insurmountable" [12]. This remains true today [13, 14].

Heart Anatomy

Wapcaplet (https://commons. wikimedia.org/wiki/ File:Diagram_of_the_ human_heart_(cropped).svg), "Diagram of the human heart (cropped)", https://creative-commons.org/licenses/ by-sa/3.0/legalcode

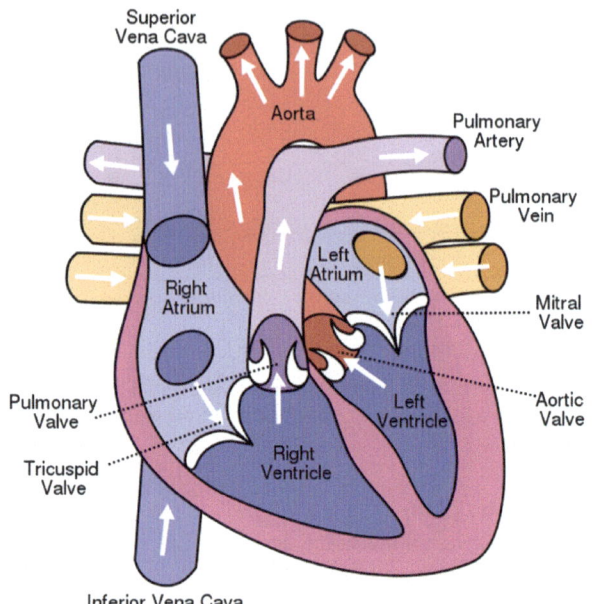

2. Several categories of disease are present:
   - Native valve endocarditis (NVE), acute or subacute [1, 2, 14–17].
     - The presentation and course of NVE is characterized by acute or subacute infection. Acute IE is aggressive and typically involves normal valves. It often is due to *Staphylococcus aureus* or group B streptococci. Subacute NVE usually involves abnormal valves and is more indolent over months.
   - Prosthetic valve endocarditis (PVE), early or late [1, 2, 14–20].
     - PVE causes 20% of IE cases. Close to 4% of mechanical or bioprosthetic valves will become infected over their lifespan (mechanical valves are infected more commonly with in the first 3 months). Early PVE occurs within 60 days of implantation, commonly due to coagulase negative staphylococci, gram-negative bacilli, or *Candida*. IE occurring after 60 days is late PVE, with *S. aureus* being the most common cause.
   - Intravenous drug abuse endocarditis (IVDA IE) [1, 2, 14–20].
     - Up to 75% of patients with IVDA and IE have no underlying cardiac defect, with 50% of infections including the tricuspid valve. These are usually infected with *S. aureus*.

 – Other types of IE include pacemaker IE and nosocomial IE (NIE). Pacemaker IE is most commonly used due to *S. aureus* and can be challenging to treat. NIE occurs after 48 hours of hospitalization or is associated with healthcare environment exposure within 4 weeks of a performed procedure.

3. IE is rare, with an annual incidence of up to 10 cases per 100,000 persons [1, 2, 10]. Approximately, 40,000–50,000 new cases occur in the US each year, with most cases occurring in urban settings (higher rates of intravenous drug use) [6, 10].

4. Risk factors include prior endocarditis (the most common risk factor), structural heart damage, IV drug abuse (IVDA), poor immune function (vasculitis, HIV, diabetes, malignancy), nosocomial factors (surgical hardware placement, poor surgical technique, hematoma development), and poor oral hygiene [1, 2, 6, 10, 20].

5. The risk of IE in IV drugs abusers is 2–5% per year, with a mean age of 30 years at time of diagnosis. In those with a history of IVDA and fever, close to 15% of patients have endocarditis [1, 2, 7–10, 17].

6. Males are more commonly affected (1.5–3:1 male to female), and adults are more commonly affected. The age of those affected has steadily increased, with currently more than 50% of patients being greater than 50 years old [1, 2, 7–10, 17].

7. Before antibiotics, this disease was associated with 100% mortality. Mortality is still high, with 1-year mortality approaching 20–40% and in-hospital mortality approaching 22% [1, 2, 7–10, 20].

Physiology/Pathophysiology

1. Normally, valvular endothelium is resistant to microbial colonization. Trauma to the endothelium can result from high-pressure flow gradients and states of turbulent flow, which occur in patients with existing valvular or cardiac structural defects (rheumatic disease, congenital heart disease, prior endocarditis, prosthetic valve). Hypercoagulable or chronic inflammatory states (vasculitis, malignancy) can also result in vegetation formation along valves. IV drug use results in particulate matter bombardment along the cardiac structures, as well as vasospasm [1, 2, 7–10, 21–23].

2. This damage to the endothelium increases the risk of sterile thrombus formation, consisting of fibrin and platelets [21–23].

3. Microbes may attach and grow on this thrombus in episodes of bacteremia, viremia, or fungemia. These episodes most commonly occur in patients with periodontal disease and other sites of infection such as pneumonia, pyelonephritis, and cellulitis. Bacteremia results in the delivery of organisms to the valve surface. However, organisms must be able to attach and adhere to the valve (Table 19.1) [1, 2, 21–23].

4. The most common valve affected is the mitral valve, followed by the aortic valve, the aortic and mitral valves combined, the tricuspid valve, and the pulmonic valve. IVDA IE most commonly affects the tricuspid valve [1, 2, 7–10, 14, 17].

Table 19.1 Most common causative organisms in IE

[2, 14–18, 24–29]

Organism	Features
S. aureus	Most common cause of IE overall (including acute, IVDA IE, PVE)
	Over half of IE cases do not have an underlying valve disorder
	35–60% of bacteremia due to *S. aureus* are complicated by IE, with increased incidence of methicillin-resistant *Staphylococcus aureus* (MRSA) associated with IE
	A large percentage of bacteremia are due to an infected peripheral or central line
	Mortality approaches 50%
Coagulase-negative *Staphylococci*	Usually presents with subacute IE
	Similar presentation to *S. viridans* (below)
	Causes 30% of PVE and < 5% of NVE
	One form is *S. lugdunensis*, which is extremely aggressive compared to other forms (positive blood culture highly suggestive of endocarditis)
Streptococcus viridans	Accounts for 50–60% of subacute IE cases
	Many of the clinical signs and symptoms are due to immunologic phenomena with this form
Streptococcus intermedius	Acute or subacute infections
	Accounts for close to 15% of IE cases due to *Streptococcus*
	May invade and form abscesses, especially in the central nervous system (CNS)
Group A, C, G strep	Resembles *S. aureus* with high mortality and acute presentation
	Group A responds to penicillin
	Group C and G require synergistic combination of antibiotics
Group B strep	Acute disease in pregnant and older patients with comorbidities
	Mortality approaches 40%
	Common complications include metastatic infection, arterial thrombi, and heart failure, which may require valve replacement
Group D strep	Most are subacute, with sources including the gastrointestinal (GI) or genitourinary (GU) tract
	Third most common cause of IE
	Often resistant to antibiotics
Nonenterococcal group D	Subacute presentation
	Often due to large bowel pathology (cancer, inflammatory bowel disease)
	Sensitive to penicillin
Bartonella	More common in homeless patients with poor hygiene
	Blood cultures may be negative
Pseudomonas	Most commonly presents in the acute form, except for right-sided disease
	Surgery typically required for treatment

Table 19.1 Continued

[2, 14–18, 24–29]

Organism	Features
HACEK (*Haemophilus aphrophilus, Actinobacillus, Cardiobacterium hominis, Eikenella corrodens, Kingella*)	Often results in subacute form Account for 5% of IE Most common gram-negative organisms in IE May cause complications such as arterial emboli and congestive heart failure Treatment often requires ampicillin, gentamicin, and surgery
Fungal	Often results in subacute form *Candida albicans* is the most common cause of NVE and PVE Fungal IVDA IE often due to *Candida parapsilosis* or *tropicalis*
Polymicrobial	*Pseudomonas* and *enterococci* are most common combination Also found in IVDA IE Cardiac surgery mortality rate higher in polymicrobial infections

Making the Diagnosis

Endocarditis is a deadly disease, but our patient presented with flu-like symptoms. Plus, there are so many risk factors for IE, many of which are extremely common! Remember Osler's quote? The key seems to be knowledge of risk factors and potential presentations…

Can't Miss Diagnoses in Patients with Flu-like Symptoms
- Endocarditis
- Myocarditis
- Spinal epidural abscess
- HIV/AIDS
- Necrotizing fasciitis
- Tickborne illness
- Encephalitis/meningitis
- Tuberculosis
- Malaria, dengue fever
- Thyroid disease (thyrotoxicosis)
- Heat stroke
- Ingestion/toxicologic—carbon monoxide

1. History and Examination Findings

- Nonspecific presentations are the norm, with most patients presenting with flu-like symptoms. Fever occurs in up to 90% of patients at some point with IE, and malaise is found in 80%. Other symptoms include weakness, chills, headache, night sweats, weight loss, and arthralgias [1, 2, 7–10].
- Time from initial disease to symptom involvement depends on the type of IE. Acute IE in IVDA is associated with severe, fulminant disease. Patients with this form more commonly demonstrate high-grade fevers and chills, as well as cardiac involvement with congestive heart failure. Subacute NVE includes a more nonspecific and subtle presentation with low-grade fever and flu-like symptoms.
- Cardiac or pulmonary symptoms may occur with valvular disease causing congestive heart failure [1, 2, 7–10]. Neurologic complications may occur with embolic disease, including stroke or vertebral osteomyelitis/spinal epidural abscess.
- Time between disease onset and diagnosis approaches 6 weeks, and less than half of patients have known valvular disease before diagnosis of IE [1, 2, 7–10, 30].
- Signs of IE result from emboli and immunologic mechanisms [1, 2, 7–10].
- Symptoms from emboli occur in 20–50% of patients. Factors associated with emboli include specific organisms (*S. aureus, Candida*, and HACEK organisms), vegetations >1 cm, mobile vegetations, and involvement of the mitral valve [1, 2, 7–10, 24–30].
  - Pulmonary emboli typically occur in IVDA, with tricuspid valve involvement and right-sided IE. These emboli may be septic or sterile, leading to pulmonary infarction, pulmonary abscess, or pneumonia [1, 2, 30].
  - Cerebral emboli can occur in 20% of cases, with mortality reaching 40% (second leading cause of death in IE). Stroke, abscess, arteritis, aneurysm, encephalomalacia, and meningitis are other CNS problems associated with IE [1, 2, 7–10, 30, 31].
  - Renal emboli result in abscess, ischemia, or infarction. Patients can present with flank pain, pyuria, or hematuria and may be confused for pyelonephritis, urinary tract infection, or urolithiasis [1, 2, 10, 30].
  - Splenic emboli may result in flank pain, but patients may be asymptomatic [1, 2, 7–10].
  - Eye involvement includes painless conjunctival/subconjunctival hemorrhage. The eye vasculature may be affected, resulting in visual field deficits. Roth spots are a classic finding but do not occur in all patients [1, 2, 7–10].

Open source. Mosby's
Medical Dictionary, 8th
edition. (2009). Retrieved
May 15, 2018

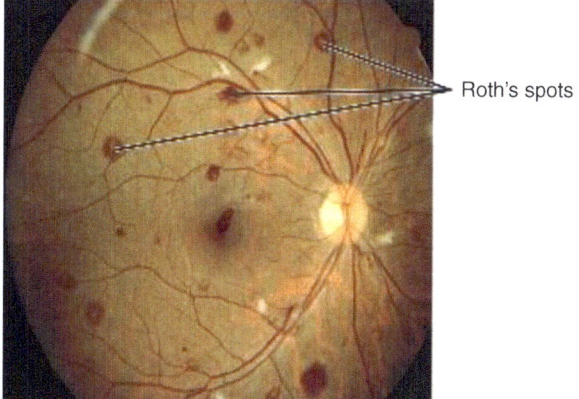

Roth's spots

- – Skin emboli are seen in 5–15% of patients. Janeway lesions are painless, hemorrhagic lesions on the hands and feet due to microemboli. Osler nodes are tender nodular red lesions on the pads of the digits, hands, and feet. These were thought to be due to immune complex deposition or allergic vasculitis [32–38], but more current literature suggests they may be due to microemboli [33, 34]. Petechiae is capillary bleeding under the skin. These skin findings may be found in bacteremia, systemic lupus erythematous, and an infected intravascular graft [32, 33].

Janeway Lesion.
Wikicommons courtesy
of Warfieldian

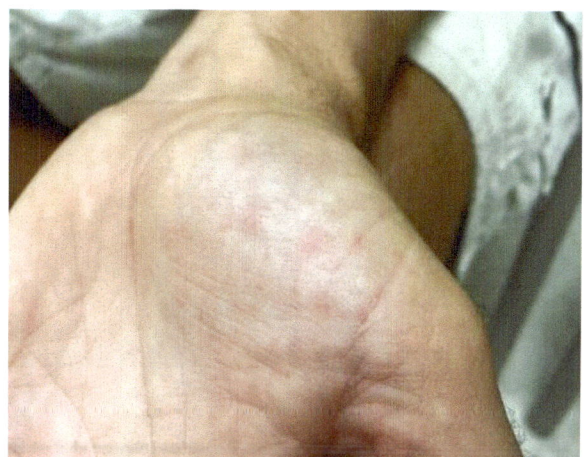

Osler Nodules courtesy
of Roberto J. Galindo

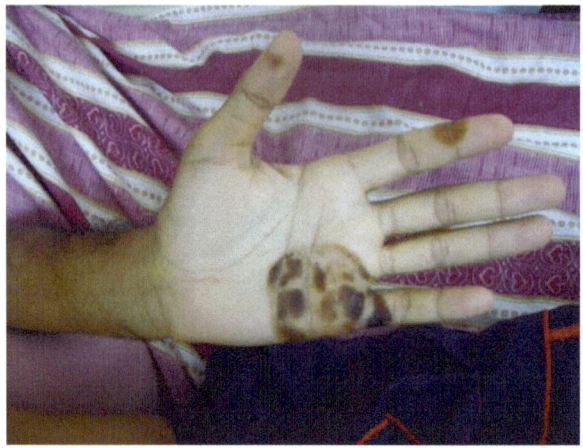

- Splinter hemorrhages are red to brown, non-blanchable, linear lesions 1–3 mm in length under the nail plate. These are also found in other disease states (vasculitis, malignancy, renal failure, trauma) [32–38].

Splinter Hemorrhages.
Public Domain Image

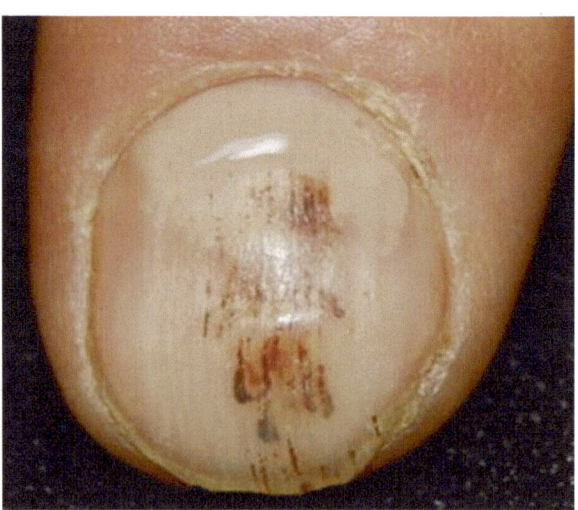

- Heart murmur is found in up to 85% of patients [1, 2, 7–10].
- Infections in more than one spot or affecting more than one organ system should trigger consideration of endocarditis, including multilobar pneumonia, or a patient with concomitant pyelonephritis and pneumonia.
- Evaluate the patient's dentition. If poor, consider IE.
- Risk factors are the key in considering IE: IVDA, instrumentation/procedures, indwelling lines, hemodialysis, known cardiac disease, or known valvular disease [1, 2, 7–10].

2. Diagnostic Criteria
   - Diagnosis typically requires fulfilling Duke Criteria, which were initially described in 1994 and modified in 2000 (Table 19.2a and b). As you read through these criteria, you will find that diagnosis in the ED is difficult using these criteria. This again emphasizes the need for careful and focused history and examination. Many times, the diagnosis is made after admission.
3. Laboratory
   - White blood cell (WBC) count may be normal, elevated, or depressed and is not sensitive or specific (elevation occurs in 50% of patients) [1, 2, 7–10].
   - Urinalysis may reveal hematuria in 50% of patients due to renal emboli [1, 2, 7–10].
   - Inflammatory markers such as CRP and ESR may be sensitive, with elevation occurring in over 90% of cases. However, these labs are not specific [1, 2, 7–10].
   - Rheumatoid factor and other testing for immune complexes may be positive in 50% of patients after 6 weeks of infection [1, 2, 7–10].
   - Electrocardiogram (ECG) does not assist in formal diagnosis of IE, but it may be used to diagnose complications such as ischemia or conduction abnormalities [1, 2, 39].
   - PCR and serologies for specific organisms may assist (Brucella, Coxiella, bartonella, legionella, chlamydia) [1, 2].
   - One important key is that if a culture from other sites reveals atypical bacteria, then endocarditis should be considered.
   - Blood cultures are required for diagnosis, with at least three sets. Though the classic recommendation is to obtain three sets at least 1 hour apart, literature suggests the volume of blood obtained per culture is more important [1–10, 40–42].
     - Toxic or critically ill patients require antibiotics and resuscitation; thus, blood cultures should be obtained over 5–30 minutes, rather than spaced apart.
     - The greater number of cultures obtained increases the sensitivity. Two cultures will demonstrate on organism in 90% of cases, with three sets demonstrating an organism in 98% [43, 44].
     - Keep in mind that blood cultures may be negative in 5–20% of patients, and prior antibiotic therapy may result in false-negative cultures [7–10].
     - After blood cultures have been obtained, they should be held for up to 21 days to evaluate for fastidious organisms.
     - Abnormal organisms, specifically one such as *S. lugdunensis,* is strongly suggestive of endocarditis [1, 2].
4. Imaging
   - Chest X-ray may demonstrate bilateral pulmonary infiltrates, which should be a clue to endocarditis. However, there is no specific finding for IE.
   - CT can evaluate for complications, including imaging of the head, chest, abdomen, or pelvis (abscess, pseudoaneurysm, distal infarction, septic emboli) [1, 8, 9].

Table 19.2 Duke criteria for diagnosis of IE

(a) [11]

Modified Duke criteria for diagnosis of IE

Major criteria:

1. Blood culture positive for IE

   Typical microorganisms consistent with IE from two separate blood cultures

   Viridans streptococci; *Streptococcus bovis*, HACEK group, *S. aureus*; or

   Community-acquired enterococci, in the absence of a primary focus

   Microorganisms consistent with IE from persistently positive blood cultures, defined by:

   ≥2 positive blood cultures of blood samples drawn >12 h apart; or

   All of three or a majority of >4 separate cultures of blood (with first and last sample drawn ≥1 h apart)

   Single positive blood culture for *Coxiella burnetii* or antiphase I IgG antibody titer >1: 800

2. Evidence of endocardial involvement

3. Echocardiogram positive for IE (Transesophageal echocardiogram (TEE) recommended in patients with prosthetic valves, rated at least "possible IE" by clinical criteria, or complicated IE [paravalvular abscess]; TTE as first test in other patients), defined as follows:

   Oscillating intracardiac mass on valve or supporting structures, in the path of regurgitant jets, or on implanted material in the absence of an alternative anatomic explanation;

   Abscess; or

   New partial dehiscence of prosthetic valve

4. New valvular regurgitation (worsening or changing or preexisting murmur not sufficient)

Minor criteria:

1. Predisposition, predisposing heart condition, or injection drug use

2. Fever, temperature > 38 °C (100.4 °F)

3. Vascular phenomena, major arterial emboli, septic pulmonary infarcts, mycotic aneurysm, intracranial hemorrhage, conjunctival hemorrhage, and Janeway lesions

4. Immunologic phenomena: Glomerulonephritis, Osler nodes, Roth's spots, and rheumatoid factor

5. Microbiological evidence: Positive blood culture but does not meet a major criterion as noted previously (excluding single positive cultures for coagulase-negative staphylococci and organisms that do not cause endocarditis) or serologic evidence of active infection with organisms consistent with IE

(b) [11]

Modified Duke criteria definitions

Definite IE

Pathologic criteria:

1. Microorganisms demonstrated by culture or histologic examination of a vegetation, a vegetation that has embolized, or an intracardiac abscess specimen; or

2. Pathologic lesions: vegetations or intracardiac abscess confirmed by histology examination showing active endocarditis

Clinical criteria: Two major criteria, one major and three minor criteria, or five minor criteria

Possible IE

1. One major criterion and one minor criterion

2. Three minor criteria

Rejected

1. Firm alternate diagnosis explaining evidence of IE

2. Resolution of IE syndrome with antibiotic therapy for <4 days

3. No pathologic evidence of IE at surgery or autopsy, with antibiotic therapy for ≤4 days

4. Does not meet criteria for possible IE, as described previously

- Transthoracic echocardiogram (TTE) is a first-line imaging modality, with sensitivity over 60% and specificity 94% [44–49]. Sensitivity increases as the vegetation size increases, with TTE detecting over 70% of vegetations >6 mm, but <25% of vegetations <5 mm [44–51]. In the setting of PVE or intracardiac device, TTE is not sensitive [47–51]. TTE is useful for diagnosis of cardiac function and complications (ejection fraction, hemodynamic severity of valve lesions, abscess).
- Transesophageal echocardiogram (TEE) is superior to TTE for diagnosis of IE and its complications [47–51].

Treating the Patient

1. Start with ABCs if sick or critical.
2. If not toxic, blood cultures should be obtained, followed by antibiotics.
3. If the patient is critical, begin resuscitation and obtain cultures while providing antibiotics.
   - Antibiotics are typically provided empirically based on the type of valve and IE (Table 19.3) [1, 2, 7–10, 52–56].
   - Adding an aminoglycoside is often recommended, especially in the setting of enterococcal infection. However, there is increased patient harm with aminoglycosides, including increased risk of renal injury, with no benefit to clearing infection [53, 56].
   - Duration of antibiotic therapy is typically 4–6 weeks to kill dormant bacteria present in the infected foci. However, patients with NVE and normal renal function may be appropriate for shorter courses, such as 2 weeks [53–56].
4. Surgery may be associated with improved outcomes versus antibiotics alone, especially for left-sided IE or *S. aureus* IE. Patients with IVDA IE usually only require medical management [52, 57].
   - Hard indications for surgery include refractory CHF, valvular insufficiency causing cardiogenic shock, persistent infection despite antibiotics, fungal or pseudomonal infection, ≥1 emboli within the first week of antibiotics, valvular complication (dehiscence, perforation, fistula, large perivalvular abscess) [1, 2, 52, 57–59].
   - Potential indications include vegetation >10 mm, early PVE (within 2 months of surgery), and recurrent embolization [1, 2, 5, 53].
   - Right-sided IE cases normally do not need surgery, in part due to high recurrence rate of IE in IVDA patients.

Table 19.3 Antibiotics for IE

Valve Status	Empiric Regimen	Severe Penicillin (PCN) Allergy
NVE	Cefepime 2 g IV	Aztreonam 2 g IV
	Vancomycin 20 mg/kg IV	Vancomycin 20 mg/kg IV
PVE	Cefepime 2 g IV	Aztreonam 2 g IV
	Vancomycin 20 mg/kg IV	Vancomcyin 20 mg/kg IV
	Gentamicin 1 mg/kg IV	Gentamicin 1 mg/kg IV
	Rifampin 300 mg IV/PO	Rifampin 300 mg IV/PO

5. Anticoagulation is not indicated in the acute management of IE, as it does not prevent formation of vegetations or embolization. If the patient is on anticoagulation when IE is diagnosed, it used to be relatively contraindicated. Recent data suggest that the risk of bleeding with anticoagulation in the setting of IE may be overstated.
   - However, a patient receiving warfarin for another indication before diagnosis of IE should receive heparin instead of warfarin [60, 61].
6. Patients with suspected or diagnosed IE should be admitted and receive early surgical and infectious disease consultation. Patients may be appropriate for outpatient treatment after several days of admission [1, 2, 5, 52].
7. Prognosis depends on the occurrence of complications, and if left untreated, IE is usually fatal. NVE mortality ranges from 16–27% with antibiotics, while PVE mortality is higher. Mortality for IE associated with a pacemaker approaches 34%. Other risk factors for high mortality include older age, aortic valve infection, congestive heart failure development, CNS complication, diabetes, and the organism involved. *S. aureus* IE is associated with a mortality up to 40% [1, 2, 5, 7–10].

Case Conclusion

The patient is admitted to the hospital ward. Cultures grow *S. aureus* within 8 hours. Comprehensive echocardiogram reveals a vegetation of 8 mm. Cardiothoracic surgery evaluates the patient and recommends continued antibiotic therapy.

Case Discussion

Endocarditis can be a difficult diagnosis, as it presents with symptoms resembling a viral-like illness. Though fever and murmur are present in the majority of cases, they may not be present at the time of initial presentation. Other findings such as Roth spots, Janeway lesions, Osler nodes, and so on are not common. Many of these patients will present multiple times to the ED with symptoms. The key is consideration of risk factors. A patient with IVDA (past or current use) and fever should trigger consideration of IE. Other keys are multiple sites of infection, poor dentition, and abnormal culture results with atypical organisms.

If a patient presents with risk factors for IE and endocarditis is on the table, admission for further evaluation is key. A bedside transthoracic echocardiogram may pick up an abnormality, but it is not diagnostic in 100% of cases.

Pattern Recognition

- Risk factors are key in flu-like symptoms and IE: prior IE, structural heart damage, IVDA, poor immune function, and poor oral hygiene
- Patients with multiple sites of infection
- Murmur, fever, and/or poor dentition with IE risk factors
- Abnormal culture results with atypical organisms

Disclosure Statement This review does not reflect the views or opinions of the US government, Department of Defense, SAUSHEC EM Program, or US Air Force.

References

1. Baddour LM, Wilson WR, Bayer AS, et al. Infective endocarditis in adults: diagnosis, antimicrobial therapy, and management of complications. Circulation. 2016;134:1435–86.
2. Cahill TJ, Prendergast BD. Infective endocarditis. Lancet. 2016;387:882–93.
3. Prendergast BD. Diagnostic criteria and problems in infective endocarditis. Heart. 2004;90:611–3.
4. Habib G, Lancellotti P, Antunes MJ. 2015 ESC guidelines for the management of infective endocarditis: the task force for the Management of Infective Endocarditis of the European Society of Cardiology (ESC). Endorsed by: European Association for Cardio-Thoracic Surgery (EACTS), the European Association of Nuclear Medicine (EANM). Eur Heart J. 2015;36(44):3075–128.
5. Baddour LM, Wilson WR, Bayer AS. Infective endocarditis: diagnosis, antimicrobial therapy, and management of complications: a statement for healthcare professionals from the Committee on Rheumatic Fever, Endocarditis, and Kawasaki Disease, Council on Cardiovascular Disease in the Young, and the Councils on Clinical Cardiology, Stroke, and Cardiovascular Surgery and Anesthesia, American Heart Association: endorsed by the Infectious Diseases Society of America. Circulation. 2005;111(23):e394–434.
6. Bor DH, Woolhandler S, Nardin R, et al. Infective endocarditis in the U.S., 1998-2009: a nationwide study. PLoS One. 2013;8(3):e60033.
7. Moreillon P. Endocarditis and enteritis, Chap. 47. In: Cohen J, editor. Infectious diseases. 3rd ed. Missouri; 2010. p. 514–28.
8. Aretz H, Krandin R. Cardiac infections, Chap. 8. In: Krandin R, editor. Diagnostic pathology of infectious disease. 1st ed. Philadelphia: Saunders; 2010. p. 189–213.
9. Tan C, Rodriguez E. Endocarditis and other intravascular infections, Chap. 11. In: Procop G, et al., editors. Pathology of infectious diseases. 1st ed. Philadelphia: Saunders; 2014. p. 229–46.
10. Nishimura RA, Otto CM, Bonow RO, et al, and the American College of Cardiology/American Heart Association Task Force on Practice Guidelines. 2014 AHA/ACC guideline for the management of patients with valvular heart disease: a report of the American College of Cardiology/American Heart Association task force on practice guidelines. J Am Coll Cardiol. 2014;63:e57–185.
11. Li JS, Sexton DJ, Mick N. Proposed modifications to the Duke criteria for the diagnosis of infective endocarditis. Clin Infect Dis. 2000;30(4):633–8.
12. Osler W. The Gulstonian lectures, on malignant endocarditis. BMJ. 1885;1:577–9.
13. Cahill TJ, Baddour LM, Habib G. Challenges in infective endocarditis. J Am Coll Cardiol. 2017;69(3):325–44.

14. Devlin RK, Andrews MM, von Reyn CF. Recent trends in infective endocarditis: influence of case definitions. Curr Opin Cardiol. 2004;19(2):134–9.
15. Selton-Suty C, Célard M, Le Moing V. Preeminence of Staphylococcus aureus in infective endocarditis: a 1-year population-based survey. Clin Infect Dis. 2012;54(9):1230–9.
16. Vogkou CT, Vlachogiannis NI, Palaiodimos L, et al. The causative agents in infective endocarditis: a systematic review comprising 33,214 cases. Eur J Clin Microbiol Infect Dis. 2016;35(8):1227–45.
17. Murdoch DR, Corey GR, Hoen B, et al., and the International Collaboration on Endocarditis-Prospective Cohort Study (ICE-PCS) Investigators. Clinical presentation, etiology, and outcome of infective endocarditis in the 21st century: the International Collaboration on Endocarditis-Prospective Cohort Study. Arch Intern Med. 2009;169:463–73.
18. Wang A, Athan E, Pappas PA, et al., and the International Collaboration on Endocarditis-Prospective Cohort Study Investigators. Contemporary clinical profile and outcome of prosthetic valve endocarditis. JAMA. 2007;297:1354–61.
19. Habib G, Thuny F, Avierinos J-F. Prosthetic valve endocarditis: current approach and therapeutic options. Prog Cardiovasc Dis. 2008;50:274–81.
20. Martín-Dávila P, Navas E, Fortún J. Analysis of mortality and risk factors associated with native valve endocarditis in drug users: the importance of vegetation size. Am Heart J. 2004;150:1099.
21. Widmer E, Que YA, Entenza JM, et al. New concepts in the pathophysiology of infective endocarditis. Curr Infect Dis Rep. 2006;8:271–9.
22. Werdan K, Dietz S, Luffler B, et al. Mechanisms of infective endocarditis: pathogen-host interaction and risk states. Nat Rev Cardiol. 2014;11:35–50.
23. Que Y-A, Haefliger J-A, Piroth L, et al. Fibrinogen and fibronectin binding cooperate for valve infection and invasion in Staphylococcus aureus experimental endocarditis. J Exp Med. 2005;201:1627–35.
24. Pasha AK, Lee JZ, Low SW, et al. Fungal endocarditis: update on diagnosis and management. Am J Med. 2016;129(10):1037–43.
25. Giamarellou H. Nosocomial cardiac infections. J Hosp Infect. 2002;50(2):91–105.
26. Revest M, Egmann G, Cattoir V, Tattevin P. HACEK endocarditis: state-of-the-art. Expert Rev Anti-Infect Ther. 2016;14(5):523–30.
27. Chu VH, Miro JM, Hoen B, et al., and the International Collaboration on Endocarditis-Prospective Cohort Study Group. Coagulase-negative staphylococcal prosthetic valve endocarditis—a contemporary update based on the International Collaboration on Endocarditis: prospective cohort study. Heart. 2009;95:570–76.
28. Nigo M, Munita JM, Arias CA, Murray BE. What's new in the treatment of enterococcal endocarditis? Curr Infect Dis Rep. 2014;16:431.
29. Das M, Badley AD, Cockerill F, et al. Infective endocarditis caused by HACEK microorganisms. Annu Rev Med. 1997;48:25–33.
30. Silverman ME, Upshaw CB Jr. Extracardiac manifestations of infective endocarditis and their historical descriptions. Am J Cardiol. 2007;100:1802–7.
31. Heiro M, Nikoskelainen J, Engblom E, et al. Neurologic manifestations of infective endocarditis: a 17-year experience in a teaching hospital in Finland. Arch Intern Med. 2000;160(18):2781–7.
32. Servy A, Valeyrie-Allanore L, Alla F, et al, and the Association Pour l'Etude et la Pr.vention de l'Endocardite Infectieuse Study Group. Prognostic value of skin manifestations of infective endocarditis. JAMA Dermatol. 2014;150:494–500.
33. Gomes RT, Tiberto LR, Bello V, et al. Dermatologic manifestations of infective endocarditis. An Bras Dermatol. 2016;91(5 suppl 1):92–4.
34. Gomes A, Glaudemans AWJM, Touw DJ. Diagnostic value of imaging in infective endocarditis: a systematic review. Lancet Infect Dis. 2017;17(1):e1–e14.
35. Chong Y, Han SJ, Rhee YJ, et al. Classic peripheral signs of subacute bacterial endocarditis. Korean J Thorac Cardiovasc Surg. 2016;49(5):408–12.

36. Haber R, Khoury R, Kechichian E, Tomb R. Splinter hemorrhages of the nails: a systematic review of clinical features and associated conditions. Int J Dermatol. 2016;55(12):1304–10.
37. Gunson TH, Oliver GF. Osler's nodes and Janeway lesions. Australas J Dermatol. 2007;48(4):251–5.
38. Marrie TJ. Osler's nodes and Janeway lesions. Am J Med. 2008;121(2):105–6.
39. Meine TJ, Nettles RE, Anderson DJ, et al. Cardiac conduction abnormalities in endocarditis defined by the Duke criteria. Am Heart J. 2001;142:280–5.
40. Lamy B, Dargère S, Arendrup MC, et al. How to optimize the use of blood cultures for the diagnosis of bloodstream infections? A State-of-the Art. Front Microbiol. 2016;7:697.
41. Riedel S, Bourbeau P, Swartz B, et al. Timing of specimen collection for blood cultures from febrile patients with bacteremia. J Clin Microbiol. 2008;46:1381–5.
42. Gould FK, Denning DW, Elliott TSJ, et al. Guidelines for the diagnosis and antibiotic treatment of endocarditis in adults: a report of the Working Party of the British Society for Antimicrobial Chemotherapy. J Antimicrob Chemother. 2012;67:269–89.
43. Lee A, Mirrett S, Reller LB, Weinstein MP. Detection of bloodstream infections in adults: how many blood cultures are needed? J Clin Microbiol. 2007;45:3546–8.
44. Cockerill FR 3rd, Wilson JW, Vetter EA, et al. Optimal testing parameters for blood cultures. Clin Infect Dis. 2004;38:1724–30.
45. Bai AD, Steinberg M, Showler A. Diagnostic accuracy of transthoracic echocardiography for infective endocarditis findings using transesophageal echocardiography as the reference standard: a meta-analysis. J Am Soc Echocardiogr. 2017;30(7):639–646.e8.
46. Fowler VG Jr, Li J, Corey GR, et al. Role of echocardiography in evaluation of patients with Staphylococcus aureus bacteremia: experience in 103 patients. J Am Coll Cardiol. 1997;30:1072–8.
47. Joseph JP, Meddows TR, Webster DP, et al. Prioritizing echocardiography in Staphylococcus aureus bacteraemia. J Antimicrob Chemother. 2013;68:444–9.
48. Habib G, Badano L, Tribouilloy C, et al. Recommendations for the practice of echocardiography in infective endocarditis. Eur J Echocardiogr. 2010;11:202–19.
49. Vieira ML, Grinberg M, Pomerantzeff PMA, et al. Repeated echocardiographic examinations of patients with suspected infective endocarditis. Heart. 2004;90:1020–4.
50. De Castro S, Cartoni D, d'Amati G, et al. Diagnostic accuracy of transthoracic and multiplane transesophageal echocardiography for valvular perforation in acute infective endocarditis: correlation with anatomic findings. Clin Infect Dis. 2000;30:825–6.
51. Daniel WG, Mügge A, Martin RP, et al. Improvement in the diagnosis of abscesses associated with endocarditis by transesophageal echocardiography. N Engl J Med. 1991;324:795–800.
52. Habib G. Management of infective endocarditis. Heart. 2006;92(1):124–30.
53. Fernández-Hidalgo N, Almirante B, Gavaldà J. Ampicillin plus ceftriaxone is as effective as ampicillin plus gentamicin for treating enterococcus faecalis infective endocarditis. Clin Infect Dis. 2013;56(9):1261–8.
54. Korzeniowski O, Sande MA. Combination antimicrobial therapy for Staphylococcus aureus endocarditis in patients addicted to parenteral drugs and in nonaddicts: a prospective study. Ann Intern Med. 1982;97:496–503.
55. Rybak MJ, Lomaestro BM, Rotschafer JC, et al. Therapeutic monitoring of vancomycin in adults summary of consensus recommendations from the American Society of Health-System Pharmacists, the Infectious Diseases Society of America, and the Society of Infectious Diseases Pharmacists. Pharmacotherapy. 2009;29(11):1275–9.
56. Fowler VG, Boucher HW, Corey GR. Daptomycin versus standard therapy for bacteremia and endocarditis caused by Staphylococcus aureus. N Engl J Med. 2006;355(7):653–65.
57. Prendergast BD, Tornos P. Surgery for infective endocarditis: who and when? Circulation. 2010;121:1141–52.
58. Mihos CG, Capoulade R, Yucel E, et al. Surgical versus medical therapy for prosthetic valve endocarditis: a meta-analysis of 32 studies. Ann Thorac Surg. 2017;103(3):991–1004.

59. Eiken PW, Edwards WD, Tazelaar HD, et al. Surgical pathology of nonbacterial thrombotic endocarditis in 30 patients, 1985-2000. Mayo Clin Proc. 2001;76(12):1204–12.
60. Snygg-Martin U, Rasmussen RV, Hassager C, et al. Warfarin therapy and incidence of cerebro-vascular complications in left-sided native valve endocarditis. Eur J Clin Microbiol Infect Dis. 2011;30(2):151–7.
61. Wilson W, Taubert KA, Gewitz M. Prevention of infective endocarditis: guidelines from the American Heart Association: a guideline from the American Heart Association rheumatic fever, endocarditis, and Kawasaki disease committee, council on cardiovascular disease in the young, and the council on clinical cardiology, council on cardiovascular surgery and anesthesia, and the quality of care and outcomes research interdisciplinary working group. Circulation. 2007;116(15):1736–54.

Excited Delirium: *"I'm So Excited … I Just Can't Hide It"*

20

M. Scott Cardone and Cynthia G. Leung

Case

Pertinent History

A 23-year-old male presents via Emergency Medical Services (EMS), restrained and chemically sedated. He had been observed running through the streets naked and screaming, which prompted bystanders to call the local police department. Officers reportedly chased the patient through the neighborhood, and the pursuit ended when the patient ran through a glass storm door. At this point, several officers were able to wrestle the patient to the ground and EMS was able to rapidly sedate the patient. The patient required multiple doses of sedative medications before he could be safely transported to the emergency department (ED). Upon arrival to the ED, the patient is unresponsive to verbal stimuli presumably due to the sedatives used on scene.

Pertinent Physical Exam

- BP 158/98, Pulse 132, and RR 32.

Except as noted below, the findings of the complete physical exam are within normal limits.

M. S. Cardone · C. G. Leung (✉)
Department of Emergency Medicine, Wexner Medical Center at The Ohio State University, Columbus, OH, USA
e-mail: Cynthia.Leung@osumc.edu

© Springer Nature Switzerland AG 2020
C. G. Kaide, C. E. San Miguel (eds.), *Case Studies in Emergency Medicine*, https://doi.org/10.1007/978-3-030-22445-5_20

- General: The patient is diaphoretic and unresponsive to verbal stimuli.
- Cardiovascular: Tachycardic. Regular rhythm. No murmurs, gallops, or rubs.
- Skin: The upper chest and extremities are covered with multiple lacerations and abrasions of differing sizes.

Pertinent Test Results

The patient's lab work revealed significant metabolic acidosis and a markedly elevated CK level.

Emergency Department Management

The patient required frequent large doses of benzodiazepines for continued sedation. He was intubated for airway protection. He was started on IV fluids for rehydration and a bicarbonate infusion to maintain a urine pH above or equal to 7.5. The patient's lacerations were irrigated, sutured, and dressed. He was admitted to the Medical Intensive Care Unit for further management.

Learning Points: The Excited Delirium Syndrome

Priming Questions
1. Describe the proposed pathophysiology of excited delirium.
2. What diagnostic evaluation is required for this type of patient presentation?
3. Why is it important to rapidly chemically restrain patient with suspected excited delirium syndrome? What are the preferred agents for chemical restraint?
4. What additional medical management is indicated for these patients?

Introduction/Background

1. The term "Excited Delirium" is a historically controversial subcategory of delirium, which describes a syndrome of altered mental status, agitation, and overactive adrenergic autonomic dysfunction, typically in the setting of acute-on-chronic drug abuse or serious mental illness [1].
   - For about 150 years, case reports have described cases with this constellation of symptoms without using the exact term "Excited Delirium," which did not gain popularity until a 1985 paper by Wetli and Fishbain describing a series of cocaine-related deaths [1, 2].

- Since 1985, the concept of Excited Delirium has been used by EMS, psychiatry, emergency medicine, and law enforcement to describe a subset of patients who are otherwise without a unifying clinical diagnosis. The term was developed to describe patients who suffered an apparent psychiatric decompensation, ultimately resulting in an unexplained death [1–3].

2. The typical or classic course for an Excited Delirium patient begins with acute drug intoxication, often cocaine, a struggle with authorities or law enforcement, physical or chemical restraint, and sudden cardiac arrest [1, 3, 4].
   - Cases of death associated with Excited Delirium Syndrome tend to share similar features. Patients are overwhelmingly young adult males, with an average age of 36 years old. There is generally a history of drug use and aggressive or strange behavior prompting law enforcement involvement. Patients often have a history of psychiatric illness. Patients are frequently nude or dressed inappropriately for the situation or environment. They often fail to recognize or respond appropriately to law enforcement officers, and struggle against officers, staff, and providers. These patients are regularly noted to have "superhuman" strength and do not seem to fatigue [1, 5].

Physiology/Pathophysiology

1. The pathophysiology of the Excited Delirium Syndrome remains unclear [1, 3, 6].
   - Illicit drug abuse, particularly cocaine, is highly associated with Excited Delirium Syndrome, though it does not appear that deaths can be attributed to simple drug overdose. Fatal cases of Excited Delirium have been found to involve serum cocaine concentrations similar to those found in recreational drug users rather than the high levels seen in acute fatal cocaine intoxication [1, 3].
2. One hypothesized mechanism involves dopaminergic pathways in the central nervous system [6].
   - Postmortem brain examination of cocaine abusers who die in police custody has shown loss of dopamine transporters in the striatum, suggesting that excessive dopaminergic activation in the striatum may underlie Excited Delirium in these patients. These changes are likely induced by chronic psychostimulant use and may predispose the patient to an episode of Excited Delirium during episodes of acute-on-chronic drug abuse [1, 6].
   - Thermoregulation is also modulated by dopaminergic pathways, and dysregulation of these pathways may explain the hyperthermia commonly seen in Excited Delirium Syndrome [1].
3. Metabolic derangements, particularly metabolic acidosis, are common in Excited Delirium [1, 4, 5].
   - Severe metabolic acidosis is strongly associated with Excited Delirium Syndrome and may contribute to the hemodynamic collapse and cardiac arrest seen in fatal cases [1, 4, 5].
   - Rhabdomyolysis and hyperkalemia are also common features [1, 4, 5].

4. Among fatal cases of Excited Delirium, bradyarrhythmia and asystole are the most common arrhythmias seen [1, 5].
   - Ventricular arrhythmias are very rare in these patients, only present in 1 out of 13 patients in an extended case series [5].

Making the Diagnosis

Differential Diagnosis

Pearl: The differential diagnosis for altered mental status can be remembered with the mnemonic "AEIOU TIPS" [7].

- A – Alcohol
- E – Endocrine, encephalopathy, and electrolytes
- I – Insulin (hypoglycemia)
- O – Oxygen (hypoxia) and opiates (or other drugs of abuse)
- U – Uremia
- T – Toxins, trauma, and temperature (hypo or hyperthermia)
- I – Infection
- P – Psychiatric and Porphyria
- S – Shock, stroke, subarachnoid hemorrhage, and space-occupying CNS mass

Excited Delirium Syndrome may involve several of the above causes of altered mental status, including drug abuse, psychiatric illness, and metabolic derangements.

1. Clinical Characteristics
   - Historical features
2. Patients are often males in their 30s and have history of mental illness and/or stimulant drug abuse.
   - Prehospital features
     - Police are typically called to the scene due to destructive, aggressive, or bizarre behavior; nudity or inappropriate dress; or running in traffic.
     - Patients usually fail to respond to verbal commands and may also demonstrate unusual strength, lack of fatigue, and seeming imperviousness to pain. They resist physical restraint and continue to struggle despite futility.
     - A small but not insignificant number of patients are reported to have exhibited fascination with mirrors or reflective surfaces such as glass.
   - Clinical features
     - Vital signs are consistent with adrenergic overstimulation and include tachypnea, tachycardia, hypertension, and hyperthermia.
     - Laboratory evaluation often reveals significant metabolic acidosis and may also show marked rhabdomyolysis [1, 4].

- Serum or urine toxicology screen is typically positive for drugs of abuse, often cocaine, but drug levels may be lower than one might anticipate.

Treating the Patient

1. Restraint is a prerequisite to further medical management in agitated and unco-operative patients.
   - Physical struggle is thought to be a major cause of catecholamine surge as well as the metabolic acidosis and other metabolic derangements associated with Excited Delirium Syndrome. However, in the interest of both patient and staff safety, physical restraint is often required, at least initially. Efficient physical restraint of the patient with multiple security personnel who are trained in safe physical control measures is therefore recommended [1, 3].
     - As physical constraint can play such a key role in the worsening of this condition, it should be discontinued as quickly and as safely as possible. Typically, this means after the patient is successfully chemically restrained.
     - Early theories of positional asphyxiation as a cause of sudden death in this patient population pointed to prolonged periods of prone restraint as a possible factor in clinical deterioration. In particular, placing the patient in a hogtie or hobble (laying prone with arms and legs tied together behind the back) was considered significantly dangerous. While this has not completely been demonstrated in the literature to be a direct cause of clinical deterioration, these positions of restraint are nonetheless not recommended if the clinician is concerned about Excited Delirium [5].
     - Sudden cessation of struggling with altered breathing patterns often occurs just prior to cardiac arrest and should be considered an ominous sign [5].
   - Chemical restraint should be administered rapidly to avoid exacerbation of the catecholamine surge to the extent possible and to facilitate further evaluation and care. However, the benefit of rapid chemical restraint has not been proven to alter outcomes [1, 3].
     - Intramuscular benzodiazepines or ketamine are the preferred agents for chemical restraint.
       o Recent literature suggests that ketamine may be preferable for a number of reasons. It is the most widely used anesthetic agent for surgical procedures worldwide, and its excellent safety profile is well described. Additionally, it has the most rapid onset of action of any of the available intramuscular agents, taking effect on average in about 3 minutes. Suggested initial dosing is 4–5 mg/kg. Case reports indicate excellent effect and safety when used in Excited Delirium [1, 8].
       o The drawbacks of ketamine include rare but possible side effects such as laryngospasm, emergence phenomena, and increased oral secretions. There is also a potential and unknown interaction with phencyclidine, or PCP, an illicit drug that may mimic the effects of cocaine or produce

symptoms similar to that of cocaine. Ketamine and PCP both act on the NMDA receptor, and it therefore may not be advisable to use ketamine in cases of suspected PCP intoxication [1, 9].

- o Benzodiazepines are extremely safe as well, though onset is longer and initial dosing is empiric, and therefore may require repeat administration before adequate sedation can be obtained [1, 8].
- o Exercise caution with antipsychotics due to QT prolongation [8].
- – Paralysis and/or intubation should be considered if sedation alone is ineffective.

2. Treatment of hyperthermia may be indicated, and it may involve either external cooling measures such as removal of clothing, cool environment, cooling blankets, and ice packs, or internal cooling such as infusion of cold saline or placement of a cooling catheter.
   - Care must be taken not to overcool the patient and induce hypothermia.
   - See the chapter on hyperthermia for more details on the differential diagnosis and management of this condition.
3. Metabolic acidosis and hypovolemia are common in Excited Delirium and should be treated when present. IV fluid resuscitation is the cornerstone of management of these metabolic issues [1, 3, 4].
   - Intravenous bicarbonate administration should be considered in severe cases of acidosis. Empiric use of bicarbonate remains controversial but is approved for use by some EMS agencies [1].
   - Avoid interfering with hyperventilation as this is the major compensatory mechanism for metabolic acidosis [1]. If the patient must be intubated, the ventilator must be set with this in mind, as too low of a respiratory rate will take away this compensatory mechanism and cause worsening acidosis [1].
4. Rhabdomyolysis and hyperkalemia are the other common metabolic problems associated with Excited Delirium. Rhabdomyolysis should be treated with intravenous fluids and urinary alkalization, and hyperkalemia should be treated with any indicated interventions such as intracellular shifters, potassium binding agents, and cardiac membrane stabilizers depending on the degree of hyperkalemia and whether there are EKG changes present [1, 10].

Case Discussion

1. Excited Delirium Syndrome is potentially a difficult diagnosis to make but is an important diagnosis to not miss, as it can be fatal. Many emergency physicians routinely see patients brought in by police, intoxicated on illicit drugs of abuse. It requires a high index of suspicion to recognize that this particular intoxicated, agitated, aggressive patient is not just behaving in an uninhibited fashion but is actually in serious danger of hemodynamic collapse and requires rapid and aggressive intervention. The young male who habitually presents to the ED with aggressive behavior after cocaine abuse and always simply requires a few hours to sober up is a particularly dangerous case, as his chronic stimulant abuse may

set the stage for a future episode of Excited Delirium Syndrome, and the physicians who know his usual presentation well may be cognitively biased to miss what separates that episode from his countless prior ones.

2. Rapid adequate sedation is recommended, though it has not been proven to alter outcomes. Patients with Excited Delirium Syndrome can struggle with seemingly bottomless strength and stamina against physical restraint, which is hypothesized to worsen their catecholamine surge and put them at further risk. When concerned for Excited Delirium, it is advisable to bring extra security personnel who can safely and efficiently restrain the patient to facilitate administration of intramuscular (IM) sedatives, preferably benzodiazepines or ketamine.

3. As soon as the patient is sedated enough for safe IV access, a broad laboratory evaluation should be conducted to look for metabolic derangements, which should be treated aggressively. Hyperthermia and hypovolemia should be corrected, and the patient should be closely monitored for signs of hemodynamic instability.

4. Be wary of patients who suddenly cease a prolonged struggle. This may be a sign of impending hemodynamic collapse and death [1, 2, 5].

Pattern Recognition

Excited Delirium
- Young adult males with a history of mental illness
- Altered mental status
- Aggressive and/or destructive behavior
- Cocaine or other psychostimulant abuse
- Struggle with or flight from police
- "Superhuman strength"
- Metabolic acidosis
- Tachycardia, hyperthemia, tachypnea, and/or hypertension

Disclosure Statement   The authors of this chapter report no significant disclosures.

References

1. Vilke GM, DeBard ML, et al. Excited Delirium Syndrome (ExDS): defining based on a review of the literature. J Emerg Med. 2012;43(5):897–905.
2. Wetli CV, Fishbain DA. Cocaine-induced psychosis and sudden death in recreational cocaine users. J Forensic Sci. 1985;30:873–80.
3. Ruttenber AJ, Lawler-Heavner J, Yin M, Wetli CV, Hearn WL, Mash DC. Fatal excited delirium following cocaine use: epidemiologic findings provide new evidence for mechanisms of cocaine toxicity. J Forensic Sci. 1997;42:25–31.
4. Hick JL, Smith SW, Lynch MT. Metabolic acidosis in restraint-associated cardiac arrest: a case series. Acad Emerg Med. 1999;6(3):239–43.

5. Stratton SJ, Rogers C, Brickett K, Gruzinski G. Factors associated with sudden death of individuals requiring restraint for excited delirium. Am J Emerg Med. 2001;19:187–91.
6. Mash DC, Duque L, Pablo J, Qin Y, Adi N, Hearn WL, Hyma BA, Karch SB, Druid H, Wetli CV. Brain biomarkers for identifying excited delirium as a cause of sudden death. Forensic Sci Int. 2009;190(1-3):e13–9.
7. Roberts JR, Siegel E. Mnemonic for diagnosis of acute mental status change (letter to the editor). Ann Emerg Med. 1990;19(2):221.
8. Scheppke KA, et al. Prehospital use of IM Ketamine for sedation of violent and agitated patients. West J Emerg Med. 2014;15(7):736–41.
9. Strayer RJ, Nelson LS. Adverse events associated with ketamine for procedural sedation in adults. Am J Emerg Med. 2008;26(9):985–1028.
10. Wetli CV, Mash D, Karch SB. Cocaine-associated agitated delirium and the neuroleptic malignant syndrome. Am J Emerg Med. 1996;14(4):425–8.

Radiology Case 4

21

Priyanka Dube and Joshua K. Aalberg

Case

Interstitial Pulmonary Edema

Indication for the Exam A 61 y/o f presents with progressive dyspnea and 5 lb weight gain over the last day. There are diffuse rales on exam.

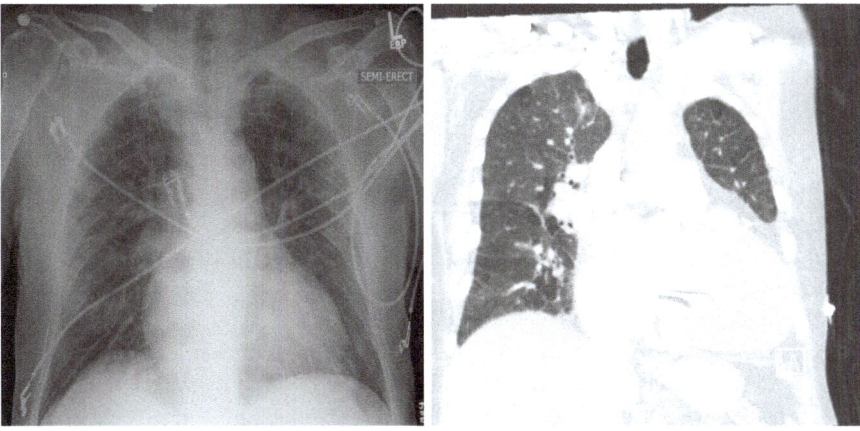

Radiographic Findings Chest radiograph (left) coronal CT (right) demonstrating interstitial pulmonary edema.

Diagnosis Congestive heart failure exacerbation.

P. Dube · J. K. Aalberg (✉)
Department of Emergency Medicine, Wexner Medical Center at The Ohio State University, Columbus, OH, USA
e-mail: Priyanka.Dube@osumc.edu; joshua.aalberg@osumc.edu

© Springer Nature Switzerland AG 2020
C. G. Kaide, C. E. San Miguel (eds.), *Case Studies in Emergency Medicine*,
https://doi.org/10.1007/978-3-030-22445-5_21

Learning Points

Priming Questions
- What are imaging findings of pulmonary edema?
- How do you differentiate between interstitial and alveolar edema?
- What are noncardiac etiologies for pulmonary edema?

Introduction/Background

Because pulmonary edema is seen most commonly in the emergency department and intensive care unit, recognition of pulmonary edema on chest radiographs is necessary to avoid acute and rapid decompensation. Extravascular fluid within the lungs is termed pulmonary edema. Edema has multiple etiologies, which are important to consider in an emergent situation. This chapter will focus on increased hydrostatic pressure resulting in interstitial pulmonary edema.

Pathophysiology/Mechanism

Pulmonary edema results from increased hydrostatic pressure, increased alveolar permeability with or without damage, or a combination of increased permeability and hydrostatic pressure. Accumulation of fluid either in the alveoli or interstitium will impact oxygenation [1].

Making the Diagnosis

- Chest radiographs are the initial imaging modalities to diagnose pulmonary edema (both alveolar and interstitial). They are quick, rapid, and highly sensitive. CT can also be utilized to evaluate pulmonary edema.
- Interstitial edema occurs when there is an increase of hydrostatic pressure within the capillaries between 15 mmHG and 25 mmHG. When there is an increase in extravascular fluid, pulmonary vessels will become indistinct, septa thicken (Kerley B lines), and fluid accumulates around the bronchi (termed peribronchial cuffing).
- When pressure exceeds 25mmHg, fluid accumulates in the alveoli which can coalesce to form basilar predominate air space opacities. This may eventually result in alveolar damage due to the increased pressure. Edema has been known to be directly associated with pulmonary capillary wedge pressures.

Common Causes

- Cardiac failure
- Valvular dysfunction
- Volume overload/renal failure
- Acute respiratory distress syndrome (ARDS)
- High altitude
- Drugs
- Head trauma/neurogenic causes

Treating the Patient

Definitive treatment is based upon correcting the cause of pulmonary edema. In the emergent setting, initial therapy is dictated by the severity of the patient's pathology. Some may do well on small amounts of supplemental oxygen or even room air while awaiting definitive treatment. This may include diuretics in the case on heart failure, hemodialysis in the setting of renal failure, or descent to a lower altitude for high-altitude pulmonary edema. There should be low threshold, however, to initiate noninvasive positive pressure (NIPPV) therapy in the form of CPAP or BiPAP, as this can direct fluid back into the vasculature. This therapy does not, however, change the underlying pathology which initially caused the increased hydrostatic pressure. Positive pressure provided from a ventilator through an endotracheal tube is perhaps even more effective than NIPPV but is clearly a more invasive process with more implicit difficulties in weaning therapy. See the chapter on flash pulmonary edema for a more detailed discussion on this topic.

Discussion

- Pulmonary edema results from increased hydrostatic pressure within the capillaries. Fluid initially accumulates within the interstitium and then can progress to fill the alveoli. Increased pressure that is long standing can eventually cause architectural distortion and damage to the alveoli.
- Pulmonary edema is due to multiple causes both cardiogenic and noncardiogenic.

Disclosure Statement   The authors of this chapter report no significant disclosures.

Reference

1. Gluecker T, Capasso P, Schnyder P, Gudinchet F, Schaller M, Revelly J, Wicky S. Clinical and radiologic features of pulmonary edema. RadioGraphics. 1999;19(6):1507–31. https://doi.org/10.1148/radiographics.19.6.g99no211507.

Flash Pulmonary Edema: *Staying Afloat in the Flash Flood*

22

Joshua Faucher, Michelle Axe, and Colin G. Kaide

Case 1

Two Cardiac Patients

Pertinent History

This patient is a 49-year-old male who presented to the emergency department (ED) by private vehicle in acute, severe respiratory distress. He has a history of poorly controlled hypertension, and he ran out of his medications a few days ago. He normally takes three medications for his blood pressure. He developed acute onset of shortness of breath after doing a few lines of cocaine. He is unable to answer any further questions at this time.

Pertinent Physical Exam

Except as noted below, the findings of the complete physical exam are within normal limits.

- Blood pressure is 240/170, heart rate is 120, and respiratory rate is 35. Temperature is 98.4 °F. SpO_2 is 78% on room air.
- General: Alert, oriented person, place, and time. Severe respiratory distress is evident with tripod positioning. The patient is diaphoretic.

J. Faucher
Rush Oak Park Hospital, Oak Park, Illinois, USA

M. Axe
Wright State University, Dayton, OH, USA

C. G. Kaide (✉)
Department of Emergency Medicine, Wexner Medical Center at The Ohio State University, Columbus, OH, USA
e-mail: Colin.kaide@osumc.edu

© Springer Nature Switzerland AG 2020
C. G. Kaide, C. E. San Miguel (eds.), *Case Studies in Emergency Medicine*,
https://doi.org/10.1007/978-3-030-22445-5_22

- Head, Eyes, Ears, Nose and Throat (HEENT): No jugular-venous distenstion (JVD) is noted.
- Cardiovascular: S1 and S2 are present. Tachycardia with regular rhythm is noted. There are murmurs.
- Lungs: Diffuse rales bilaterally and some mild expiratory wheezing are noted.
- Extremities: Peripheral pulses intact with no pitting edema.

Past Medical History
Hypertension.

Medications
- Lisinopril
- Hydrochlorothiazide
- Metoprolol
- Nifedipine

Social History
- Smokes cigarettes, one pack per day
- Endorses daily alcohol use and cocaine use.

Family History
Hypertension.

Pertinent Test Results
EKG   Sinus tachycardia with nonspecific ST and T wave changes.

Chest X-ray (CXR)   No cardiomegaly. Diffuse interstitial edema.

Emergency Department Management
The patient was brought back from triage with signs of severe respiratory distress. He was able to provide a brief history of not taking his blood pressure medication for the past few days. His symptoms began immediately after insufflating multiple lines of cocaine. Given his high blood pressure, severe dyspnea, and hypoxia, along with diffuse rales, the diagnosis of flash pulmonary edema was entertained. The patient was placed on supplemental oxygen via nonrebreather, and respiratory therapy was contacted. While waiting for their arrival, a point-of-care ultrasound was performed, demonstrating diffuse bilateral B-lines consistent with pulmonary edema. He simultaneously received two doses of sublingual nitroglycerin, and a nitroglycerin drip was ordered. Respiratory therapy placed him on noninvasive positive pressure ventilation (NIPPV) using bilevel pressures (BiPAP®) starting at 15 mmHg/5 mmHg. The patient kept stating that he "was tired of breathing and felt like he was going to die." One milligram of IV nitroglycerin was pushed over 30 seconds. The nitroglycerin drip was started at 100 mcg/min. NIPPV was titrated to 20/10. The patient reported improvement

within 2 minutes of the push dose of nitroglycerin. Two milligrams of IV loraze-pam was also administered to help him tolerate NIPPV and to mitigate some of the catecholamine effect of the cocaine.

Updates on Emergency Department Course

Thirty minutes after starting the nitroglycerin infusion, the patient's blood pressure was 140/70. He said that his symptoms were completely relieved.

Case 2

Pertinent History

This patient is a 65-year-old female who presented to the emergency department with complaints of severe shortness of breath. The patient had been significantly short of breath for the past 3 days. She reported a history of congestive heart failure secondary to ischemic cardiomyopathy. She reports a weight gain of 20 pounds over the past week. She is on 40 mg twice a day of furosemide.

Pertinent Physical Exam

Except as noted below, the findings of the complete physical exam are within normal limits.

- Blood pressure is 140/74, heart rate is 90, and respiratory rate is 25. Temperature is 97.8 °F. SpO$_2$ is 83% on room air.
- General: Alert and oriented ×3 in severe respiratory distress.
- HEENT: Significant JVD is noted.
- Cardiovascular: S1 and S2 present, tachycardic regular rhythm without murmurs.
- Lungs: Diffuse crackles bilaterally and some mild expiratory wheezing are noted.
- Extremities: Pulses intact with 3+ pitting edema.

PMH
- Myocardial infarction
- Ischemic cardiomyopathy
- Congestive heart failure

Medications
- Furosemide
- Carvedilol
- Warfarin
- Sertraline

SH
- Smokes one pack of cigarettes per day
- Denies alcohol or other drugs.

FH
- Hypertension
Coronary artery disease

Pertinent Test Results
ECG Sinus tachycardia with nonspecific ST-T wave changes.

CXR Cardiomegaly. Diffuse interstitial edema.

Emergency Department Course
The patient was immediately brought back to the treatment area. She was placed on a nonrebreather mask and her SpO2 rose to 85%. She was given 80 mg of IV furosemide and was placed on BiPAP®. The patient repeatedly attempted to remove the NIPPV mask. She was given 0.5 mg/kg of IV ketamine at which time she tolerated the mask. Her SpO2 remained in the mid 80s. She had minimal diuresis with the furosemide.

Update 1
After 60 minutes of BiPAP, she had mild improvement. After shift change, the new attending physician started the patient on an IV nitroglycerin infusion at a rate of 100 mcg/m. The patient had substantial clinical improvement after the nitroglycerin and then she began to diurese after another 80 mg of IV furosemide.

Learning Points

Priming Questions
1. What is the major difference between case 1 and case 2?
2. What is the role of nitroglycerin in the management of pulmonary edema?
3. Why is morphine for pulmonary edema dead?
4. What clinical scenarios produce the most emergent presentations of decompensated heart failure?

Introduction/Background

1. Heart failure has a tremendous burden on emergency departments, and the health care system at large. The disease has a prevalence of nearly six million patients in the US, approaching 2% of the total population, with an annual incidence of over half a million new patients [1]. Flash pulmonary edema results in over 650,000 emergency department visits annually, and 80% of these patients will be admitted to the hospital [1, 2]. It is imperative that emergency medicine (EM) physicians understand how to treat the most dangerous complication of acute decompensated heart failure: Respiratory distress due to flash pulmonary edema.

2. While pulmonary edema, secondary to heart failure, was traditionally viewed as a manifestation of volume overload, more contemporary paradigms are classifying decompensated heart failure into presentations of variable acuity, with variable contributions from volume status, acute increases in afterload, and acute insults to cardiac function.

3. Flash pulmonary edema manifests as the result of an acute rise in left ventricular filling pressures superimposed on diastolic dysfunction, such as during an acute surge of sympathetic tone [3] The one-year mortality for patients admitted with flash pulmonary edema has been estimated to be as high as 40% [4].

4. It is crucial to differentiate subacute decompensated congestive heart failure from flash pulmonary edema and cardiac injury causing acute cariogenic shock. Treatment regimens differ depending on the underlying pathology, and expeditious diagnosis and treatment of flash pulmonary edema is imperative.

Physiology/Pathophysiology

1. Decompensated heart failure can manifest with distinct patterns of presentation in different patients. Contemporary understandings of the pathophysiology of heart failure exacerbations distinguish between subacute presentations of volume overload, hyperacute presentations of flash pulmonary edema and respiratory failure, and the more uncommon patients with acute cardiogenic shock [1, 3].

   • Patients with simple volume overload present subacutely over days to weeks and are more likely to be younger, have heart failure with reduced ejection fraction, or have established coronary artery disease [5]. Nonadherence to diet and medical therapy is thought to be the primary contributor to their weight gain and peripheral edema.

   Rates of nonadherence are estimated as high at 60% [3]. Heart failure exacerbations with simple volume overload are nonetheless associated with poor prognosis and high near-term mortality [1].

   • Heart failure manifesting as cardiogenic shock, with hypotension and signs of extensive end organ failure or hemodynamic instability is the most rare manifestation of decompensated heart failure, comprising less than 5% of presentations [2]. High suspicion should be held for acute cardiac insults such as myocardial infarction, tachydysrhythmias, or valvular pathology (e.g., acute mitral regurgitation) as precipitants of acute systolic failure.

2. The most common presentation of decompensated heart failure requiring emergent management, flash pulmonary edema, is more complex than a case of simple volume overload. Up to 50% of patients may have no evidence of whole-body fluid retention or weight gain, and flash pulmonary edema can be a sentinel occurrence in patients without an established diagnosis of heart failure [3].

   • Flash pulmonary edema can instead be viewed as a mismatch between acute increases in systemic vascular resistance (SVR), creating discordance with cardiac contractility. Patients presenting acutely hypertensive with fluid shifts, rather than retention, as a consequence [3].

   • Risk factors creating the contractility-afterload mismatch and resulting pulmonary edema include increased arterial stiffness (with older age), states of acute inflammation (e.g., sepsis) [3], and sympathetic activation (e.g., pheochromocytoma, stimulant abuse) [6]. If patients have no evidence of valvular disease or preexisting cardiomyopathy causing increased left ventricular filling pressures, a likely culprit may be renal artery stenosis causing activation of the renin-angiotensin-aldosterone axis and elevated SVR [7]. Even unilateral renal artery stenosis, in the setting of acute volume contraction, appears capable of causing flash pulmonary edema due to sympathetic activation [8].

- A study of patients with acute hypertensive crises and flash pulmonary edema undergoing echocardiogram demonstrated that, compared to controls, global systolic function in these patients was preserved, but that they had worse left ventricular diastolic stiffness, ventricular-arterial coupling, and overall adaptive capacity to respond to high filling pressures [9]. Other observations of heart failure patients experiencing flash pulmonary edema have not demonstrated weight gain as a predictor of acute exacerbations [10].

- As hypertension and increased afterload increases left ventricular pressures, they are translated to the left atrium, and pulmonic veins undergo recruitment and distension in response. This causes intracapillary hypertension in the alveolar vascular bed, and increases transcapillary filtration normally balanced by hydrostatic pressure, oncotic pressure, and vascular flow. Once intracapillary pressure exceeds 20–25 mmHg, fluid floods the alveoli and impairs gas exchange, with resultant hypoxia, tachypnea, and severe dyspnea experienced by the patient [6].

Making the Diagnosis

Differential Diagnosis
- *Decompensated heart failure*
- *COPD exacerbation*
- *Pulmonary embolism*
- *Pneumothorax*
- *Acute myocardial infarction*
- *Arrhythmia*
- *Acute valvular pathology (e.g. mitral regurgitation)*
- *Pneumonia*

1. Diagnosis begins with the history and physical examination, and a patient with flash pulmonary edema will present in acute respiratory distress. They will be dyspneic, hypoxic, tachycardic, and will usually have systolic pressures greater than 160 mm Hg (and often above 180 mm Hg). Rales may be heard on auscultation, and often the patient will be utilizing accessory muscles to facilitate breathing (e.g., with tripoding posture) [11].

- An extra heart sound (S3) or gallop is highly specific for elevated left ventricular end diastolic pressure but is likely challenging to detect in the critical patient [11].
- Minimal empiric data exist on the sensitivity or specificity of exam findings, such as jugular venous distension, rales, hepatosplenomegaly, or peripheral edema for acute exacerbations of heart failure [11]. Other factors with the highest likelihood ratio allowing for clinical diagnosis include overall clinical suspicion, and an established history of heart failure [12].

2. Specialty society recommendations for initial testing include complete blood counts (e.g., to evaluate for contributing anemia), a basic metabolic panel, electrocardiogram (ECG) and troponin (to detect ischemia or arrhythmia), and liver and thyroid function if indicated based on concern for volume overload due to cirrhosis or myxedema [1].

    - Brain natriuretic peptide (BNP) and its inactive metabolite NT-pro BNP are comparable laboratory markers released by cardiac myocytes in relation to dilation and increased fluid pressure [1]. A BNP less than 100 pg/mL is highly sensitive for excluding acute heart failure as a cause of respiratory distress [1], with values less than 80 pg/mL having a negative likelihood ratio of 0.05 [13].
    - The utility of BNP is limited by low specificity of elevations for establishing acute heart failure. Possible confounding conditions include pulmonary embolism and sepsis [13], and a rise in chronically elevated BNP has not been found to precede acute exacerbations of heart failure [10]. BNP may be disproportionately lower in patients with comorbid obesity, a large segment of heart failure patients [1]. BNP measurement has been associated with small benefits in more nebulous domains such as reduced hospital costs [14] and decreased lengths of stay [15, 16].

3. Chest radiography is a longstanding standard component of the evaluation of acute dyspnea. Pulmonary venous congestion on chest X-ray has a fairly high likelihood ratio for the diagnosis of flash pulmonary edema [12] and has the obvious benefit of visualizing associated cardiomegaly or alternative diagnoses (e.g., pneumothorax, pleural effusion, pneumonia) in a single view. The bilateral interstitial infiltrates characteristic of flash pulmonary edema can have other causes, but findings increasing the likelihood of decompensated heart failure as the etiology include Kerley B lines (thin horizontal peripheral opacities from edematous interlobular septa), and opacities that are more predominant centrally rather than peripherally [11] (Fig. 22.1).

4. Point-of-care lung ultrasound is a highly useful and expeditious imaging modality in the assessment of flash pulmonary edema. Evident benefits over chest X-ray as the first-line choice of imaging include ultrasound taking place at the bedside in tandem with other clinical tasks (compared to unprotected staff leaving the room during X-ray), and the concurrent evaluation of cardiac anatomy, function, and volume status via a view of the heart and inferior vena cava (IVC).

    - The lung ultrasound in a patient with flash pulmonary edema will show B-lines, which are vertical, hyperechoic lines extending from the near field and pleura to the far field of the screen without fading [17]. These may be

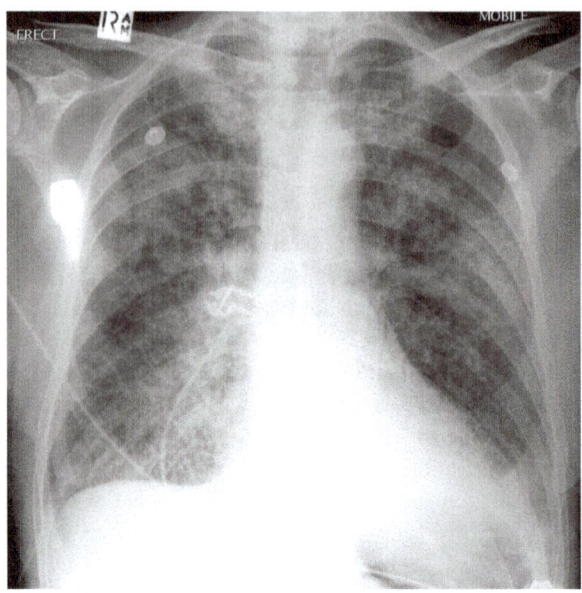

more prominent in the lateral and basilar windows of the lungs. Detecting at least three B-lines in bilateral lung fields has a specificity over 97% for detecting alveolar interstitial fluid, and a sensitivity in the mid 80s percentwise [17].

- Lung ultrasound has been shown to enhance diagnostic accuracy of heart failure when combined with the initial clinical assessment [18]. When combined with evidence of fluid overload via visualization of the IVC and/or reduced ejection fraction, the sensitivity of ultrasound for excluding decompensated heart failure as a cause of pulmonary edema and dyspnea approaches 100% [19]. Ultrasound can be reliably used to exclude pulmonary edema as a contributor to, for instance, a patient with dyspnea and an additional diagnosis of chronic obstructive pulmonary disease (COPD) (Fig. 22.2).

Treating the Patient

1. Positive Pressure Ventilation
    - Flash pulmonary edema causes severe dyspnea and respiratory distress. Upon arrival to the ED, the first step in management should be assisting proper ventilation. Proper ventilation can both improve hypoxemia preventing end-organ damage and relieve symptoms of dyspnea that are contributing to catecholamine surge and increased afterload.
    - While endotracheal intubation may be required for refractory patients, the safety and efficacy of noninvasive ventilation (NIV) for initial management of respiratory distress is widely recognized by clinical authorities [1, 20]. This consists of either continuous positive airway pressure (CPAP) or noninvasive positive pressure ventilation (NIPPV, with bilevel positive airway pressure

Fig. 22.2 An example of B-lines indicating the presence of interstitial fluid (such as from pulmonary edema) on lung ultrasound. (Case courtesy of Dr Maulik S Patel, Radiopaedia.org, rID: 35793. Published with kind permission of © Colin G. Kaide 2019. All Rights Reserved)

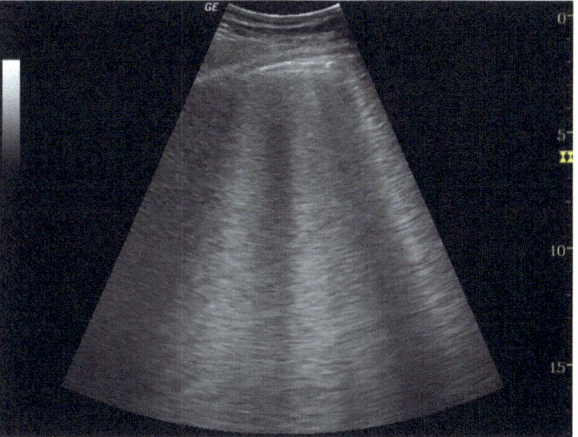

commonly referred to by the trade name BiPAP). NIV has been associated with reduced risk of in-hospital mortality and endotracheal intubation, and shortened ICU stays [20, 21]. It also produces observable improvement in dyspnea, tachycardia, tachypnea, and respiratory acidosis [22].

- NIV manufacturers are diverse, and appropriate initial settings vary by machine. You should be familiar with options available at your institution, and ideally utilize NIV with appropriate support from a respiratory therapist. As rules of thumb, CPAP is typically titrated from 5 cm H_2O to a maximum of 15 cm H_2O, and BiPAP is started at 10/5 cm H_2O and titrated up to 15 or 20/10. Patients who do not tolerate NIV may require low doses of anxiolytics such as benzodiazepines or ketamine, with caution to avoid respiratory depression.

2. Vasodilator and Antihypertensive Therapy
   - Vasodilator therapy, which can be used to reduce both preload and afterload, is viewed as a key component of emergent management for cardiogenic flash pulmonary edema [2, 23]. It reduces left ventricular end diastolic pressure, thereby reducing third spacing of fluids across the alveolar membrane and increasing cardiac output [2].
   - Nitroglycerin is the preferred vasodilator agent in the ED, with easily administered sublingual and IV formulations, a wide therapeutic range, and the avoidance of the cyanide toxicity encountered with the previously favored sodium nitroprusside [2]. Nitroglycerin use in hypoxic heart failure patients has been associated with decreased rates of intubation, mortality, and myocardial infarction (MI) [24].
   - Nitroglycerin is typically initiated as an infusion at 100 µg/min and titrated upward to effect or lower to avoid hypotension, but doses of 400 µg can be administered sublingually (perhaps while wetting the dry mouth of a dyspneic patient) while access is being obtained [2]. Bolus doses of up to 2000 µg IV every 3 minutes have been shown to reduce the need for intubation, NIV, and ICU admission without significant adverse effects [25, 26].

- Angiotensin-converting-enzyme inhibitors (ACE-Is) are another antihypertensive therapy that may be beneficial in hypertensive patients with decompensated heart failure and flash pulmonary edema. Captopril administration has been associated with a decrease in ICU admission [26, 27]. IV enalapril can be considered for administration in patients with refractory hypertensive crisis after vasodilator therapy, but caution should be used due to the risk of first-dose hypotension and shock [2].

3. Volume Reduction
   - For patients presenting with subacute decompensated heart failure, with volume overload as the primary finding and no significant dyspnea or hypertensive crisis on exam, diuresis with loop diuretics like furosemide may be the primary component of therapy, with the goal to return the patient to their baseline dry weight [2, 23]. Typical dosing strategies recommend an IV-dose equivalent to a patient's oral dose of furosemide, effectively double in strength due to the increased bioavailability of the IV form, with furosemide-naïve patients receiving a max initial dose of 40 mg IV [2, 23].
   - For patients presenting with hypertensive flash pulmonary edema, however, the main priority is reducing afterload to redistribute fluid, and patients may not be markedly fluid overloaded [2]. The urgency of diuresis in these patients is less clear, with cohort observations, when furosemide is administered to patients with signs of increased vascular congestion within 1 hour possibly demonstrating reduced mortality [29, 30]. Other studies demonstrate acute adverse effects such as decreased cardiac output, increased LV filling pressures, worsening renal function, and worsening activation of the renin-angiotensin-aldosterone neurohormonal axis [31, 32].

4. Treatment of Shock
   - As mentioned earlier, patients with decompensated heart failure, flash pulmonary edema, and hypotension are the exception rather than the norm and are more likely to experience an acute insult causing cardiogenic shock such as valve pathology or myocardial infarction [2]. Definitive management via thrombolytic therapy, catheterization, or cardiac surgery may be the only effective way to manage their condition.
   - Temporizing management of cardiogenic shock in the ED may involve the standard approach of fluid resuscitation and pressor support [2]. Small boluses (250–500 ml) of fluid may be employed, monitoring for responsiveness while avoiding large infusions that could contribute to volume overload and ironically, worsening pulmonary edema. Dobutamine, with its inherent ionotropic support, is a reasonable choice as the first pressor [2], with dopamine and milrinone also capable of producing vasodilatory effects that may improve cardiac output [5].

5. To Be Avoided: Morphine
   - While historically used for its potent reduction of dyspneic symptoms, morphine is no longer recommended for routine management of flash pulmonary edema in decompensated heart failure [2]. On reflection, the lack of utility of opiates that decrease the respiratory drive is not surprising given the benefits we now appreciate from positive pressure ventilation.

- Morphine administration has been associated with increases in intubations and ICU admissions [27], worsening symptoms of dyspnea [28], and overall mortality [30]. Opiate administration for dyspnea should be avoided in decompensated failure

Case Conclusion

Both patients did very well with the strategies that were used.

In case 1, the patient was able to be weaned off of NIPPV, and the nitroglycerin was slowly titrated down. He was given doses of his regular medications and admitted for observation with the diagnosis of flash pulmonary edema. He was discharged the next day.

In case 2, the patient was weaned off of BiPAP and admitted to step-down. After 3 days of diuresis and medication adjustment, she was discharged home in good condition.

Discussion

Acute severe dyspnea with hypoxia has a wide range of etiologies, each with variable management required of EM physicians ranging from a chest tube for a tension pneumothorax to NIV and vasodilator infusions for flash pulmonary edema. Flash pulmonary edema from decompensated heart failure can present in patients without a history of CHF, and quick diagnosis with the use of clinical suspicion, an astute exam, and bedside ultrasound can allow for timely institution of positive-pressure ventilation to improve patient symptoms and hemodynamics.

Acute decompensated heart failure exists with a spectrum of presentations, from subacute volume overload needing only inpatient or outpatient diuresis to acute cardiogenic shock needing procedural intervention. Flash pulmonary edema from heart failure is the most common emergent presentation physicians will encounter, and they must be familiar with the need for ventilatory support and high-dose nitroglycerin for afterload reduction to take priority over aggressive diuresis.

The following is from the senior author's personal experience treating patients with flash pulmonary edema who have impending respiratory failure.

If you manage the flash pulmonary edema patient correctly and aggressively there is a very low chance that you will need to intubate. If you delay, hesitate or use techniques designed to manage garden-variety chronic heart failure the patient will end up on the ventilator or dead. **You should stand at the bedside until the initial sequence of orders is carried out and the patient is beginning to improve.** *Be ready to intubate if the patient won't tolerate the treatments or they tire out. By being very aggressive with medical therapy, I have only rarely had to intubate a flash pulmonary edema patient. I teach the mnemonic BONED! Bi-level Oxygen, Nitroglycerin, Enalapril, Diuretics/Dobutamine.*

- *The first drug is oxygen. It should be delivered by BiPAP. You should start at 10/5 and work your way quickly up to 15 or 20/10. If the normal intrathoracic pressure during breathing is -40 and his MAP is around 160, and then a transthoracic pressure gradient is around 200. This represents the difference between the pressure in the chest and the pressure in the rest of the body. It also represents a workload the heart has a work against to push blood forward. If you give somebody a positive pressure during BiPAP of around +10, the transthoracic pressure gradient drops to 150. A lower transthoracic pressure gradient means the heart can pump more efficiently in the "forward direction." Judicious use of small doses of midazolam (Versed®) or ketamine may facilitate the BiPAP and tone down the catecholamine release associated with the cocaine use. It may help in general with decreasing the catecholamine surge that can happen from the stress of the event.*
- *Nearly simultaneous to the BiPAP and prior to the respiratory therapist initiating the BiPAP, nitroglycerin needs to be given. Please note that the starting dose your nurses are familiar with is 10–20 mcgs per minute. **This is nowhere near the correct dose for flash pulmonary edema.** While you are waiting for the nitroglycerin drip to be started at around 100 mcgs per minute, you can give 2–4 sublingual nitroglycerin. Remember that this catecholamine-charged patient who is breathing dry, high-low oxygen will probably have a dry mouth and you might want to stick a few ice chips or some water under the patient's tongue with the nitroglycerin, so it actually dissolves. If you have nitroglycerin spray, that works even better because it doesn't require dissolving. A single sublingual dose of nitroglycerin contains 400 mcg. Since the bioavailability is around 40%, if you give one sublingual every 5 minutes, it delivers ~30 mcg/min (400 mcg × 40% is 160 mcg; 160 mcg over 5 minutes is 32 mcg/min). You should even consider putting 2 sublingual nitroglycerin at a time into the patient's mouth. (~60 mcg/min), and even up to 4.*
- *The minimum dose of nitroglycerin that you should start IV for flash pulmonary edema is 50 mcg per minute, but preferably 100 mcg/min). You should be aggressive and consider doubling this number very quickly in the course of the resuscitation. You can then double it again if needed. At lower doses, nitroglycerin is a pre-load reducing agent. At higher doses it acts as an afterload reducing agent also.*
- *An alternative "bolus approach" involves using IV NTG boluses. Nitroglycerin comes in a concentration of 200 mcg/ml or 400 mcg/ml. You can draw up a 1 mg (5 ml or 2.5 ml, depending on the concentration) into a syringe and deliver it as a bolus. This can be followed by a drip at 100 mcg/min*
  - *In the rare patient who is still hypertensive after very high doses of nitroglycerin, you can consider adding IV enalapril. The dose is 0.625 mg IV up to 2.5 mg IV. My personal experience is that you mostly don't need it, but if you do use it, you should start at the very low end and add more if needed. When I have used high doses of nitroglycerin + high doses of enalapril, I have made some patients hypotensive!*
- *The next step in this process is to think about using some diuretics. This is less effective in flash pulmonary edema when the total body volume of fluid is normal but maldistributed to the lungs instead of the rest of the circulation owing to high afterload.*

- *If you think that contractility is an issue and the patient is not responding to the other aggressively administered treatments, consider adding dobutamine to increase squeeze. Increasing the contractility of the heart while simultaneously causing some vasodilation is a good thing in some patients.*
- *Forget morphine! It doesn't help and likely harms!*

Pattern Recognition

Flash Pulmonary Edema
- Acutely hypertensive and severe dyspnea and hypoxia
- A history of CHF, with poor compliance
- Afterload-rising precipitants: stimulants, dehydration, and other illness

Disclosure Statement   Colin Kaide—Callibra, Inc.,-Discharge 123 medical software company. Medical Advisory Board Portola Pharmaceuticals. I have no relationship with a commercial company that has a direct financial interest in subject matter or materials discussed in article or with a company making a competing product.

Joshua Faucher—I have no disclosures.

References

1. Weintraub N, et al. Acute heart failure syndromes: emergency department presentation, treatment, and disposition: current approaches and future aims. Circulation. 2010;122:1975–96.
2. Long B, Koyfman A, Gottlieb M. Management of heart failure in the emergency department setting: an evidence-based review of the literature. J Emerg Med. 2018;55(5):635–46.
3. Cotter G, et al. The pathophysiology of acute heart failure – is it all about fluid accumulation? Am Heart J. 2008;155:9–18.
4. Roguin A, et al. Long-term prognosis of acute pulmonary oedema – an ominous outcome. Eur J Heart Fail. 2012;2(2):137–44.
5. Collins S, et al. Beyond pulmonary edema: diagnosis, risk stratificaition, and treatment challenges of acute heart failure management in the emergency department. Ann Emerg Med. 2008;51(1):45–57.
6. Rimoldi SF, et al. Flash pulmonary edema. Prog Cardiovasc Dis. 2009;52(3):249–59.
7. Messerli FH, et al. Flash pulmonary oedema and bilateral renal artery stenosis: the Pickering Syndrome. Eur Heart J. 2011;32:2231–7.
8. Cimen T, et al. Flash pulmonary edema: a rare cause and possible mechanisms. Turkish J Emerg Med. 2017;17:65–7.
9. Margulescu AD, et al. Cardiac adaptation in acute hypertensive pulmonary edema. Am J Cardiol. 2012;109:1472–81.
10. Lewin J, et al. Clinical deterioration in established heart failure: what is the value of BNP and weight gain in aiding diagnosis? Eur J Heart Fail. 2005;7:953–7.
11. Ware LB, Matthay MA. Acute pulmonary edema. N Engl J Med. 2005;353(26):2788–96.
12. Wang CS, et al. Does this dyspneic patient in the emergency department have congestive heart failure? JAMA. 2005;294(15):1944–56.

13. Schwam E. B-type natriuretic peptide for diagnosis of heart failure in emergency department patients: a critical appraisal. Acad Emerg Med. 2004;11(6):686–91.
14. Trinquart L, et al. Natriuretic peptide testing in EDs for managing acute dyspnea: a meta-analysis. Am J Emerg Med. 2011;29:757–67.
15. Ray P, et al. Differential diagnosis of acute dyspnea: the value of B natriuretic peptides in the emergency department. Q J Med. 2008;101:831–43.
16. Lam LL, et al. Meta-analysis: effect of B-type natriuretic peptide on clinical outcomes in patients with acute dyspnea in the emergency setting. Ann Intern Med. 2010;153:728–35.
17. Volpicelli G, et al. Bedside lung ultrasound in the assessment of alveolar-interstitial syndrome. Am J Emerg Med. 2006;24:689–96.
18. Pivetta E, et al. Lung ultrasound-implemented diagnosis of acute decompensated heart failure in the ED. Chest. 2015;148(1):202–10.
19. Anderson KL, et al. Diagnosing heart failure among acutely dyspneic patients with cardiac, inferior vena cava, and lung ultrasonography. Am J Emerg Med. 2013;31(8):1208–14.
20. Vital FMR, Ladeira MT, Atallah AN. Non-invasive positive pressure ventilation (CPAP or bilevel NPPV) for cardiogenic pulmonary oedema (Review). Cochrane Database Syst Rev. 2013;5:CD005351.
21. Pang D, et al. The effect of positive pressure airway support on mortality and the need for intubation in cardiogenic pulmonary edema. Chest. 1998;114(4):1185–92.
22. Gray A, et al. Noninvasive ventilation in acute cardiogenic pulmonary edema. N Engl J Med. 2008;359:142–51.
23. Yancy CW, et al. 2013 ACCF/AHA guideline for the management of heart failure: a report of the American College of Cardiology Foundation/American Heart Association Task Force on Practice Guidelines. J Am Coll Cardiol. 2013;62:e147–239.
24. Carlson MD, Eckman PM. Review of vasodilators in acute decompensated heart failure: the old and new. J Card Fail. 2013;19:478–93.
25. Cotter G, et al. Randomised trial of high dose isosorbide dinitrate plus low-dose furosemide versus highdose furosemide plus low-dose isosorbide dinitrate in severe pulmonary oedema. Lancet. 1998;351:389–93.
26. Levy, et al. Treatment of severe decompensated heart failure with high-dose intravenous nitroglycerin: a feasibility and outcome analysis. Ann Emerg Med. 2007;50(2):144–52.
27. Sacchetti A, et al. Effect of ED management on ICU use in acute pulmonary edema. Am J Emerg Med. 1999;17(6):571–4.
28. Hoffman JR, Reynolds S. Comparison of nitroglycerin, morphine, and furosemide in treatment of presumed pre-hospital pulmonary edema. Chest. 1987;92(4):586–93.
29. Peacock WF, et al. Morphine and outcomes in acute decompensated heart failure: an ADHERE analysis. Emerg Med J. 2008;25:205–9.
30. Masue Y, et al. Time-to-furosemide treatment and mortality in patients hospitalized with acute heart failure. J Am Coll Cardiol. 2017;69(25):3042–51.
31. Francis GS, et al. Acute vasoconstrictor response to intravenous furosemide in patients with chronic congestive heart failure. Ann Intern Med. 1985;103(1):1–6.
32. Butler J, et al. Relationship between heart failure treatment and development of worsening renal function among hospitalized patients. Am Heart J. 2004;147(2):331–8.

Guillain–Barré Syndrome: *"I May Be Weird, but I Still Can't Walk!"*

23

Travis Sharkey-Toppen and Colin G. Kaide

LEARNing Rounds

Learn, Evaluate, Adopt…Right Now!

Case

Tingling and Difficulty Walking

Pertinent History

This patient is a 26-year-old male who presents with progressive leg pain, numbness, and weakness. Starting a little over a week ago, the patient began having numbness and tingling in his left leg. This turned into painful tingling, which then progressed to involve the left fingertips. It spread to include his right leg and now right fingertips as well. It is painful but also feels very numb. He previously was active and states it took him 15 minutes to walk just from a store to the church next door where he sleeps at a homeless shelter. He reports getting a flu shot about 2 weeks ago and shortly after began developing coryza, cough, sore throat, and very foul-smelling diarrhea. He also endorses a couple spells of blurry vision in the past couple weeks that resolved on their own. He denies any fevers. He presented to another Columbus, Ohio, hospital yesterday and had a chest X-ray and head CT done, which he was told were negative and that there may be a psychogenic component to his symptoms. He felt he was being kicked out because he was homeless and had no insurance. He takes no medications except ibuprofen and acetaminophen recently to try to help the pain, which had no effect. He has a history of heroin use.

T. Sharkey-Toppen · C. G. Kaide (✉)
Department of Emergency Medicine, Wexner Medical Center at The Ohio State University, Columbus, OH, USA
e-mail: Colin.kaide@osumc.edu

© Springer Nature Switzerland AG 2020
C. G. Kaide, C. E. San Miguel (eds.), *Case Studies in Emergency Medicine*,
https://doi.org/10.1007/978-3-030-22445-5_23

Notes from Outside Hospital

Nursing Note

"The patient presents with numbness and tingling to the left side starting a few weeks ago. He states that yesterday it went into his right arm and fingertips. It feels like my body is asleep. He also complains of a stabbing left-sided chest pain that came on suddenly 2 days ago. He cannot relate specific activity to pain. He has associated shortness of breath with chest pain. Patient has pain behind his right calf. No redness or swelling. Palpable pulses noted. Patient ambulated with a limp complaining of numbness in his legs. He also states he gets muscle spasms and sometimes feels like he's going to fall over. He has no respiratory distress noted. He answers questions appropriately he has no facial droop or slurred speech. He admits to a history of heroin use but he has been clean for a long time."

Clinician Note

"This is a 26-year-old male with a history of heavy polysubstance drug abuse including meth, crack, heroin, alcohol who presents with body numbness. It started in his left leg like and felt it was going to sleep. The feeling has now progressed to his whole body on both sides. The patient also states that yesterday he had terrible chest pain that went on all day and brought him to his knees but today he hasn't had any. He has never had this before and has had no headaches or vision change. Physical exam findings showed the following: Alert and oriented to person place and time. Cranial nerves II through XII are intact. No motor deficits. No sensory deficits. No extremity tenderness. No edema. Mood and affect are normal. Remainder of exam is unremarkable."

Pertinent Physical Exam

Except as noted below, the findings of the complete physical exam are within normal limits.

- Neurologic Exam: He displays abnormal reflexes (no reflexes noted bilaterally in the lower extremities, even with distraction.
- He displays no atrophy.
- A sensory deficit is present as he reports decreased sensation to light touch in the left lower extremity up to hip; right lower extremity up to knee; fingertips feel numb bilaterally to light touch).
- No cranial nerve deficits, with II–XII intact.
- He exhibits abnormal muscle tone (strength 3/5 bilaterally in the hip flexors, 3/5 bilaterally biceps, triceps). I question this effort because during interview, gross strength appeared 4/5 if not normal.
- Gait (knees buckling, shuffling, nearly falling multiple times).
- Romberg positive (abnormal).
- Lungs: Clear bilaterally to auscultation.

PMH   Hypertension and diet-controlled type 2 diabetes mellitus.

SH   Smokes tobacco. History of heroin abuse, but clean for the last 4 years.

FH   No pertinent history.

Pertinent Test Results

Lumbar puncture results			
Test	Result	Units	Normal values
Glucose	66	mg/dL	40–80 mg/dL or < 40% of simultaneously measured plasma level if that plasma level is abnormal
Protein	140	mg/dL	15–60 mg/dL
WBCs	1	Leukocyte/mcL	0–5 leukocytes/mcL
RBCs	0	RBC/mcL	0–10 erythrocytes/mcL

Toxicology Results: Positive for cotinine (nicotine metabolites)
Thyroid studies: Within normal limits
CBC: Within normal limits
Chem 7: Within normal limits
Immunology: Hepatitis C positive (later result)

ED Management

Updates on ED Course
When attempting to ambulate the patient, he fell to his knees and was unable to stand on his own afterwards. Given concerns for ascending areflexia, numbness, and painful tingling with associated weakness demonstrated on examination, the differential diagnosis highly favored Guillain–Barré Syndrome (GBS) and also included multiple sclerosis, transverse myelitis, and (less likely) psychomotor/conversion disorder.

Learning Points

Priming Questions
1. What key features of Guillain–Barré syndrome should increase suspicion for GBS, and which should make you consider alternative diagnoses?
2. How is the diagnosis made and what role do CSF studies play in the diagnosis?
3. What is the expected progression of disease and anticipatory guidance we should be giving our patients who are going to be admitted for GBS?

Introduction/Background

1. Basic Epidemiology [1, 2]
   - Occurs at the rate of nearly one to two cases per 10,000 person years.
   - Men:women ratio is 2:1
   - Two-thirds of cases are preceded by URI symptoms or diarrhea [3].
     - Thirty percent are associated with *Campylobacter jejuni*.
     - Ten percent are associated with CMV.
     - Other known associations are with Epstein-Barr virus, varicella-zoster virus, and *Mycoplasma pneumoniae*.
   - There are fairly recent cases of GBS associated with peginterferon (PEG) therapy for Hep C, as well as neuropathies with Hep C [4, 5].
2. According to data from the 2009 Pandemic of Influenza A (H1N1), some studies demonstrated an increased risk of GBS after vaccination. However, given the rarity of the diagnosis itself, it is difficult to interpret the precise risk the vaccine has on the population. This mainly occurred in older patients [6].

Physiology/Pathophysiology

1. Cross reactivity between neural antigens and antibodies to specific infectious agents is believed to be the cause of the inflammatory neuropathy. This causes multifocal mononuclear cell infiltration in peripheral nerves causing segmental demyelination, often causing secondary axonal degeneration. This is seen in spinal nerve roots as well as in large and small motor and sensory nerves [1].
2. There are demyelinating and axonal subtypes – acute inflammatory demyelinating polyneuropathy and acute motor axonal neuropathy. The classification is based on nerve conduction studies. The details of this are too in-depth for this review.
3. Prognosis is variable and difficult to predict for any given individual [1, 2].
   - Three to five percent of patients with GBS die, usually from medical complications such as sepsis, pulmonary emboli, or unexplained cardiac arrest possibly related to dysautonomia.
   - GBS symptoms progress for up to 1–3 weeks after the onset of symptoms.
   - Two-thirds of patients are unable to walk independently when maximum weakness is reached.
   - Respiratory insufficiency occurs in 25% of patients, and major complications including pneumonia, sepsis, pulmonary embolism, and gastrointestinal bleeding develop in 60% of intubated patients.
   - Among severely affected patients, 20% remain unable to walk 6 months after the onset of symptoms.
4. Serious and potentially fatal autonomic dysfunction occurs in 20% of patients with GBS [1, 2]. Symptoms include:
   - Arrhythmia.
   - Labile BPs with hypertension or hypotension.
   - Bradycardia may be so marked that it can cause asystole.

Making the Diagnosis

Differential Diagnosis
- Guillain–Barré Syndrome, including variants (Miller Fisher)
- Botulism
- Acute flaccid paralysis from a spinal cord injury
- Hypokalemia with hypokalemic paralysis
- Infectious myelitis such as poliomyelitis
- Multiple sclerosis (transverse myelitis)
- Myasthenia gravis

1. The hallmark presentation of Guillain–Barré syndrome is relatively symmetric, progressive, ascending motor weakness, which progresses over 12 hours to as long as 28 days [7]. Other common associated symptoms include:
   - Paresthesia and pain in the affected limbs. The presence of distal paresthesias makes the diagnosis of GBS more likely!
     - *The **absence** of paresthesias should suggest other diagnoses such as hypokalemia, botulism, or myasthenia gravis.*
   - Areflexia or hyporeflexia in affected areas.
     - Normal reflexes may be present in up to 10% of patients.
   - History of URI symptoms or diarrhea 3 days to 6 weeks prior to onset of neurological symptoms.
   - Late symptoms can include respiratory difficulty, typically presenting in about 25% of patients, but usually manifests after hospitalization.
   - If the CNS is involved, symptoms can manifest as vivid dreams, hallucinations, or psychosis.
     - In one study, this was reported to happen in one-third of patients.
2. The Brighton criteria were developed as a diagnostic tool to identify a level of certainty for the diagnosis of GBS, including physical and laboratory findings [7].
   - Bilateral and flaccid weakness of limbs.
   - Decreased or absent deep tendon reflexes in weak limbs.
   - Monophasic course with the time between onset and nadir being 12 hours to 28 days.
   - CSF WBC count <50 cells/mL.
   - CSF protein concentration > normal value.
   - Nerve conduction findings consistent with one of the subtypes of GBS.
   - Absence of alternative diagnosis for weakness.
3. The common teaching is that the patient will have "albuminocytologic dissociation" (high CSF protein in the absence of WBCs). In reality, this finding is unreliable, as it is present in only 50% of patients by the first week of symptoms and expected to rise to only up to 88% after week 2 [7].
4. Nerve conduction studies can be helpful to confirm the diagnosis [7].

5. There are subtypes of GBS that can involve specific nerves and muscle groups. The Miller Fisher variant affects the head and neck and has abnormal muscle coordination and paralysis of the eye muscles and absence of tendon reflexes. Most patients have complete recovery [1]
   - Rare (3% of GBS cases in the United States)
   - Bilateral ophthalmoplegia
   - Ataxia
   - Areflexia
   - Facial, bulbar weakness occurs in 50% of cases
Trunk, extremity weakness occurs in 50% of cases

Treating the Patient

1. General care to prevent pulmonary embolism, super-infections, and other complications.
2. Vigilance for the need to intubate if the patient's respiratory status deteriorates.
   - You can measure a NIF to help investigate diaphragmatic strength.
   - You can watch for difficulty handling secretions.
3. Pain control: Opioids, gabapentin, or carbamazepine may help.
4. Plasma exchange (PLEX) removes offending antibodies and causes improvement in symptoms.
5. Immunotherapy with IVIG is as effective as PLEX and has replaced PLEX in many cases.
6. The combination of PLEX and IVIG is *not* more effective than either one alone.

Case Conclusion

Despite IVIG therapies, the patient's symptoms did progress to diaphragmatic weakness, respiratory failure, and intubation. His course was complicated by presumed pneumonia. He was treated with antibiotics. He eventually regained strength compatible with extubation. He was then transferred to a step-down unit and finally to the floor. He was discharged home with plans for outpatient rehab therapy for minor neurological deficits. In final follow-up, he made a full recovery.

Discussion

Given the lack of sensitivity of lumbar puncture studies for GBS, especially early on or in the acute setting, this is primarily a clinical diagnosis. This is a diagnosis that is very hard to make early in the course unless you are thinking about it. It can only be made with a high level of suspicion and identification of key features in history and physical examination as described above. It is not uncommon to have patients presenting after multiple visits either for past infectious symptoms preceding neurological symptoms or for worsening progression of the disease.

Do not forget to overlook other diagnoses as discussed, especially those which have easily reversible causes such as hypokalemia.

Pattern Recognition

- Ascending paralysis
- Pain and paresthesias (almost always seen in GBS).
- Albuminocytologic dissociation (may be seen in only 50% of cases of early GBS).
- Autonomic dysfunction (dangerous and can cause rapid BP swings, profound bradycardia, and arrhythmias).
- Symptoms preceded by a URI or diarrhea (two-thirds of cases).
- The Miller Fisher Syndrome involves primarily the head and neck, along with muscular incoordination, bulbar paralysis, and areflexia.

Disclosure Statement Travis Sharkey-Toppin: No disclosures.

Colin Kaide: Callibra, Inc.-Discharge 123 medical software company. Medical Advisory Board Portola Pharmaceuticals. I have no relationship with a commercial company that has a direct financial interest in subject matter or materials discussed in article or with a company making a competing product.

References

1. Walling AD, Dickson G. Guillain-Barre syndrome. Am Fam Physician. 2013;87:191–7.
2. Yuki N, Hartung H. Guillain-Barre syndrome. NEJM. 2012;366:2294–304.
3. Sejvar JJ, Baughman AL, Wise M, Morgan OW. Population incidence of Guillain-Barré syndrome: a systematic review and meta-analysis. Neuroepidemiology. 2011;36(2):123–33.
4. Vigani AG, Macedo-de-Oliveira A, Pavan MH, Pedro MN, Goncales FL. Hepatitis C virus infection, cryoglobulinemia, and peripheral neuropathy: a case report. Braz J Med Biol Res. 2005;38:1729–34.
5. Marzo ME, Tintore M, Fabregues O, Montalban X, Codina A. Chronic inflammatory demyelinating polyneuropathy during treatment with interferon-alpha. J Neurol Neurosurg Psychiatry. 1998;65:604.
6. Vellozi C, Igbal S, Broder K. Guillain-Barre syndrome, influenza, and influenza vaccination: the epidemiologic evidence. Clin Infect Dis. 2014;58(8):1149–55.
7. Fokke C, van den Berg B, Drenthen J, Walgaard C, van Doom PA, Jacobs BC. Diagnosis of Guillain-Barre syndrome and validation of Brighton criteria. Brain. 2014;137:33–43.

HELLP Syndrome: *"I Need Somebody HELLP, Not Just Anybody…"*

24

Yuxuan (Tony) Qiu and Simiao Li-Sauerwine

Case

Pregnant, Hypertensive, and in Pain

Pertinent History

A 32-y/o G4P3 EGA 33-week patient presented to the ED with 3 days of epigastric discomfort, malaise, and nausea. She recently moved to the area and had no documented OB visits for this pregnancy but stated that her last three pregnancies were unremarkable. Her pain in the epigastric region, dull and nonradiating, had been getting worse. She reported that her nausea did not resolve with ondansetron at home. She denied other GI symptoms. She tolerated oral fluids this morning. She reported mild headache for the last 2 days and denied neck pain, trauma, fever, photophobia, or weakness.

Pertinent Physical Exam

Except as noted below, the findings of the complete physical exam are within normal limits.

- Vitals: HR 92 beats per minute, BP 132/90 mmHg, RR 22, SaO_2 96% on RA, afebrile.
- General: Sitting in bed, appears uncomfortable.
- Cardiac, pulmonary, and neurological exams were unremarkable.
- Abdominal exam showed normal BS, tenderness in epigastrium and RUQ, negative Murphy's sign, and no rebound or guarding.
- Generalized edema is noted.
- Fetal heart tones on Doppler were within normal limits.

Y.(T.) Qiu (✉) · S. Li-Sauerwine
Department of Emergency Medicine, Wexner Medical Center at The Ohio State University, Columbus, OH, USA
e-mail: yuxuan.qiu@osumc.edu; simiao.li-sauerwine@osumc.edu

© Springer Nature Switzerland AG 2020   247
C. G. Kaide, C. E. San Miguel (eds.), *Case Studies in Emergency Medicine*,
https://doi.org/10.1007/978-3-030-22445-5_24

PMH GERD, iron-deficiency anemia, G4P3000

SH Denies use of alcohol, tobacco, and other recreational drugs

FH Hypertension in both mother and father

Pertinent Test Results

Test	Result	Units	Normal range
WBC	12.3	K/μL	3.8–11.0 10^3/mm^3
Hgb	11	g/dL	(Male) 14–18 g/dL
			(Female) 11–16 g/dL
Platelets	45	K/μL	140–450 K/μL
Sodium	140	mEq/L	135–148 mEq/L
Potassium	4.9	mEq/L	3.5–5.5 mEq/L
Chloride	103	mEq/L	96–112 mEq/L
Bicarbonate	24	mEq/L	21–34 mEq/L
BUN	20	mg/dL	6–23 mg/dL
Creatinine	1.85	mg/dL	0.6–1.5 mg/dL
Glucose	98	mg/dL	65–99 mg/dL
ALT	140	IU/L	8–32 IU/L
AST	160	IU/L	6–21 IU/L
Alk Phos	88	IU/L	32–110 IU/L
Total Bili	1.3	mg/dL	0.2–1.4 mg/dL
INR	1.0	–	≤1.1
LDH	1586	U/L	50–150 U/L

Urine protein/SCr: 0.8∗
(∗Ratio < 0.15 is normal, > 0.7 is significant proteinuria, in between warrants 240 h urine collection to quantify proteinuria)
UA: 2+ protein

Emergency Department Management

High-flow O_2 was initiated with improvement of SpO_2 to 100%; 2 units of platelets was given in anticipation of C-section, and the repeat platelet count was 75 K/μL. Antihypertensive medications were held due to consistent SBP < 150 mmHg. Six grams of magnesium sulfate were given, followed by a 2 g/h infusion. OB was consulted emergently.

Updates on ED Course

OB evaluated the patient and recommended immediate delivery. OB anesthesia was consulted for neuro-axial anesthesia and epidural was inserted. The patient was taken emergently to the OR for C-section.

Learning Points

Priming Questions
1. At what stages of pregnancy can HELLP present?
2. In terms of pathophysiology, how is HELLP different from pre-eclampsia or eclampsia, and from TTP/HUS?
3. What treatment of HELLP should be initiated in the ED?

Introduction/Background

1. Hemolysis, elevated liver enzymes, low platelet (HELLP) syndrome is considered a severe clinical variant of pre-eclampsia [1]. It is associated with significant maternal morbidity and mortality.
   - Diagnosis of HELLP requires all three components, but having all three components is associated with higher rate of complications.
   - Partial HELLP contains one or two components of H/EL/LP.
   - HELLP is often misdiagnosed at initial presentation.
2. HELLP can occur at any time from 20 weeks of pregnancy to postpartum period (30% of all HELLP) [2]. While the critical period for developing post-partum eclampsia is the first week after delivery, postpartum pre-eclampsia can occur from 2 days to 6 weeks after delivery [3]. While HELLP occurs in 0.5–0.9% of all pregnancies, 10–20% of all HELLP cases occur with patients with severe pre-eclampsia [1].
3. Risk factors for HELLP syndrome are slightly different from those of pre-eclampsia. They include multi-parity, advanced maternal age, Caucasian race, and previous history of pre-eclampsia or HELLP syndrome. Additionally, some studies have shown an association between antiphospholipid antibody syndrome and early-onset HELLP [4, 5].

Physiology/Pathophysiology

1. While some consider HELLP as a clinical variant of pre-eclampsia, 10–20% can present without hypertension or preceding proteinuria.
2. The pathophysiology of HELLP is mainly unknown, but its presentation may be related to the pathogenesis seen in pre-eclampsia as well as the consequent thrombotic microangiopathies.
3. H and LP: Maternal factors and certain genetic mutations induce the placenta to release bioactive substances that lead to endothelial dysfunction and activation of the complement system and the coagulation cascade. Similar to thrombotic microangiopathy, endothelial cells release von Willebrand Factor, leading to platelet aggregation and endothelial microthrombi formation, which explains the classic microangiopathic hemolytic anemia (MAHA) feature of HELLP.

4. EL: The bioactive substances and the hemolytic microangiopathy can both cause hepatocellular damage. Some speculate that elevated liver enzymes are due to fibrin deposits in sinusoid obstructing hepatic flow. This may explain the hepatic hemorrhage and necrosis seen in HELLP complications [5].
5. Additionally, the direct glomerular endothelial damage from bioactive substances and arterial hypertension may contribute to proteinuria [4, 6].

Making the Diagnosis

Differential Diagnosis
- *Hematologic: Thrombotic Thrombocytopenia Purpura* (TTP), Hemolytic Uremic Syndrome (HUS), idiopathic thrombocytopenia purpura (ITP)
- *GI*: Hepatitis, cholangitis, cholecystitis, pancreatitis, gastritis
- *Renal*: Pyelonephritis
- *Pregnancy-related complications*: Acute fatty liver of pregnancy, benign thrombocytopenia of pregnancy
- *Others: Systemic lupus erythematosus* (SLE), antiphospholipid syndrome, and hemorrhagic or septic shock

1. Clinical presentation: peak presentation between the 27th and 37th EGA, although HELLP can occur postpartum.
   - The course of the illness can be progressive or lead suddenly to maternal–fetal deterioration [7].
   - Classic signs and symptoms that are "red flags" for HELLP include right upper quadrant (RUQ)/epigastric pain, N/V, and headache/visual symptoms. It is important to note that hypertension and proteinuria are absent in 10–20% of all cases [1].
   - Often the presentation can be vague. Other symptoms that should raise your suspicion include flu-like presentation, malaise, excessive weight gain, and generalized edema [1].
   - Past history that should raise clinical suspicion includes previous pre-eclampsia, previous HELLP, and multiparity.
2. ED evaluation should include CBC, smear, LFTs, bilirubin, LDH, urine protein or protein:SCr ratio, uric acid, and coagulation panel.
3. There are different diagnostic classifications for HELLP syndrome [1]. The main laboratory abnormalities are categorized into hematologic and hepatic abnormalities [8].
   - Hematologic abnormalities (Fig. 24.1): Platelet ≤100,000–150,000 cells/μL, labs suggestive of microangiopathic hemolytic anemia (LDH ≥ 600 U/L, schistocytes on smear, haptoglobin <25), abnormal coagulation panel.
   - Hepatic abnormalities: AST or ALT >70, total bilirubin >1.2 mg/dL.

Fig. 24.1 Schistocytes on Peripheral Smear. (By Erhabor Osaro (Associate Professor) – Own work, CC BY-SA 3.0, https://commons.wikimedia.org/w/index.php?curid=32131623)

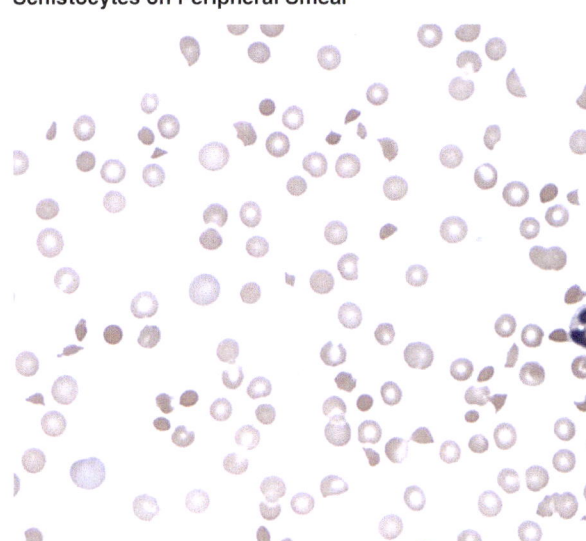

Schistocytes on Peripheral Smear

Treating the Patient

1. Initial stabilization in the ED for patients with HELLP is similar to treatments for pre-eclampsia. ABCs, IV magnesium, BP control, reversal of coagulopathy, and definitive OB management are the mainstay treatments. An "ABCDEF" approach is outlined below:
   - Airway:
     - Airway anatomy changes during pregnancy: (1) anterior displacement of larynx, (2) increased laryngeal edema [9], and (3) further upper airway narrowing associated with pre-eclampsia in small studies (potentially complicating intubation) [10].
     - Failed intubation is more common and has greater consequences in pregnant patients. Difficult airway should be anticipated [11, 12].
     - High-flow O$_2$ should be used early to avoid fetal hypoxia and maternal hypoxemia.
     - Neuromuscular blockade agents can be used in conventional doses without significant transplacental passage [9].
     - The choice of induction agents should be based on maternal hemodynamic status.
   - Breathing: Anatomical changes of pregnant women alter physiological reserve.
     - Due to gravid uterus and increased intra-abdominal pressure, pregnant women have decreased functional residual capacity and chest wall compliance. They also have an increased risk for aspiration.
     - Antiemetics and early intubation are recommended.

- Circulation: BP control and reversal of coagulopathy and thrombocytopenia are important.
  - If the patient is hypertensive, the approach is the same as that for treating hypertension in pre-eclampsia.

Drugs to Treat Hypertension in Pre-eclampsia			
	Agent	Initial dose	Repeat dose
First line	IV Labetalol	20 mg over 2 min	20–80 mg q10–30 min (max 300 mg)
	IV Hydralazine	5 mg over 2 min	5–10 mg q 20 min
Alternative	PO Nifedipine	10–20 mg	10–20 mg q 30 min (max 50 mg in 1 h)
Goal BP: <160/105 mmHg			

  - IV labetalol or IV hydralazine are great first-line therapies with PO nifedipine as an alternative.
- IV labetalol 20 mg over 2 min can be given initially, followed by 10–30 min interval doses of 20–80 mg (maximum 300 mg).
- Hydralazine can be given as 5 mg IV over 1–2 min with repeat doses of 5–10 mg after 20 min (maximum 20 mg).
- Immediate-release nifedipine is an oral agent with typical dose of 10–20 mg, which can be repeated in 30 min up to 50 mg in 1 h.
  - The ideal BP goal should be <160/105 mmHg.
- Disability: Administer IV magnesium sulfate for fetal neuroprotection and maternal seizure prophylaxis.
  - Similar to treating pre-eclampsia, a loading dose of 4–6 g over 15–20 min of IV magnesium sulfate should be administered, followed by 1–2 g/h infusion with hourly assessment for magnesium toxicity.
  - Magnesium toxicity can cause weakness, areflexia, visual disturbance, or pulmonary edema. The antidote is calcium, which can be used in patients experiencing significant cardiopulmonary compromise.
- ED characteristics: It is ideal to bring OB and pediatric colleagues to the bedside immediately. If the patient presented to a community hospital without OB service, stabilization discussed in this section must be performed before transferring to definitive OB care.
- Fetal consideration: Fetal monitoring should commence as soon as possible. Regardless of the gestational age, for women with HELLP, immediate delivery is warranted.
2. OB management of patients
- The only definitive treatment for HELLP is delivery.
- There have been controversies on the usage of corticosteroids for HELLP. Randomized controlled trial provided no evidence of improved maternal/fetal outcome, although there may be some benefit of increased platelet count [7, 13]. However, delivery should not be delayed for steroid administration.
- For women with EGA ≤ 24 weeks or ≥ 34 weeks, the recommendation is for immediate delivery after stabilization.

- For women with EGA between 24 and 34 weeks, some have advocated for delaying delivery for 24–48 h in order to complete a course of corticosteroid for fetal considerations if the maternal–fetal condition is stable. However, the evidence for such practice is not robust, and the risk of complications from HELLP significantly outweighs the theoretical benefit of corticosteroid [1, 7].

3. Complications of HELLP [1, 2]
   - The most common complications include *eclampsia, abruptio placentae*, disseminated intravascular coagulation (*DIC*), postpartum bleeding, acute renal failure secondary to MAHA, and pulmonary edema.
     - Platelet transfusion is warranted for patients with thrombocytopenia and active bleeding. It has also been shown that patients with intrapartum platelet count <40,000 cells/μL are associated with increased risk of postpartum bleeding. However, the same retrospective study suggested that prophylactic platelet transfusion does not significantly reduce the risk of postpartum hemorrhage [14].
   - Hepatic complications are rare: *Subcapsular liver hematoma with possible rupture* is life threatening. Liver infarction and hepatic vein thrombosis are also possible.
     - Neurological and ophthalmologic complications include retinal detachment and cerebral hemorrhage and infarction.
     - Neonatal complications include intrauterine growth restriction (IUGR), preterm delivery, thrombocytopenia, and respiratory distress syndrome (RDS).

4. Special considerations in communities without OB service.
   - Given the high maternal and fetal morbidity, the most ideal disposition is a hospital with maternal–fetal medicine specialists and NICU capacity.
   - Transferring the patients to appropriate tertiary care center should be initiated early, and communication with the receiving provider should occur at the same time as ED stabilization. Timely transfer for delivery should occur immediately after initial stabilization.

Case Conclusion

The patient was stabilized in the ED and the on-call maternal–fetal medicine specialist performed a C-section. The patient did not have significant bleeding and recovered without complications. The baby was delivered prematurely at 33 weeks of gestation and admitted to NICU for prematurity. After an uneventful NICU stay, the baby was discharged home to her parents.

Discussion

The clinical course can deteriorate rapidly for patients with HELLP. In any patient between EGA 20 weeks to postpartum, a low threshold to assess for HELLP syndrome is necessary.

Evaluation of HELLP includes basic HELLP labs and early communication with OB. If a transfer to a tertiary care center is necessary, transport should be arranged with OB and NICU of the receiving hospital as early as possible.

Although there have been discussions on benefit versus harm of early delivery between 24 and 34 weeks, the risk of maternal deterioration without prompt delivery outweighs the weak evidence of using corticosteroids. Delivery and definitive management of HELLP should not be delayed.

Pattern Recognition

- A pregnant patient after 20 weeks of gestation or in the postpartum period (2 days to 6 weeks) with the features given below:
- Progressively worsening or rapid deterioration
- Abdominal pain, edema, neurological symptoms, and/or hypertension
- All three features of H/EL/LP may not be present

Disclosure Statement   The authors of this chapter report no significant disclosures.

References

1. Haram K, Abildgaard U, et al. The HELLP syndrome: clinical issues and management. A review. BMC Pregnancy Childbirth. 2009;9:8.
2. Sibai BM, Friedman SA, et al. Maternal morbidity and mortality in 442 pregnancies with hemolysis, elevated liver enzymes, and low platelets (HELLP syndrome). Am J Obstet Gynecol. 1993;169(4):1000–6.
3. Al-Safi Z, et al. Delayed postpartum preeclampsia and eclampsia: demographics, clinical course and complications. Obstet Gynecol. 2011;118(5):1102–7.
4. Abildgaard U, Heimdal K. Pathogenesis of the syndrome of hemolysis, elevated liver enzymes, and low platelet count (HELLP): a review. Eur J Obstet Gynecol Reprod Biol. 2013;166(2):117–23.
5. Padden M O'h. HELLP syndrome: recognition and perinatal management. Am Fam Phys. 1999;60(3):829–36.
6. Kappler S, Graham A, et al. Thrombotic microangiopathies (TTP, HUS, HELLP). Hematol Oncol Clin North Am. 2017;31(6):1081–103.
7. The American College of Obstetricians and Gynecologists. Hypertension in pregnancy. Task Force and Work Group Report. 2013.
8. Tintinalli JE, et al. Tintinalli's emergency medicine a comprehensive study guide. 8th ed. New York: McGraw-Hill; 2016.
9. Bouchard S. Trauma in the obstetric patient: a bedside tool. ACEP Now. July 1 2010. https://www.acepnow.com/article/trauma-obstetric-patient-bedside-tool/.
10. Izci B, Douglas NJ, et al. The upper airway in pregnancy and pre-eclampsia. Am J Respir Crit Care Med. 2003;167(2):137.

11. McDonnell NJ, et al. Difficult and failed intubation in obstetric anesthesia: an observational study of airway management and complications associated with general anaesthesia for cae-sarean section. Int J Obstet Anesth. 2008;17(4):292–7.
12. Barnardo PD, et al. Failed tracheal intubation in obstetrics: a 6-year review in a UK region. Anaesthesia. 2000;55(7):690–4.
13. Woudstra DM, Dowswell T et al. Corticosteroid for HELLP syndrome in pregnancy. Cochcrane Database Syst Rev. 2010.
14. Robert WE, Martin JN Jr, et al. The intrapartum platelet count in patients with HELLP (hemo-lysis, elevated liver enzyme, and low platelet) syndrome: is it predictive of later hemorrhagic complications? Am J Obstet Gynecol. 1994;171(3):799–804.

Hemolytic Uremic Syndrome: *Another FAT RN?*

25

Seth Klein and Colin G. Kaide

Case 1

Bad Burger-Barn

Pertinent History

A 23-year-old male presents with complaints of abdominal pain and diarrhea. His symptoms started 5 days ago. He began to notice some blood in his stool not only on the toilet paper but also in the toilet. He complains of significant cramping and a low-grade fever up to 100.5 °F for a few days. He was seen in an urgent care 2 days ago and received a single dose of levofloxacin for persistent diarrhea. Since then, the diarrhea had become a bit worse. He complains of associated fatigue, lightheadedness, and dizziness. He reported decreased appetite despite his attempt to eat. He denies any other symptoms at this time. He said his girlfriend had similar symptoms but improved significantly after a few days.

PMH Type 1 diabetes mellitus (T1DM)–well controlled

SH No tobacco, recreational alcohol, or drug use

FH T1DM, HTN

S. Klein · C. G. Kaide (✉)
Department of Emergency Medicine, Wexner Medical Center at The Ohio State University, Columbus, OH, USA
e-mail: Seth.klein2@osumc.edu; Colin.kaide@osumc.edu

© Springer Nature Switzerland AG 2020
C. G. Kaide, C. E. San Miguel (eds.), *Case Studies in Emergency Medicine*,
https://doi.org/10.1007/978-3-030-22445-5_25

Pertinent Physical Exam

- Vital Signs: BP 160/95 mmHg, HR 110 beats per minute, Temp 99.4 °F (37.4 °C), RR 18

Except as noted below, the findings of the complete physical exam are within normal limits.

- General: Ill-appearing male who appears uncomfortable.
- Abdomen: Soft with diffuse tenderness and mild guarding. No rebound.
- Rectal Exam: Grossly bloody stool noted
- Skin: Pale appearing but warm and dry. No rash noted.

Pertinent Diagnostic Testing

Test	Result	Units	Normal range
WBC	11.7 ↑	K/μL	3.8–11.0 10³ cells/ mm³
Hgb	10.1 ↓	g/dL	(Male) 14–18 g/dL
			(Female) 11–16 g/dL
Platelets	68 ↓	K/μL	140–450 K/μL
Sodium	143	mEq/L	135–148 mEq/L
Potassium	4.9	mEq/L	3.5–5.5 mEq/L
Chloride	110	mEq/L	96–112 mEq/L
Bicarbonate	22	mEq/L	21–34 mEq/L
BUN	65 ↑	mg/dL	6–23 mg/dL
Creatinine	4.3 ↑	mg/dL	0.6–1.5 mg/dL
Glucose	231 ↑	mg/dL	65–99 mg/dL
ALT	45 ↑	IU/L	8–32 IU/L
AST	36 ↑	IU/L	6–21 IU/L
Alk Phos	88	IU/L	32–110 IU/L
Albumin	4.0	g/dL	3.5–5.0 g/dL
Total Bili	5.1 ↑	mg/dL	0.2–1.4 mg/dL
Direct Bili	1.1 ↑	mg/dL	0.0–0.4 mg/dL
INR	1.1	–	≤1.1
PTT	28 s	seconds	21–35 s

Emergency Department Course

The patient appeared dehydrated and received 2 L of normal saline. When the initial labs returned showing thrombocytopenia, low hemoglobin, and renal failure, suspicion was raised for thrombotic thrombocytopenic purpura (TTP) or HUS. Additional questions were asked regarding possible food exposures for the diarrhea and patient recalled eating at a "farmer's market" hamburger stand that advertised locally grown beef, processed on site. He and his girlfriend both ate hamburgers from the vendor. Additional testing was done showing the following results.

Test	Result	Units	Normal range
LDH	1586	U/L	50–150 U/L
Haptoglobin	<30	mg/dL	30–200 mg/dL

Update 1

An internal medicine resident, rotating in the ED, volunteered to look at the peripheral smear since there was no pathologist on call to verify a manual differential on the CBC. The findings are given below.

Schistocytes on Peripheral Smear

Image courtesy of Colin Kaide, MD. (Published with kind permission of © Colin G. Kaide 2019. All Rights Reserved)

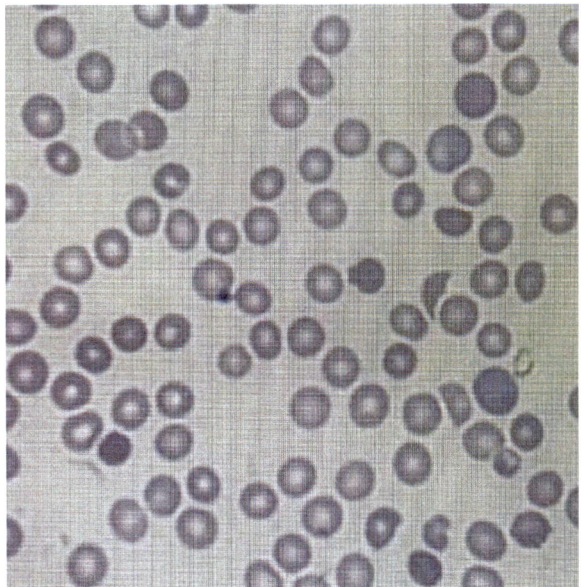

Update 2

Given the findings of thrombocytopenia, hemolytic anemia with schistocytes (microangiopathic hemolytic anemia), and new renal failure, presumptive diagnosis of hemolytic uremic syndrome was given. The bloody diarrhea in conjunction with HUS suggested a shiga toxin–producing bacteria as the cause. Stool was sent for shiga toxin assay and culture.

Case 2

Pertinent History

A 21-year-old female presents with nausea and vomiting. She states she has not been feeling well for the last few days and threw up seven times yesterday and two times this morning. The vomit was nonbilious. She has not been able to eat or drink. Patient does not remember eating anything that triggered her nausea. Patient denies pain but does complain of stomach cramps. She also had watery diarrhea prior to her current symptoms one to two times over the past 4 days. She noticed new "red dotted" rashes over her chest and extremities. She denies any known sick exposures but was around a lot of people at an outdoor festival 5 days ago. She denies eating anything unusual recently. She started taking birthcontrol pills 2 months ago but did not have any other new medications, recent travel, or animal exposure. She is not sexually active and has never had any STIs. She has never done recreational drugs and does not have any tattoos. She denies personal or family history of known hematological processes.

- PMH: Asthma, migraines
- SH: No tobacco or drug use. Social drinker of alcohol.
- FH: Breast cancer in her maternal grandmother. Prostate cancer in her father. Thyroid cancer in her paternal grandmother.

Pertinent Physical Exam

- Vital Signs: BP 157/87 mmHg, HR 95 beats per minute, Temp 98.1 °F (36.7 °C), RR 18

Except as noted below, the findings of the complete physical exam are within normal limits.

- General: Oriented to person, place, and time. Appears well developed and well nourished. No distress.
- Cardiovascular: Normal rate, rhythm, and heart sounds.
- Pulmonary/Chest: Effort and breath sounds normal.
- Abdominal: Soft. No distension or mass. No tenderness. Hypoactive bowel sounds.
- Musculoskeletal: Normal range of motion. No edema or deformity.
- Neurological: Alert and oriented to person, place, and time.
- Skin: Warm and dry. Petechiae over chest/stomach/back/extremities.

Diagnostic Studies

Test	Result	Units	Normal range
WBC	10.2	K/µL	3.8–11.0 10^3 cells/mm^3
Hgb	8.8 ↓	g/dL	(Male) 14–18 g/dL
			(Female) 11–16 g/dL
Platelets	35 ↓	K/µL	140–450 K/µL
Sodium	136	mEq/L	135–148 mEq/L
Potassium	4.4	mEq/L	3.5–5.5 mEq/L
Chloride	104	mEq/L	96–112 mEq/L
Bicarbonate	20 ↓	mEq/L	21–34 mEq/L
BUN	69 ↑	mg/dL	6–23 mg/dL
Creatinine	5.0 ↑	mg/dL	0.6–1.5 mg/dL
Glucose	105 ↑	mg/dL	65–99 mg/dL
ALT	19	IU/L	8–32 IU/L
AST	46 ↑	IU/L	6–21 IU/L
Alk Phos	37	IU/L	32–110 IU/L
Albumin	3.5	g/dL	3.5–5.0 g/dL
Total Bili	2.5 ↑	mg/dL	0.2–1.4 mg/dL
Direct Bili	0.5 ↑	mg/dL	0.0–0.4 mg/dL
INR	1.1	–	≤1.1
PTT	28 s	seconds	21–35 s
HcG	Negative	–	Negative
LDH	1629 ↑	U/L	50–150 U/L
Haptoglobin	< 30 ↑	g/dL	30–200 mg/dL

Emergency Department Course

The patient's lab work showed thrombocytopenia, anemia, and acute renal failure. She had no neurological symptoms or fever. All these symptoms were suspicious for HUS or possibly TTP. Given her history of GI illness with diarrhea, concern for shiga toxin–producing organism as the cause of HUS was high. Stool studies were sent, and the patient was admitted to hematology service.

Update 1

The peripheral smear was reported to contain schistocytes. The presumptive diagnosis was HUS.

Image 1 Schistocytes on peripheral smear

Image courtesy of Nicholas Nowacki, MD. (Published with kind permission of © Colin G. Kaide 2019. All Rights Reserved)

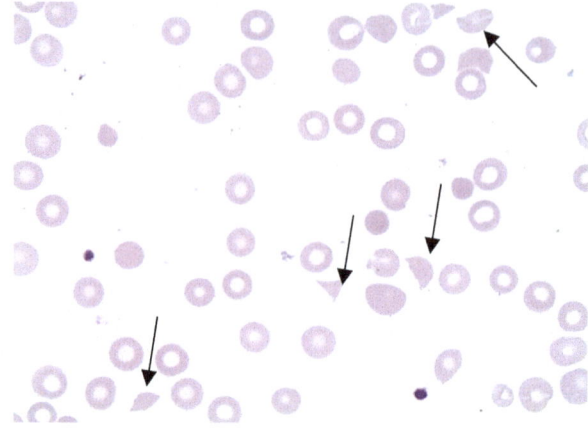

Learning Points

Priming Questions
1. What is the differential diagnosis of acute bloody diarrhea?
2. What is the classic triad of HUS?
3. What diagnostic steps and treatment should be provided?
4. What is atypical HUS and how does it differ from HUS?

Introduction/Background

1. Thrombotic-microangiopathy (TMA) is a collection of pathological changes that ultimately lead to multisystem organ injury. These processes include endothelial swelling and injury, platelet activation, and accumulation of fibrin and platelet thrombi that occlude microvascular lumen and cause shearing destruction of red blood cells. TMA can affect the brain, heart, lungs, and GI tract but has a predilection for causing the greatest injury to the kidneys [1].
2. The incidence of HUS is about 1.5/100,000 persons/year. Atypical HUS accounts for about 10% of cases [2, 3].
3. TMAs are classified into four groups [1].
   - *Group I*: Includes thrombotic thrombocytopenia purpura (TTP), caused by a deficiency of ADAMTS13 (*A Disintegrin And Metalloproteinase with a ThromboSpondin type 1 motif, Member 13—for any nerds who care*). This can be due to autoimmune inhibitors or genetic mutations.
   - *Group II*: Includes atypical HUS. Caused by abnormal complement activity typically as the result of genetic mutations or autoantibodies to the activators/regulators of the pathway.

- *Group III*: Includes HUS. Can be toxin associated or drug related.
- *Group IV*: Includes fibrin-platelet thrombosis such as disseminated intravascular coagulation (DIC), HELLP syndrome (Hemolysis, Elevated Liver Enzymes, Low Platelets), catastrophic antiphospholipid syndrome, or heparin-induced thrombocytopenia (HIT).

4. HUS is a rare TMA characterized by a triad of hemolytic anemia, acute kidney failure, and thrombocytopenia. It is the most common cause of acute renal failure in children [4]. Adults are much less commonly affected. Systemic thrombotic microangiopathy stems from endothelial damage, leukocyte activation, platelet activation, widespread inflammation, and multiple thromboses in the blood, which leads to organ damage, failure, and even death. This disorder is separated into two categories based on the pathophysiology: typical versus atypical.

- Typical HUS—due to shiga toxin–producing bacteria, most often *Escherichia coli*, *Shigella dysenteriae*, or *Streptococcus pneumoniae* [4, 5].
  - This is the more common form (up to 90% of cases) and affects mainly children from 6 months to 4 years old. It is typically preceded by an episode of infectious bloody diarrhea due to a foodborne illness or a contaminated water supply.
  - Since enterohemorrhagic *E. coli* is non-invasive, bacteremia and fever are uncommon.
  - Mortality approaches 5% with permanent renal injury developing in about 25% of cases [2].
- Atypical HUS—due to genetic defects leading to chronic, uncontrolled complement activation [3].
  - Represents about 5–10% of cases and is much more severe, with 33–40% of patients dying or developing end-stage renal disease from their first clinical bout. With subsequent relapses, one article reported that 65% of patients died, required dialysis, or had permanent renal damage within the first year of diagnosis regardless of treatment.

Physiology/Pathophysiology

1. The pathophysiology of HUS, atypical HUS, and TTP is complicated, making differential diagnosis difficult at times. There is some overlap in how each one causes damage, but each has distinct etiology. The following explanation is basic and designed to hit the highlights of only distinguishable characteristics of each disease and should not be considered definitive [1].
2. Both typical and atypical HUS are members of the thrombotic microangiopathic hemolytic anemias (MAHA) along with TTP and DIC. While both disease states present with the same symptoms, the underlying pathophysiology differs greatly [1, 3].

Simplified Etiologies of HUS, Atypical HUS and TTP

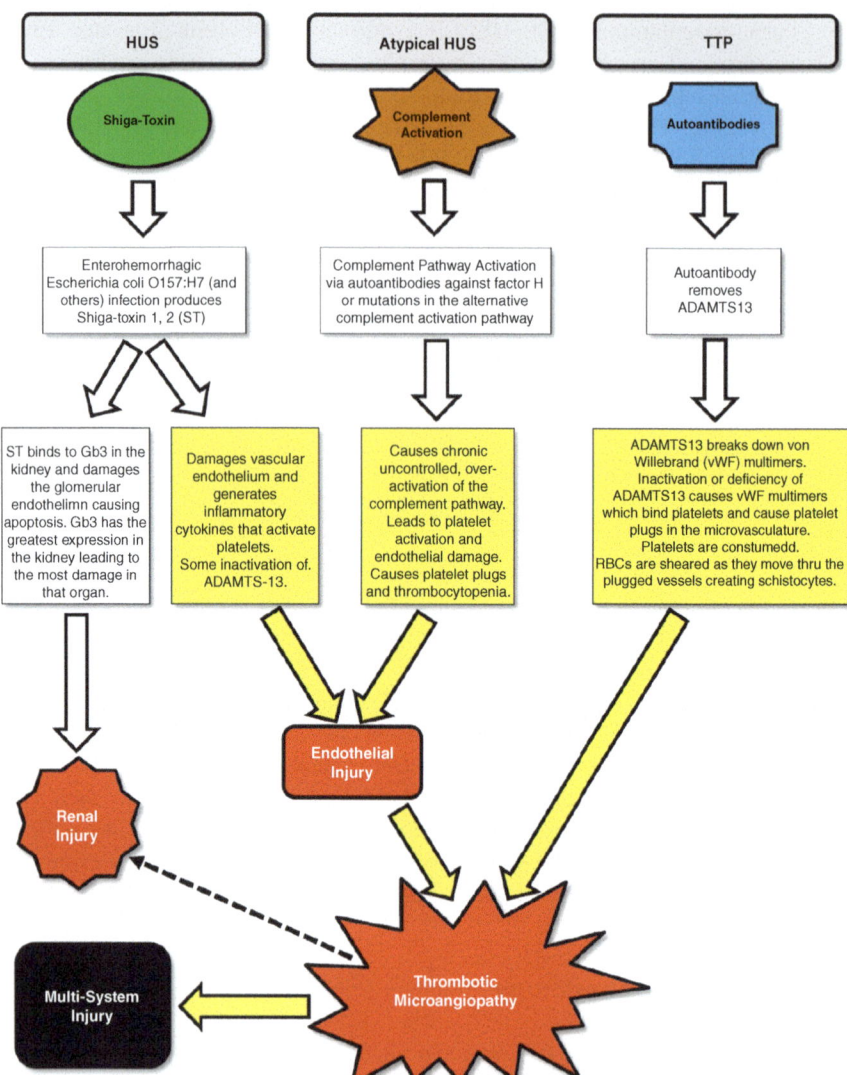

Figure Courtesy of Colin Kaide. (Published with kind permission of © Colin G. Kaide 2019. All Rights Reserved)

3. Typical HUS involves binding of shiga toxin (stx1 and 2) to various receptors mainly in the glomerular cells of the kidneys and endothelial cells of the vasculature [6].
   - Renal—Shiga toxin binds to the globotriaosylceramide (Gb3) receptor on the glomerular endothelium which leads to apoptosis of the endothelial cells and subsequent renal failure.

- Vasculature—Shiga toxin releases cytokines and chemokines involved in platelet aggregation and becomes thrombogenic in blood vessels, although the full mechanism is unknown. Furthermore, the binding of shiga toxin to platelets inactivates ADAMTS13, the protein deficient in TTP. This leads to multimers of von Willebrand factor to form and initiate platelet activation. The result is microthrombus formation in the arterioles and capillaries of the body, which destroy red blood cells as they squeeze through the vasculature causing microangiopathic anemia (MAHA) with schistocytes [6].
- Complement pathway—Shiga toxin activates the alternative complement pathway by binding to complement factor H, an inhibitor of the cascade. Activation of the complement pathway produces cell damage through opsonization and formation of membrane attack complexes. For we clinicians farther removed from basic science, opsonization refers to the immune process that targets something (bacteria, etc.) for destruction by phagocytosis.

4. Atypical HUS involves activation of the complement system due to mutation in regulatory proteins or acquisition of autoantibody inhibitors to system components. Some of the components suggested to be implicated are factor H, I, and B; complement C3; and thrombomodulin [3, 7].

- Unlike *typical* HUS, activation of complement is the central disease process of atypical HUS.
- Complement system is thought to be activated in two ways in atypical HUS: autoantibodies against factor H or mutations in the alternative complement activation pathway.
- Complement pathway activation leads to platelet activation, endothelial cell damage, and white blood cell activation.

von Willebrand Multimers

Image Courtesy of Colin Kaide. (Published with kind permission of © Colin G. Kaide 2019. All Rights Reserved)

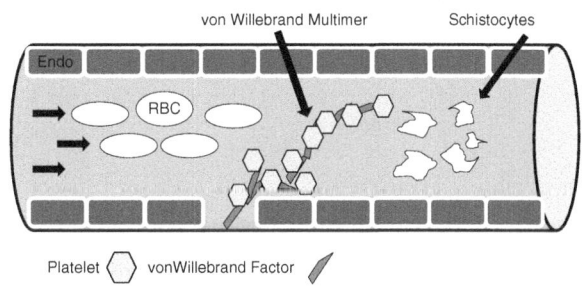

Making the Diagnosis

Differential Diagnosis
- TTP
- HUS
- Atypical HUS
- DIC

1. Start with a thorough history and physical exam.
   - Diarrhea—usually starts as watery and progresses to bloody diarrhea with abdominal cramps. Fever is typically absent with enterohemorrhagic *E. coli* infection [4].
   - Nausea and vomiting are common.
   - HUS develops 5–10 days later (if it is going to happen).
     - Decreased urine output
     - Blood in urine
     - Hypertension
     - Edema
     - Neurological symptoms – confusion, encephalopathy
     - May lead to organ system failure
   - If sudden onset of symptoms + acute renal failure in the absence of diarrhea—more likely atypical HUS.
     - More severe symptoms
     - May present with myocardial infarction, stroke, pancreatitis, or liver necrosis
   - Characteristics of systemic thrombocytopenic MAHA.
     - Thrombocytopenia + microangiopathic hemolysis
     - Plus one of the following:
       - Neurological symptoms—confusion, cerebral convulsions, and seizures
       - Renal impairment—elevated creatinine, decreased GFR, abnormal urinalysis
       - GI symptoms—diarrhea, nausea, vomiting, abdominal pain, and gastroenteritis

Classic findings in thrombotic angiopathies

Findings	HUS and atypical HUS	TTP
Fever	Rare	Rare
Anemia	MAHA with schistocytes	MAHA with schistocytes
Thrombocytopenia	Present	Present
Renal Abnormalities	+++	+
Neurologic Abnormalities	One-third of patients	Two-thirds of patients

Courtesy of Colin Kaide, MD

2. Lab testing
    - Stool sample—screens for shiga toxin–producing *E. coli* but can be negative.
    - Atypical HUS specific—screens for complement mutations and antibodies (These tests are not widely available, especially in the ED and may be requested by consultants).
    - Common abnormal lab values for both typical and atypical HUS:

Abnormal findings in HUS, atypical HUS, TTP, and DIC

Lab/findings	HUS	Atypical HUS	TTP	DIC
INR/PTT	Normal	Normal	Normal	Elevated
Platelets	Low	Low	Low	Low
Schistocytes	Present	Present	Present	Present
Renal abnormalities	+++	+++	+	NA[a]
Hemoglobin	Decreased	Decreased	Decreased	Decreased
LDH	Increased	Increased	Increased	Increased
Haptoglobin	Decreased	Decreased	Decreased	Decreased
ADAMTS 13	Normal	Normal	Low	Normal
Increased D-dimers	No	No	No	Yes
Decreased fibrinogen	No	No	No	Yes
Platelet plugs	Yes	Yes	Yes	No
Fibrin plugs	No	No	No	Yes

Courtesy of Colin Kaide, MD

[a]Not unless the DIC specifically clots either renal or cerebral vessels or causes bleeding intrarenally or intracranially

Treating the Patient

1. Typical HUS
    - The mainstay of treatment is supportive care [1, 8].
        - Fluid replacement and volume management if oliguric renal failure develops.
        - Renal care paying close attention to electrolyte management.
        - Management of neurological manifestations
    - Antibiotics are controversial—current recommendation is not to use them due to evidence that they may increase shiga toxin production or release [1].
        - Experience during an outbreak of *E. coli* in Germany showed no worsening of the disease and a decrease in long-term carriage of *E. coli* when macrolide antibiotics were used [9].
        - For now, the answer is probably not to give antibiotics.
    - Other treatments have not been proven to be beneficial including steroids, antiplatelet agents, eculizumab (used in atypical HUS successfully) and plasma exchange (PLEX) [2–4].
    - Platelet transfusion is rarely needed, as bleeding is rare and platelet counts usually do not fall into the critical range. Due to the theoretical concern that platelets may worsen the HUS reaction, transfusion should be considered only in life-threatening bleeding situations [10].

2. Atypical HUS
   • Plasma exchange (PLEX) was considered the most effective treatment until eculizumab was introduced. If used, it should be started as soon as diagnosis is suspected [3, 7].
     – Replaces defective and overactive proteins.
     – Replaces one to two plasma volumes in adults with each treatment.
     – Some will require continued treatment for the rest of their lives to maintain remission.
   • Eculizumab (Soliris®)—a terminal complement inhibitor first shown in 2009 to be effective in more than 80% of patients [2].
     – It improves renal function, hematological parameters, and platelet counts, allowing for the discontinuation of plasma exchange or dialysis in some patients.
     – Beware of discontinuation of the medication, as this has been associated with relapse.
     – A black box warning was issued owing to *Neisseria meningitidis* infection—all patients should be vaccinated and be considered for antibiotic prophylaxis [11].
       o Studies have shown 2000-fold increased risk of meningococcal disease, thought to be related to impaired antimeningococcal antibodies [11].
       o Penicillin is recommended. If allergic, consider macrolides.

Case Conclusion

Case 1

The stool studies showed the presence of shiga toxin, and the culture grew *E. coli* 0157:H7. The local health department was contacted, and the hamburger stand where the patient and his girlfriend ate was investigated. Two samples of meat were contaminated with *E coli*. Four other shiga toxin–positive diarrhea cases were identified, but no additional cases of HUS were reported.

The patient went on to need dialysis for approximately a month. He recovered his renal function mostly with a new baseline creatinine of 2.45 mg/dL.

Case 2

The patient's tests showed no growth of pathogenic *E. coli,* and shiga toxin assay was negative.

Given her acute hemolytic anemia, thrombocytopenia, nonoliguric AKI, and schistocytes seen on smear suggestive of thrombotic microangiopathy combined with diarrhea and negative enteric panel, she was diagnosed with atypical HUS. She failed plasmapheresis three times and was started on hemodialysis. She received long-acting eculizumab as part of a clinical trial. Upon discharge, her LDH was trending down. She will continue to follow up for the clinical trial.

After 3 months, her renal function improved significantly, returning to nearly baseline.

Discussion

Typical HUS is seen in about two cases per 100,000 person-years in the United States and has been a major source of morbidity from meat and fast food industries. As seen in our first case, FDA quickly identifies the source of infection and quarantines the food to prevent further infection. Although acute renal failure occurs in 55–70% of patients with typical HUS, 70–85% recover their normal renal function. With aggressive early treatment, more than 90% of patients survive the acute phase and about 9% may develop end-stage renal disease [3].

Atypical HUS is considered an ultra-rare disease with a prevalence of about three cases per million worldwide. It can be either inherited or acquired and does not appear to vary by race, gender, or geographic location. Patients with the disease have an extremely poor prognosis, with permanent kidney damage, need for dialysis within the first year occurring in about 70% of cases, or death. Quality of life is poor for these patients with a majority being burdened with fatigue, hypertension, neurological impairment, and chronic dialysis for the rest of their lives. As seen in our second case, she was in the lucky minority with full recovery of renal function and discontinuation of dialysis.

Pattern Recognition

Hemolytic Uremic Syndrome
- *General*
  - Anemia with schistocytes (MAHA)
  - Thrombocytopenia
  - Renal failure
- *Typical HUS*
  - Diarrhea, especially bloody with nausea/vomiting and abdominal pain
  - Mental status change
  - More common in childhood
- *Atypical HUS*
  - Sudden onset
  - No history of diarrhea
  - Worse course and outcomes

Disclosure Statement Klein—Nothing to disclose

Kaide—Callibra, Inc.-Discharge 123 medical software company. Medical Advisory Board Portola Pharmaceuticals. I have no relationship with a commercial company that has a direct financial interest in subject matter or materials discussed in article or with a company making a competing product.

References

1. Tsai HM. Autoimmune thrombotic microangiopathy: advances in pathogenesis, diagnosis, and management. Semin Thromb Hemost. 2012;38:469–82.
2. Cody EM, Dixon BP. Hemolytic uremic syndrome. Pediatr Clin N Am. 2019;66(1):235–46. https://doi.org/10.1016/j.pcl.2018.09.011.
3. Noris M, Remuzzi G. Atypical hemolytic-uremic syndrome. N Engl J Med. 2009;361(17):1676–87.
4. Scheiring J, Andreoli SP, Zimmerhackle LB. Treatment and outcome of Shiga-toxin-associated hemolytic uremic syndrome (HUS). Pediatr Nephrol. 2008;23:1749–60.
5. Besbas N, Karpman D, Landau D, Loirat C, Proesmans W, Remuzzi G, Rizzoni G, Taylor CM. A classification of hemolytic uremic syndrome and thrombotic thrombocytopenic purpura and related disorders. Kidney Int. 2006;70:423–31.
6. Nolasco LH, Turner NA, Bernardo A, Tao Z, Cleary TG, Dong J, Moake JL. Hemolytic uremic syndrome-associated Shiga toxins promote endothelial-cell secretion and impair ADAMTS13 cleavage of unusually large von willebrand factor multimers. Blood. 2005;106:4199–209. https://doi.org/10.1182/blood-2005-05-2111.
7. Hodgkins KS, Bobrowski AE, Lane JC, Langman CB. Clinical grand rounds: atypical hemolytic uremic syndrome. Am J Nephrol. 2012;35:394–400.
8. Noris M, Remuzzi G. Hemolytic uremic syndrome. J Am Soc Nephrol. 2005;16(4):1035–50.
9. Nitschke M, Sayk F, Härtel C, et al. Association between azithromycin therapy and duration of bacterial shedding among patients with Shiga toxin-producing enteroaggregative Escherichia coli O104:H4. JAMA. 2012;307(10):1046–52.
10. Tarr PI, Gordon CA, Chandler WL. Shiga-toxin-producing Escherichia coli and haemolytic uraemic syndrome. Lancet. 2005;365(9464):1073–86.
11. McNamara LA, Topaz N, Wang X, Hariri S, Fox L, MacNeil JR. High risk for invasive meningococcal disease among patients receiving eculizumab (Soliris) despite receipt of meningococcal vaccine. MMWR Morb Mortal Wkly Rep. 2017;66:734–7.

Radiology Case 5

26

Priyanka Dube and Joshua K. Aalberg

Indication for the Exam A 4-y/o female fell on her outstretched right hand and now has pain and swelling of the distal forearm.

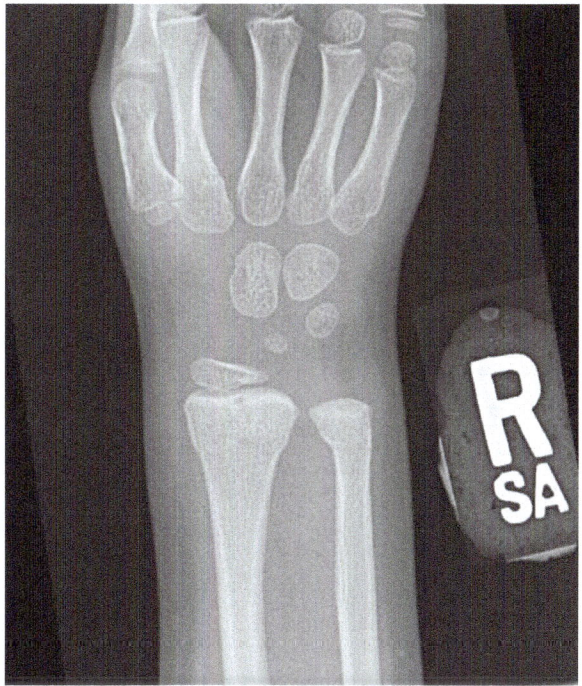

P. Dube · J. K. Aalberg (✉)
Department of Emergency Medicine, Wexner Medical Center at The Ohio State University, Columbus, OH, USA
e-mail: Priyanka.Dube@osumc.edu; joshua.aalberg@osumc.edu

© Springer Nature Switzerland AG 2020
C. G. Kaide, C. E. San Miguel (eds.), *Case Studies in Emergency Medicine*,
https://doi.org/10.1007/978-3-030-22445-5_26

Radiographic Findings There is buckling of the cortical margins of the distal radius and ulna. There is mild soft tissue swelling overlying the fractures.

Diagnosis Buckle fractures of the right radius and ulna.

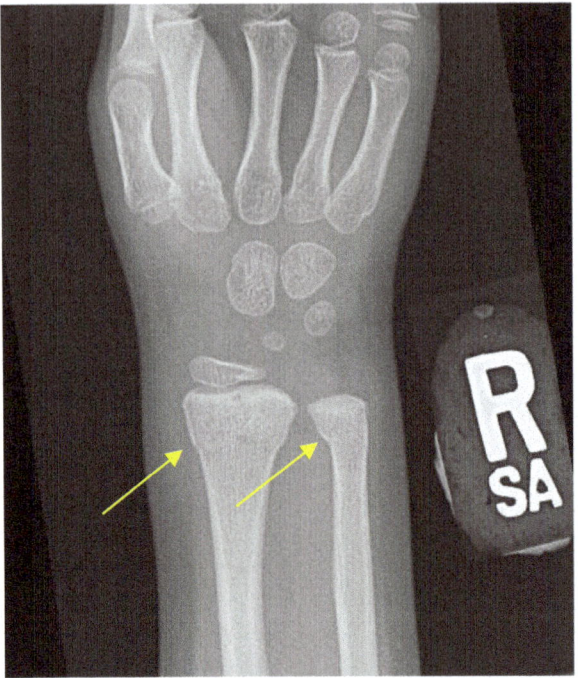

Learning Points

Priming Questions
1. What is the mechanism of a buckle fracture?
2. How are buckle fractures treated?
3. What follow-up is required?

Introduction

A buckle fracture, also known as a torus fracture, is an incomplete fracture seen in skeletally immature patients. It usually involves the metaphysis. The most common locations include the distal radius and ulna, metacarpals, metatarsals, phalanges, and tibia [1].

Pathophysiology/Mechanism

Buckle fractures are caused by focal compression of the cortex by an axial load. Pediatric bones have higher water content than adult bones, which allows them to buckle instead of break [2].

Making the Diagnosis

Buckle fractures can be very subtle on radiographs. The cortex should normally be smooth with gentle curvature. A sudden change in angulation of the cortex is suspicious for a buckle fracture. Generally, the opposite side of the bone is unaffected. Sometimes, a buckle fracture is evident only on one view. Soft tissue swelling may also help identify the area of interest in patients who are unable to localize the site of injury. Radiographs of the contralateral extremity can be helpful for comparison if there is any question on the initial images [1]. A similar fracture that is commonly seen in children is a greenstick fracture.

	Buckle fracture	Greenstick fracture
Affected (tension) side of the bone	Buckled or bent	Cortical disruption
Opposite side of the bone	Unaffected	Buckled or bent
Treatment	Conservative management with gentle immobilization; a removable splint is generally ok	Strict immobilization with a cast for 6 weeks, generally

Treating the Patient

Buckle fractures heal with conservative treatment. There is no consensus on the type and length of immobilization [3]. Usually the patient is immobilized in a cast or splint for several weeks, with some authors advocating for the use of removable splints. These fractures do not require emergent orthopedic surgery consultation. Radiographic follow-up is not necessary routinely if the patient is clinically improving [4].

Discussion

- Buckle fractures are very common injuries, and the radiographic findings can be subtle. Thankfully, the consequences for missing a buckle fracture are generally minimal as these fractures are stable [5].

- Distinguishing these fractures from unstable ones such as greenstick fractures is important to ensure proper treatment and follow-up. If in doubt, the fracture site can be fully immobilized using a splint or cast, following local ED practices, and the patient can be referred to orthopedics.

References

1. Donnelly L. Fundamentals of pediatric imaging. 2nd ed. Philadelphia: Elsevier; 2017.
2. Manaster BJ, May DA, Disler DG. Musculoskeletal imaging: the requisites. 4th ed. Philadelphia: Elsevier; 2013.
3. Williams BA, et al. Buckling down on torus fractures: has evolving evidence affected practice. J Child Orthop. 2018;12(2):123–8.
4. van Bosse HJP, et al. Minimalistic approach to treating wrist torus fractures. J Pediatr Orthop. 2005;25:495–500.
5. Little JT, et al. Pediatric distal forearm and wrist injury: an imaging review. Radiographics. 2014;34(2):472–90.

Hyperthermia: *"I'm Hot Blooded; Check It and See"*

27

Benjamin Smith and Matthew Michalik

Case #1

Found altered at bus stop

Pertinent History A 58-year-old male brought to the ED by EMS after bystanders found him at a bus stop on a 100 °F day. He smells of alcohol and is unable to supply a history due to his altered mental status. He has no visible signs of trauma. He is homeless and well known to the emergency department with multiple visits for alcohol intoxication.

PMH Alcoholic cirrhosis, hypertension, hepatitis C

Social History Homeless, smoker, chronic alcohol abuse, distant history of IV heroin use.

Pertinent Physical Exam

- BP 103/62 mmHg, Pulse 130 beats per minute, Temp 102.4 °F (39.1 °C) axillary, RR 18 breaths/minute, SpO2 95%

Except as noted below, the findings of the complete physical exam are within normal limits.

- General: Intoxicated, minimally responsive.
- HEENT: Normocephalic, atraumatic, pupils 3 mm ERRL.
- Back: Blistering and superficial burns noted to the upper back and buttocks.

B. Smith (✉) · M. Michalik
Department of Emergency Medicine, University of North Carolina at Chapel Hill School of Medicine, Chapel Hill, NC, USA
e-mail: benjamin_smith@med.unc.edu; Matthew.Michalik@unchealth.unc.edu

© Springer Nature Switzerland AG 2020
C. G. Kaide, C. E. San Miguel (eds.), *Case Studies in Emergency Medicine*,
https://doi.org/10.1007/978-3-030-22445-5_27

- Extremities: No deformities or edema. Burns with blistering noted over posterior calves and posterior arms.
- Neuro: Moans and opens eyes to painful stimuli, withdraws from pain, moves all extremities equally.

Pertinent Diagnostic Testing

Test	Result	Units	Normal range
WBC	16.2 ↑	K/μL	3.8–11.0 10^3 cells/mm³
Hgb	12.8 ↓	g/dL	(Male) 14–18 g/dL
			(Female) 11–16 g/dL
Hematocrit	39.2	%	34.9–44.3%
Platelets	105 ↓	K/μL	140–450 K/μL
Sodium	136	mEq/L	135–148 mEq/L
Potassium	4.8	mEq/L	3.5–5.5 mEq/L
Chloride	100	mEq/L	96–112 mEq/L
Bicarbonate	18 ↓	mEq/L	21–34 mEq/L
BUN	31 ↑	mg/dL	6–23 mg/dL
Creatinine	1.2	mg/dL	0.6–1.5 mg/dL
Glucose	120 ↑	mg/dL	65–99 mg/dL
ALT	41 ↑	IU/L	8–32 IU/L
AST	62 ↑	IU/L	6–21 IU/L
Alk Phos	121 ↑	IU/L	32–110 IU/L
INR	1.3 ↑	–	≤1.1
CK	1340 ↑	U/L	30–220 U/L
pH	7.34	–	7.320–7.420
pCO_2	32	mmHg	36.1–52.1 mmHg
pO_2	256 ↑	mmHg	46.1–71.1 mmHg
Lactate	2.5 ↑	mmol/L	<2.0 mmol/L
Alcohol	380 ↑	mg/dL	<10 mg/dL
UA – specific gravity	1.040 ↑	–	1.001–1.035
UA – Leukesterase	Negative	–	Negative
UA – Nitrites	Negative	–	Negative
UA – Blood	Positive	–	Negative
UA – Ketones	Positive	–	Negative
UA – Protein	Negative	–	Negative

CXR No focal opacities, no pneumothorax, stable from prior exams.

CT Head No evidence of trauma, no intracranial hemorrhage.

CT C-Spine No fracture or dislocation.

EKG Sinus tachycardia, rate 132, no ectopy, normal ST segments.

Plan Observation pending sobriety.

ED Update The nurse obtained rectal temperature measuring 107.2 °F (41.8 °C). Active cooling measures with cold saline IV and evaporative cooling were initiated. The patient was intubated using rapid sequence intubation (RSI) and after

30 minutes of cooling had a core temperature of 39 °C. He was admitted to the ICU for further care.

Case #2 Partied Too Hard

Pertinent History   A 26-year-old male is brought to the ED by EMS at 4 a.m. after partying all night. His friends state that they had been drinking and went to a "rave." When they were ready to leave, they went looking for their friend and found him altered and lying in the parking lot outside of the party. They immediately called EMS. They are unsure if he used any drugs but say that he "probably" did.

Social History   Nonsmoker, binge drinks, and occasionally uses party drugs per friends.

Pertinent Physical Exam

- BP 115/62 mmHg, pulse 145 beats per minute, Temp 107.4 °F (41.9 °C) rectal, RR 24 breaths/minute, SpO$_2$ 98%

Except as noted below, the findings of the complete physical exam are within normal limits.

- General: Diaphoretic, minimally responsive.
- HEENT: Normocephalic, atraumatic, pupils 8 mm ERRL.
- CV: Tachycardic, regular, no murmurs appreciated. 2+ capillary refill
- Neuro: Minimal moaning to painful stimuli, does not open eyes, moves all extremities equally, withdraws from pain. Slightly increased muscle tone with six beats of clonus.

Pertinent Diagnostic Testing

Test	Result	Units	Normal range
WBC	18.3 ↑	K/μL	3.8–11.0 10³ cells/mm³
Hgb	14.2	g/dL	(Male) 14–18 g/dL
			(Female) 11–16 g/dL
Hematocrit	44.5 ↑	%	34.9–44.3%
Platelets	284	K/μL	140–450 K/μL
Sodium	135	mEq/L	135–148 mEq/L
Potassium	4.7	mEq/L	3.5–5.5 mEq/L
Chloride	105	mEq/L	96–112 mEq/L
Bicarbonate	10 ↓	mEq/L	21–34 mEq/L
BUN	31 ↑	mg/dL	6–23 mg/dL
Creatinine	1.1 ↑	mg/dL	0.6–1.5 mg/dL
Glucose	105 ↑	mg/dL	65–99 mg/dL
ALT	29	IU/L	8–32 IU/L
AST	34 ↑	IU/L	6–21 IU/L
Alk Phos	115 ↑	IU/L	32–110 IU/L

Test	Result	Units	Normal range
INR	1.0	–	≤1.1
CK	2445 ↑	U/L	30–220 U/L
pH	7.24 ↓	–	7.320–7.420
pCO_2	25 ↓	mmHg	36.1–52.1 mmHg
pO_2	312 ↑	mmHg	46.1–71.1 mmHg
Lactate	4.1 ↑	mmol/L	<2.0 mmol/L
Alcohol	80 ↑	mg/dL	<10 mg/dL
UA – specific gravity	1.042 ↑	–	1.001–1.035
UA – Leukesterase	Negative	–	Negative
UA – Nitrites	Negative	–	Negative
UA – Blood	Positive	–	Negative
UA – Ketones	Negative	–	Negative
UA – Protein	Negative	–	Negative

CXR No focal opacities, no pneumothorax, stable from prior exams.

CT Head No evidence of trauma, no intracranial hemorrhage.

CT C-Spine No fracture or dislocation.

EKG Sinus tachycardia, rate 146, no ectopy, normal ST segments.

Plan The Patient was intubated immediately upon arrival using versed and rocuronium. Active cooling was initiated with cold saline bolus, evaporative cooling, ice packs in the groin and axilla, and he was kept sedated with fentanyl and versed drips. He was admitted to the ICU after cooling to 39 °C.

Learning Points: Hyperthermia

Priming Questions
1. What is the pathophysiology behind hyperthermia and the development of heat stroke?
2. What is the differential diagnosis for a patient with hyperthermia?
3. What are the complications of hyperthermia and heat stroke?
4. How is hyperthermia managed and what are the recommendations on cooling measures?

Introduction/Background

1. Hyperthermia can be the result of environmental exposure, physical overexertion, drug/medication use, or a combination of any of the above.
2. Heat stroke and hyperthermia can have various presentations based on the underlying etiology and can present on a broad spectrum from simple heat cramps to alteration in mental status.

3. About 618 people are killed by environmental heat–related illness in the United States every year according to the CDC [1].
   - Fluctuations in weather can lead to increased deaths. For instance, during a heat wave in France in 2003, there were an estimated 14,800 deaths from heat-related illness [2].
   - Heat related illness is almost always preventable with public education on the dangers of extreme heat exposure and common sense.
4. Illicit drugs use, particularly sympathomimetics such as MDMA, cocaine, and methamphetamine can cause significant hyperthermia, particularly when used in a warm environment and combined with physical activity (i.e., dancing for a prolonged period).

Physiology/Pathophysiology

1. The body's temperature is regulated through multiple mechanisms of heat dissipation and heat production and is maintained at the hypothalamic thermoregulatory center.
   - Hyperthermia occurs when the mechanisms of heat dissipation are overwhelmed, when the body generates excessive heat, or a combination of both. In essence, the body's natural cooling mechanisms are unable to bring the body temperature down to the (intact) hypothalamic "set point."
     - In contrast, a fever occurs when the hypothalamic set point is increased, typically in response to either infection or inflammation. Patients with a fever feel cold and shiver because the actual body temperature is below the set point. The body is acting the same way at 37 °C (98.6 °F) when the set point is 39 °C (102.2 °F) as it normally would at 35 °C (95 °F) when the set point is 37 °C (98.6 °C), because in both cases the body's actual temperature is 2 °C below the "set point." When the "set point" returns to normal, the patient begins to feel warm and sweat. A fever "breaking" is the body's natural response to lower the body temperature down to the newly reset, set point. This chapter focuses on hyperthermia, not fevers.
     - In rare cases, injury to the hypothalamus may also cause temperature dysregulation.
   - The core temperature is normally maintained between 36 and 38 °C (96.8–100.4 °F), and temperature regulation mechanisms become much less effective at temperatures >40 °C (104 °F) [3].
   - When the body's temperature rises, there are primarily four physiological responses: dilation of blood vessels, increased sweat production, decreased heat production, and behavioral changes.
   - The mechanisms of heat transfer away from the body are:
     - Radiation: transfer of heat from warmer object to cooler object by electromagnetic waves
     - Conduction: heat exchange between two surfaces in direct contact
     - Convection: heat transfer by air/liquid that is moving across the surface of another object
     - Evaporation: heat is lost by vaporization of water or sweat [4].

2. Heat stroke is severe hyperthermia (>40 °C (104 °F)) from heat exposure with altered mental status. Injury is directly related to how high the body temperature is and how long the temperature has been elevated [5].
    - Hyperthermia leads to a secondary increase in release of endotoxins, increase in vascular permeability, and a systemic inflammatory response that can lead to multiorgan failure [5, 6].
    - Elevated body temperature then leads to denaturing of proteins. Many proteins begin to denature at or above temperatures of 41 °C (105.8 °F) [7].
    - Prolonged hyperthermia overwhelms the body's natural thermoregulatory mechanisms, which leads to cellular death, resulting in excessive release of endotoxins causing multiorgan dysfunction and even death if not rapidly identified and treated.
    - Elderly patients have a decreased ability to compensate by the above mechanisms and are much more susceptible to hyperthermia when exposed to heat.
3. Hyperthermia may also be caused by increased metabolism and heat production by the body. This is most commonly due to physical exertion during sports, but other metabolic mechanisms can result in hyperthermia.
    - Sympathomimetic drugs, particularly amphetamines and cocaine, can increase the body's temperature by increased release and decreased reuptake of catecholamines:
        - Increased norepinephrine leads to a sympathomimetic toxidrome, which consists of tachycardia, hypertension, diaphoresis, anxiety, hyperreflexia, mydriasis, paranoia, seizures, etc.
        - Increased serotonin levels can lead to a clinical picture similar to serotonin syndrome, which consists of hyperthermia, agitation, hyperreflexia, tremor, diaphoresis, mydriasis, ataxia, and muscle rigidity [8, 9].
        - In addition, environments where these drugs are consumed (concerts, clubs, raves, etc.) are often warm and humid with poor ventilation and involve ongoing physical activity.
    - Serotonin syndrome, thyrotoxicosis, malignant hyperthermia, and neuroleptic malignant syndrome can also cause severe hyperthermia due to significantly increased metabolism.

Making the Diagnosis

Anything that can cause increased core body temperature with central nervous system dysfunction should be included in the differential.

The Differential Diagnosis
- Infectious: sepsis, meningitis, encephalitis, malaria, etc.
- Endocrinopathy: thyroid storm, pheochromocytoma, DKA
- Neurological: CVA, ICH, Status epilepticus
- Toxicological: anticholinergic, sympathomimetic, neuroleptic malignant syndrome, serotonin syndrome, salicylate overdose, etc.

1. The diagnosis of heat stroke should be suspected based on history and physical exam. While context clues can help with the diagnosis (high ambient temperatures, found in warm environment, etc.), the other possible causes listed above should be considered and excluded prior to making the diagnosis of heat stroke.
   - The prototypical non-exertional heat stroke patient will be an elderly patient with underlying chronic medical diseases such as cardiovascular disease, neurological disease, obesity, etc. These comorbidities limit the ability of the body to thermoregulate and often limit patient's ability to remove themselves from an excessively hot environment. They may have anhidrosis as well, but this is not a sensitive finding in heat stroke [5, 10].
   - Patients with heat stroke will often present with abnormal vital signs such as tachycardia, tachypnea, hypotension, and, of course, elevated temperature.
   - IMPORTANT: It is vital that an accurate temperature be recorded in these patients. Central monitoring probes should be used. Rectal thermometers will be most practical for the ED physician on initial assessment, but Foley catheters with temperature probes are very useful and easy to place for continuous temperature monitoring. For intubated patients, esophageal probes are also an option.
   - Central nervous system findings in heat stroke can vary and may be as minimal as confusion and/or irritability or as severe as seizures and coma, thus a high index of suspicion is key to prompting measurement of the core temperature as other methods may not reflect the true degree of hyperthermia [5].
   - History and physical exam should also focus on identification of possible toxidromes. Hyperreflexia and clonus may point toward serotonin syndrome or overdoses of drugs with serotonergic effects such as MDMA. Hyperreflexia may also be seen in thyrotoxicosis. Skin should be examined for moisture; dry flushed skin may point toward an anticholinergic toxidrome whereas diaphoresis may indicate sympathomimetic toxidromes.
2. Laboratory workup in hyperthermia should be broad and targeted at diagnosing complications of hyperthermia, primarily end organ damage, as well as identifying underlying etiologies if the clinical picture is unclear.
   - It is important to check CBC, CMP, ABG, coagulation studies, CK, urinalysis/UDS, EKG, and CXR. Other studies such as TSH may be indicated in the appropriate clinical setting.
   - If the patient's presentation is not clear, a CT of the head and LP to rule out CNS infection or hemorrhage may be indicated as well.

Treating the Patient

1. Like any critically ill patient, resuscitation should begin with the ABCs.
   - Airway: Patients who are unable to protect their airway should be intubated for airway protection similar to most patients presenting to the ED. Hyperthermic patients may gain additional benefit from intubation with paralytic agents as paralysis will reduce heat generation and prevent shivering.

- Breathing: Poor oxygenation may be due to aspiration, underlying infection, or poor respiratory effort. This can be assessed with CXR, ABG/VBG, and clinical exam.
- Circulation: Patients with heat stroke are often volume depleted due to excessive sweating and vasodilation. Fluid resuscitation should begin immediately in these patients. Avoid alpha agonists such as phenylephrine due to the fact that the peripheral vasodilation is needed to help with heat dissipation.
  - In contrast, patients with hyperthermia due to drug use may present hypertensive. Treatment of the hypertension should begin with benzodiazepines and if necessary, escalated to a titratable drip such as nicardipine.
2. All patients with hyperthermia will need rapid cooling.
   - Do not forget to remove the patient from the hot environment. If you are practicing in the ED, this is typically already accomplished by virtue of the patient's presence in the ED.
   - There is no evidence for any particular temperature endpoint, though endpoints as high as 39.4 °C (102.9 °F) have been used in the literature with good outcomes [11]. The ultimate goal is normothermia.
   - One of the most practical and effective methods of cooling in the ED is evaporative and convective cooling by exposing patients as much as possible and spraying tepid water on them with fans blowing air across their body.
   - A systematic review in 2009 showed immersive cooling is the most rapid method; however, this is rarely available in the ED. Additionally, immersive cooling may complicate monitoring and intravenous access. Lastly, the studies of immersive cooling have been conducted primarily in young healthy adults with no comorbidities, so generalization to elderly non-exertional heat stroke patients with multiple medical problems is unknown [5, 12, 13].
   - Other adjuncts include cooled oxygen, cooling blankets, cool IV fluids, bladder irrigation, intravenous temperature management systems, and gastric lavage. Often, many of these modalities are slow to initiate and the patient can be cooled to a safe temperature by other methods faster. In addition, gastric lavage may even cause water intoxication.
   - In a limited resource environment, simple ice packs can be used to help with cooling. Traditionally, it is taught that the most effective placement is in the groin, neck, and axilla. However, a randomized controlled trial with ten healthy adults showed that applying ice packs to the cheeks, palms, and soles in exercise-induced hyperthermia was more effective [14].
3. Other complications from hyperthermia and heat stroke that will need to be managed include respiratory dysfunction, arrhythmias, seizures, rhabdomyolysis, and end organ damage such as kidney and liver damage.
   - Respiratory complications: aspiration, noncardiogenic pulmonary edema, Acute Respiratory Distress Syndrome (ARDS), and pulmonary hemorrhage. These patients are often acidotic as well and will need intubation not only for airway protection but also for respiratory failure.
     - A study in India of 28 patients admitted for heat stroke found that 86% of the patients developed respiratory failure [15].

- Cardiac dysfunction: sinus tachycardia is the most common finding. Acute heart failure and elevated biomarkers with ST changes on EKG can be seen, but cases of stress-induced cardiomyopathy as a complication from heat stroke exist only as case reports [16].
- CNS dysfunction: patients present on a spectrum of CNS dysfunction from slightly altered cognition to seizures. While cooling is the definitive management, short-acting benzodiazepines can be used while cooling measures are being initiated.
- Other injuries to consider while managing these patients:
  - Rhabdomyolysis
  - Acute kidney injury
  - Hepatic injury
  - Coagulopathies such as DIC.
  - Hyponatremia from excessive water intake or drug effects [17].
  - Adverse effects from the underlying cause of hyperthermia
    - A case series in 2012 described three cases of intracranial hemorrhage in the setting of MDMA use. These patients were all in their twenties, and none were found to have underlying aneurysms [18].
    - There is also a case report of an aortic dissection that was "likely related" to the ingestion of ecstasy in a 29-year-old at a rave [19].

Case 1 Conclusion

The patient was admitted to the ICU with a normal temperature and extubated on hospital day 2. His mental status returned to his baseline, and he was discharged from the hospital on day 4 with normalizing labs and vital signs.

Case 2 Conclusion

The patient was admitted to the ICU, and his temperature continued to normalize. He was extubated the following day. His CK rose to 31,470 without evidence of AKI. He left the hospital against medical advice on hospital day 5.

Case Discussion

As presented in the cases above, hyperthermia may be fairly obvious on presentation but may also be somewhat subtle without high suspicion. Any altered patient brought from a hot environment, especially the elderly or otherwise impaired patient or patients suspected of using illicit drugs should have an accurate *core* temperature measured. Once identified, hyperthermia should be aggressively treated to reduce the core temperature to a safe range as underlying pathology and complications are managed.

Pattern Recognition

- Altered mental status
- Hyperthermia
- Hot ambient temperatures and/or
- Known drug abuse

Disclosures The authors of this chapter report no significant disclosures.

References

1. Extreme Heat (5/20/2018). Retrieved from https://www.cdc.gov/disasters/extremeheat/index.html.
2. Argaud L, Ferry T, Le QH, et al. Short- and long-term outcomes of heatstroke following the 2003 heat wave in Lyon, France. Arch Intern Med. 2007;167:2177.
3. Charkoudian N. Skin blood flow in adult human thermoregulation: how it works, when it does not, and why. Mayo Clin Proc. 2003;78:603.
4. Stapczynski JS, Tintinalli JE. Tintinalli's emergency medicine: a comprehensive study guide. 8th ed. New York: McGraw-Hill Education LLC; 2016.
5. Bouchama A, Knochel JP. Heat stroke. N Engl J Med. 2002;346:1978.
6. Lim CL, Mackinnon LT. The roles of exercise-induced immune system disturbances in the pathology of heat stroke: the dual pathway model of heat stroke. Sports Med. 2006;36:39.
7. Fagain CO. Protein stability and stabilization of protein function. Georgetown: Landes Bioscience; 1997.
8. Kalant H. The pharmacology and toxicology of "ecstasy" (MDMA) and related drugs. CMAJ. 2001;165(7):917.
9. Rochester JA, Kirchner JT. Ecstasy (3,4-methylenedioxymethamphetamine): history, neuro-chemistry, and toxicology. J Am Board Fam Pract. 1999;12(2):137.
10. Bross MH, Nash BT Jr, Carlton FB Jr. Heat emergencies. Am Fam Physician. 1994;50(2):389.
11. Bouchama A, Cafege A. Et. Al. ineffectiveness of dantrolene sodium in the treatment of heat-stroke. Crit Care Med. 1991;19(2):176–80.
12. McDermott BP, et al. Acute whole body cooling for exercise induced hyperthermia: a system-atic review. J Athl Train. 2009;44(1):84–93. https://doi.org/10.4085/1062-6050-44.1.84.
13. Smith JE. Cooling methods used in the treatment of exertional heat illness. Br J Sports Med. 2005;39:503.
14. Lissoway JB, Lipman GS, Grahn DA, Cao VH, Shaheen M, Phan S, Weiss EA, Heller HC. Novel application of chemical cold packs for treatment of exercise-induced hyperthermia: a randomized controlled trial. Wilderness Environ Med. 2015;26(2):173. Epub 2015 Mar 12.
15. Varghese GM, John G, Thomas K, Abraham OC, Mathai D. Predictors of multi-organ dysfunc-tion in heatstroke. Emerg Med J. 2005;22(3):185–7.
16. Chen WT, et al. Stress-induced cardiomyopathy caused by heat stroke. Ann Emerg Med. 2012;60(1):63. Epub 2011 Dec 7.
17. Hartung TK, Schofield E, Short AI, Parr MJ, Henry JA. Hyponatraemic states following 3,4-methylenedioxymethamphetamine (MDMA, 'ecstasy') ingestion. QJM. 2002;95(7):431.
18. Kahn DE, Ferraro N, Benveniste RJ. Three cases of primary intracranial hemorrhage asso-ciated with "Molly", a purified form of 3,4-methylenedioxymethamphetamine (MDMA). J Neurol Sci. 2012;323(1–2):257. Epub 2012 Sep 19.
19. Duflou J, Mark A. Aortic dissection after ingestion of "ecstasy" (MDMA). Am J Forensic Med Pathol. 2000;21(3):261.

Coarctation of the Aorta: *Open Your Heart to Me, Baby*

28

Christopher Jones and Jennifer Mitzman

Case

A 9-Day-Old Male Presenting with Difficulty Feeding

Pertinent History

This patient was a 9-day-old, former full-term male who presented to the emergency department for difficulty with feeding. The mother stated that he typically breast-feeds for 15 minutes on each breast every 2 hours. Today kept falling asleep while trying to eat. She stated he started sweating with feeding today as well. Right before arrival, the mother noticed his breathing was faster. The mother denied fevers, weight loss, vomiting, or diarrhea.

Pertinent Physical Exam

Except as noted below, the findings of the complete physical exam are within normal limits.

- *General:* Lethargy with poor tone.
- *Heart:* 2/6 systolic heart murmur heard at the left upper sternal border that radiates to the back.
- *Abdomen:* Liver edge down 3 cm below the costal margin.
- *Vascular:* Absent femoral pulses. Delayed capillary refill of 6 seconds.
- *Skin:* Mottled skin.

C. Jones
Nationwide Children's Hospital, Columbus, OH, USA

J. Mitzman (✉)
Nationwide Children's Hospital, Columbus, OH, USA

Department of Emergency Medicine, Wexner Medical Center at The Ohio State University, Columbus, OH, USA

© Springer Nature Switzerland AG 2020
C. G. Kaide, C. E. San Miguel (eds.), *Case Studies in Emergency Medicine*,
https://doi.org/10.1007/978-3-030-22445-5_28

Past Medical History

- The child was born at 39 weeks to a Gravida 2 Para 2 Mother. Prenatal screening for Group B strep was negative. The patient was born via spontaneous vaginal delivery without complication. The patient passed congenital heart disease pulse oximetry screening in the newborn nursery at 24 hours of age.
- No medications or allergies.

ED Management

The patient was examined, and the murmur was detected along with other signs of poor perfusion. Lab tests including a venous blood gas, complete blood count, chemistry, ammonia, glucose, and lactate were obtained given the patient's overall critically ill appearance. A 12-lead electrocardiogram and chest radiograph were obtained to evaluate heart size and rhythm. Four extremity blood pressures are indicated in patients in whom coarctation is suspected. In this patient's case, the pressures were obtainable only after fluid resuscitation.

Based on the murmur and decreased overall perfusion with absent femoral pulses, fluid resuscitation was initiated. We elected to use serial aliquots of 10 mL/ kg normal saline rather than 20 mL/kg to avoid fluid overload.

Since the first item on the differential diagnosis for a critically ill patient of this age is most commonly sepsis, empiric antibiotic coverage was initiated. This included ampicillin and gentamicin. Due to age less than 14 days, acyclovir to cover for risk of neonatal herpes infection was given as well.

The patient's overall presentation was very suggestive of ductal dependent congenital heart lesion. As a result, we initiated prostaglandin E1 at 0.1 mcg/kg/min. The main risks associated with prostaglandin are apnea and hypotension. This is most commonly seen at initiation, so we were prepared to intubate if necessary. Our patient did develop apnea and was intubated using a 3.5 endotracheal tube and a medication regimen of atropine, ketamine, and rocuronium. Cardiology was consulted when the diagnosis was suspected. However, initiation of prostaglandin was not delayed given its critical nature.

Updates on ED Course

Lab results			
Lab	Result	Units	Normal range
Lactate	6	mmol/L	<2.0 mmol/L
pH venous	7.25	–	7.32–7.42
pvO_2	94	mmHg	Not well-established
pCO_2	55	mmHg	35–45
HCO_3	16	mEq/L	21–34 mEq/L
Glucose	40	mg/dL	65–99 mg/dL

Once resuscitation and prostaglandins were initiated, we were able to obtain four extremity blood pressures as follows: right arm: 84/44, left arm 82/40, right leg 62/38, left leg 64/40. The chest X-ray showed cardiomegaly and pulmonary edema. The electrocardiogram showed right ventricular hypertrophy for age.

Chest X-ray

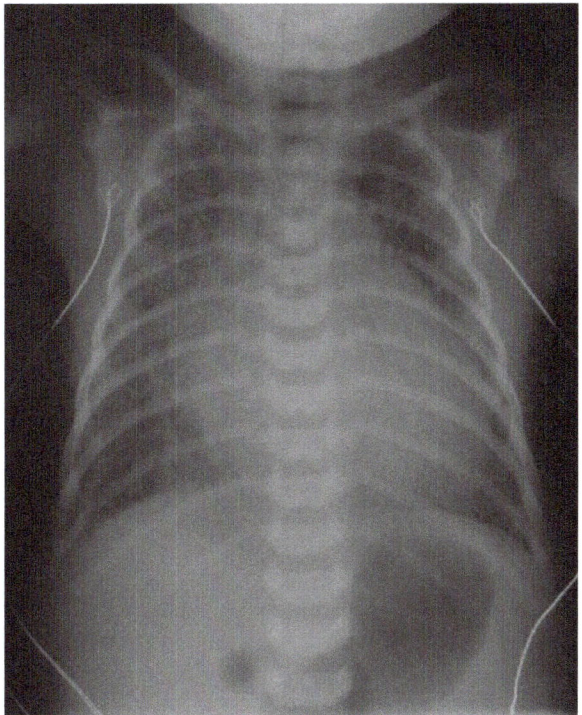

http://www.adhb.govt.nz/newborn/TeachingResources/Radiology/CXR/HLHS/CXR-HLHS-
congested.jpg

EKG Showing Right Ventricular Hypertrophy

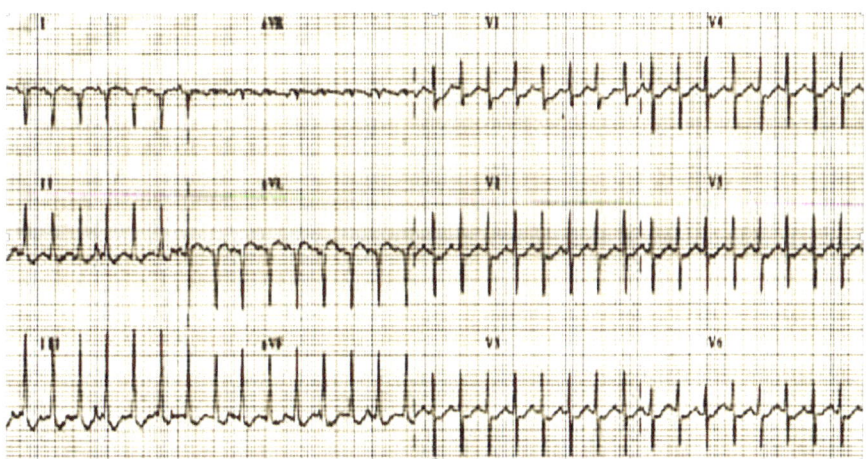

Image courtesy of Colin Kaide, MD

Learning Points

Priming Questions
1. What pathophysiology leads to the diagnosis of critical coarctation of the aorta in the first weeks of life?
2. What exam features suggest this diagnosis? What laboratory or imaging studies can help solidify your clinical suspicion of this problem?
3. What treatment should be initiated in the emergency department for this diagnosis and what are the anticipated complications of that therapy?

Introduction/Background

1. Coarctation of the Aorta (COA) occurs in up to 10% of all congenital heart disease diagnoses.
   - There is a 2:1 male predominance.
2. Females with coarctation should be worked-up for Turner's syndrome, as 30% of patients with TS have coarctation.
3. Most common associated anomaly is bicuspid aortic valve, which occurs in >50% of patients with COA [1].
4. There is a bimodal distribution of presentation of newly diagnosed COA. The first patients have critical coarctation with ductal dependence. They present within the first weeks of life often with shock and heart failure. The other group is asymptomatic without ductal dependence and found in infants and children undergoing evaluation for unexplained hypertension.
5. Patients with a history of coarctation can also have re-stenosis later in life, which will present with new blood pressure discrepancies and hypertension [2].

Physiology/Pathophysiology

1. Coarctation of the aorta is a narrowing of the descending aorta that occurs opposite of the site of the ductus arteriosus (PDA).
2. Coarctation occurs as either a localized constriction of the aorta or a tubular hypoplasia of the aorta [3].
3. Coarctation of the aorta presents in a bimodal age distribution depending on the extent of the lesion and the dependence on a patent ductus arteriosus [4].
   - Critical coarctation in an infant presents when the PDA closes. Closure causes a mechanical obstruction and sudden increase in afterload, which results in the left ventricle having to pump harder. This often results in heart failure due to decreased cardiac output. These patients will present ill and in shock. They can often be worsening, so quickly it seems to literally happen before your eyes.
   - With patients in shock due to critical coarctation, sometimes there is uniform hypotension in all limbs until resuscitation occurs. Once the patient has been adequately resuscitated the difference between upper and lower blood pressures is more apparent.

- The weak/absent femoral pulses come from poor blood flow distal to the coarctation.
- Noncritical coarctation can be diagnosed throughout childhood and into adulthood. It is generally found by evaluation of persistent hypertension [1].

Coarctation of the Aorta

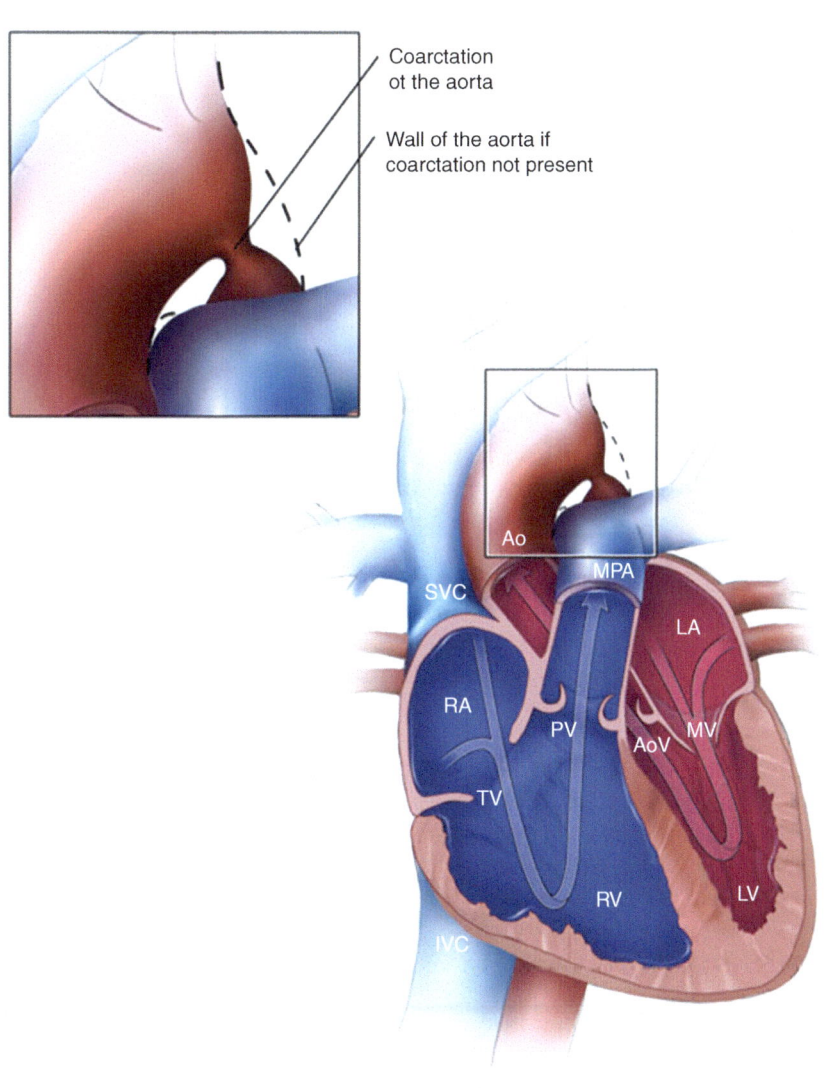

Coarctation
ot the aorta

Wall of the aorta if
coarctation not present

RA. Right Atrium	SVC. Superior Vena Cava	TV. Tricuspid Valve
RV. Right Ventricle	IVC. Inferior Vena Cava	MV. Mitral Valve
LA. Left Atrium	MPA. Main Pulmonary Artery	PV. Pulmonary Valve
LV. Left Ventricle	Ao. Aorta	AoV. Aortic Valve

Image public domain courtesy of Centers for Disease Control and Prevention, National Center on Birth Defects and Developmental Disabilities

Making the Diagnosis

Differential Diagnosis
- Ductal dependent Congenital Heart Disease includes cyanotic lesions such as hypoplastic left heart, pulmonary atresia, tricuspid atresia, transposition of the great vessels, tetralogy of Fallot or total anomalous pulmonary venous return as well as acyanotic lesions such as coarctation of the aorta, aortic stenosis, ventricular septal defect or atrial septal defect
- Sepsis
- Inborn error of metabolism
- Non-accidental trauma

1. A good history and physical exam will guide you in the correct diagnosis of many ill-appearing infants.
2. Examination will often show systolic ejection murmur radiating to the back, hypotension in lower extremities, weak/absent femoral pulses, and an overall listless baby with tachypnea.
3. Blood gas will often show an acidosis with high lactate levels.
4. Chest X-ray will often show cardiomegaly.
5. EKG will often show RVH, which is somewhat common in the neonatal period already. The reason is hypothesized to be that the right ventricle in utero is the dominant ventricle and pumps blood through the PDA to the descending aorta. In addition to this normal physiology, if there is also a coarctation of the aorta, there will be increase in the afterload of the RV and worsen RVH [5].
6. Echocardiogram helps confirm the diagnosis, but depending on where you are practicing, you may not have the capabilities of a formal echocardiogram prior to transfer. Echocardiogram will be needed prior to surgery, however.

Treating the Patient

1. Hypoglycemia should be managed with dextrose-containing fluids.
2. Hypotension can be managed with normal saline while awaiting the prostaglandin E1 (PGE) administration. It is important to monitor for response to fluids to avoid over-resuscitation; however, given the poor feeding that is associated with coarctation, some fluids are usually warranted.
3. PGE should be ordered quickly and started as soon as possible. PGE is a natural vasodilator that will keep the PDA open, which allows appropriate oxygen delivery and blood flow for ductal-dependent congenital heart disease. This is a temporizing measure until cardiac surgery fixes the lesion. The risks of PGE initiation in patients this critically ill with suspected congenital heart disease are low. Therefore, do not wait for an echocardiogram or cardiology consult to start this medication. If the patient is ill-appearing and has any findings from the above section, the physician should have a low threshold for starting PGE.

4. Apnea is associated with PGE administration, particularly at initiation or dose increases. Patients do NOT need to be prophylactically intubated due to PGE therapy, but close airway monitoring is essential. The patient should be transported by a team qualified in newborn airway management.
5. Antibiotics are often started when the patient arrives to the ED based on the suspicion for sepsis in your differential. This is appropriate given the degree of shock and overall ill appearance of these children. Once coarctation is confirmed, antibiotics may be discontinued. Initial antibiotics can include ampicillin and gentamicin. Cefotaxime and ampicillin is another appropriate regimen in this age group.

Case Conclusion

The patient was admitted to the cardiac ICU. As the PDA opened due to PGE1, he showed a marked improvement of his lactic acidosis. The patient remained intubated due to the risk of apnea with PGE administration. The patient was taken to the operating room for correction of the coarctation by excision and end-to-end anastomosis of the unaffected aorta. He had an uneventful postoperative course and was subsequently discharged.

Care must be taken with the way the aortic anastomosis is repaired, as patients will be at risk for re-coarctation from scar tissue.

Discussion

It is difficult to make the diagnosis of critial coarctation of the aorta in the neonatal period. In most cases, the first thought should be sepsis, sepsis, sepsis. One must be broad with their differential diagnosis including congenital heart disease with superimposed sepsis, inborn errors of metabolism, and nonaccidental trauma. When starting a broad workup, certain lab results and physical exam findings should prompt consideration of the diagnosis of coarctation of the aorta. On physical exam, most patients will have a 2–3/6 systolic ejection murmur heard at the LUSB with radiation to the back. This is a valuable diagnostic clue. Hepatomegaly in the setting of tachypnea and overall ill appearance also places heart failure much higher on the differential. Of all findings, the weak/absent femoral pulses and hypotension in lower extremities should help to solidify a diagnosis of coarctation. Once the diagnosis is suspected, begin prostaglandin therapy. Do not wait for definitive echocardiography for diagnosis. The risks of PGE initiation in patients this critically ill with suspected congenital heart disease are low [6, 7].

Apnea is a risk with prostaglandin, and one must be vigilant with airway management. Often due to the critical status of the patient, they have already been intubated during the diagnostic period. However, given the goal of resuscitation prior to intubation, this is not always the case. If the patient's respiratory status is stable, it is not mandatory to intubate prior to starting PGE [8]. It is imperative that the child be continuously monitored and that the team be ready to provide bag valve mask ventilation and proceed to intubation promptly if necessary.

Pattern Recognition

- Difficulty with feeding
- Hypertension in upper extremities
- Absent/weak femoral pulses
- Systolic murmur that radiates to the back
- Cardiomegaly on CXR

Disclosure Statement   The authors of this chapter report no significant disclosures.

References

1. Bohan JS, Kosowsky JM, Dolbec K, Mick NW. Congenital heart disease. Emerg Med Clin North Am. 2011;29(4):811–27.
2. Tanous D, Benson LN, Horlick EM. Coarctation of the aorta: evaluation and management. Curr Opin Cardiol. 2009;24:509–15.
3. Hastings LA, Nichols DG. 27: Coarctation of the aorta and interrupted aortic arch. In: Critical heart disease in infants and children. 2nd ed. Philadelphia: Mosby; 2006. p. 625–49.
4. Head CE, Jowett VC, Sharland GK, Simpson JM. Timing of presentation and postnatal outcome of infants suspected of having coarctation of the aorta during fetal life. Heart. 2005;91:1070.
5. Johnson WH, Moller JH. Conditions affecting blood flow in children. In: Pediatric cardiology: the essential pocket guide. 3rd ed. Oxford: Wiley; 2014. p. 150–8.
6. Horeczko T, Inaba AS. Cardiac disorders. In: Marx JA, Hockberger RS, Walls RM, Biros MH, et al., editors. Rosen's emergency medicine: concepts and clinical practice. 8th ed. Philadelphia: Saunders, an imprint of Elseiver Inc; 2009.
7. Park MD. Obstructive lesions. In: Park's pediatric cardiology for practitioners. 6th ed. Philadelphia: Elsevier Saunders; 2014. p. 184–206.
8. Meckler GD, Lowe C. To intubate or not to intubate? Transporting infants on prostaglandin E1. Pediatrics. 2009;123(1):e 25–30.

In-Flight Emergencies: *Medical Mile High Club*

29

Erica Ross and Christopher E. San Miguel

Your flight for Honolulu has just taken off from Los Angeles when you notice some commotion at the front of the passenger cabin. After a few minutes, you hear the flight attendant's voice over the intercom, "Is there a doctor onboard?"

Learning Points

Priming Questions
1. What are the legal/ethical obligations and risks of a health-care provider assisting with an in-flight emergency?
2. What are the environmental factors present during air travel that put passengers at a higher risk of medical issues?
3. What support and medical supplies are available onboard an aircraft?
4. What are the most common in-flight emergencies, and how should one approach diagnosing and treating a patient at 40,000 ft?
5. When and how are planes diverted due to medical emergencies?
6. What are the challenges of in-flight medical care?

Introduction/Background

1. The true incidence of in-flight medical events is unknown given that there are no standards or minimal requirements for reporting by airlines. The US National

E. Ross · C. E. San Miguel (✉)

Department of Emergency Medicine, Wexner Medical Center at The Ohio State University, Columbus, OH, USA

e-mail: erica.ross@osumc.edu; christopher.sanmiguel@osumc.edu

© Springer Nature Switzerland AG 2020

C. G. Kaide, C. E. San Miguel (eds.), *Case Studies in Emergency Medicine*, https://doi.org/10.1007/978-3-030-22445-5_29

293

Transportation Safety Board requires medical emergencies to be reported if the event requires 48 hours of hospitalization, involves injury to internal organs, or fractures (excluding nose, finger, or toe fractures) [1]. Most studies that evaluate in-flight emergencies acquire data from on-ground medical communication center records. According to one study, significant medical emergencies occur in one passenger per 10,000–40,000 passengers [2]. Another study found that the incidence of reported medical emergencies was one per 604 flights [3]. As the median age of the general population continues to rise and airlines can carry more people per aircraft over further distances, the incidence of in-flight emergencies will likely increase in frequency and severity. Medical professionals should be prepared to face this situation.

2. Prior to World War II, most American flight attendants were nurses who were able to handle nearly all in-flight medical emergencies [5]. When this standard changed, the need for medical professional volunteers became increasingly important. Emergency Medicine providers undergo training that allows them to be particularly effective in managing undifferentiated medical problems that may require immediate intervention. This does not mean that the in-flight environment is not still very challenging, as access to diagnostic and treatment modalities is very limited. Fortunately, most medical problems that occur on flights are self-limited and resolve without major treatment or diversion of flight [3]. The mortality rate for in-flight emergencies is ~0.3–1.3% [3].

3. Aviation agencies generally provide either mandates or guidelines as to the medical equipment that must be available on commercial airline flights. In the United States, it is mandated that all commercial airline flights that require the presence of a flight attendant and have a payload greater than 7500 lbs have onboard at least one first aid kit, an emergency medical kit, supplemental oxygen, and an automated external defibrillator (AED) [4].

Do I Have to Help, and if I Do, Will I Get Sued?

1. There is no legal requirement in the United States, Canada, or the United Kingdom for medical professionals to volunteer when the flight crew requests assistance with an ill passenger. However, Australia and multiple countries within the European Union require medical professionals to assist with in-flight emergencies [5, 6]. The question of which country's laws apply is a very complicated one without a clear answer. The country in which the airline is based, the flight departure country, and the flight arrival country all have a potential argument to support their laws' applicability. Many argue that medical professionals have an ethical obligation to assist as able, but as above, this obligation is largely not codified.

2. Providers may hesitate to volunteer to help with in-flight medical emergencies due to concern for malpractice liability when offering assistance. However, this concern should not dissuade medical professionals from assisting in these situations. The 1998 Aviation Medical Assistance Act Good Samaritan Provision largely protects health-care professionals from legal liability (at least within the United States).

LIABILITY OF INDIVIDUALS—An individual shall not be liable for damages in any action brought in a Federal or State court arising out of the acts or omissions of the individual in providing or attempting to provide assistance in the case of an in-flight medical emergency unless the individual, while rendering such assistance, is guilty of gross negligence or willful misconduct [7].

This statute is much more protective of the medical provider than typical malpractice standards [5]. Examples of actions that are generally thought to rise to the level of gross negligence include rendering aid while intoxicated and practicing beyond their professional scope of practice. Therefore, medical professionals should not assist if they have recently ingested alcohol or CNS depressants.[8.] Further, medical professionals should practice only within their scope of knowledge and openly communicate with the flight crew their credentials and skill set.

- There is considerable debate whether receiving a token of gratitude or compensation for medical services voids the protection granted by this federal law. Indeed, many "Good Samaritan" laws explicitly contain language prohibiting the medical professional from receiving any sort of compensation. As you can read, this law does not include any such explicit prohibition. Small tokens of gratitude such as a seat upgrade or frequent flier points are generally thought to be ok, although this has, as far as we are aware, never been confirmed as part of a judicial case. Larger value gifts or cash compensation is thought to be less likely to stand up to judicial review should the medical professional be sued.
  - Perhaps the most telling case law is *Baillie v. MEDAIRE INCORPORATED*. A man on a British Airlines flight from London to Phoenix complained of chest pain. The crew consulted Medaire Inc., a company who contracted with the airline to provide medical consultation. At their request, a fellow passenger who was a physician examined the man, obtained a history, and reported his findings to the flight crew and the ground-based medical consultants. Ultimately, the medical consultation team did not recommend diversion. Unfortunately, after arrival in Phoenix, the patient was taken to the hospital where it was found that he had suffered a myocardial infarction. He subsequently died 3 months later while awaiting a heart transplant.
    - The man's wife, on behalf of his estate, sued British Airlines, the physician onboard, the medical consultation company (Medaire Inc.), and the two individual physicians who provided consultation as part of their role with the consultation company.
    - Both British Airlines and the physician onboard reached a settlement with the man's estate.
    - Medaire Inc. and the two physicians who provided consultation from the ground were eventually both dismissed on legal grounds that are beyond the scope of this chapter. That dismissal is currently being appealed.
    - Most revealing, however, is a federal's judge's ruling on a Motion for Judgment on the Pleadings filed by the defendants. Medaire Inc. and the

two consultation physicians argued that they should be protected under the 1998 Aviation Medical Assistance Act Good Samaritan Provision. The judge ruled that their relationship as contractors with the airline to provide medical consultation was fundamentally different than that described in the provision; namely, that they were not volunteers and they were not present on the aircraft. The judge further states, "For clarification, here the individuals that would be immune from liability under the Act are the crewmembers and the physician who provided aide to Mr. Baillie while in the air, not Defendants." [9] Unfortunately, in this case, the onboard physician had already reached a settlement agreement.

- A 2002 review stated that the authors were unaware of any legal action ever being brought against a physician who assisted with an in-flight medical emergency [10]. We are similarly unaware of any cases brought against a physician who assisted with in-flight medical emergency going to trial. This does not, however, take into account physicians who may have been named in a lawsuit and subsequently dismissed or those who may have settled outside of court, as in the above case. While we believe the risk of being named in a lawsuit from assisting in an in-flight medical emergency is very low (and the risk of losing is even lower), we cannot say that the risk is nonexistent.

3. Airlines are not considered a covered entity as defined by HIPAA, and so medical providers are able to legally speak to the flight crew and ground-based consultants about the patient's medical issues [11]. However, the provider should still attempt to protect the patient's privacy and modesty as much as possible during an in-flight emergency.

Physiology/Pathophysiology

1. Most commercial airlines have a cruising altitude of ~30,000–45,000 feet above sea level. This altitude allows for better fuel efficiency, less turbulence, and lower chance of inclement weather [11]. For perspective, Mount Everest is ~29,000 feet above sea level. The passenger cabin is pressurized to be equivalent to approximately 6000–8000 feet above sea level [1]. This is comparable to a small peak by mountain standards but is still significantly higher than the elevation at which most people live. An aircraft structure made suitable to allow a passenger cabin to be pressurized to sea level pressure would be too heavy to fly [11].

2. The low cabin atmospheric pressure affects the partial pressure of gasses. The low pulmonary artery oxygen tension that is present during flight decreases the affinity of hemoglobin for oxygen, to the point where even healthy individuals can have arterial oxygen saturations as low as 89%. The body compensates by increasing minute ventilation and cardiac output with mild hyperventilation and tachycardia. Patients who are chronic smokers or have conditions such as COPD and congestive heart failure may be unable to illicit or handle the body's natural compensation mechanisms [1].

3. At the low barometric pressures within the passenger cabin, gas expands (per Boyle's Law). Gas expanding within closed body cavities can cause pain, and passengers may complain of ear, sinus, and bowel discomfort [12]. Further, passengers must be careful about traveling within certain timeframes post intra-abdominal, eye, neurologic, and middle ear surgical procedures, as these surgeries can introduce small amounts of air into these cavities. If passengers are unaware or do not heed these restrictions, complications such as pain, wound dehiscence, or worse conditions may occur [11]. Gas expansion at low pressure can also affect air-filled medical devices such as tracheostomy tubes, feeding tubes, urinary catheters, and pneumatic splints, causing discomfort and malfunction [11].

4. Other circumstances present in-flight can cause a variety of medical issues. Low cabin humidity, which helps prevent airplane corrosion, can cause dry eyes and dehydration and exacerbate reactive airway disease [11, 12]. Immobility and cramped seating can put passengers at risk for thrombus formation [16]. Decompression sickness is a risk for those who have recently been scuba diving. Moreover, close contact places passengers at a higher risk of contracting communicable respiratory infections [1, 11].

Making the Diagnosis

1. General approach to any patient [3, 5, 8]

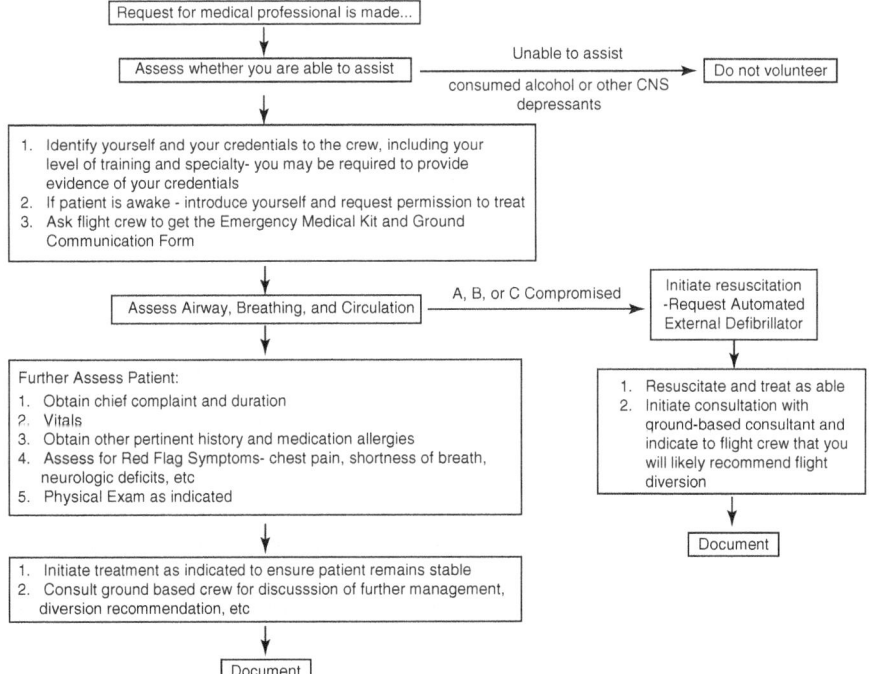

2. The most valuable diagnostic tool at your disposal is the one that you carry with you everywhere; your brain! History and physical exam are the major diagnostic clues for in-flight emergencies. However, completing a high-quality physical exam can be difficult due to limited space, poor light, and a noisy cabin [11]. In the United States, emergency medical kits must be equipped with a stethoscope and sphygmomanometer, but that is the extent of mandated diagnostic tools. Some airlines may carry medical kits with other supplies such as a glucometer or a thermometer, but this is not required. Further, some automated external defibrillators (AED) carried by airlines may have telemetry capabilities that can be used for cardiac monitoring in a nonarrest situation, but the sophistication of the AED is not standardized between airlines. It may be possible to utilize equipment such as a glucometer from another passenger, but always consider the cleanliness of the device and the possibility of blood-borne pathogen risk [13, 16].
3. Maintaining open lines of communication with the consultant ground-based medical crew is essential. Many airlines require consultation with these providers prior to use of the emergency medical kit. These ground-based consultants have more familiarity with the austere environment encountered during in-flight emergencies, are well versed in the medical resources available, understand airline operational concerns, and may have knowledge of passenger pre-existing conditions [3, 11].
4. The most common in-flight medical issues (in order of decreasing incidence) include syncope/presyncope, respiratory symptoms, nausea/vomiting, cardiac symptoms, and seizure. In one study, these symptoms accounted for >70% of reported in-flight medical events [3]. For pediatric patients, the most common emergencies included infectious symptoms (fever and otitis media), neurologic symptoms (seizure and syncope), respiratory symptoms (asthma), and allergic reactions [14]. The most common surgical emergencies include appendicitis and thrombosis [6].
5. Remember that coming to a clear final diagnosis is not the vital priority. During in-flight emergencies, the medical provider volunteer's primary objective is to assess the patient, stabilize, and provide treatment as able, and communicate with the ground-based crew health consultant/pilot to assist with the decision to divert the plane or continue to the original destination.

Treating the Patient

1. The medical provider volunteer should provide only treatments that they are qualified to provide, within their scope of training [11].
2. Typically, the safest place to treat the passenger is in their seat. Sometimes, moving the patient to the galley can assist with effective treatment. Avoid treating the patient in the aisle, as this impairs the flight crew from performing their duties and can affect other passengers [12].

3. Flight attendants are required to be trained in CPR and AED use every 2 years, although some airlines have yearly training [1]. Flight attendants are trained to intervene in minor medical issues and have access to a basic first aid kit. Flight attendants also carry manuals with helpful information on many common medical conditions and emergencies. Flight attendants are not sanctioned to use advanced medical equipment and medications unless under the guidance of a licensed medical provider [11]. The medical volunteer should request that a flight attendant remain with them at all times while providing care.

4. The medical volunteer should use every resource available. While many airlines require communication between the in-flight medical volunteer and the ground-based medical consultant; it is wise for the volunteer to utilize this extra provider's knowledge of flight medicine and the aircraft's medical equipment to their advantage. Further, do not hesitate to request further assistance from other medical professionals onboard. A physician may struggle with placement of an IV, as it is not a procedure that they frequently complete, while a passenger who is a nurse may be able to complete this procedure effectively and efficiently [11]. You may also request medical equipment and medications from other passengers but do so with caution [11].

5. Below is the medical equipment that has been mandated to be present on United States-based airline flights since 2004. The shelf life of emergency medical kit medications is ~1 year, and the FAA recommends replacement annually [11]. Many airlines supplement these basic supplies, but the additions are not mandated or standardized. Additionally, international flights do not have the same standard equipment; emergency medical kits on international flights may vary significantly between airlines, and medications may have different names on international flights [5]. Moreover, challenges arise in the care of pediatric patients, since the formulations and doses of medicines in the emergency medical kit medication are based on adult dosing and may not be provided in child-friendly administration forms (e.g., tablet vs. liquid form) [14]. Overall, the most commonly used medical supplies were oxygen, IV fluids, and aspirin [3].

Medical supplies mandated to be available on every United States airplane [9]		
Category	Equipment	Quantity
Personal protective equipment	Nonpermeable gloves	1 pair
Diagnostic	Sphygmomanometer	1
	Stethoscope	1
Airway management	CPR masks – 1 pediatric, 1 small adult, 1 large adult	3 in total
	Oropharyngeal airways – 1 pediatric, 1 small adult, 1 large adult	3 in total
	Self-inflating manual resuscitation device with three masks – 1 pediatric, 1 small adult, 1 large adult	1:3 total masks

Medical supplies mandated to be available on every United States airplane [9]		
Category	Equipment	Quantity
Medications	Analgesic, nonnarcotic – 325 mg	4
	Antihistamine injectable – 50 mg	2
	Antihistamine tablets – 25 mg	4
	Aspirin tablet – 325 mg	4
	Atropine – 0.5 mg, 5 cc	2
	Basic instructions for use of medications included in medical kit	1
	Bronchodilator, inhaled (metered dose inhaler or equivalent)	1
	Dextrose – 50%/50 cc injectable	1
	Epinephrine 1:10,000–2 cc injectable (thought to be an error in the federal regulation; essentially all airlines carry the 10 cc code vials) [15]	2
	Epinephrine 1:1000–1 cc injectable	2
	Lidocaine 20 mg/ml – 5 cc	2
	Nitroglycerin tablets – 0.4 mg	10
	Saline solution – 500 cc	1
Other	Adhesive tape, 1 inch standard	1
	Alcohol sponges	2
	Automated external defibrillator	1
	Bandage and tape scissors	1
	IV tubing with 2 Y connectors	1
	Needles (2–18 ga., 2–20 ga., 2–22 ga., or sizes necessary to administer required medications)	6 in total
	Supplemental oxygen	Varies
	Syringes (1–5 cc, 2–10 cc, or sizes necessary to administer required medications)	4 in total
	Tourniquet	1
First aid kit contents	Adhesive bandage compresses, 1-inch	16
	Antiseptic swabs	20
0–50 passengers – 1 kit	Ammonia inhalants	10
	Bandage compresses, 4-inch	8
51–150 passengers – 2 kits	Triangular bandage compresses, 40-inch	5
	Arm splint, noninflatable	1
151–250 passengers – 3 kits	Leg splint, noninflatable	1
	Roller bandage, 4-inch	4
>205 passengers – 4 kits	Adhesive tape, 1-inch standard roll	2
	Bandage scissors	1

6. One of the major roles of the in-flight medical volunteer is to provide insight and advice to the pilot and ground-based medical consultant on whether plane diversion is necessary. Aircraft diversion occurs in ~7% of in-flight medical emergencies. The pilot makes the final decision on whether the flight will be diverted due to a medical emergency [5]. There are many factors that are considered when making the decision to divert. If the plane is to be diverted, the pilot must find a diversion location that meets the needs of the aircraft (suitable runway length and weather conditions) and the patient (nearby presence of full-service hospitals and the availability of prehospital health-care providers). Logistically, the decision to divert does not produce immediate results because descent, landing,

and shuttling to the gate will take approximately 40 minutes under the best conditions. The most common conditions that lead to the decision to divert include unstable vital signs, CPR in progress, conditions requiring urgent treatment (including myocardial infarction, respiratory distress, and stroke), unconsciousness, and obstetric emergencies [12]. The decision to divert is a costly one; the cost of diversion can range from $30,000 to $725,000 depending on the size of the aircraft and result from the need to possibly dump fuel in order to meet landing weight requirements and passenger rerouting [2, 6].

7. Tips for dealing with common in-flight medical emergencies: Do not forget to follow the general approach to any patient already discussed in this chapter [3, 8, 5, 16, 17, 18].

Syncope

If still symptomatic, place patient in the galley, supine with legs elevated

Provide oxygen

Assess for and treat hypoglycemia if able (this may require borrowing a glucometer from another patient)

Administer fluids (oral or IV) and cold compresses

Carefully assess for neurologic deficits

If passenger fails to regain consciousness, consider recommendation for flight diversion

Chest pain

Provide oxygen

If you suspect cardiac chest pain, give 325 mg of aspirin

If the patient is normotensive or hypertensive, consider administering sublingual nitroglycerin; however, be aware that if the passenger has a right-sided myocardial infarction, nitroglycerin may cause further decompensation

Some AEDs have telemetry capabilities – if applicable, utilize AED to assess for dysrhythmia or ST elevations

Consider pneumothorax – needles are available for needle decompression if indicated

If a pneumothorax is confirmed or suspected, consider recommendation of descent to lower altitude and flight diversion

Consider recommendation for flight diversion for unrelenting chest pain or cardiac chest pain

Gastrointestinal issues – nausea/vomiting/abdominal pain

Most often benign, but consider and assess for more serious diagnoses such as myocardial infarction or bowel obstruction

No antacids or antiemetics are mandated medical supplies, but enhanced medical kits or fellow passenger may have these medications (always be careful about accepting unmarked medications)

Fluids and analgesics as indicated

In severe cases of bowel obstruction, you can request a reduction in altitude to decrease bowel gas expansion

Cardiac arrest

Initiate cardiopulmonary resuscitation (CPR) and other basic life support resuscitation efforts

Immediately obtain the onboard AED, place pads on the patient, and allow for the machine to assess the patient's rhythm (remember that the flight attendants should be trained in using this device and can assist you)

Code concentration epinephrine (1:10,000) is available and 1 mg (10 mL) should be given for cardiac arrest

If the AED advises a shock, presumably due to a ventricular arrhythmia, consider administering 100 mg (5 mL) of lidocaine

If the patient is symptomatically bradycardic, consider administering 0.5 mg atropine

Administer naloxone, if available

Avoid declaring death, particularly on international flights, even if CPR is ceased, because legal implications of the declaration of death vary between countries [11]. Only a physician can pronounce death during flight.

Recommend flight diversion unless there is cessation of resuscitative efforts

Trauma

The most common injuries are caused by blunt force trauma from turbulence

Consider patient-specific factors that lead to more serious injuries – age, use of anticoagulants, and other medical conditions

Emergency medical kits include various wound-cleaning supplies, bandages and splints, tourniquet, and analgesics, which can be used to treat wounds and injuries

Depending on the severity of injury and patient-specific factors, consider recommendation for flight diversion for severe bleeding, open fractures, severe pain, unstable vital signs, need for tourniquet use, and/or neurological deficits (including ongoing confusion)

Suspected stroke

Give supplemental oxygen

Check blood glucose if able: if low or unable to test, administer dextrose

Avoid aspirin administration, as there is no way to distinguish hemorrhagic versus ischemic stroke

Recommend flight diversion for neurological deficits

Altered mental status

Wide differential

Consider hypoglycemia, opiate overdose, and hypoxia and provide treatment as necessary

If unable to resolve, recommend flight diversion

Obstetric emergencies

Pregnant women are told not to fly after the 35th week of pregnancy, none-the-less this does not preclude the possibility of an in-flight precipitous delivery

Gather equipment and prepare yourself as well as any assistants (including flight attendants) to manage a neonatal resuscitation (blankets for warming and tactile stimulation as well as supplemental oxygen) and postpartum bleeding (IV access, fluids, and bandages/material for potential packing)

Recommend flight diversion

Dyspnea

Past medical history will allow you to assess if the symptoms are likely due to an exacerbation of an underlying condition or a new acute process

Administer supplemental oxygen

Consider using the bronchodilator meter dosed inhaler (10–12 puffs is roughly equivalent to a nebulized breathing treatment)

Consider pneumothorax and perform needle thoracostomy, if indicated

Descent to a lower altitude may improve symptoms

Some aircraft may have intubating equipment available, but all should have equipment for bagging the patient

For persistent symptoms recommend flight diversion

Seizure

Do not place anything in the patient's mouth and place patient in an area that they will not be physically injured by seizure activity (this will likely mean leaving the patient in their seat and providing some surrounding padding with blankets)

Seizure abortive medications are not part of the FAA requirements but may be available on longer haul flights and those in Europe

Assess for and treat hypoglycemia if able

If unable to resolve, recommend for flight diversion

Anaphylaxis

If concerned for anaphylaxis, give the allergy/IM-concentrated epinephrine 1:1000, give 0.5 mg (0.5 mL); this can be redosed in 10 minutes if symptoms persist

Emergency medical kit will also contain an antihistamine and bronchodilators, which can be administered

Give IV fluids for hypotension

Consider recommendation for flight diversion

Acute infections

If this is a potentially contagious disease, make every effort to isolate the patient

Consider giving ASA, acetaminophen, or ibuprofen as an antipyretic

Administer fluids for tachycardia and/or hypotension

Communicate with pilot, as they are required to convey concern for communicable disease to the receiving airport

Decompression illness [19]

Occurs when the atmospheric pressure decreases, such as returning to the surface of the water after a dive or during ascent in an airplane

The decrease in atmospheric pressure causes dissolved gasses to escape from solutions within the body and form air bubbles

Technically, this could occur with any change in atmospheric pressure but is unlikely to happen on commercial aircraft with pressurized cabins except in the setting of recent SCUBA diving

SCUBA diving causes there to be increased amounts of various gasses including nitrogen in the body, making this process of gas bubble creation more likely to occur

Depending on the depth and time of diving, it is generally recommended to avoid flying for 12–24 hours after returning to the surface

This should be suspected in divers who board aircraft shortly after diving or who have dove extensively in the days before the flight

The most commonly affected organ system is the musculoskeletal system, as patients complain of deep, achy pain in their joints. This is known as "the bends."

The nervous system can also be involved, and this should be in the differential for any SCUBA diver who suddenly develops any neurological symptom, such as focal deficit, ataxia, word finding difficulties, or vision changes

Finally, involvement of the cardiovascular or pulmonary system can cause chest pain and shortness of breath.

If any type of decompression illness is suspected, place the patient on 100% O_2 (or as close to it as possible), give a bolus of fluid, and discuss altitude reduction and diversion with ground-based medical control and the pilot.

Discussion

1. In-flight emergencies are common, and medical professionals should be pre-pared to encounter them while traveling. Due to a lack of standardized or mandated incident reporting, the incidence of medical emergencies that is currently reported in the literature is likely a gross underestimate. Emergency medical providers have a skill set that can allow them to be particularly help-ful in the event of an in-flight emergency, but having an understanding of the constraints of this practice environment is also key for providing optimal medical care. In the United States, volunteer medical providers are protected under the Good Samaritan Provision of the 1998 Aviation Medical Assistance Act from legal liability unless the provider is guilty of "gross negligence or willful misconduct." Even when a medical provider is the only medical pro-vider available, it is important that they practice within the scope of their training.

2. In-flight medicine presents many challenges. This includes limited space, poor light, and a loud environment hindering physical exam assessment. Further, medical equipment, diagnostic testing, and available treatment options are severely limited in this environment. In the United States, there is standardiza-tion on mandated basic medical supplies and training of flight crew, but this is not true on international flights. Pediatric and pregnant patient present particular difficulties as provided equipment and medications are often not specific for these populations.

3. Communication with the flight crew and ground-based medical consultants is vital. The major role of the volunteer medical provider is to assess and stabilize the patient, communicate with flight crew and ground-based medical consultants, and provide advice regarding if flight diversion is indicated. The ultimate decision regarding diversion rest with the pilot of the aircraft alone.

Disclosure Statement The authors of this chapter report no significant disclosures.

References

1. Riou B. Management of in-flight medical emergencies. Anesthesiology. 2008;108(4):749–55.
2. Hon K. Review of issues and challenges of practicing emergency medicine above 30,000-feet altitude: 2 anonymized cases. Air Med J. 2017;36:67–70.
3. Peterson D. Outcomes of medical emergencies on commercial airline flights. N Engl J Med. 2013;368(22):2075–83.
4. Emergency medical equipment. 14 U.S.C. § 121.803, 2011.
5. Nable J. Is there a doctor on board? In-flight medical emergencies. Cleve Clin J Med. 2017;84(6):457–62.
6. Sand M. Surgical and medical emergencies on board European aircraft: a retrospective study of 10189 cases. Crit Care. 2009;13(1):R3.
7. Aviation Medical Assistance Act of 1998 49 U.S.C. § 44701, 1998.
8. Nable J. In-flight medical emergencies during commercial travel. N Engl J Med. 2015;373(10):939–45.
9. Baillie v. MEDAIRE INCORPORATED, No. CV-14-00420-PHX-SMM (D. Ariz. Dec. 8, 2015).
10. Gendreau MA, Dejohn C. Responding to medical events during commercial airline flights. N Engl J Med. 2002;346:1067–73.
11. Donner H. Is there a doctor onboard? Medical emergencies at 40,000 feet. Emerg Med Clin North Am. 2017;35(2):443–63.
12. Ho S. What to do during inflight medical emergencies? Practice pointers from a medical ethicist and an aviation medicine specialist. Singap Med J. 2017;58(1):14–7.
13. (2018) Appendix A to Part 121-first aid kits and emergency medical kits. Electronic code of federal regulations.
14. Moore B. Pediatric emergencies on a US based commercial airline. Pediatr Emerg Care. 2005;21(11):725–9.
15. Thompson CA. Know what's in airplane's emergency medical kit, two pharmacists say. In: American Society of Health-System Pharmacists; 2015. https://www.ashp.org/news/2015/01/13/know_what_s_in_airplane_s_emergency_medical_kit__two_pharmacists_say. Accessed 26 Feb 2019.
16. Silverman D. Medical issues associated with commercial flights. Lancet. 2008;373:2067–77.
17. Badawy S. In-flight emergencies: medical kits are not good enough for kids. J Paediatr Child Health. 2016;52:363–5.
18. Isakov A. Management of inflight medical events on commercial airlines. UpToDate. 2018.
19. Bowers RC, Vivolo JC. Disorders due to physical & environmental agents. In: Stone C, Humphries RL, editors. Current diagnosis & treatment: emergency medicine. 8th ed. New York, NY: McGraw-Hill; 2017.

Pediatric Intussusception: *Not Galileo's Telescope*

30

Jennifer E. Melvin

Case 1

Constipation and Abdominal Pain

Pertinent History

A 5-year-old female presents to the emergency department (ED) with constipation for the past month, as well as abdominal pain for the past 3 days that worsened on the day of arrival. The patient is unable to pinpoint an exact location of the pain. The pain is sharp and intermittent, often coming in waves. The patient last had passed a small, hard stool 4 days ago. She has not had any fevers, vomiting, diarrhea, dysuria, cough, or rashes. There has not been any recent trauma.

Pertinent Physical Exam

- BP 118/87, Pulse 142, Temp 98.1 °F (36.7 °C), RR 21, SpO$_2$ 98% on room air

Except as noted below, the findings of a complete physical exam are within normal limits.

- Cardiovascular: Tachycardia with regular rhythm, normal heart sounds with no murmurs, rub nor gallop appreciated. Distal pulses including femoral and radial pulses are intact and symmetric. Capillary refill is less than 3 seconds.
- Abdomen: Abdomen is soft and nondistended with normoactive bowel sounds. There is mild tenderness to palpation diffusely. No hepatosplenomegaly is appreciated.

J. E. Melvin (✉)
Nationwide Children's Hospital, Columbus, OH, USA
e-mail: Jennifer.melvin@nationwidechildrens.org

© Springer Nature Switzerland AG 2020
C. G. Kaide, C. E. San Miguel (eds.), *Case Studies in Emergency Medicine*,
https://doi.org/10.1007/978-3-030-22445-5_30

Past Medical History

Constipation
    Up to date on immunizations

Family History

Paternal grandfather: Hodgkin lymphoma

Pertinent Test Results

Test	Result	Units	Normal range
WBC	6.02	K/μL	3.8–11.0 10^3/mm^3
Hgb	11.9	g/dL	(Male) 14–18 g/dL
			(Female) 11–16 g/dL
Lactate	0.2	mmol/L	<2.0 mmol/L
AST	32 ↑	IU/L	6–21 IU/L
ALT	31	IU/L	8–32 IU/L

Abdominal Plain Radiograph Mild stool retention without signs of obstruction or impaction.

Limited Abdominal Ultrasound (US) Ileocolic intussusception noted without any identifiable lead points, no free air appreciated.

ED Management

Once the US was obtained, the patient subsequently underwent a pneumatic enema reduction of her ileocolic intussusception. This procedure was successful with resolution of the intussusception, and there were no complications.

Updates on ED Course

After the successful reduction of her intussusception, the patient had resolution of her abdominal pain. After a period of observation, she continued to remain asymptomatic and tolerated an oral food challenge without complications. She was subsequently discharged home in stable condition with outpatient follow-up.

Case 2: Lethargy in an Infant

Pertinent History

A 10-month-old male presents to the ED with lethargy that started on the day of presentation. The patient's mother notes the patient slept later than usual this morning and continued to be abnormally tired throughout the day. He has taken several prolonged naps despite usually only taking one short afternoon nap. She denies any recent fevers, vomiting, diarrhea, or rashes. There has been no known trauma. She denies concern for accidental ingestion, with the only medications in the home being acetaminophen and ibuprofen.

Pertinent Physical Exam

- BP 105/84, Pulse 158, Temp 98.1 °F (36.7 °C), RR 21, SpO_2 97% on room air

Except as noted below, the findings of a complete physical exam are within normal limits.

- General Appearance: Patient is tired, although easy to arouse. He is well nourished, well appearing, and in no acute distress with normal color.
- Musculoskeletal: He is moving all extremities; there are no obvious deformities, swelling, lesions, or bruising.
- Neurologic: Sleeping. Arouses with mild stimulation but continues to fall back asleep throughout examination. Anterior fontanelle is open, soft, and flat. Strength and sensation are intact throughout. There are no obvious focal neurologic deficits.

Past Medical History

The patient was born at full term via spontaneous vaginal delivery. There were no complications with the pregnancy or delivery. The patient is up to date on immunizations.

Social History

The patient lives with his mom, dad, and four-year-old brother. He attends daycare 3 days a week and is occasionally babysat by his maternal grandmother.

Family History

Mom, vitamin B12 deficiency

Pertinent Test Results

Laboratory work-up including a complete blood count, comprehensive metabolic panel, hepatic function panel, and urinalysis was normal. A urine drug screen was negative.

EKG Normal sinus rhythm, with no concerning findings

CT Non-contrast Head Unremarkable

Limited Abdominal US Ileocolic intussusception noted without an identifiable lead point and with no free air appreciated.

ED Management

After the US findings were discovered, the patient was taken for a pneumatic enema reduction. This was successful and completed without complications.

Updates on ED Course

After the successful reduction of his intussusception, the patient was awake and acting appropriately. After a period of observation, he continued to remain asymptomatic and tolerated an oral food challenge without complications. He was discharged home in stable condition with outpatient follow-up.

Learning Points

Priming Questions
1. What is intussusception, and what are the common and uncommon clinical manifestations of intussusception?
2. How can the diagnosis of intussusception be made?
3. What are the different treatment options for intussusception, and what clinical circumstances would preclude each?

Introduction

1. Intussusception is one of the most common causes of acute intestinal obstruction in children [1, 2].
2. Intussusception refers to the invagination of one segment of bowel into a more distal segment. This can occur across different areas of the bowel causing several different types of intussusception.
   - Ileocolic intussusception involves the ileocecal junction and accounts for 90% of all cases [1].
   - Small-bowel intussusception, such as ileo-ileal and jejuno-jejunal or jejuno-ileal, has also been described [3].
   - Other types include ileocecal and colo-colic intussusceptions, although these are less common.
3. Intussusception in children typically presents between 6 and 36 months of age, with 80–90% of children being less than 2 years old.
   - Approximately 10% of cases occur in children over 5 years old and 1% occur in children younger than 3 months.
4. There is a slight male-to-female preponderance of cases [1, 2, 4].
5. Historically, intussusception has been related to oral administration of the live rotavirus vaccine [5]. This vaccine has since been removed from the market.

Pathophysiology

1. Intussusception occurs when bowel invaginates into a more distal segment; this can occur for several reasons.
   - Intussusceptions caused by lead points are much less common in the pediatric population; however, they may be seen in relation to underlying disease processes or other conditions.
     - Underlying diseases may include enlarged mesenteric lymph nodes, cystic fibrosis (thick inspissated stool acts as the lead point), Henoch-Schonlein purpura (small-bowel wall hematoma acts as the lead point), lymphoma, and Crohn's disease (due to strictures and inflammation acting as lead points) [4, 6].
     - Other conditions that may act as lead points include a Meckel's diverticulum, polyp, duplication cyst, vascular malformations, bacterial enteritis, or the presence of a G tube [4, 7].
   - In approximately 75% of cases, no clear disease trigger or lead point can be identified; these are termed "idiopathic intussusception." Increasing evidence suggests viral triggers may play a role. This is thought to be secondary to stimulation of lymphatic tissue in the intestinal tract, specifically, hypertrophy of Peyer patches in the terminal ileum, which may act as a lead point for an ileocolic intussusception [8, 9].

2. Invagination of the bowel onto itself may lead to impairment of venous and lymphatic return; this will eventually lead to bowel wall ischemia. If left untreated, this may further progress to incarceration and bowel necrosis [7, 10].

Making the Diagnosis

Differential Diagnosis
The differential diagnosis depends on the clinical presentation.
Fussiness or lethargy

1. Trauma, including nonaccidental trauma
2. Toxins
3. Sepsis
4. Metabolic derangement

Crampy abdominal pain

1. Appendicitis
2. Gastroenteritis
3. Malrotation with volvulus
4. Ovarian torsion

Hematochezia

1. Meckel diverticulum
2. Colitis
3. Polyp
4. Inflammatory bowel disease

1. The well-described classic triad of symptoms includes abdominal pain, a palpable sausage-shaped abdominal mass, and currant jelly stool. Unfortunately, this classic triad is seen in less than 15% of patients [11], although some studies state that up to 40% of patients may present with these symptoms [12–15]. The most common presentation, however, is episodic, colicky abdominal pain, followed by a drawing up of the legs. Emesis is also often seen in these patients. Stool is grossly bloody in about 50% of cases. At times, the only presenting symptom may be lethargy or altered consciousness [16].
2. Laboratory Testing
   • Although there is no specific laboratory test to diagnose intussusception, blood and urine tests may be beneficial to assess for other etiologies of the presenting symptoms.
3. Imaging
   • Intussusception is most commonly diagnosed by ultrasound although it may also be recognized on plain abdominal radiograph or abdominal computed tomography.

- Ultrasound is often the first-line method to detect intussusception. Sensitivity, specificity, and negative predictive value begin to approach 100% when performed by an experienced sonographer [10, 17]. Ultrasound may also be able to detect lead points and allows for further evaluation of other causes of symptoms if indicated.
- The classic appearance of intussusception on ultrasound is caused by the formation of alternating echogenic and hypoechogenic bands of intestine telescoping on itself. This classically resembles a target or bullseye and is usually visible in the right lower quadrant.
- Abdominal radiographs should be obtained in patients presenting with symptoms concerning for intussusception. Not only will this allow for evaluation for other pathology, it also allows for assessment of a perforation. If a perforation was present, the intussusception would require operative management instead of nonoperative reduction.
  - Findings concerning intussusception include lack of air in the ascending colon [1], obscured liver margin, and an intraluminal mass that may manifest as a target or meniscus sign [18].
  - As a diagnostic tool, when used alone, abdominal radiography has a sensitivity ranging from 29% to 89% [18–20].

Treating the Patient

1. Nonoperative reduction: Definitive treatment for most intussusceptions is by nonoperative reduction using hydrostatic (contrast or saline) or pneumatic enema, performed under sonographic or fluoroscopic guidance.
   - In the subgroup of patients in whom the initial enema fails, the next step in management depends on the clinical picture. Stable, nontoxic patients who had partial resolution after the initial treatment may undergo a delayed repeat enema; however, unstable, toxic patients and those with no improvement after an initial treatment should proceed to surgical management [21–23].
2. Surgery: In patients who are acutely ill, have signs of perforation, or have failed nonoperative reduction techniques, operative management is required.
3. Observation: In certain cases, such as transient and benign small-bowel intussusception, definitive interventions may not be indicated beyond a period of observation [3].

Case Conclusion

Both patients in the presenting cases underwent pneumatic enemas with successful reduction of the intussusceptions. Neither had return of the intussusception and neither went on to be diagnosed with any underlying pathology or illness that may have predisposed them to having lead points. Access to pediatric ultrasound examination and radiologists capable of performing nonoperative reduction techniques played an important role in the early diagnosis and management of these cases.

Discussion

1. Classically, intussusception is described in the young toddler who presents with episodic abdominal pain, bloody stools, and a palpable abdominal mass. This presentation is not often the case, however, and an increased awareness of intussusception in patients with crying, lethargy, or other nonspecific complaints is essential to ensuring timely diagnosis and treatment.

2. Although patients are commonly diagnosed by ultrasound, a diagnosis may be possible on abdominal plain radiography or abdominal computed tomography scan as well. Most hemodynamically stable patients will be amenable to nonoperative reduction techniques using either hydrostatic or pneumatic enema. Patients who are acutely ill, however, usually require surgery as they often have bowel wall ischemia. A small percentage of patients will have repeat episodes of intussusception.

3. Overall, appropriate diagnostic awareness and evaluation for intussusception in the pediatric population can reduce morbidity and mortality in this population.

Pattern Recognition

Intussusception
1. Young infants and toddlers with episodic abdominal pain, bloody stools and palpable abdominal mass.
2. Young infants and toddlers with crying, fussiness, and pulling their legs up to their chest.
3. Young infants and toddlers with unexplained lethargy.

Disclosure Statement The authors of this chapter report no significant disclosures.

References

1. Mandeville K, Chien M, Willyerd FA, Mandell G, Hostetler MA, Bulloch B. Intussusception: clinical presentations and imaging characteristics. Pediatr Emerg Care. 2012;28(9):842–4.
2. Weihmiller SN, Buonomo C, Bachur R. Risk stratification of children being evaluated for intussusception. Pediatrics. 2011;127(2):e296–303.
3. Melvin JE, Zuckerbraun NS, Nworgu CR, Mollen KP, Furtado AD, Manole MD. Management and outcome of pediatric patients with transient small bowel-small bowel intussusception. Pediatr Emerg Care. Epub ahead of print 2018.
4. Lochhead A, Jamjoom R, Ratnapalan S. Intussusception in children presenting to the emergency department. Clin Pediatr (Phila). 2013;52(11):1029–33.
5. Rotavirus vaccine for the prevention of rotavirus gastroenteritis among children. Recommendations of the advisory committee on immunization practices (ACIP). MMWR Recomm Rep. 1999;48(RR-2):1–20.

6. Navarro O, Intussusception DA. Part 3: diagnosis and management of those with an identifiable or predisposing cause and those that reduce spontaneously. Pediatr Radiol. 2004;34(4):305–12; quiz 69.
7. Nylund CM, Denson LA, Noel JM. Bacterial enteritis as a risk factor for childhood intussusception: a retrospective cohort study. J Pediatr. 2010;156(5):761–5.
8. Arbizu RA, Aljomah G, Kozielski R, Baker SS, Baker RD. Intussusception associated with adenovirus. J Pediatr Gastroenterol Nutr. 2014;59(5):e41.
9. Bhisitkul DM, Todd KM, Listernick R. Adenovirus infection and childhood intussusception. Am J Dis Child. 1992;146(11):1331–3.
10. Carroll AG, Kavanagh RG, Ni Leidhin C, Cullinan NM, Lavelle LP, Malone DE. Comparative effectiveness of imaging modalities for the diagnosis and treatment of Intussusception: a critically appraised topic. Acad Radiol. 2017;24(5):521–9.
11. Yamamoto LG, Morita SY, Boychuk RB, Inaba AS, Rosen LM, Yee LL, et al. Stool appearance in intussusception: assessing the value of the term "currant jelly". Am J Emerg Med. 1997;15(3):293–8.
12. Harrington L, Connolly B, Hu X, Wesson DE, Babyn P, Schuh S. Ultrasonographic and clinical predictors of intussusception. J Pediatr. 1998;132(5):836–9.
13. Klein EJ, Kapoor D, Shugerman RP. The diagnosis of intussusception. Clin Pediatr (Phila). 2004;43(4):343–7.
14. Kuppermann N, O'Dea T, Pinckney L, Hoecker C. Predictors of intussusception in young children. Arch Pediatr Adolesc Med. 2000;154(3):250–5.
15. Waseem M, Rosenberg HK. Intussusception. Pediatr Emerg Care. 2008;24(11):793–800.
16. Pumberger W, Dinhobl I, Dremsek P. Altered consciousness and lethargy from compromised intestinal blood flow in children. Am J Emerg Med. 2004;22(4):307–9.
17. Hryhorczuk AL, Strouse PJ. Validation of US as a first-line diagnostic test for assessment of pediatric ileocolic intussusception. Pediatr Radiol. 2009;39(10):1075–9.
18. Saverino BP, Lava C, Lowe LH, Rivard DC. Radiographic findings in the diagnosis of pediatric ileocolic intussusception: comparison to a control population. Pediatr Emerg Care. 2010;26(4):281–4.
19. Daneman A, Intussusception NO. Part 1: a review of diagnostic approaches. Pediatr Radiol. 2003;33(2):79–85.
20. Hooker RL, Hernanz-Schulman M, Yu C, Kan JH. Radiographic evaluation of intussusception: utility of left-side-down decubitus view. Radiology. 2008;248(3):987–94.
21. Curtis JL, Gutierrez IM, Kirk SR, Gollin G. Failure of enema reduction for ileocolic intussusception at a referring hospital does not preclude repeat attempts at a children's hospital. J Pediatr Surg. 2010;45(6):1178–81.
22. Lautz TB, Thurm CW, Rothstein DH. Delayed repeat enemas are safe and cost-effective in the management of pediatric intussusception. J Pediatr Surg. 2015;50(3):423–7.
23. Navarro OM, Daneman A, Chae A. Intussusception: the use of delayed, repeated reduction attempts and the management of intussusceptions due to pathologic lead points in pediatric patients. AJR Am J Roentgenol. 2004;182(5):1169–76.

Radiology Case 6

31

Caitlin Hackett and Joshua K. Aalberg

Case 6a

Indication for the Exam

77-year-old man arrives after a motorcycle accident with positive loss of consciousness. He had obvious facial trauma, but seemed neurologically intact.

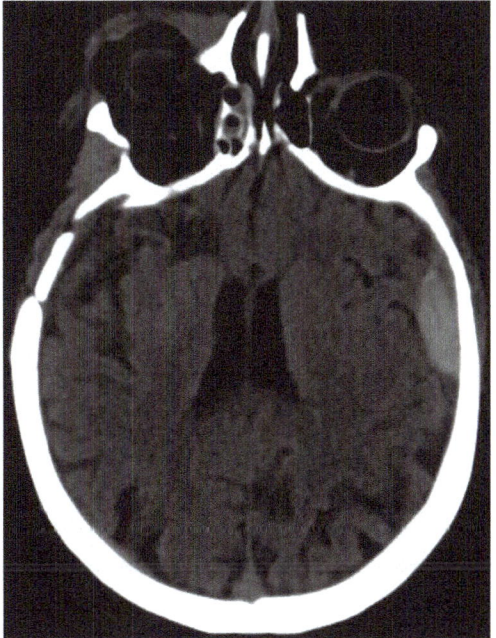

C. Hackett · J. K. Aalberg (✉)
Department of Emergency Medicine, Wexner Medical Center at The Ohio State University, Columbus, OH, USA
e-mail: Caitlin.Hackett@osumc.edu; joshua.aalberg@osumc.edu

© Springer Nature Switzerland AG 2020
C. G. Kaide, C. E. San Miguel (eds.), *Case Studies in Emergency Medicine*,
https://doi.org/10.1007/978-3-030-22445-5_31

Radiographic Findings Lentiform hyperdense collection along the left frontotemporal convexity with mild mass effect.

Diagnosis Epidural Hematoma

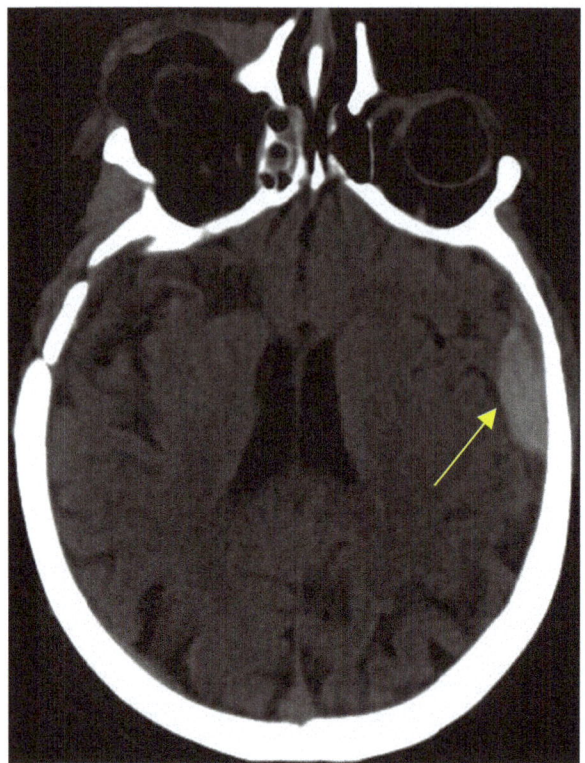

Case 6b Indication for the Exam

19-year-old male presents after being kicked in the face by a bull. He had extensive trauma to the face with a Glasgow Coma Score of 5.

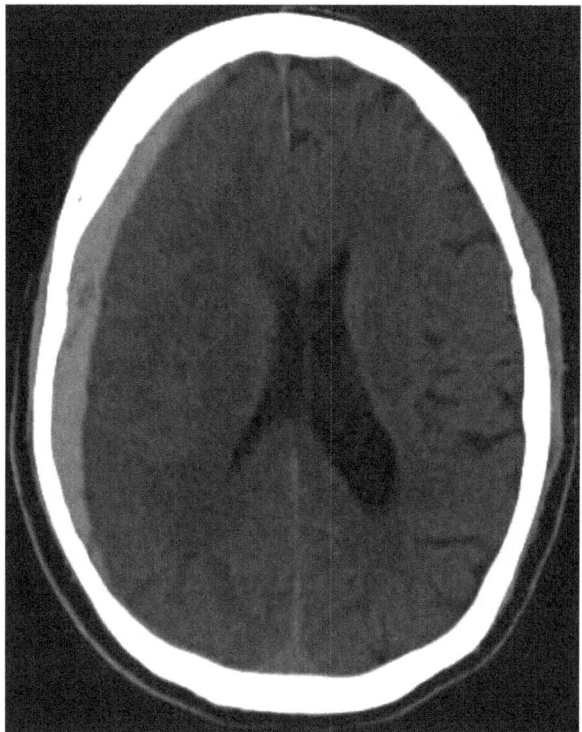

Radiographic Findings He had crescentic hyperdense collection along the right frontal convexity compatible with acute subdural hematoma. There is mass effect and midline shift. The irregular area of hypodensity in the central portion of the hematoma is concerning for active bleeding (swirl sign).

Diagnosis Subdural hematoma

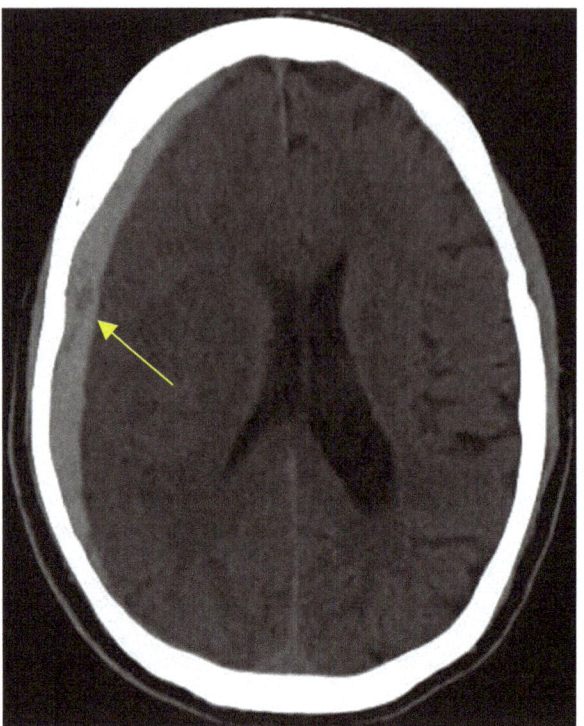

Learning Points

Priming Questions
- How do the radiologic findings differentiate epidural and subdural hematomas?
- How do the treatments differ?
- What are common associated injuries?

Introduction

Extra-axial hemorrhage is defined as bleeding within the cranial vault outside of brain tissue.

- An epidural hematoma (EDH) is bleeding between the inner table of calvarium and outer layer of dura.
- A subdural hematoma (SDH) is bleeding between the inner layer of dura and the arachnoid membrane [1].

Pathophysiology/Mechanism

- EDH is usually caused by shear injury to an artery from a skull fracture. The most commonly injured vessel is the middle meningeal artery. Less than 10% of EDH are venous, most commonly from the middle meningeal vein, diploic vein, or venous sinus. The most common cause is trauma. Occasionally, EDH can be spontaneous from coagulopathy, thrombolysis, vascular malformation, neoplasm, epidural anesthesia, and Paget's disease of the skull. They are rarely bilateral [2].
- Tearing of the bridging veins causes SDH. It is more common in patients with cerebral atrophy, as this increases the length that the bridging veins have to traverse. The most common cause is trauma, though the trauma can be relatively minor. SDH can also be spontaneous, particularly in patients on anticoagulation. Other causes include vascular malformations and hemorrhage of dural metastatic lesions. Up to 20% are bilateral in the elderly [1].

Making the Diagnosis

The classic presentation seen in 50% of patients with EDH is a lucid interval after the initial head injury and loss of consciousness. This can deceive clinicians into believing that the injury is less serious than it is. However, loss of consciousness can also be seen with SDH. Both types of bleed can also have seizures and other signs of mass effect.

The initial test of choice is the noncontrast computed tomography (CT) of the head. Acute blood should be hyperdense (brighter) compared to brain parenchyma. Hyperacute blood that has not clotted can be of low density. Therefore, a low-density area in an acute bleed implies active bleeding as seen in Case 6b above. As blood ages, it becomes less dense and can have a layered appearance. Collections that are subacute and isodense to brain can be easily missed. Isodense collections can also be seen acutely in patients with anemia. Chronic blood products approach CSF density. There can be septations and calcifications within chronic collections [1].

- EDH has a biconvex or lentiform appearance. The collection may cross midline but should not cross sutures, since the dura attaches at the sutures. The exception to this rule is venous bleeds. Ninety to 95% have an associated skull fracture [3].
- SDH is crescent shaped and can cross sutures. Blood can track along the falx and tentorium but should not cross midline overlying cerebral hemispheres.

Secondary signs of hematoma can be helpful if the collection is isodense. These include mass effect, sulcal effacement, sulci that do not extend to the skull, and asymmetry of the lateral ventricles and midline structures [3].

Treating the Patient

Both epidural and subdural hematomas have better outcomes if identified quickly and treated appropriately.

- EDH requires prompt neurosurgery evaluation. Most are treated with craniotomy and evacuation. Mortality rate is 5–8% for surgically treated EDH. The prognosis depends on the extent of the bleed. Infratentorial hematomas, which comprise 5% of EDH, have a worse prognosis. Smaller hematomas <10 mm with no cerebral edema may be managed conservatively. Hematomas usually expand and reach maximal size at 36 hours [4]. One third to one half of patients have another significant neurological injury such as a SDH or parenchymal contusion. EDH in the anterior middle cranial fossa is almost always venous and has an indolent course [5].
- Traumatic SDH has worse prognosis than EDH due to commonly associated parenchymal injuries such as diffuse axonal injury. Acute SDH >2 cm with other parenchymal injuries is associated with >50% mortality. Midline shift exceeding 2 mm is also associated with a worse prognosis [6]. Spontaneous and chronic SDH have a better prognosis. Treatment may involve surgical decompression or drain placement versus observation.

Discussion

- Extra-axial bleeds are common findings in patients with head trauma, though the physical exam may be deceptively normal initially.
- Prompt diagnosis and surgical evaluation is key to improve mortality.
- If there is high clinical suspicion and the initial CT is negative, consider MRI for further evaluation, as this is more sensitive. MRI should also be considered if the degrees of mass effect or symptoms are greater than expected for size of the bleed [1].

Disclosure statement The authors of this chapter report no significant disclosures.

References

1. Yousem DM, Grossman RI. Neuroradiology: the requisites. 3rd ed. Philadelphia: Elsevier; 2010.
2. Weissleder R, et al. Primer of diagnostic imaging. 5th ed., 3rd ed. Philadelphia: Elsevier; 2011.
3. Mirvis SE, et al. Emergency medicine case review. 1st ed. Philadelphia: Elsevier; 2009.
4. Hamilton M, Wallace C. Nonoperative management of acute epidural hematoma diagnosed by CT: the neuroradiologist's role. Am J Neuroradiol. 1992;13(3):853–9.
5. Gean AD, et al. Benign anterior temporal epidural hematoma: indolent lesion with a characteristic CT imaging appearance after blunt head trauma. Radiology. 2010;257(1):212–8.
6. Dent DL, et al. Prognostic factors after acute subdural hematoma. J Trauma. 1995;39(1):36–42.

Lemierre's Syndrome: *A Real Pain in the Neck*

32

Patrick Sylvester and Creagh Boulger

Case

Sore Throat

Pertinent History

Patient presents to the emergency department with 1 month of sore throat. She had sought care twice already at the student health center of her local university and had been prescribed two rounds of oral antibiotics (amoxicillin and azithromycin, respectively). Both times, she says she had a rapid-strep test done, which was positive, and on the second encounter, she reports she had been tested for mono, which was negative. She had finished her last dose of azithromycin 5 days prior to arrival without significant improvement. In addition to the sore throat, she had persistent fevers up to 104 ° F, as well as palpable swelling of her right anterior neck, and pain with lateral rotation of her neck.

PMH

Reports frequent streptococcal pharyngitis, no chronic medical conditions, or daily medications.

SH

College student, never-smoker, occasional ETOH use.

P. Sylvester (✉) · C. Boulger
Department of Emergency Medicine, Wexner Medical Center at The Ohio State University, Columbus, OH, USA
e-mail: Patrick.Sylvester@osumc.edu; Creagh.Boulger@osumc.edu

© Springer Nature Switzerland AG 2020
C. G. Kaide, C. E. San Miguel (eds.), *Case Studies in Emergency Medicine*,
https://doi.org/10.1007/978-3-030-22445-5_32

Pertinent Physical Exam

- Blood pressure 118/61, pulse 137, temperature 101.4 °F (38.6 °C), temperature source Oral, resp. rate 16, height 1.6 m (5′ 3″), SpO2 94%.

Except as noted below, the findings of the complete physical exam are within normal limits.

- General: No obvious distress. Appears to be handling secretions without issue.
- HEENT: Three finger trismus. She has erythema and fullness of right soft palate, uvula midline. There is a palpable 3 × 3 cm mass in right anterior neck at level of cricoid cartilage, tender to palpation with induration and central fluctuance. She reports pain and limited ROM on rightward lateral rotation of neck.
- Respiratory: Trachea midline. No respiratory distress. Breath sounds clear to auscultation bilaterally.

Pertinent Test Results

Lab results			
Lab	Result	Units	Normal range
WBC	40.7	K/uL	3.8–11.0 10³/mm³
Hgb	14	g/dL	(Male) 14–18 g/dL
			(Female) 11–16 g/dL
Platelet	365	K/uL	140–450 K/uL
Creatinine	0.63	mg/dL	0.6–1.5 mg/dL
Lactate	2.6	mmol/L	< 2.0 mmol/L
ESR	31	mm/hr	0–22 mm/hr (male)
			0–29 mm/hr (female)
CRP	187.7	mg/L	< 8 mg/L

ED Management

A soft-tissue CT scan of the neck with IV contrast was ordered to evaluate for peritonsillar abscess versus retropharyngeal abscess. Given the high suspicion for infection, empiric IV ampicillin/sulbactam and clindamycin were started.

Updates on ED Course

Update 1: (1210) CT of the neck resulted showing a right peritonsilar abscess (1.4 cm × 2.1 cm × 2.0 cm) as well as complex cervical abscess of the right anterior neck (1.8 cm × 3.3 cm × 4.0 cm). The right internal jugular vein appears to be occluded throughout its cervical course.

- Heparin was started with a bolus and an infusion.
- Otolaryngology was consulted.

Abscess on Soft Tissue Neck CT

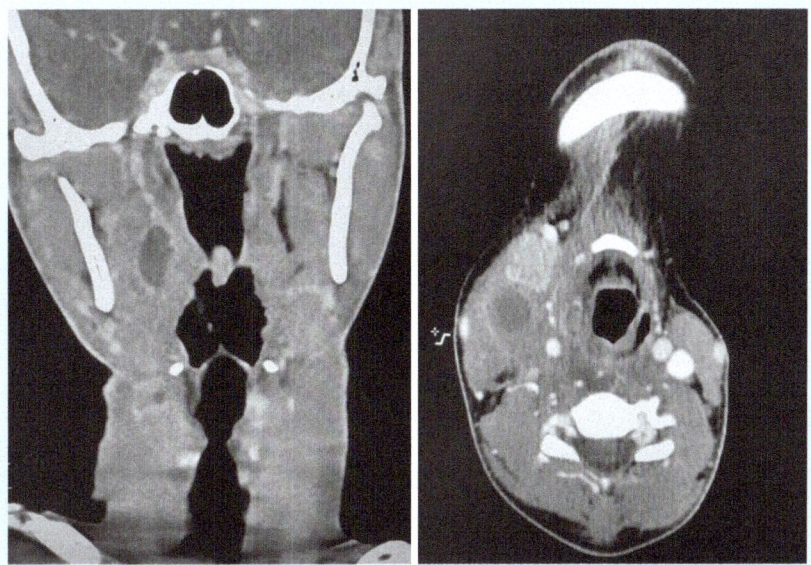

Images courtesy of Patrick Sylvester, MD and Colin Kaide, MD

Update 2: (1415) She was evaluated by otolaryngology and admitted to their service. They requested the heparin infusion to be stopped in preparation for surgery.

– Nothing by mouth
– Maintenance IV fluid

Learning Points

Priming Questions
1. Which pathogens are implicated in this disease process?
2. How does this diagnosis fit in the differential of other ENT infections?
3. What is the role of anticoagulation in this disease, and should it be started in the emergency department?

Introduction/Background

1. Sore throat is a common chief complaint in the emergency department (ED) and primary care offices. The presentation can be acute, subacute, or chronic. Additionally, the etiology can range from the benign such as postnasal drip to

life-threatening such as anaphylaxis, or a mass (infectious, malignant, or traumatic) causing airway compromise.

2. In the emergency department (ED), one is more often looking for serious complications of pharyngitis including peritonsillar and retropharyngeal abscesses. Lemierre's syndrome, which describes a septic thrombophlebitis of the internal jugular vein, should be another diagnosis to add to that list.

3. Admittedly, it is a relatively rare, occurring in less than 1 in one million cases in the general population.1 However, this disease entity can have significant complications if missed.

Physiology/Pathophysiology

1. Lemierre's syndrome classically occurs in the context of an oropharyngeal infection (i.e., tonsillitis or pharyngitis), although it can be associated with odontogenic (dental) infections and rarely lower respiratory tract infections.
   - This typically occurs within 1–2 weeks of an untreated oropharyngeal infection.2
   - The disease was much more prominent prior to the use of penicillin, and we may anticipate a slight increase in incidence as we become more guarded with the use of antibiotics in undifferentiated pharyngitis.3

2. The precise mechanism of developing venous thrombosis is not entirely clear and is likely multifactorial with the following playing a role:
   - Direct extension of infection from pharyngeal space posterolaterally to the carotid sheath.
   - Transient bacteremia.
   - Hypercoagulable state in the setting of ongoing inflammation1.

3. The most common pathogen implicated in Lemierre's syndrome, particularly in presentation with concomitant pharyngitis/tonsillitis is *Fusobacterium necrophorum*.4
   - Interestingly, this anaerobic bacterium is part of the normal oropharyngeal flora and can be found in healthy individuals. However, it is frequently identified in peripheral blood cultures and on operative cultures. There is some body of evidence to suggest that most cases are polymicrobial.
   - Additional pathogens implicated include *Streptococcus* sp., Eikenella corrodens, and *Bacteroides*.

Not All Exudative Pharyngitis Is Strep!

In 2015, a study by Centor, R.M., et al. looked at throat specimens of 312 university students presenting to a University of Alabama campus clinic with sore throat compared to 180 asymptomatic controls. The study looked at the prevalence of *F. necrophorum* versus other bacterial causes such as Mycoplasma pneumoniae, groups A and C/G beta-hemolytic Streptococci. They also looked at the ability of the Centor criteria to predict bacterial infection.

Surprisingly, *F. necrophorum* was the most common cause of pharyngitis. It was detected in 20.5% of symptomatic patients versus 9.4% of controls. Group A Strep was identified in 10.3% of symptomatic patients and 1.1% of asymptomatic controls. Other bacteria including Group GCS/GGS was found in 9.0% of symptomatic patients and 3.9% of controls. Mycoplasma comprised a negligible component of both symptomatic and control patients.

The higher the Centor score, the more likely the PCR (polymerase chain reaction) test for a pathogenic bacteria would test positive.

Centor RM, Atkinson TP, Ratliff AE, et al. The clinical presentation of Fusobacterium-positive and streptococcal-positive pharyngitis in a university health clinic: a cross-sectional study. Ann Intern Med. 2015;162(4):241.

Chapter Author's Comments: Not all exudative pharyngitis is Strep. If the Strep test is negative and the patient has persistent or worsening symptoms (especially in the face of a negative Mononucleosis test, done in the appropriate time frame), think of other bacterial pathogens!

Making the Diagnosis

Differential Diagnosis
- Streptococcal pharyngitis
- Peritonsillar abscess
- Retropharyngeal abscess
- Epiglottitis
- Infectious mononucleosis
- Lymphoma
- Allergies
- Malignancy
- Esophagitis

1. Lemierre's syndrome may be clinically suspected in a patient with a history recent dental, pharyngeal, or tonsilar infection who presents with persistent fevers, sore throat, and neck pain despite conventional oral antibiotic treatment.[12]
   - It may also be suspected clinically based upon identification of a palpable cord in anterior neck. However, this finding may be subtle and may be difficult to discern from reactive lymphadenopathy associated with an oropharyngeal infection.
2. Laboratory testing frequently shows the presence of leukocytosis and inflammatory markers (ESR/CRP) may be elevated; however, these do not have a significant role in the diagnosis of this syndrome.
3. When a thrombus is suspected, it can be most readily confirmed by a vascular ultrasound of the neck, although with the caveat that this is limited with regards to the visualization of vascular structures below the clavicle.

- A CT study of the neck with IV contrast, therefore, is a reasonable alternative and likely the most readily available. Not only can a CT of the neck examine the vasculature of the neck, but it will be helpful in evaluating for concomitant peritonsilar or retropharyngeal abscesses or deep space infection.5
- If a thrombus is detected with suspicion for septic etiology, further imaging of the chest should be considered to evaluate for extension of the clot and septic emboli.
4. If the primary source is not clear, in addition to careful examination of the oropharynx, additional imaging such as panoramic x-ray of the teeth can be helpful in identifying an underlying source. Blood cultures are also useful at the time of diagnosis and may yield a basis for antibiotic selection.

Treating the Patient

1. The treatment of Lemierre's syndrome first and foremost involves assessment of the airway for possible compromise due to soft tissue edema.
   - Symptoms such as drooling, dysphonia, or strider should prompt early consultation with otolaryngology, and if there are any signs of respiratory compromise, preparations should be made for intubation with equipment necessary for a predicted difficult airway.
   - Steroids have little role in the treatment of Lemierre's syndrome; however, if there is concern for life-threatening inflammation of the upper airway, they may be considered as a temporizing measure prior to definitive airway management.
2. Empiric antibiotics should be started with coverage for Gram-positive and anaerobic bacteria.
   - Typical first-line regimens include ampicillin-sulbactam, piperacillin-tazobactam, or clindamycin delivered intravenously.6 Antibiotics may be subsequently tailored based on the availability of culture data.
   - Duration of antibiotics is variable and depends on the ability to achieve source control. Most common treatment plans include IV antibiotics for approximately 4 weeks. Imaging may be utilized at the conclusion of this therapy to determine if an extension of therapy is necessary—particularly if there is persistent phlegmonous collection, thrombosis, or vascular inflammation noted on imaging.
3. Otolaryngology consultation should be obtained if there is the presence of a drainable abscess within the soft tissue of the neck or in the deeper pharyngeal or perivascular spaces as a means of achieving source control.
4. With the presence of an occlusive thrombus, much concern is spent on the question of whether anticoagulation is necessary. There are no randomized, prospective studies looking at the efficacy of this treatment. However, on review of retrospective studies in both children and adults with Lemierre's syndrome, the use of anticoagulation (such as unfractionated heparin or low-molecular-weight heparin) appears unclear. The outcomes were similar for those who underwent systemic anticoagulation and those who did not.

- Expert opinion at this time suggests that in patients who have persistent bacteremia or fevers despite appropriate antibiotic treatment, anticoagulation should be considered as a means of expediting resolution of the infectious nidus within the thrombus. In rare circumstances, vascular intervention such as thrombectomy may be considered; however, there is no data to support this routine practice. Overwhelmingly, treatment of the underlying infection can demonstrate resolution of the thrombus within a period of 1–2 months.7

Case Conclusion

The patient was taken to the OR for I & D of both the neck abscess as well as the peritonsilar abscess. Intraoperative cultures grew *Fusobacterium necrophorum* as well as *Staphylococcus hominis.* Blood cultures on admission and on hospital day 2 showed no growth. Infectious disease was consulted and recommended 4 weeks of ertapenem, with a follow-up CT scan of the neck at the time of completion. No anticoagulation was recommended given the rapid improvement. The patient was discharged at 48 hours with a PICC line and 4 weeks of Ertapenem. By 10 days post-op, the incision had healed and patient was asymptomatic. Follow-up CT showed visualization of the right internal jugular vein as well as resolution of soft tissue inflammation and abscess.

Case Discussion

For the patient with significant lateralized neck pain, persistent fevers, and decreased range of motion of the neck, most ED physicians are going obtain cross-axial imaging of the neck looking for extension of tonsilar/pharyngeal infection. Coincidentally, this same study would also identify the presence of Lemierre's syndrome with visualization of the internal jugular vein. And given that the treatment for this is IV antibiotics and source control, similar to other deep space oropharyngeal infections, it is likely that you will stumble upon the diagnosis at some point!

That being said, identifying the presence of septic thrombophlebitis of the internal jugular vein should place the patient in a higher class of acuity than the average oropharyngeal infection and prompt hospital admission for further monitoring and workup. There should be consideration of further investigation of thromboembolic phenomenon. The need for systemic anticoagulation is rather unclear, but currently available evidence supports anticoagulation in the setting of treatment failure or worsening embolic phenomenon. Thus, in the emergency department, the role of anticoagulation is almost nonexistent. This can be something that may be decided upon later in the patient's hospital course.

REMEMBER: "Not all exudative pharyngitis is Strep. If the Strep test is negative and the patient has persistent or worsening symptoms (especially in the face of a negative Mononucleosis test, done in the appropriate time frame), think of other bacterial pathogens!"

Pattern Recognition

- Pharyngitis that is refractory to multiple rounds of antibiotics
- Sore throat + palpable cord on examination
- Occlusion of internal jugular vein
- If persistent fevers despite appropriate treatment, look for propagation/embolization

Disclosure Statement The authors of this chapter report no significant disclosures.

References

1. Sibai K, Sarasin F. [Lemierre syndrome: a diagnosis to keep in mind]. Rev Med Suisse Romande. 2004;124(11):693–5.
2. Golpe R, Marín B, Alonso M. Lemierre's syndrome (necrobacillosis). Postgrad Med J. 1999;75(881):141–4.
3. Ramirez S, Hild TG, Rudolph CN, et al. Increased diagnosis of Lemierre syndrome and other Fusobacterium necrophorum infections at a Children's Hospital. Pediatrics. 2003;112(5):e380.
4. Holm K, Bank S, Nielsen H, Kristensen LH, Prag J, Jensen A. The role of Fusobacterium necrophorum in pharyngotonsillitis - a review. Anaerobe. 2016;42:89–97.
5. Gottlieb M, Long B, Koyfman A. Clinical mimics: an emergency medicine-focused review of streptococcal pharyngitis mimics. J Emerg Med. 2018;54(5):619–29.
6. Desmet K, Claus PE, Alliet G, Simpelaere A, Desmet G. Lemierre's syndrome: a case study with a short review of literature. Acta Clin Belg. 2018:1–5.
7. Cupit-link MC, Nageswararao A, Warad DM, Rodriguez V. Lemierre syndrome: a retrospective study of the role of anticoagulation and thrombosis outcomes. Acta Haematol. 2017;137(2):59–65.

Lightning Strike: Thunderbolts and Lightning, Very, Very Frightening… The Cosmic DC Countershock

33

David Hartnett and Colin G. Kaide

Case

Lightning Strike

Pertinent History

A 54-year-old man is brought in by EMS after a cardiac arrest. He is unable to provide any history; however, bystanders report he was struck by lightning and was immediately unresponsive. Bystander CPR was initiated and performed for 5 minutes prior to EMS arrival. On arrival, EMS continued CPR and placed a King LT airway. The patient's initial rhythm was asystole, and he received an additional 4 minutes of CPR and 1 mg of IV epinephrine. On the next rhythm check, he was in ventricular tachycardia. Defibrillation was performed a total of three times with progressively increasing joules. He received an additional dose of epinephrine; and two amps of sodium bicarb before he had return of spontaneous circulation (ROSC). He was then transported to the emergency department (ED) without incident.

Pertinent Physical Exam

- Blood pressure 86/42, pulse 42, temperature 94 degrees F, respiratory rate 20, SpO2 98%.

Except as noted below, the findings of the complete physical exam are within normal limits.

- Eyes: Pupils are 2 mm in diameter, round, and nonreactive.

D. Hartnett (✉) · C. G. Kaide
Department of Emergency Medicine, Wexner Medical Center at The Ohio State University, Columbus, OH, USA
e-mail: David.Hartnett@osumc.edu

© Springer Nature Switzerland AG 2020
C. G. Kaide, C. E. San Miguel (eds.), *Case Studies in Emergency Medicine*,
https://doi.org/10.1007/978-3-030-22445-5_33

329

- Cardiovascular: Bradycardia with regular rhythm, palpable pulses throughout.
- Respiratory: King airway in place with color change colorimetry, clear bilateral breath sounds with manual ventilation.
- Spine: Cervical collar in place, no step offs or deformities in the cervical, thoracic, or lumbar spine.
- Neurologic: Unresponsive, GCS 3 T.
- Skin: Four centimeter laceration with no active bleeding to the chin. Violaceous discoloration to the entire chest, shoulders, and right flank with an associated 1% total body surface area burn on the low midline chest over the sternum.
- The patient's past medical, social, and family history are unknown.

Pertinent Test Results

EKG – Junctional escape rhythm with a rate of 30
CT head, face, cervical/thoracic/lumbar spine, chest, abdomen, and pelvis – no significant traumatic injuries

ED Management

The 54-year-old male patient presented as a level 1 trauma alert after a lightning strike with associated cardiac arrest after prehospital ROSC. On arrival, a King LT airway was in place and he had palpable pulses. He was bradycardic and hypotensive on presentation and intravenous fluid resuscitation was begun. An EKG was obtained which showed a bradycardic junctional escape rhythm, and temporary cardiac pacing was initiated as well as an epinephrine infusion. These interventions increased his heart rate to the mid 80s and his blood pressure was improving. A repeat EKG was obtained and continued to show a junctional rhythm. Central access and arterial monitoring lines were placed. He was initiated on a therapeutic hypothermia protocol.

CT imaging was obtained to evaluate for associated traumatic injuries. The patient was then admitted to the surgical intensive care unit (SICU) in critical condition.

Learning Points

Priming Questions
1. What is the pathophysiology of lightning-related injuries and are these similar to other electrical injuries?
2. What are the first steps after a lightning strike?
3. How does cardiac arrest occur and are there any special considerations for treatment following a lightning strike?

Introduction/Background

1. In the United States, there are approximately 25 million lightning strikes per year with an average of 47 deaths per year from lightning strikes. Lightning strikes are one of the leading causes of weather-related death with an approximately 10% mortality rate in the United States. The lifetime risk of being struck by lightning in the United States is approximately 1 in 14,600 [1].

2. Lightning is a rapid discharge of electricity between two opposite charges. Initially, the air acts as an insulator between positive and negative charges between the clouds or a cloud and the ground. When the difference in charge becomes too great, there is a unidirectional (in one direction) discharge of electrons. The potential difference that results may exceed two million volts/m. This is most similar to a DC current exceeding 50,000 amps, which when converted to heat, can generate a temperature of over 50,000 °F [2].

3. There are five main types of lightning strike injuries [3].

   - *Direct Strike*: This happens when a patient is directly struck by lightning without the lightning first contacting another object. Direct strikes have the highest fatality rates.

     - Upward Streamers: A less common type of direct lightning injury (sometimes called the 5th mechanism) was described in the early 2000s [4, 5]. Injury happens when a person is caught in an upward streamer. Upward streamers are induced by the downward lightning leader as it approaches the ground. Multiple upward streamers can develop but usually only one connects with the downward stroke, completing the circuit. Even if the individual is not part of the completed lightning channel, the discharging of the streamer can cause injury or death. Although the upward streamers are much less powerful than a completed lightning stroke, they can still deliver hundreds of amps. The frequency of this type of lightning injury is likely underestimated.

   - *Contact Injury:* This occurs when the lightning strikes an object that the patient is touching. The current travels through the object and then into the patient.

   - *Side-Splash:* This is a phenomenon where the lightning strikes an object near a patient, and then, as it is traveling through that object, the current jumps through the air to the patient.

   - *Ground Current Injury:* This occurs when the lightning strikes the ground near a patient and travels through the ground. It then travels up into the patient through the legs, or whichever body part is touching the ground.

   - *Blast Injury:* This can occur due to a thermoacoustic blast wave that occurs from rapid superheating of the surrounding air-thunder, and can create an overpressure as high as 100 atmospheres of pressure surrounding the lightning.

Types of Lightning Strikes

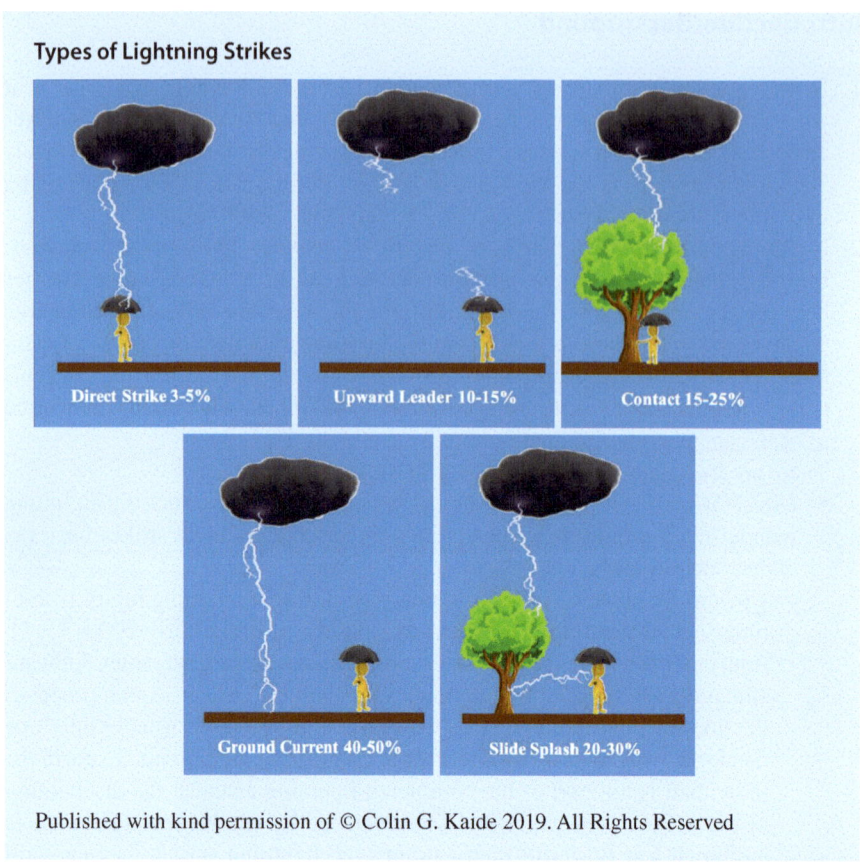

Physiology/Pathophysiology

1. As lightning travels through the heart, it acts as a massive countershock, causing simultaneous depolarization of the entire heart, followed by a period of asystole. This is most common with a direct strike. The intrinsic automaticity of the heart may restart, leading to spontaneous return of normal cardiac rhythm. However, respiratory arrest may persist longer and hypoxia can lead to further cardiac decompensation and repeat arrest. There are numerous ongoing manifestations of lightning injury [6].
   - Although the immediate effects of a lightning strike are difficult to study, a patient with an implanted loop recorder had been struck with a rhythm strip recorded "live" during the event. When this patient was struck, there was immediately a large spike of electricity, followed by ventricular fibrillation for a few seconds and then ventricular tachycardia. Although he spontaneously returned to a sinus rhythm, two friends with him at the time, died immediately [7].

- There are also case reports of multiple patients (with implanted cardiac devices (ICDs)) who have been struck or have been very near to lightning that have been defibrillated. Unfortunately, about half of the reports have been inappropriate shocks delivered by the ICDs. The magnetic field produced by the lightning has the ability to disrupt normal function of the ICDs [8].
- In the first 3 days following lightning strikes, there may be a severely reduced ejection fraction of less than 15% and ongoing cardiogenic shock. This cardiomyopathy typically resolves within 1–2 weeks.
- In a direct lightning strikes, there may also be electrocardiographic changes consistent with myocardial injury, such as ST elevation, QTc prolongation, or pericardial effusion. The source of these changes is not entirely clear and while some patients do have underlying ischemia, other patients have had normal cardiac enzymes and no evidence of myocardial infarction despite these EKG changes [8].

2. One cause of cellular damage from lightning strikes is electroporation where the lipids of the cell membrane reorganize into pores, altering the cell membrane potentials. As ATPase fails to compensate for the rapid exchange of ions across the membrane through these large pores, cell death occurs. This has the greatest effect on skeletal muscle and nerve cells due to their large size and thus large cellular membranes [3].

3. While the cardiac manifestations are the best studied, several other organ systems have important effects of lightning strike.
   - Respiratory arrest is common in lightning strike and is thought to be due to a combination of central medullary depression and chest wall muscle paralysis [3]. Direct pulmonary damage is rarely described [6].
   - Neurologic effects are widely varied. Most victims will lose consciousness. These effects are classified into four groups [3].
     - Group 1 neurologic effects are immediate and transient. These are the most common effects and include loss of consciousness, confusion, paresthesias, and transient paralysis—often of the lower extremities.
     - Group 2 neurologic effects are also immediate, but are either prolonged or permanent. This group includes hypoxic injuries, intracerebral hemorrhage, postcardiac arrest cerebral infarction, and cerebellar syndromes.
     - Group 3 neurologic effects are delayed syndromes such as motor neurodiseases and movement disorders.
     - Group 4 neurologic effects are injuries from the associated fall or blast such as subdural or epidural hematoma and subarachnoid hemorrhage.
   - Otic complications are very common, with up to 80% of lightning strike victims having tympanic membrane rupture [6].

Making the Diagnosis

If there was a witnessed lightning strike, or the patient is conscious and able to report the event, the diagnosis may be obvious. However, the alternative may be a patient in cardiac arrest without any history of the event.

Differential Diagnosis
- Lightning strike
- Associated traumatic injuries
- Thermal burns
- Seizure
- Stroke
- Subarachnoid hemorrhage
- Other causes of cardiac arrest

1. Often times, the patient may have been witnessed as having been struck by lightning and the diagnosis is clear. In these cases, the objective is to identify any related injuries. Other times, the diagnosis is less obvious, but can be assumed – the patient was found down unconscious in a field immediately following a storm would likely raise suspicion. But occasionally, there is no context to raise suspicion for a lightning strike.
2. The skin lesions seen in a lightning injury can often be very revealing. While the pathognomonic finding may or may not be present, there are additional skin findings that can also be seen [3].
   - Linear streaking burns occur due to the rapid heat of the lightning causing vaporization of sweat on the body. These are typically small and seen in areas likely to have accumulated sweat – under the arms, middle of the chest, etc. [9].
   - Punctate burns may also occur that are small, usually less than 1 cm. These burns have been described as occurring on the tips of the toes and the sides of the feet in lightning patients—a so-called tip toe sign [10].
   - Thermal burns may occur from the patient's clothing or other nearby structures catching fire.
   - The pathognomonic skin finding in lightning strikes is the Lichtenberg figure. This skin finding is not a burn, but rather occurs from extravasation of blood in the subcutaneous tissue. They are often not present in lightning strike patients, and when they are present, last for only a few hours [11].

Lightning Strike "Feathering" or Lichtenberg Pattern

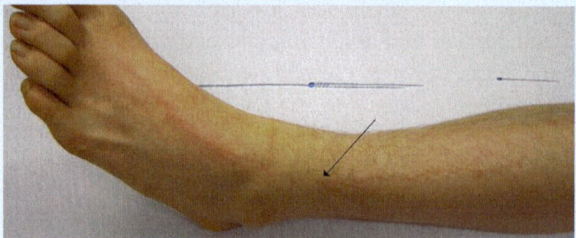

By James Heilman, MD – Own work, CC BY-SA 3.0, https://commons.wikimedia.org/w/index.php?curid=11110313

Lightning Strike "Feathering" or Lichtenberg Pattern

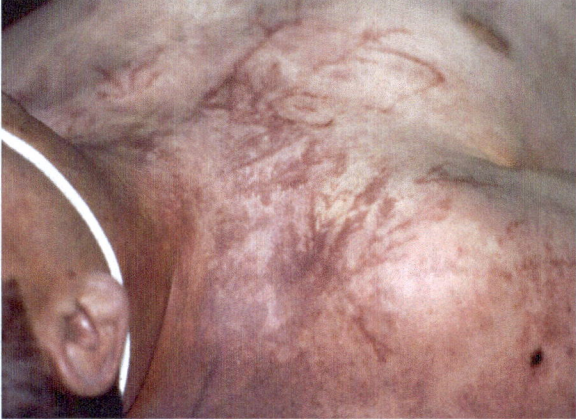

Image courtesy of David Effron MD, FACEP

Burns from a Direct Lightning Strike

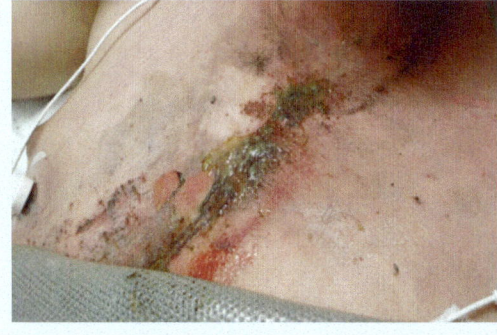
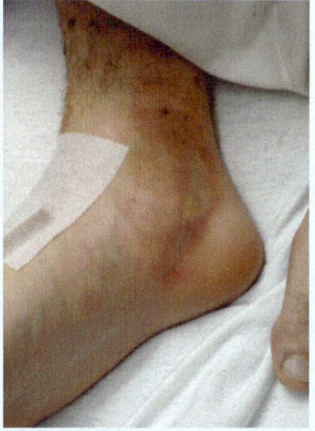

Image courtesy of Brittany Carver, DO

3. Transient paralysis of the lower extremities following a lightning strike is common and termed keraunoparalysis [12]. This abnormality typically resolves without any further intervention. However, lower extremity paralysis could also be caused by associated spinal trauma, and thus any lightning strike victim with neuro deficits will likely require CT imaging of the head and spine and MRI of the full spine. Additional neurologic injuries such as cerebral edema require the same supportive care measures as other etiologies of these injuries.

4. Finally, the thermoacoustic pressure that occurs from the superheated air surrounding the lightning strike may result in blast injuries to the patient. You must investigate for primary injuries from the barotrauma, including otic, pulmonary, and viscous injuries, as well as tertiary injuries from blunt trauma. Similar to other trauma patients, the physical exam will likely guide your imaging choices. However, if the patient is obtunded or unable to provide a reliable exam, then you should assume there was a high mechanism of injury and pursue broad imaging.

Treating the Patient

1. The average patient struck by lightning is in their late teens to early thirties, male, and otherwise relatively healthy. As such, when a patient is struck by lightning and suffers from a combined cardiac and respiratory arrest, he or she may often survive with early intervention. The patients who are struck and do not immediately suffer from respiratory arrest are unlikely to experience significant decompensation and die. Therefore, a reverse triage system is appropriate at the scene of a lightning strike, focusing first on any patients who are not spontaneously breathing with or without a pulse [13].
   - Initiation of usual BLS, ACLS, and defibrillation should be provided to lightning victims. Once return of spontaneous circulation has been obtained, respiratory arrest may persist due to the central depression and chest wall paralysis. Therefore, ventilatory support may need to continue to prevent a secondary arrest due to hypoxia [14].
   - Due to the patient's potential lack of comorbidities or underlying pathology of the heart, prolonged resuscitations can often lead to successful outcomes [15].
2. Due to the cardiac stunting that may occur with lightning strike, patients are at risk for developing ongoing cardiomyopathy with similarities to takotsubo cardiomyopathy. Many of these patients resolve spontaneously in the course of weeks. However, they may require significant cardiovascular support for acutely decompensated heart failure involving inotropic support and aggressive volume management [8].
3. Lightning strike victims who suffer a cardiac arrest are likely to require comprehensive trauma care in a regional trauma center in order to provide ongoing support for all possible associated injuries. However, many patients are discharged from the emergency department if they have a reassuring evaluation.

Why Your Car Protects You from Lightning Strikes

When you are in your car, you are protected from lightning! The car acts like a Faraday Cage and the current passes around the outside of the vehicle and disperses into the ground. The rubber tires have no role in this effect.

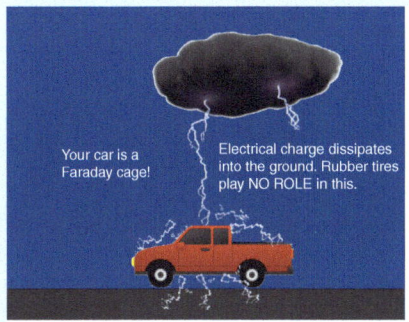
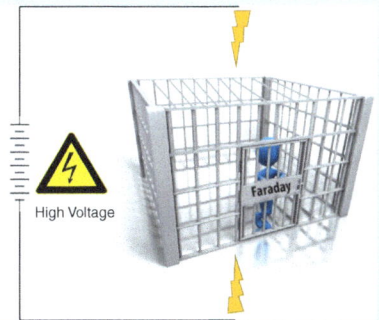

Position of Safety in Anticipated Strike

The position of safety has been advocated by some wilderness medicine experts when a person is caught in a lightning storm and can't reach safe shelter. It is based on sound theory, but for obvious practical reasons, no randomized trials exist proving that it works. The thought is that if your hair stands on end and you feel tingling in your skin, a lightning strike is imminent!

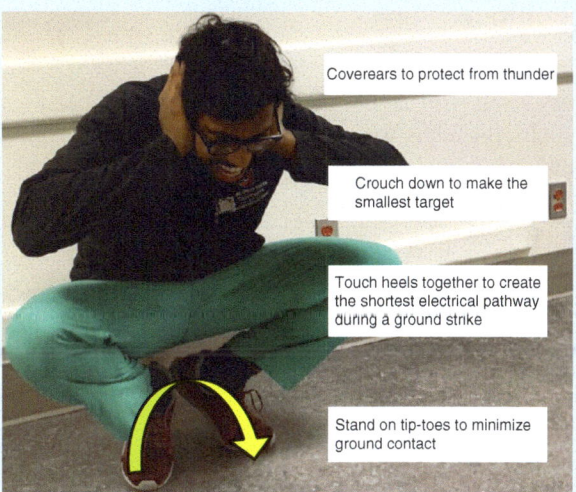

Case Conclusion

The patient's mental status slowly improved, and he was extubated on hospital day 2. He had an elevated troponin during hospitalization and underwent cardiac catheterization, showing no significant occlusive disease. He was discharged to home on hospital day 4 and has returned to his baseline physical status after undergoing physical and occupational therapy. He continues to have skin discoloration changes over his chest and flank as a reminder of the event.

Discussion

Morbidity and mortality from lightning strikes have significantly decreased over the past 100 years, and victims of lightning strikes are now much more likely to be participating in recreational activity rather than agriculture. While the overall number of deaths per year has declined, many of these deaths can still be avoided with further proactive measures. The national weather service and many other national organizations have focused on layperson awareness of the dangers of lightning. Simple common sense practices of staying inside a stable building or in a car during storms has the most impact. When there is no safe shelter during a storm, the proposed body position is to crouch down close to the ground to reduce the risk of a direct strike, stand on your toes with heels touching to reduce the likelihood of ground current injury, and cover your ears to protect them from primary blast injury. While this may be good in theory, hopefully you will never need to use the lightning crouch.

Pattern Recognition

- Respiratory arrest with cardiac activity
- Neuro deficits, including fixed and dilated pupils or paralysis, can be common and often transient
- Lichtenberg pattern on skin
- Potential blunt trauma

Disclosure Statement David Hartnett: No disclosures

Colin Kaide: Callibra, Inc.-Discharge 123 medical software company. Medical Advisory Board Portola Pharmaceuticals. I have no relationship with a commercial company that has a direct financial interest in subject matter or materials discussed in article or with a company making a competing product.

References

1. National Weather Service. How dangerous is lightning. [Online] [Cited: June 18, 2018]. https://www.weather.gov/safety/lighting-odds.
2. National Weather Service. Understanding lightning. [Online] [Cited: June 18, 2018]. https://www.weather.gov/safety/lightning-science-scienceintro.
3. Ritenour AE, Morton MJ, JG MM, Barillo DJ, Cancio LC. Lightning injury: a review. Burns. 2008;34:585–94.
4. Anderson RB. Does a fifth mechanism exist to explain lightning injuries? IEEE Eng Med Biol. 2001;20:105–16.
5. Cooper MA. A fifth mechanism of lightning injury. Acad Emerg Med. 2002;9:172–4.
6. Conrad L. Clinical update on lightning injuries. Wilderness Environ Med. 1998;9:217–22.
7. Atalhi A, Al-Manea A, Alqweai N, Alothman M. Cardiac rhythm recorded by implanted loop recorder during lightning strike. Ann Saudi Med. 2017;37:401–2.
8. Christophides T, Khan S, Ahmad M, Fayed H, Boggle R. Cardiac effects of lightning strikes. Arrhythm Electrophysiol Rev. 2017;6:114–7.
9. O'keefe Gatewood M, Zane RD. Lightning injuries. Emerg Med Clin North Am. 2004;22:369–403.
10. Fahmy FS, Brinsden MD, Smith J, Frame JD. Lightning: the multisystem group injuries. J Trauma. 1999;46:937–40.
11. Bartholome CW, Jacoby WD, Ramachand SC. Cutaneous manifestatiosn of lifhtning injury. Arch Dermatol. 1975;111:1466–8.
12. ten Duis HJ, Klasen HJ, Reenalda PE. Keraunoparalysis, a 'specific' lightning injury. Burns. 1985;12:54–7.
13. Taussig HB. "Death" from lightning – and the possibility of living again. Ann Intern Med. 1968;68:1345–53.
14. ECC Committee, ECC Subcommittees, and ECC Task Forces; and Authors of Final Evidence Evaluation Worksheets 2005. International Consensus on Cardiopulmonary Resuscitation and Emergency Cardiovascular Care With Treatment Recommendations Conference Part 10.9: electric shock and lightning strikes. IV. Circulation. 2005;112:154–5.
15. Marcus MA, Thigis N, Meulemans AI. A prolonged but successful resuscitation of a patient struck by lightning. Eur J Emerg Med. 1994;1:199–202.

Loperamide Toxicity: *"I'm in Love ... I'm All Stopped Up"*

Bridget Onders and Kurt Neltner

Case

Pertinent History

The patient arrived to the emergency department (ED) via EMS at 0600. He reported he took 400 tablets of loperamide at 2200 the previous evening in an attempt to get high. He awoke this morning with lightheadedness, right-sided abdominal pain, nausea, and dyspnea. The initial EKG by EMS was concerning for widened QRS and extremely prolonged QTc.

PMH Depression, panic disorder

SH Denies a history of illicit drug use, but states he has been taking loperamide to get high. He reports taking 100 tablets every 1–2 days for the past 2 months. Denies current tobacco use but has a history of smokeless tobacco.

Pertinent Physical Exam

- BP 119/66, pulse 82, temperature 98.1 °F (36.7 °C), RR 17, SpO2 100%

  Except as noted below, the findings of a complete physical exam are within normal limits.

- Cardiovascular: Normal rate, irregular rhythm. No murmur heard. Normal heart sounds.

B. Onders · K. Neltner (✉)
Department of Emergency Medicine, Wexner Medical Center at The Ohio State University, Columbus, OH, USA
e-mail: bridget.onders@osumc.edu; kurt.neltner@osumc.edu;

© Springer Nature Switzerland AG 2020
C. G. Kaide, C. E. San Miguel (eds.), *Case Studies in Emergency Medicine*, https://doi.org/10.1007/978-3-030-22445-5_34

Pertinent Diagnostic Testing

Test	Result	Units	Normal Range
Sodium	135	mEq/L	135–148 mEq/L
Potassium	2.9 ↓	mEq/L	3.5–5.5 mEq/L
Chloride	102	mEq/L	96–112 mEq/L
Bicarbonate	22	mEq/L	21–34 mEq/L
BUN	14	mg/dL	6–23 mg/dL
Creatinine	1.64 ↑	mg/dL	0.6–1.5 mg/dL
Calcium	8.4 ↓	mg/dL	8.6–10.5 mg/dL
Phosphate	5.0 ↑	mg/dL	2.2–4.6 mg/dL
Magnesium	1.5 ↓	mg/dL	1.6–2.6 mg/dL
Salicylate	< 5	mg/dL	<30.0 mg/dL
Acetaminophen	<10	mcg/mL	<32.0 mcg/mL
Alcohol	380 ↑	mg/dL	<10 mg/dL
Troponin	0.01	mg/dL	< 0.04 ng/dl

EKG on Arrival

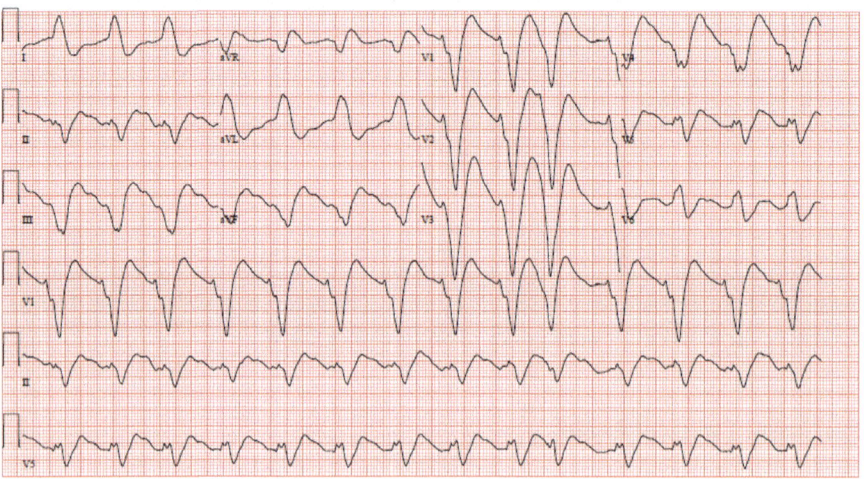

Plan

The patient arrived alert and oriented, but lightheaded. He was placed on a cardiac monitor, given IV fluids. Given the patient's EKG with QRS widening and QT prolongation, he was given IV magnesium, IV calcium, and IV bicarbonate.

The poison center was contacted regarding the patient's case. The patient's symptoms, including cardiac dysrhythmias were felt to be consistent with massive loperamide overdose. As the patient was found to be hypokalemic and hypomagne-semic, these electrolytes were replaced. After speaking with the poison center, it was thought the widened QRS was primarily a potassium channel event and there-fore would not respond to naloxone. The patient was admitted to the ICU.

Learning Points: Loperamide Overdose

Priming Questions
1. How does loperamide work as an anti-diarrheal agent?
2. How does loperamide toxicity present?
3. How do you treat and stabilize a loperamide toxicity?

Introduction/Background

1. Loperamide is a synthetic opioid, sold over the counter as an antidiarrheal agent. At therapeutic doses, it acts at the μ-opioid receptor to inhibit peristaltic activity of the mesenteric plexus of the large intestine [1].
2. It has been considered low risk for abuse due to its peripheral activity and lack of central effects at therapeutic doses.
   - This is due to both the low bioavailability and active excretion at the blood–brain barrier by P-glycoprotein, a multidrug efflux pump [2].
   - Although this drug has been considered to have a wide margin of safety and considered low risk for abuse, there is growing evidence that misuse and abuse of loperamide for its opioid effects are growing.
     - A study looking at the National Poison Data System found a 91% increase in reported loperamide exposures from 2010 to 2015 [3].

Physiology/Pathophysiology

1. Loperamide is a phenylpiperidine opioid, similar to meperidine. By stimulating μ-opioid receptors in the myenteric plexus, it acts to slow the intestinal transit time. The medication also possesses antisecretory properties and blocks intesti-nal calcium channels [2].
2. It has been considered safe and low risk for abuse due in part to its low bioavailability.
   - Predominant metabolism is by intestinal and hepatic cytochrome P450 enzymes, which metabolize the drug to inactive metabolites [4].
   - Absorbed loperamide as well as its metabolites undergo biliary excretion.
3. In addition to its low bioavailability, the presence of P-glycoprotein (P-gp) at the blood–brain barrier decreases this medication's abuse potential. P-gp is a

multidrug efflux pump that is found in several different areas of the body. Its importance in loperamide is due to its active role in limiting the passage of loperamide into the brain [5].

4. There are several known drug interactions with loperamide which can influence its concentration within the blood and brain.
   - Because the low bioavailability of loperamide is in part due to its metabolism by cytochrome P450 enzymes, any inhibitor of these enzymes has the potential to increase bioavailability [2].
   - P-gp inhibitors also act to increase loperamide concentration by not only increasing the absorption of loperamide from the intestine but also by inhibiting efflux pumping of loperamide out of the brain.
     - In both humans with genetic polymorphisms resulting in decreased P-gp activity, as well as knock out mice with no functional P-gp, decreased activity of this pump led to increased plasma and brain concentrations of loperamide [6, 7].

5. At the maximum recommended dose of 16 mg/day, the effects of loperamide are limited to the gut; however, increased dosages are noted to have central nervous system effects
   - Saturation of the P-gp enables loperamide to cross the blood–brain barrier and activate central opioid receptors.

6. Loperamide has a well-demonstrated cardiotoxicity. The FDA issued a warning on June 7, 2016, about the serious cardiac events, which can result from abuse and misuse of loperamide [8].
   - Mechanisms of the pro-arrhythmic effects of loperamide are likely related to the inhibition of the sodium/potassium transmembrane ion channels in the cardiac cells.
     - QRS prolongation is likely related to delays in depolarization while QT prolongation is reflective of delays in repolarization [9].
     - Studies have demonstrated that loperamide has an ability to inhibit all three of the most abundant cardiac sodium channels at different affinities.
     - One of the sodium channels for which loperamide has demonstrated the highest affinity is the hERG channel. Inhibitory action on this channel is thought to be responsible for the EKG changes of a loperamide toxicity. Inhibition at this channel can affect both depolarization as well as repolarization, therefore causing both QRS prolongation as well as QT prolongation [9].

Making the Diagnosis

Differential Diagnosis – Consider Loperamide Toxicity in these Situations
- Cardiac dysrhythmias in patients with a significant history of opioid abuse.
- self-treating opioid withdrawal,
- chronic diarrheal illness (IBS, post cholecystectomy, etc.) and self-treating with over-the-counter remedies.

1. Loperamide toxicity presentations can vary with many different presenting complaints.
   - Although many of the toxicities secondary to loperamide are cardiotoxicities, these are not the only presentation.
   - In our case, the patient reported lightheadedness, abdominal pain, and nausea. These symptoms are very ambiguous, and if the patient is not forthcoming with loperamide use, there can be a significant delay to diagnosis.
   - Loperamide toxicity can also manifest as somnolence with respiratory depression that is classically seen in other opioid overdoses.
   - Other case reports have found presentations for syncope, cardiac arrest, weakness, slurred speech, tachycardia, and near syncope [10–15].
2. Because loperamide is available over the counter, patients may think its use to be unimportant and therefore be less forthcoming with reporting its use. It is also used by patients in many different ways and with different intentions.
   - Patients have taken large and inappropriate loperamide doses as a means to treat diarrhea from a wide range of causes, without the intention of abuse [10, 11].
   - Patients may be taking this medication in order to treat opioid withdrawal symptoms [12].
   - Some patients are taking loperamide with the intention of an opioid-like high [14].
3. The EKG is your best friend in loperamide toxicities. Because cardiac toxicity is the dangerous element of a loperamide toxicity, the EKG is an imperative step in evaluation.
   - Loperamide toxicities significant enough to cause cardiac toxicities will often have QRS as well as QT prolongation.
4. Evaluate for co-ingestion (intentional or unintentional) of cytochrome p450 and P-gp inhibitors, as these can increase loperamide concentration [16].
5. History! History! History!
   - Asking specific questions about loperamide abuse is the best way to identify this toxicity. Loperamide does not come up positive on routine drug testing and therefore can be difficult to identify if the patient does not endorse taking it [16].

Treating the Patient

1. Treatment for loperamide overdose is mostly supportive with most treatment recommendations extrapolated from toxicological principles and anecdotal experience.
   - Naloxone is indicated in cases presenting with signs and symptoms of opioid overdose such as respiratory depression or somnolence with risk of compromising the airway.
     - As with naloxone use in other opioid overdoses, the lowest effective dose should be used, but repeated dosing should also be expected due to loperamide's slow elimination [2].

- Activated charcoal is a possible treatment in the setting of a large overdose as long as the patient's mental status is intact.
    - The case for administration of activated charcoal in the setting of loperamide overdose is based on the belief that a clinically important amount of drug would still remain in the GI tract and its adsorption to charcoal might favorably influence the patient's clinical course [17].
2. Cardiotoxicity secondary to loperamide should be treated with standard advanced cardiac life support (ACLS) therapy when applicable.
    - Initial stabilization with ACLS treatment of any cardiac arrest including cardioversion or defibrillation for shockable rhythms as well as intravenous magnesium for polymorphic ventricular tachycardia should be the first priority.
        - Repeated shocks may be required, as demonstrated in several case reports [10, 11, 18].
    - Overdrive pacing using transvenous electrical pacing and isoproterenol have been used to suppress ventricular ectopy and prevent recurrent dysrhythmias in patients with torsades de pointes secondary to loperamide [11–14].
    - Although there is no specific treatment for the QT prolongation induced by loperamide, it is reasonable to ensure that other reversible factors that can contribute to QT prolongation have been addressed such as hypokalemia, hypomagnesemia, and other medication effects [2].
    - Treatment of the widening of the QRS complex caused by loperamide sodium channel blockade can be addressed with a trial of intravenous sodium bicarbonate; however, it is unclear if this will effectively improve conduction [2].
        - Cases have demonstrated multiple concomitant treatments including magnesium, potassium chloride, sodium bicarbonate, and antiarrhythmic medications such as lidocaine and amiodarone with minimal EKG improvement reported [11, 12, 15, 19, 20].
3. Intravenous lipid emulsion is a reasonable consideration for patients with significant cardiotoxicity with limited published cases using this modality [18, 21].
4. Hemodialysis is not considered a possible treatment, as loperamide is a lipophilic, highly protein bound medication (97%).
5. Venoarterial extracorporeal membrane oxygenation (ECMO) is a potential treatment for severe loperamide cardiotoxicity refractory to other measures; however, there is very limited experience and literature to support ECMO in this setting [21, 22].
6. In patients with loperamide toxicity, an effort to determine the reason for loperamide use and abuse should be made.
    - Consideration should be given to appropriate management of an underlying opioid use disorder or other psychiatric disorder.
    - In cases of accidental overdose, patient education is paramount to prevent recurrence.

Case Conclusion

This patient was admitted to the ICU. Throughout his first 24 hours of admission, he was on IV dopamine and IV isoproterenol and was in and out of multiple different cardiac rhythms including sinus bradycardia, ventricular tachycardia, and an accelerated junctional rhythm with bundle branch block. Over the next several days of hospitalization, his QRS narrowed, but his QT remained prolonged and he had multiple episodes of ventricular tachycardia and torsades de pointes. Each of these episodes self-resolved and he did not receive any cardiac defibrillation. Eventually, his QTc gradually shortened. The patient remained hemodynamically stable and his QTc improved to 450 ms. On hospital day 10, the patient was discharged to a psychiatric facility as there was concern for intentional ingestion.

Discussion

1. Loperamide has been available without a prescription since 1988 due to low concern for abuse. This was largely based on its pharmacokinetics when taken at therapeutic doses, but does not take into account the change in pharmacokinetics when taken at higher doses and in toxic ingestions [3].
2. Loperamide abuse has been increasing and is projected to continue to increase in the age of the opioid epidemic [9]. This has been demonstrated through epidemiologic studies, which demonstrate a 91% increase in nonmedical use of loperamide from 2010 to 2015 [3]. This is likely multifactorial, but contributing factors are thought the be the ease of access to the drug over-the-counter, low price, and increased knowledge of illicit uses of this medication [2]. Increased Internet interest in the illicit use of loperamide has also been seen, demonstrating the ease of access to information as well as the rapid nature in which this information can be spread via the Internet [23].
3. Treatment of loperamide toxicity is largely supportive with a focus on stabilization from a cardiac standpoint. Data are limited on the best methods for treatment of cardiac toxicity secondary to loperamide and most information in the literature is from case studies [9–15, 19, 20].

Pattern Recognition

- Suspected loperamide abuse by report or history of opioid abuse, withdrawal, or chronic diarrhea.
- Nonspecific symptoms vs syncope vs palpitations vs respiratory depression.
- Cardiac dysrhythmias, particularly widened QRS and prolonged QT.

Disclosure Statement The authors of this chapter report no significant disclosures.

References

1. Mackerer CR, Clay GA, Dajani EZ. Loperamide binding to opiate receptor sites of brain and myenteric plexus. J Pharmacol Exp Ther. 1976;199:131–40.
2. Wu PE, Juurlink DN. Clinical review: loperamide toxicity. Ann Emerg Med. 2017;70:245–52. https://doi.org/10.1016/j.annemergmed..2017.04.008.
3. Vakkalanka JP, Charlton NP, Holstege CP. Epidemiologic trends in loperamide abuse and misuse. Ann Emerg Med. 2017;69:73–8. https://doi.org/10.1016/j.annemergmed.2016.08.444.
4. Kim KA, Chung J, Jung DH, Park JY. Identification of cytochrome P450 isoforms involved in the metabolism of loperamide in human liver microsomes. Eur J Clin Phamacol. 2004;60:575–81.
5. Regnard C, Twycross R, Mihalyo M, Wilcock A. Loperamide. J Pain Symptom Manag. 2011;42:319–23. https://doi.org/10.1016/j.jpainsymman.2011.06.001.
6. Skarke C, Jarrar M, Schmidt H, Kauert G, Langer M, Geisslinger G, Lotsch J. Effects of ABCB1 (multidrug resistence transporter) gene mutations on disposition and central nervous effects of loperamide in healthy volunteers. Pharmacogenetics. 2003;13:651–60.
7. Schinkel AH, Wagenaar E, Mol CA, van Deemter L. P-glycoprotein in the blood-brain barrier of mice influences the prain penetration and pharmacological activity of many drugs. J Clin Invest. 1996;97:2517–24.
8. FDA warns anbout serious heart problems with high doses of the antidiarrheal medicine loperamide (Imodium), including from abuse and misuse; 2016. https://www.fda.gov/Drugs/DrugSafety/DrugSafetyPodcasts/ucm506835.htm. Accessed 1 June 2018.
9. Akel T, Bekheit S. Loperamide cardiotoxicity: "a brief review". Ann Noninvasive Electrocardiol. 2018;23:e12505. https://doi.org/10.1111/anec.12505.
10. Upadhyay A, Bodar V, Malekzadegan M, Singh S, Frumkin W, Mangla A, Doshi K. Loperamide induced life threatening ventricular arrhythmia. Case Rep Cardiol. 2016;2016:5040176. https://doi.org/10.1155/2016/5040176.
11. Spinner HL, Lonardo NW, Mulamalla R, Stehlik J. Ventricular tachycardia associated with high-dose chronic loperamide use. Pharmacotherapy. 2015;35:234–8. https://doi.org/10.1002/phar.1540.
12. Mukarram O, Hindi Y, Catalasan G, Ward J. Loperamide induced torsades de pointes: a case report and review of the literature. Case Rep Med. 2016;2016:1. https://doi.org/10.1155/2016/4061980.
13. Rasla S, Parikh P, Hoffmeister P, St Amand A, Garas MK, El Meligy A, Minami T, Shah NR. Unexpected serious cardiac arrhythmias in the setting of loperamide abuse. R I Med J. 2017;100:33–6.
14. Salama A, Levin Y, Jha P, Alweis R. Ventricular fibrillation due to overdose of loperamide, the "poor man's methadone". J Community Hosp Intern Med Perspect. 2017;7:222–6. https://doi.org/10.1080/20009666.2017.1351290.
15. Wightman RS, Hoffman RS, Howland MA, Rice B, Biary R, Lugassy D. Not your regular high:cardiac dysrhythmias caused by loperamide. Clin Toxicol. 2016;54:454–8. https://doi.org/10.3109/15563650.2016.1159310.
16. Bishop-Freeman SC, Feaster MS, Beal J, Miller A, Hargrove RL, Brower JO, Winecker RE. Loperamide-related deaths in North Carolina. J Anal Toxicol. 2016;40:677–86.
17. Juurlink DN. Activated charcoal for acute overdose: a reappraisal. Br J Clin Pharmcol. 2016;81:482–7. https://doi.org/10.1111/bcp.12793.
18. Marraffa JM, Jolland MG, Sullivan RW, Morgan BW, Oakes JA, Wiegand TJ, Hodgman MJ. Cardiac conduction disturbance after loperamide abuse. Clin Toxicol. 2014;52:952–7. https://doi.org/10.3109/15563650.2014.969371.
19. Katz KD, Cannon RD, Cook MD, Amaducci A, Day R, Enyart J, Burket G, Porter L, Roach T, Janssen J, Williams KE. Loperamide-induced torsades de pointes: a case series. J Emerg Med. 2017;53:339–44. https://doi.org/10.1016/j.jemermed.2017.04.027.

20. Kozak PM, Harris AE, McPherson JA, Roden DM. Torsades de pointes with high-dose loperamide. J Electrocardiol. 2017;50:355–7. https://doi.org/10.1016/j.jelectrocard.2017.01.011.
21. Enakpene EO, Riaz IB, Shirazi RM, Raz Y, Indik JH. The long QT teaser: loperamide abuse. Am J Med. 2015;128:1083–6. https://doi.org/10.1016/j.amjmed.2015.05.019.
22. Johnson NJ, Gaieski DF, Allen SR, Perrone J, DeRoos F. A review of emergency cardiopulmonary bypass for severe poisoning by cardiotoxic drugs. J Med Toxicol. 2013;9:54–60. https://doi.org/10.1007/s13181-012-0281-8.
23. Borron SW, Watts SH, Tull J, Baeza S, Diebold S, Barrow A. Intentional misuse and abuse of loperamide: a new look at a drug with "low abuse potential". J Emerg Med. 2017;53:73–84. https://doi.org/10.1016/j.jemermed.2017.03.018.

LVAD Woes: *Lub-Dub, Lub-Dub, Lub-Dub…or Maybe Not!*

35

Nick Kman and Leslie Adrian

Case 1

A 57-year-old male with history of ischemic cardiomyopathy eventually necessitating LVAD placement presented with shortness of breath. He complained of progressively worsening orthopnea for 2–3 days, now with dyspnea at rest, with worsening bilateral lower extremity swelling. He takes warfarin daily and has not missed any doses. He also takes atorvastatin and insulin daily.

Pertinent Physical Exam

Except as noted below, the findings of the complete physical exam are within normal limits.

- Vital signs: Mean arterial pressure (MAP) 63, temperature 98.6 °F/37C
- General: Pale, appears ill but in no acute distress, awake, and alert
- Cardiovascular: Whir of LVAD auscultated, unable to palpate extremity pulses
- Respiratory: Bibasilar crackles, diminished breath sounds bilaterally
- Extremities: Cool and dry, with 2+ pitting edema bilaterally to knees, no rashes or wounds

PMH

Ischemic cardiomyopathy s/p LVAD placement 2 years prior and an internal cardioverter-defibrillator (ICD) placement

Insulin-dependent diabetes mellitus, type II

Hyperlipidemia

N. Kman (✉) · L. Adrian
Department of Emergency Medicine, Wexner Medical Center at The Ohio State University, Columbus, OH, USA
e-mail: Nicholas.Kman@osumc.edu; leslie.adrian@osumc.edu

© Springer Nature Switzerland AG 2020
C. G. Kaide, C. E. San Miguel (eds.), *Case Studies in Emergency Medicine*,
https://doi.org/10.1007/978-3-030-22445-5_35

SH

Former 1.5 pack per day smoker; quit 2 years ago

FH

Father with CAD at age 45; death from myocardial infarction at age 66

ED Management

Patient placed on cardiac monitoring; 2 large bore IVs placed

Pertinent Test Results

EKG showed sinus tachycardia with heart rate of 103 and no ST segment changes or T wave inversions
CXR: small bilateral pleural effusions and mild interstitial pulmonary edema

Test	Result	Units	Normal range
Hgb	10.1 ↓	g/dL	(Male) 14–18 g/dL
			(Female) 11–16 g/dL
Sodium	132	mEq/L	135–148 mEq/L
Creatinine	1.1	mg/dL	0.6–1.5 mg/dL
Troponin	0.06	ng/ml	<0.04 ng/ml
INR	2.4	–	≤1.1

Plan

Serial EKGs, troponins, and bedside and formal echocardiogram (echo) were performed and a consult to open heart surgery was placed. If the patient were to become hypotensive or to deteriorate clinically, we planned for administration of vasopressors.

Updates on ED Course

Bedside echo showed a dilated right ventricle and functioning LVAD. A CT pulmonary angiogram (CTPE) was ordered based on symptoms and right heart dilatation on echo and was negative for pulmonary embolism.
Open heart surgery came to see the patient and recommended medical management for right heart failure and admission to congestive heart failure service.

Repeat troponin trended up, now at 0.94 ng/ml 3 hours after the original troponin, concerning for subendocardial ischemia.

Case 2

A 61-year-old male with a history of ischemic cardiomyopathy, status-post LVAD placement 3 years prior as destination therapy, presented with chest pain and repeated ICD firing. His LVAD team recommended calling EMS for transport to the nearest LVAD center. EMS reported that his heart rhythm as ventricular tachycardia. They administered 150 mg of amiodarone prior to arrival without conversion to sinus rhythm. Home medications include dobutamine, torsemide, spironolactone, warfarin, amiodarone, hydralazine, and aspirin [1].

Pertinent Physical Exam

Except as noted below, the findings of the complete physical exam are within normal limits.

- Vital signs: BP 122/80 (automatic cuff), RR 18, temperature 98.6 °F/37 °C, LVAD motor speed 10,000 rpm
- General: Well-appearing, no distress, but anxious
- Cardiovascular: Whir of LVAD auscultated, thrill palpated on arterial pulse examination
- Respiratory: Clear breath sounds bilaterally
- Extremities: Warm and dry, no edema

PMH

Ischemic cardiomyopathy with LVAD placement 3 years prior
  ICD placement, with hospitalization within the last 2 weeks for CHF exacerbation
  Chronic kidney disease, stage III

SH

No history of smoking or drug use; occasional alcohol use

FH

No family history of cardiac disease

ED Management

An EKG was obtained showing polymorphic ventricular tachycardia with a heart rate of 300 bpm. Amiodarone drip and prophylactic magnesium infusion were administered. Chemistries, CBC, troponin, and CXR were ordered.

Pertinent Test Results

CXR – LVAD and PICC line in proper position, cardiomegaly and bibasilar atelectasis with interstitial edema (similar to previous)

Test	Result	Units	Normal range
WBC	4.2	K/uL	3.8–11.0 K/uL
Hgb	10.6	g/dL	(Male) 1418 g/dL
			(Female) 11–16 g/dL
Platelets	146	K/uL	140–450 K/uL
Sodium	134	mEq/L	135–148 mEq/L
Potassium	3.6	mEq/L	3.5–5.5 mEq/L
Bicarbonate	24	mEq/L	21–34 mEq/L
BUN	28	mg/dL	6–23 mg/dL
Creatinine	2.1	mg/dL	0.6–1.5 mg/dL
Glucose	146	mg/dL	65–99 mg/dL
Magnesium	2.3	mg/dL	1.6–2.6 mg/dL
INR	2.4	–	≤1.1
Troponin	0.06	ng/ml	<0.04 ng/ml

Plan

An electrophysiology consult was placed and synchronized cardioversion with procedural sedation was planned.

Updates on ED Course

Patient was sedated with propofol and was successfully cardioverted with 360 J 1 hour after his presentation to ED. The postcardioversion EKG showed normal sinus rhythm with QTc prolongation (588 ms). Postcardioversion LVAD display showed 10,000 RPM and cardiac output of 4.7 L/min. The patient was admitted to the heart failure service after remaining hemodynamically stable postcardioversion.

Learning Points

Priming Questions
1. How do you evaluate patients with LVADs? How do you assess vital signs?
2. What kind of complications do patients experience with LVADs?
3. How is management of a coding patient with an LVAD different from standard ACLS?

Introduction/Background

1. Types of LVADs:
   - All LVADs are designed to assist left ventricular output in patients with severe cardiomyopathy. In each case, the implanted pump, which is powered by an external power source and controller, transfers blood from the left ventricular apex to the aortic outflow tract. The controller is connected to the pump via the driveline, a surgically implanted tunneled power cable [2].

LVAD

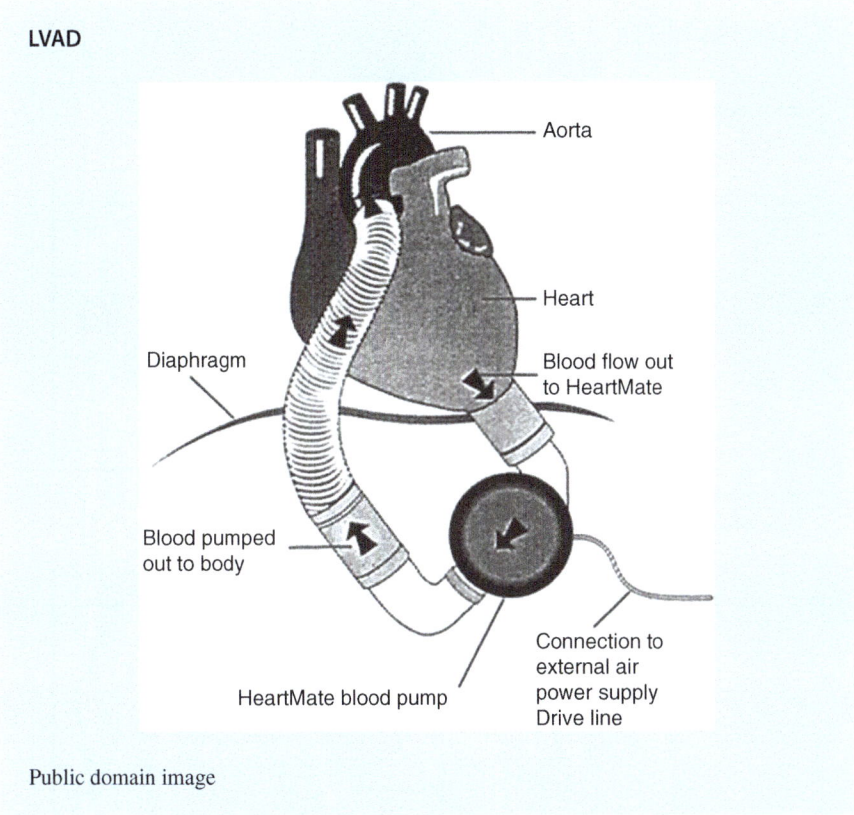

Public domain image

- There are two general types of LVADs: Pulsatile flow and continuous flow. Pulsatile flow LVADs mimic a physiologic systole and diastole, while continuous flow (as it sounds) continuously moves blood from the LV to the aorta. Continuous flow increases diastolic pressure and decreases pulse pressure. Continuous flow models are most often used for their improved safety profile compared to pulsatile flow devices [2].
   - Axial flow pump devices (including the commonly used HeartMate II®, Thoratec Corporation, Pleasanton, CA) use a curved rotor blade (impeller), which draws blood in a nonpulsatile fashion from the LV to the aortic outflow tract.

- Centrifugal pump devices use "centrifugal force" to generate continuous, nonpulsatile flow. The newest devices, such as the HeartMate III® (Thoratec Corporation, Pleasanton, CA) rely on an electromagnet to suspend the rotor and thus decrease rotor contact with the pump casing, with the goal of reducing shear flow and hemolysis. A two-year follow-up study in patients with HeartMate III® implantation showed lower rates of reoperation for pump malfunction and pump thrombosis but no difference in survival compared to axial flow devices [3].

Types of LVADS

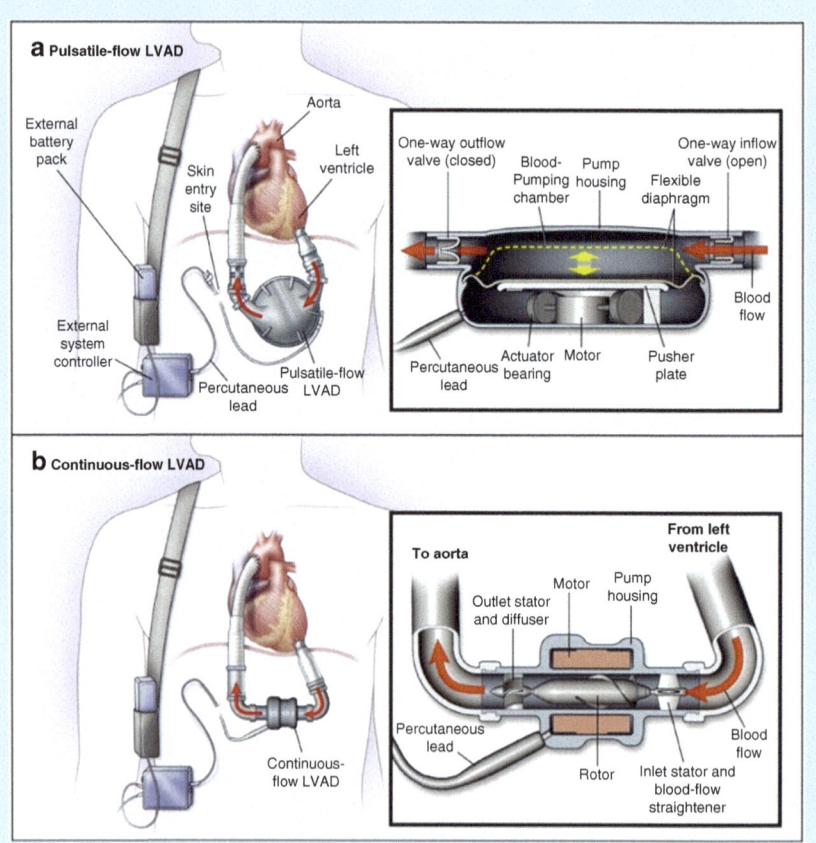

From New England Journal of Medicine: Mark S. Slaughter, M.D., Joseph G. Rogers, M.D., Carmelo A. Milano, M.D. et al. Advanced Heart Failure Treated with Continuous-Flow Left Ventricular Assist Device. 361;23, p 2244 Copyright © 2009, Massachusetts Medical Society. Reprinted with permission from Massachusetts Medical Society

2. Indications for LVAD placement:
   - End-stage heart failure that cannot be further treated by medications or surgical procedures.
     – May be due to ischemic heart disease or more commonly nonischemic cardiomyopathy from infection, toxic medications, etc.
   - Temporary support during left ventricular recovery after acute insult, bridge to eventual transplantation, or "destination therapy," which is becoming more common given the lack of availability of heart transplantation [1].
3. Scope of the problem:
   - There are 5.8 million cases of heart failure in the USA as of 2015, and an estimated 100,000–200,000 have heart failure refractory to medical management [2, 4]. The mortality rate is above 50% annually for these patients without further intervention [5].
4. Natural course of disease post-LVAD placement:
   - As reported in a 2014 systematic review on clinical outcomes post-LVAD placement, survival rates were 56–87% at 1 year, 43–84% at 2 years, and 47% at 4 year, with a 5-year mean survival of 54% after implantation. This is greatly improved compared to survival of end-stage heart failure patients who cannot undergo LVAD placement and are receiving medical management alone (6% at 1 year), making the number needed to treat to save one life 2 years after LVAD placement as less than 2 patients. Quality of life also improved after LVAD placement in most patients, with 80% going from NYHA class IIIB or IV symptomatology to NYHA class I or II symptomatology, representing a tremendous improvement in functional capacity [6, 7].
   - Readmission rate was reported as 55% (for any cause) in the first year after implantation from 2007 to 2013. This and the following numbers can be quoted to patients to facilitate a risk benefit discussion prior to LVAD placement [6].
     – 50%, major bleeding event (not including hemorrhagic stroke).
     – 10%, hemorrhagic or ischemic stroke.
     – 20%, serious device related infections.
     – 18%, ongoing heart failure symptoms.
     – 5%, pump thrombosis and device malfunction.

Physiology/Pathophysiology

Types of Complications
1. Ventricular arrhythmias
   - Ventricular arrhythmias are common in LVAD patients. Observational studies have shown that the events are most common in the first 2–3 months after LVAD placement with an incidence rate of 22–52%. Ventricular arrhythmias within 30 days of placement are associated with higher mortality than arrhythmias that occur later [8–10].

- Interestingly, patients can be awake and perfusing during these rhythms! This is because LVADs are still perfusing the periphery even if the native heart rhythm is not generating a perfusing rhythm. What is tricky is that the LVAD only augments blood flow from the left side of the heart and does not have any positive effect on the right ventricle. Therefore, if the nonperfusing rhythm is sustained, severe damage can occur from right heart failure.
    - One study from The Cleveland Clinic showed that ventricular fibrillation decreased cardiac output by 1 L/min [11]. It is currently unknown how long patients can withstand the decrease in cardiac output. However, it is certain that these patients will eventually need cardioversion or defibrillation to regain a normal perfusing rhythm.

2. Bleeding
    - The most common types of bleeding are gastrointestinal (GI) and intracranial bleeds. These are thought to be secondary to arteriovenous malformations, which develop in the setting of reduced pulse pressure (increased diastolic pressure) typically in the upper GI tract and small bowel. In addition, these patients are on anticoagulation to prevent pump thrombosis.
    - It is also possible, although much rarer, to have bleeding from mechanical device leaks. This can be significantly worsened by an acquired Von Willebrand's type syndrome produced by shearing force created by the pump itself, causing a reduction in the number of large von Willebrand (vW) multimers and subsequent decrease in vW-platelet binding capacity [12].
    - Bleeding is the most common reason for an LVAD patient to present to the ED, and recent estimates show an occurrence rate of 1.5 bleeding events per patient per year, with the highest risk in the first 2 weeks after implantation [6, 13].

3. Ischemic and hemorrhagic stroke – leading cause of death in LVAD patients
    - The internal components of the LVAD can serve as a nidus for thrombosis just like any implanted device. Even with anticoagulation, ischemic (embolic) strokes are relatively common.
        - In one study that included 183 LVAD patients in a single center, 21% suffered a stroke after placement (13% ischemic and 10.3% hemorrhagic). Hemorrhagic stroke had higher all-cause mortality than ischemic stroke [14].
    - Another single-center study found that strokes occurred in 19% of LVAD patients, 49% of which were ischemic, 37% hemorrhagic, and 14% ischemic with hemorrhagic conversion. There was a higher ischemic stroke burden in patients with CAD, and higher hemorrhagic stroke burden in patients with diabetes mellitus [15]. Incidence of stroke increased the longer the patients had LVADs [6].

4. Right heart failure
    - LVADs do not assist the right ventricle (RV) with blood flow to the pulmonary circuit, and subsequent right heart failure is common after LVAD implantation. If the LV cannot get blood flow from the lungs and RV, it cannot provide systemic flow. This is more likely if the patient had the LVAD placed for ischemic cardiomyopathy.
        - More common in males or patients who were older in age at placement [16].
        - Tachyarrhythmias will affect LVAD patients more severely than patients without heart failure symptoms.

- Twenty to twenty-five percent of patients will end up needing persistent inotropic support. Right heart failure is an independent mortality risk factor after LVAD placement [6].
5. Infection
   - Driveline infection is the overall most common infection site in LVAD patients. Risk factors include obesity and younger age, as shown in a large meta-analysis. Fortunately, this is an easier infection to treat in these patients, using a combination of local debridement and antibiotics.
     - Driveline infection is shown to be responsible for bacteremia in about 40% of cases [17]. One proposed mechanism of driveline infections is patients accidentally dropping the controller and accidently pulling the drive line out of the skin slightly, introducing skin flora deeper into the driveline site [18].
   - Bacteremia is less common than driveline infection. However when it does happen, resistant *Pseudomonas* infections can develop along with an increased incidence of stroke [17]. Between 2005 and 2016, a study of 164 patients showed that the incidence of bacteremia was 29% at 1 year and 36% at 2 years after implantation.
     - The incidence of hemorrhagic stroke was 22% without bacteremia and 32% with bacteremia at 1 year, and 22% without bacteremia and 44% with bacteremia at 2 years. This study showed that bacteremia was an independent risk factor for hemorrhagic stroke <90 days after LVAD implantation [19].
   - Severe infections were shown to increase 2-year mortality after placement by 14% [6].
6. Pump Thrombosis
   - As with any implanted foreign body, LVAD pump can be a nidus for thrombosis, leading to embolic complications and failure of the pump itself. For this reason, patients need to be on systemic anticoagulation, unless severe bleeding complications occur. The incidence of pump thrombosis is around 8% for all LVAD patients during their lifetime.

Making the Diagnosis

Differential Diagnosis of the Unstable LVAD Patient
- LVAD power loss/connection failure
- Pump failure
- Acute coronary syndrome
- Arrhythmia
- Pulmonary embolism
- Hyper or hypokalemia
- LVAD thrombosis
- Sepsis/hypovolemia
- Right heart failure

1. The most important aspect of the initial assessment is the same as every other patient in the ED – sick or not sick? In the LVAD patients, however, one must rely on clinical indicators rather than focusing solely on vital signs. Patients will not have a reliable pulse due to the continuous flow of the LVAD. Instead, capillary refill, mental status, urine output, and skin color will provide a more reliable assessment of perfusion. You may be able to feel a thrill at the central or distal arterial sites, but this will not tell you the heart rate. The only thing that will assess the heart rate is the EKG or cardiac monitor.

2. Blood pressure measurement in these patients can be tricky! Automatic blood pressure cuffs are often unreliable as the pulse pressure is reduced. You will need to use a manual blood pressure cuff, and while you may be able to auscultate one sound representing mean arterial pressure (MAP), more likely you will need to use doppler to assess return of blood flow to the extremity while letting the cuff pressure down.
   - The MAP should be between 70 and 80, with 80 being the upper limit of normal. Higher MAP will require an assessment as to why the pump has increased power requirement. If LV afterload is too high, then the pump will not be able to efficiently deliver flow [18].

3. An arterial line will give you an actual systolic and diastolic blood pressure, and can also be used for measuring SPO_2, as the pulse oximetry monitor can be unreliable (there is no pulse). Again, with these patients, clinical picture is the key – if they look like their work of breathing is increased and poorly perfused, then they are poorly perfused.

4. Always auscultate for the "whir" of the LVAD on your cardiopulmonary exam. It should be a gentle mechanical whir, without high-pitched noises or grinding sounds. This will tell you if the pump is on, working and connected to power. Also, check the following:
   - Cables connecting the driveline to the controller.
   - Controller does not feel too hot.
   - Batteries have adequate charge.
   - Any device alarms – can help you determine what kind of malfunction could be occurring.
   - Pump pocket on the lower chest or upper abdomen and the driveline site for signs of infection.

5. If the pump is stopped for longer than 30 minutes to an hour, restarting the pump could theoretically lead to device clotting and emboli. Whether or not to restart the VAD in this scenario depends on the clinical context, as there is no evidence-based consensus on how long the pump can be stopped before the risk of clotting is high. If the patient is unstable, then pump should be restarted immediately. You may need to augment the VAD by giving vasopressors or inotropes while starting a heparin drip to stabilize any clots that may have formed [20].

6. There are many complications that you need to be familiar with when sick patients present with an LVAD. However, do not forget the forest for the trees! Patients with LVADs can get all the same illnesses and injuries as any other patients. Do not just focus on LVAD and forget everything else.

- The diagnosis of bleeding in LVAD patients is the same with any other patient. You will need to assess the source of bleeding and get a CBC to assess hemoglobin and platelet count.
  - Hemoglobin goal should be 7 mg/dl or above.
- Device infection is relatively straightforward to detect with a thorough exam of the driveline site and pump pocket. Do not forget to fully expose the patient and assess for more common infections. A CT scan of the chest or abdomen may be indicated to diagnose internal infections.
- Pump thrombosis is a diagnosis that requires the emergency physician to have a high clinical suspicion. Clues include.
  - High flow alarms on the LVAD, as the LVAD cannot efficiently transfer blood from the LV to the aorta if thrombosis is present.
  - The RPM and power requirement can increase either suddenly or gradually, indicating that there is greater resistance in the circuit and greater power is needed to overcome this phenomenon.
  - Increased hemolysis as measured by increased free hemoglobin (>40 mg/dl), increased LDH (2.5× above normal, significantly increased from patient's baseline, or above 600 IU), decreased haptoglobin, and reddish-brown urine (free hemoglobin in urine secondary to hemolysis) [18, 20].
- Right heart failure in LVAD patients will look very similar to right heart failure in patients without an LVAD including peripheral signs of volume overload, such as peripheral edema, increased jugular venous pressure and decreased exercise tolerance. Be sure to look for acute MI and pulmonary embolism. A low flow alarm may go off if there is not enough preload from the right ventricle to produce appropriate flow.

Treating the Patient

1. Resuscitation of the patient in shock with malignant arrhythmia
   - Nonperfusing and unresponsive patients who have LVADs deserve special consideration when undergoing resuscitation. The number one difference compared to standard ACLS has been the warning (from device manufacturers) not to do chest compressions for fear of dislodging the device, resulting in irreversible hemorrhage into the mediastinum. The issue is that the patient is already technically dead in this scenario.
     - There have been several small studies demonstrating that the risk versus benefit analysis is in favor of doing early chest compressions. In one of these studies, there was no device dislodgement after CPR and 50% recovered neurologically after cardiac arrest [18, 21].
     - In 2017, the American Heart Association published a guideline recommending chest compressions as part of ACLS in LVAD patients, if end tidal CO_2 is <20 mmHg after successful intubation [22]. A recent case report, written by one of the authors of this recommendation, demonstrated successful resuscitation with meaningful neurologic recovery after following

this recommendation [23]. Apart from assessing the mechanical components of the LVAD, the resuscitating physician will otherwise follow ACLS
protocols.
- Patients who look ill with mental status changes or other clinical evidence of
poor perfusion with a ventricular arrhythmia should be immediately cardioverted to restore perfusion immediately. Those patients who are awake, alert,
and are otherwise relatively well despite a ventricular arrhythmia should be
cardioverted with assistance from cardiology, electrophysiology, or LVAD
service. In some cases, if you are not at an LVAD center, it may be appropriate
to transfer a patient prior to cardioversion [1].
- As with every patient, one should assess WHY the LVAD patient is experiencing dysrhythmia and treat the underlying cause. Most common causes in
this population are myocardial ischemia and electrolyte disturbances (most
are on medications that can affect potassium, magnesium, and the QTc).
Right heart failure leading to cardiogenic shock is also common.
2. Diagnosis-specific treatments.
- *Severe bleeding* should be treated with volume resuscitation (blood products)
and reversal of anticoagulation. Consult with your LVAD team and cardiothoracic surgery prior to moving forward. Depending on the scenario, tranexamic
acid, 4-factor prothrombin complex concentrate, desmopressin, or fresh frozen
plasma can be utilized. The harm–benefit ratio of reversing anticoagulation in
life-threatening bleeding is favorable, with a recent small study showing 96%
effectiveness in INR reversal with PCC without any thrombotic events [24].
- *Pump thrombosis* should be treated with anticoagulation (heparin) and in
some cases with thrombolytics based on the recommendations of the LVAD
team. These events often require replacement of the LVAD.
  - Recent evidence shows that surgical device exchange is nearly twice as
  successful in eliminating thrombosis than medical management [25].
- *Right heart failure* should be treated with inotropy if the patient is in cardiogenic shock. Milrinone and dobutamine are first line depending on the prefer-
ence of the LVAD team. There may also be a role for inhaled nitric oxide and
epoprostenol as well as oral medications such as sildenafil, which decrease
pulmonary vascular resistance and lead to increased right ventricular ejection
fraction [6, 26].
- *Left heart failure* secondary to aortic regurgitation may be transiently treated by
increasing the pump speed. However, if severe aortic regurgitation is present,
the patient will need surgery evaluation for an aortic valve replacement [27].
- *Sepsis and dehydration* are typically treated in the same was as any patients.
The difference here is that LVAD patients are preload dependent. Dehydration
or distributive shock can lead to "low-flow" alarms and decreased cardiac
output, as the rotor does not have enough volume to perfuse the rest of the
body. This can ultimately lead to a "suction event," in which LV myocardium
overrides the inflow device [28]. With the advice from the LVAD team, this
may be temporarily resolved with IVF boluses, but ultimately require surgical
intervention.

Case Conclusion

Case 1

The patient was admitted to the heart failure service, underwent 7 L of diuresis, and was discharged after 1 week with an increased dose of home furosemide [1].

Case 2

While on the heart failure service, ICD interrogation showed that patient's ICD had fired six times prior to ED arrival without successful cardioversion. One of the leads was replaced and the generator charge was adjusted. The patient was then discharged after 3 days in the hospital [1].

Discussion

As you may have noticed throughout this chapter, we have stressed communicating early on with the LVAD coordinator or team during the patient's ED visit. If your hospital is not an LVAD center, you will be able to find an LVAD coordinator's phone number on a tag attached to the exterior controller. If this is not present, ask the patient or family for the contact information. They will be invaluable in helping you manage the complications.

As always, you need to be an advocate for the patient. Their care may involve one or several consulting services with potentially different priorities. It is your job to put it all together and recognize the safest and most appropriate treatment and disposition for each and every patient. You may need to gently remind the consultants that you have concerns about safety and discuss potential plans thoroughly. Do not be afraid to escalate to a more senior member of the consulting team if your safety concerns are not being addressed.

Pattern Recognition

LVAD Malfunction
1. Presence of an LVAD
2. Altered Mental Status
3. LVAD Alarms
4. Diaphoresis, tachydysrhythmia, dyspnea and/or other signs of poor perfusion

Disclosure Statement   The authors of this chapter report no significant disclosures.

References

1. Fitzgibbon J, Kman NE, Gorgas D. Asymptomatic sustained polymorphic ventricular tachycardia in a patient with a left ventricular assist device: case report and what the emergency physician should know. J Emerg Med. 2016;50:E135–41.
2. Baughman K, Jarcho J. Bridge to life - cardiac mechanical support. N Engl J Med. 2007;357(9):846–9.
3. Mehra MR, Goldstein DJ, Uriel N, et al. Two-Year outcomes with a magnetically levitated cardiac pump in heart failure. N Engl J Med. 2018;378:1386–95.
4. Ammar K, Jacobsen S, Mahoney D, Kors J, Redfield M, Burnett J, et al. Prevalence and prognostic significance of heart failure stages - application of the American College of Cardiology/American Heart Association heart failure staging criteria in the community. Circulation. 2007;115(12):1563–70.
5. Al Danaf J, Butler J, Yehya A. Updates on device-based therapies for patients with heart failure. Curr Heart Fail Rep. 2018;15(2):53–60.
6. McIlvennan C, Magid K, Ambardekar A, Thompson J, Matlock D, Allen L. Clinical outcomes after continuous-flow left ventricular assist device: a systematic review. Circ Heart Fail. 2014;7(6):1003–237.
7. Miller L, Rogers J. Evolution of left ventricular assist device therapy for advanced heart failure: a review. JAMA Cardiol. 2018;3(7):650–8.
8. Bedi M, Kormos R, Winowich S, McNamara D, Mathier M, Murali S. Ventricular arrhythmias during left ventricular assist device support. Am J Cardiol. 2007;99(8):1151–3.
9. Andersen M, Videbaek R, Boesgaard S, Sander K, Hartsen P, Gustafsson F. Incidence of ventricular arrhythmias in patients on long-term support with a continuous-flow assist device (HeartMate II). J Heart Lung Transplant. 2009;28(7):733–5.
10. Greet BD, Pujara D, Burkland D, Pollet M, Sudhakar D, Rojas F, Costello B, Postalian A, Hale Z, Jenny B, Lai C, Igbalode K, Wadhera D, Nair A, Ono M, Morgan J, Simpson L, Civitello A, Cheng J, Mathuria N. Incidence, predictors, and significance of ventricular arrhythmias in patients with continuous-flow left ventricular assist devices: a 15-year institutional experience. JACC Clin Electrophysiol. 2018;4(2):257–64.
11. Cantillon D, Saliba W, Wazni O, Kanj M, Starling R, Tang W, et al. Low cardiac output associated with ventricular tachyarrhythmias in continuous-flow LVAD recipients with a concomitant ICD (LoCo VT Study). J Heart Lung Transplant. 2014;33(3):318–20.
12. Kataria R, Jorde UP. GI bleeding during CF-LVAD support: state of the field. Cardiol Rev. 2018;27:8. https://doi.org/10.1097/CRD.0000000000000212.
13. Bunte MC, Blackstone EH, Thuita L, Fowler J, Joseph L, Ozaki A, Starling RC, Smedira NG, Mountis MM. Major bleeding during HeartMate II support. J Am Coll Cardiol. 2013;62(23):2188–96.
14. Izzy S, Rubin DB, Ahmed FS, Akbik F, Renault S, Sylvester KW, Vaitkevicius H, Smallwood JA, Givertz MM, Feske SK. Cerebrovascular accidents during mechanical circulatory support: new predictors of ischemic and hemorrhagic strokes and outcome. Stroke. 2018;49(5):1197–203.
15. Tahsili-Fahadan P, Curfman DR, Davis AA, Yahyavi-Firouz-Abadi N, Rivera-Lara L, Nassif ME, LaRue SJ, Ewald GA, Zazulia AR. Cerebrovascular events after continuous-flow left ventricular assist devices. Neurocrit Care. 2018;29:225. https://doi.org/10.1007/s12028-018-0531-y.
16. Asleh R, Hasin T, Briasoulis A, Schettle SD, Borlaug BA, Behfar A, Pereira NL, Edwards BS, Clavell AL, Joyce LD, Maltais S, Stulak JM, Kushwaha SS. Hemodynamic assessment of patients with and without heart failure symptoms supported by a continuous-flow left ventricular assist device. Mayo Clin Proc. 2018;93:895. https://doi.org/10.1016/j.mayocp.2018.01.031.
17. O'Horo JC, Abu Saleh OM, Stulak JM, Wilhelm MP, Baddour LM, Rizwan Sohail M. Left ventricular assist device infections: a systematic review. ASAIO J. 2018;64(3):287–94.
18. DeVore AD, Patel PA, Patel CB. Medical management of patients with a left ventricular assist device for the non-left ventricular assist device specialist. JACC Heart Fail. 2017;5(9):621–31.

19. Yoshioka D, Sakaniwa R, Toda K, Samura T, Saito S, Kashiyama N, et al. Relationship between bacteremia and hemorrhagic stroke in patients with continuous-flow left ventricular assist device. Circ J. 2018;82(2):448–56.
20. Vierecke J, Schweiger M, Feldman D, Potapov E, Kaufmann F, Germinario L, Hetzer R, Falk V, Krabatsch T. Emergency procedures for patients with a continuous flow left ventricular assist device. Emerg Med J. 2017;34(12):831–41.
21. Mabvuure N, Rodrigues J. External cardiac compression during cardiopulmonary resuscitation of patients with left ventricular assist devices. Interact Cardiovasc Thorac Surg. 2014;19(2):286–9.
22. Peberdy M, Gluck J, Ornato J, Bermudez C, Griffin R, Kasirajan V, et al. Cardiopulmonary resuscitation in adults and children with mechanical circulatory support a scientific statement from the American Heart Association. Circulation. 2017;135(24):E1115–34.
23. Ornato JP, Louka A, Grodman SW, Ferguson JD. How to determine whether to perform chest compressions on an unconscious patient with an implanted left ventricular assist device. Resuscitation. 2018;129:e12. https://doi.org/10.1016/j.resuscitation.2018.05.024.
24. Rimsans J, Levesque A, Lyons E, Sylvester K, Givertz MM, Mehra MR, Stewart GC, Connors JM. Four factor prothrombin complex concentrate for warfarin reversal in patients with left ventricular assist devices. J Thromb Thrombolysis. 2018;46:180. https://doi.org/10.1007/s11239-018-1680-8.
25. Luc JGY, Tchantchaleishvili V, Phan K, Dunlay SM, Maltais S, Stulak JM. Medical therapy compared with surgical device exchange for left ventricular assist device thrombosis: a systematic review and meta-analysis. ASAIO J. 2018;65:307. https://doi.org/10.1097/MAT.0000000000000833.
26. Loforte A, Grigioni F, Marinelli G. The risk of right ventricular failure with current continuous-flow left ventricular assist devices. Expert Rev Med Devices. 2017;14(12):969–83.
27. Sayer G, Sarswat N, Kim GH, Adatya S, Medvedofsky D, Rodgers D, Kruse E, Ota T, Jeevanandam V, Lang R, Uriel N. The hemodynamic effects of aortic insufficiency in patients supported with continuous-flow left ventricular assist devices. J Card Fail. 2017;23(7):545–51.
28. Dang G, Epperla N, Muppidi V, Sahr N, Pan A, Simpson P, Baumann Kreuziger L. Medical management of pump-related thrombosis in patients with continuous-flow left ventricular assist devices: a systematic review and meta-analysis. ASAIO J. 2017;63(4):373–85.

Radiology Case 7

36

Caitlin Hackett and Joshua K. Aalberg

Case 7a Indication for Exam 19-year-old male wrestler presents with shoulder pain during a match. The right shoulder is painful with a low lying humeral head and the arm held in slight abduction and internally rotated.

AP view   Scapular Y view

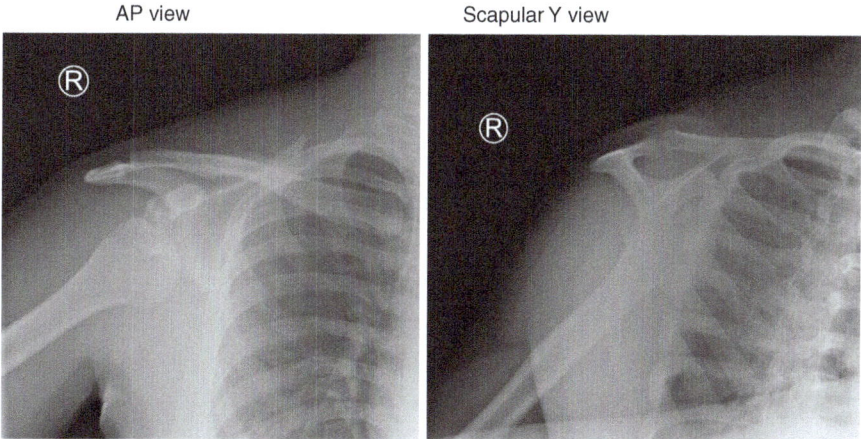

Radiographic Findings Humeral head is displaced anteriorly, medially, and inferiorly compatible with anterior subcoracoid glenohumeral dislocation.

Diagnosis Anterior Shoulder Dislocation

C. Hackett · J. K. Aalberg (✉)
Department of Emergency Medicine, Wexner Medical Center at The Ohio State University, Columbus, OH, USA
e-mail: Caitlin.Hackett@osumc.edu; joshua.aalberg@osumc.edu

© Springer Nature Switzerland AG 2020
C. G. Kaide, C. E. San Miguel (eds.), *Case Studies in Emergency Medicine*,
https://doi.org/10.1007/978-3-030-22445-5_36

Case 7b Indication for Exam 26-year-old male presents with shoulder pain after an assault. The left shoulder is painful, deformed, and fixed in internal rotation.

AP view   Scapular Y view

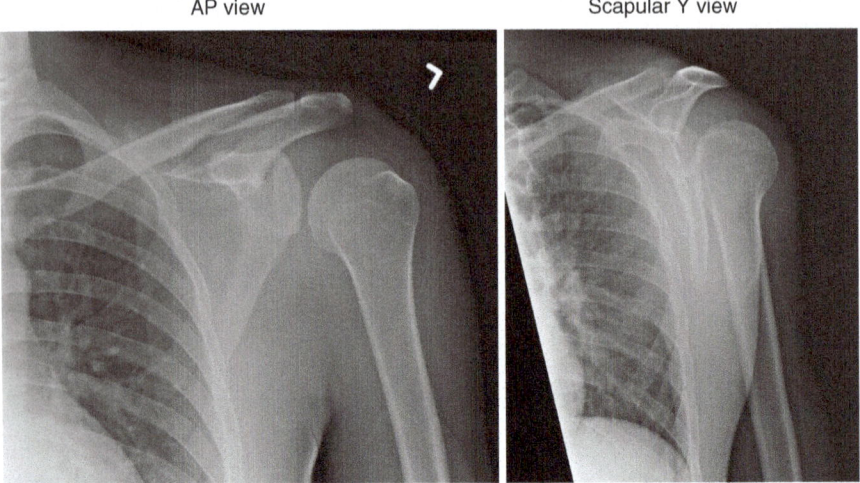

Radiographic Findings The AP view shows widening of the glenohumeral joint. The scapular Y view shows posterior displacement of the humeral head relative to the glenoid compatible with posterior dislocation.

Diagnosis Posterior Shoulder Dislocation

Learning Points

Priming Questions
- How are anterior and posterior dislocations different?
- What are the common associated injuries?
- Does the management differ for anterior vs. posterior dislocations?

Introduction

The shoulder is the most commonly dislocated joint in the body.

- Anterior shoulder dislocations account for 95% of shoulder dislocations. In those cases, the humeral head is displaced anteriorly, inferiorly, and medially. The peak age is 15–25 years, and it is more common in males. The four types of anterior dislocation are subcoracoid, subclavicular, subacromial, and intrathoracic. [1]

- Posterior shoulder dislocations account for 2–4% of glenohumeral dislocations. The humeral head usually dislocates straight posteriorly (subacromial). Rarely, the humeral head may dislocate subglenoid or subspinous. The peak age is 35–55 years, and it is more common in males. It can occasionally be bilateral depending on the mechanism [2].

Pathophysiology/Mechanism

The most common mechanism of anterior dislocation is an anterior blow to the distal arm when the arm is held in abduction/external rotation. It can also be caused by direct blow to the back of the shoulder or violent arm traction [3].

The most common mechanism of posterior shoulder dislocation is seizure. It is also classically described with electrocution patients. Posterior dislocation can also be seen with a fall on outstretched hand or blow to flexed, adducted, internally rotated shoulder. The risk is increased if the glenoid is hypoplastic [4].

Making the Diagnosis

The diagnosis is often clinically apparent. Radiographs can confirm the diagnosis, exclude fracture, and assist with treatment. As with all musculoskeletal injuries, multiple views should be obtained.

If the dislocation is obvious on the frontal/AP view, it is most likely an anterior dislocation [5].

Posterior dislocation is apparent on axillary and scapular Y views but is missed 50% of the time on the AP view [6]. Signs of posterior dislocation on the AP view include

- Incongruency of the joint: joint may appear narrow or wide depending on the position of the humeral head.
- Rim sign: shoulder joint width > 6 mm, loss of normal overlap of humeral head and glenoid.
- Some authors report a "light bulb sign." The internal rotation of the humeral head in a posterior dislocation has a more rounded appearance compared to a typical AP view of the shoulder.
- Clinically, patients with posterior dislocations are unable to externally rotate their arm beyond 90 degrees in relation to their torso.

Treating the Patient

Closed reduction should be performed promptly to avoid muscle spasm and worsening of associated injuries. There are numerous different techniques described for anterior dislocations ranging from direct traction-countertraction to the Stimson maneuver, which involves hanging a weight from the affected arm while the patient lies supine on the bed. There are fewer options described for posterior dislocations, and patients may require open reduction if closed reduction is unsuccessful. In general axial traction is applied to the arm along with forced adduction and internal rotation of the joint. Of note, closed reduction by the Emergency Physician is generally contraindicated if there is an associated humeral fracture, nerve injury, or major vascular injury (assuming the limb is still being perfused while the humerus is dislocated).

Postreduction radiographs should be obtained to confirm successful reduction as well as to look for associated injuries that may have been overlooked on the initial radiographs. Thirty-five percent of fractures are visible only after reduction [3]. If there is a sizeable effusion or hematoma in the joint, the shoulder may appear slightly inferiorly subluxed on the postreduction radiographs.

After successful reduction, patients should be placed in slings for up to 4 weeks and referred to orthopedic surgery to monitor their recovery, assess for concomitant injuries to the joint, and to discuss surgical options in the event they become chronic dislocators.

For anterior dislocations, patients younger than 20 have a 90% chance of recurrence. In patients older than 40, 10–15% have recurrence. Chronic dislocators should be taught to avoid positions when dislocation occurs and to strengthen dynamic stabilizers [7]. Nonemergent cross-sectional imaging may be helpful to determine whether additional injuries are present and to assist with surgical planning. Younger patients often eventually require surgery to repair labral tears that can cause instability. Bone grafts may be required if there are large defects in the glenoid rim or humeral head [8]. Below are some of the possible concominant injuries to the joint.

Anterior dislocations [9]
- Hill–Sachs lesion: 80%, impaction fracture of the posterolateral humeral head
- Bankart lesion: 75% have labral tear, 15% have fractures; tear or separation of the anterior inferior glenoid labrum, sometimes has fracture of adjacent glenoid rim (bony Bankart).
- Greater tuberosity fractures: in older patients.
- Glenohumeral ligament tears.
- Coracohumeral ligament tears.
- Subscapularis tears with possibly subluxation of long head of the biceps tendon or avulsion of the lesser tuberosity.
- Stripping of anterior joint capsule from glenoid attachment [6].

Posterior dislocations [6]
- Reverse Hill–Sachs: 75%, vertical compression fracture of the anterior humeral head due to anteromedial humeral head impaction on the posterior glenoid rim. The size of the reverse Hill–Sachs lesion is the best predictor of recurrence.
- Reverse Bankart: 30%.
- Posterior labrocapsular periosteal sleeve avulsion (POLPSA).

- Glenohumeral ligament tears.
- Teres minor tear.
- Lesser tuberosity fractures.

Discussion

- Glenohumeral dislocation may be obvious clinically, but radiographs can be used to confirm the type of dislocation and aid with reduction.
- Arguably, the more important radiologic findings in glenohumeral dislocation are the associated injuries as these contribute to future instability, though they rarely change management in the emergency department, as long as the patient is able to follow up with an orthopedic surgeon.

Disclosure Statement   The authors of this chapter report no significant disclosures.

References

1. Manaster BJ, May DA, Disler DG. Musculoskeletal imaging: the requisites. 4th ed. Philadelphia: Elsevier; 2013.
2. Jacobs RC, Meredyth NA, Michelson JD. Posterior shoulder dislocation. BMJ. 2015;350:h75.
3. Yu J. Musculoskeletal radiology case review. 3rd ed. Philadelphia: Elsevier; 2017.
4. Tannenbaum E, Sekiya JK. Evaluation and management of posterior shoulder instability. Sports Health. 2011;3(3):253–63.
5. Bencardino JT, Gyftopoulos S, Palmer WE. Imaging in anterior glenohumeral instability. Radiology. 2013;269(2):323–37.
6. Saupe N, et al. Acute traumatic posterior shoulder dislocation: MR findings. Radiology. 2008;248:185–93.
7. Dumont GD, Russell RD, Robertson WJ. Anterior shoulder instability: a review of patho-anatomy, diagnosis and treatment. Curr Rev Musculoskelet Med. 2011;4(4):200–7.
8. Sandstrom CK, Kennedy SA, Gross JA. Acute shoulder trauma: what the surgeon wants to know. Radiographics. 2015;35(2):475–92.
9. Gyftopoulos S, Albert M, Recht MP. Osseous injuries associated with anterior shoulder instability: what the radiologist should know. Am J Roentgenol. 2015;202:W541–50.

Malaria: *Mosquitos Suck!*

37

Nkeiruka Orajiaka and Hani Abou Hatab

Case 1

"My child keeps having fevers and won't eat!!"

Pertinent History

A 4-year-old girl presented to the emergency department (ED) due to fever and decreased appetite for 1 week. The child migrated to the USA from Burkina Faso 18 days ago. The parents reported intermittent shivering and vomiting and how on some days, she seemed fine without any symptoms. They also complained that she had been less active and playful. She had no past medical history.

Physical Exam

- Vitals: Temperature 101.9 ° F; HR 132 bpm; BP 115/67 mmHg; RR 24; SPO$_2$ 99%

Except as noted below, the findings of the complete physical exam were within normal limits.

- Constitutional: Ill but non-toxic in appearance
- Hydration: Dry skin and mucous membranes

N. Orajiaka (✉)
Department of Emergency Medicine, Wexner Medical Center at The Ohio State University, Columbus, OH, USA
e-mail: Nkeiruka.Orajiaka@nationwidechildrens.org

H. A. Hatab
Harlem Hospital Center, New York, NY, USA

© Springer Nature Switzerland AG 2020
C. G. Kaide, C. E. San Miguel (eds.), *Case Studies in Emergency Medicine*,
https://doi.org/10.1007/978-3-030-22445-5_37

- Eyes: Pale without conjunctival injection nor scleral icterus
- Abdomen: Full and soft with splenomegaly; no hepatomegaly or abdominal tenderness
- Skin: Warm and dry without rashes

ED Course

The patient was evaluated and laboratory work was ordered. The differential diagnosis included sepsis, malaria, viral infection, and typhoid fever. She received acetaminophen for her fevers. Due to a concern for dehydration, patient received a 20 cc/kg bolus of normal saline (NS) and was started on maintenance rate of D5W 0.45NS. The WBC was normal and cultures were pending. Antibiotics were not initiated due to low concern for sepsis. She was admitted for further management of malaria.

Pertinent Laboratory Findings

Preliminary blood smear: Malaria parasite on thick smear. Thin smear pending.

Due to stable respiratory stats and lack of URI symptoms, CXR was not obtained.

Test	Result	Units	Normal Range
WBC	8.2	K/uL	3.8–11.0 $10^3/mm^3$
Hgb	8.2	g/dL	(Male) 14–18 g/dL
			(Female) 11–16 g/dL
Platelets	146	K/uL	140–450 K/uL

Case 2: Severe Malaria

Pertinent History

A 14-year-old male presented to the ED with vomiting, headache, stomach pain, and subjective fevers. Symptoms started 4 days ago with frontal, non-radiating headaches without associated photo- or phono-phobia. He was evaluated in the ED 2 days ago and was tested and treated for a *Streptococcal* pharyngitis with 1.2 million units of IM penicillin G benzathine.

The patient's symptoms progressively worsened over the next 2 days with persistent headaches, multiple non-bilious and non-bloody vomiting, epigastric pain, and episodes of chills and warmth without temperature checks at home. He had used acetaminophen and bismuth subsalicylate at home with minimal to no improvement. He had lived in Ivory Coast for the past year and arrived back in the USA 2 weeks ago to visit his parents.

Physical Exam

- Vitals: Temperature 100.9 °F (38.3°C); HR 100 bpm; RR 22; BP 106/52 mmHg; SpO2 96% RA

  Exam findings are as noted below:

- General Appearance: Ill-appearing, crying due to headaches
- Eyes: Scleral icterus
- Mouth: Dry cracked lips and tacky mucous membranes
- Neck: Normal and full range of motion with no meningismus
- Abdominal: Flat with mild epigastric tenderness
- Neurological: Crying in discomfort but alert and oriented to place, person and time, GSC 15, negative Kernig's and Brudzinski signs

Significant Laboratory Findings

Test	Result	Units	Normal Range
WBC	3.3	K/uL	3.8–11.0 $10^3/mm^3$
Hgb	8.9	g/dL	(Male) 14–18 g/dL
			(Female) 11–16 g/dL
Platelets	43	K/uL	140–450 K/uL
Total Bilirubin/Direct Bilirubin	6.7/3.8	mg/dL	0.2–1.4 mg/dL/0.0–0.4 mg/dL
Albumin	2.9	g/dL	3.5–5.0 gm/dL

Preliminary blood smear: Positive for malaria parasite

ED Course

The patient received acetaminophen while in triage. During further evaluation, the patient was noted to feel hotter, sleepier, and more ill.

Repeat Vitals: Temperature 103.2F (39.6°C); HR 130 bpm; BP 82/44 mmHg.

Due to a concern that the patient may be decompensating and might be septic, an IV line was established, labs were drawn, and 2 boluses of 20 cc/kg NS were given. At the same time, IV Vancomycin and Ceftriaxone were started. Vitals improved to BP 111/65 mmHg and HR 105 bpm, but the patient remained somnolent. With preliminary smear report of malaria parasite and labs significant for anemia and thrombocytopenia, patient was also started on IV quinidine, and clindamycin. EKG was performed prior to IV quinidine which showed NSR and a QTc of 390 ms. Patient was then transferred to PICU for continued management for severe malaria.

Learning Points: Malaria in Children

Priming Questions
- What are the different manifestations of malaria in children?
- How is severe malaria diagnosed?
- When should the treatment for malaria start and what adjunct treatments must be considered in the ED?

Introduction

1. Malaria is a parasitic mosquito-borne infection of red blood cells. The word "malaria" translated from Italian is "bad air:" From *mala* "bad" + *aria* "air."
2. It is estimated that nearly 300,000 children under the age of 5 died of malaria in 2016, equivalent to nearly 800 young lives lost each day. Most of these deaths occur in the WHO African region (92%), South-East Asian region (6%), and the WHO Eastern Mediterranean region (2%) [1].
3. Although previously uncommon in the USA, malaria cases are increasing due to immigrants and travel trends. According to CDC, 1517 confirmed malaria cases were reported in the USA in 2015 [2].

Areas Where Malaria is Endemic

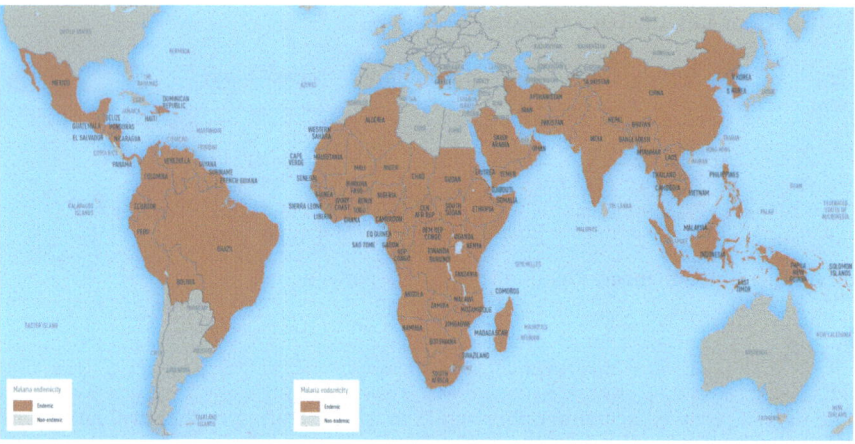

Images Courtesy of Centers for Disease Control and Prevention

Pathology/Pathophysiology

1. Malaria is transmitted through bites of carrier female anopheles mosquitos.
2. People who did not travel to endemic regions may be exposed or infected if the mosquitoes traveled in the luggage to nonendemic areas [3–5].
3. Other possible modes of transmission include blood transfusion [6], organ transplantation [7], and congenital transmission (mother to newborn) [8].
4. Life cycle:
   - After a vector mosquito bites the host, malaria parasites (sporozoites) get into the bloodstream and reach the hepatocytes.
   - These sporozoites replicate in hepatocytes forming hepatic schizonts, which eventually rupture and release parasites into the bloodstream (merozoites).

- Some sporozoites remain dormant in the liver in the form of hypnozoites, which might cause malaria relapse later. There forms are only seen in *P. vivax* and *P. ovale*.
- Merozoites infect red blood cells and either undergo asexual multiplication forming erythrocyte schizonts or develop into sexual stage gametocytes.
- Schizonts rupture releases the contents of merozoites to bloodstream, which infect other red blood cells. Schizonts are the cause of active disease.
- Gametocytes circulate in blood until ingested by the vector anopheles mosquito biting the human host [9]

Malaria Life-Cycle

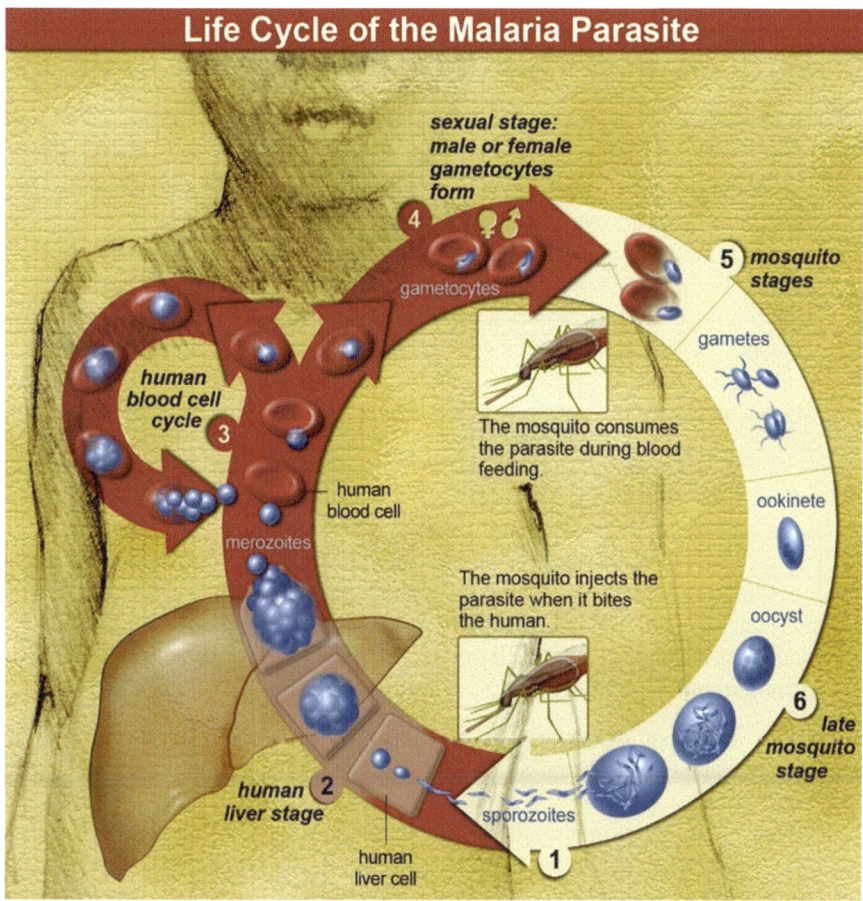

National Institutes of Health (NIH) Public Domain Image

5. Species.
   - Different species of *Plasmodium* exist:
   - *Plasmodium falciparum* is the most common and pathogenic malaria species and is associated with severe illness and death, typically among children <5 years of age.

	P. Falciparum	P. Vivax	P. Ovale	P. Malaria	P. Knowlesi (rarely affects humans)
Average Incubation [10]	9–14 days	12–17 days	16–18 days	18–40 days	9–12 days [11]
Erythrocyte cycle [12]	48 hours	48 hours	48 hours	72 hours	24 hours
Hypnozoites (liver forms)	Absent	Present	Present	Usually absent	Absent
Severe Malaria	Yes, most common	Yes [13]	No	No	Yes [14]
Relapse	No	Yes	Yes	No	No
Special Features	Cerebral malaria	Splenic rupture	Least common	Mildest and most chronic	Nephrotic syndrome (steroid resistant)

6. Symptoms
   - Initial symptoms of malaria are generally nonspecific, but fever is present in almost all patients. Fever can be persistent or periodic, and depending on species, fever appears every other day or every third day.
   - Other symptoms may include headache, fatigue, weakness, generalized muscular pain, chills, sweating, dry cough, abdominal pain, or vomiting.
   - In young children, poor feeding and lethargy may be noted.
   - In cases of severe malaria, neurological symptoms such as dizziness, confusion, disorientation, and seizures may occur [15].
   - Physical signs may include pallor, jaundice, and hepatosplenomegaly.

Cerebral Malaria

This is a medical emergency and the most severe neurological complication of infection with *P. falciparum*. This is hypothesized to occur as a result of sequestration of infected red blood cells in the brain vasculature [16]. Cerebral malaria is usually a rapid-onset illness, occurring within 24–48 hours of the initial malaria symptoms. In addition to other symptoms of malaria, seizures, prostration, or altered mental status may occur.

- Abnormal tone is common and may present in the form of decerebrate, decorticate, or opisthotonic posturing [17].
- Seizures occur in up to 70–80% of children with severe malaria. Generalized seizures are common in children with uncomplicated *P. falciparum* malaria. However, seizures may be a prodrome of cerebral malaria and any patient with more than 2 seizures within a 24 hour period should be managed as severe malaria [18].
- Meningeal signs such as neck stiffness, Kernig's sign, and photophobia are rare but could be present.

Making the Diagnosis

There is no combination of signs and symptoms that can distinguish malaria from other causes of fever.

1. History is very important: Malaria should be suspected in a child with fever and travel history to an endemic zone.
2. Laboratory testing
   - Parasite identification can be done via microscopy or rapid diagnostic tests.
     - Smear examination using light microscopy is the standard diagnostic tool. Thick smears are used to confirm presence of malaria parasites in blood and thin smears are used to identify and quantify parasite species [19].
     - Parasitemia refers to the quantitative content of circulating red cells that contain malaria parasites in the blood. This should be interpreted in the context of symptoms and endemicity. According to WHO [20]:
       - Parasitaemia <4% is considered as uncomplicated malaria.
       - Parasitaemia ≥4% is considered as hyperparasitaemia and should be an indicator for high risk requiring supervised management.
       - Parasitaemia >10% is considered severe malaria in children even without evidence of vital organ dysfunction (>5% is considered as severe malaria by CDC) [18, 21].
     - Antigen-based rapid diagnostic tests can provide results within 15–20 minutes and can be used while microscopy is pending. This is ideal in resource-limited settings.
     - Patients who do not have immunity, such as patients in the USA, may be symptomatic at a very low parasite density that may be undetectable on the smear. Parasite identification testing should be repeated every 12 hours at least 3 times before malaria is ruled out.
   - Other nonspecific laboratory findings include:
     - Anemia
     - Thrombocytopenia
     - Hyperbilirubinemia
     - Elevated transaminases
     - Elevated BUN
3. Lumbar puncture (LP):
   - LP is recommended in suspected cases of cerebral malaria. This can help rule out or rule in other differential diagnosis such as meningitis or encephalitis.
   - Patients with abnormal respiration and/or papilledema due to increased intracranial pressure should not have an LP.
   - CSF studies in malaria are usually within normal limits or may show a slightly elevated total protein and white cell count [22].
4. Fundoscopy
   - Malarial retinopathy reliably distinguishes malarial coma from nonmalarial coma and significantly improves diagnostic specificity without compromising sensitivity [23].

- Malarial retinopathy is best seen by indirect ophthalmoscopy and includes patchy whitening of the macula, whitening of the peripheral retina, discoloration of the retinal vessels to pale orange or white, and multiple (predominantly white-centered) retinal hemorrhages [23, 24].
- Though not specific to malaria, papilledema may also be seen.

5. Imaging
   - In a case of suspected severe malaria and positive chest findings, a CXR may be done to rule out pulmonary edema.
   - There are currently no strong recommendations to do a head CT in cases of suspected cerebral malaria. Results may be normal or show signs of cerebral edema [25].

Complicated/Severe Malaria

In the absence of any other identified cause, severe *falciparum* malaria is defined as positive *P. falciparum* smear and one or more of the following [18]:

Impaired consciousness	GCS <11 in adults or Blantyre coma scale <3 in children
Prostration	Generalized weakness so that a person is unable to sit, stand, or walk without assistance
Multiple Convulsions	More than two episodes within 24 hours
Acidosis	A base deficit of >8 mEq/L, a plasma bicarbonate level of <15 mmol/L, or venous plasma lactate ≥5 mmol/L; clinical indicators of acidosis include rapid, deep, labored breathing
Hypoglycemia	Blood glucose <40 mg/dL (<2.2 mmol/L) for children ≥5 years and adults; blood glucose <54 mg/dL (<3 mmol/L) for children <5 years
Severe anemia	Hemoglobin ≤5 g/dL or hematocrit ≤15% in children <12 years of age (<7 g/dL and < 20% in adults) with parasite count >10,000/μL (0.2% parasitemia)
Renal impairment	Serum creatinine >3 mg/dL (265 μmol/L) or blood urea >20 mmol/L
Jaundice	Bilirubin >50 μmol/L (3 mg/dL) with a parasite count >100,000/μL (0.2% parasitemia)
Pulmonary edema	Radiographically confirmed or oxygen saturation < 92% on room air with respiratory rate > 30/minutes, often with chest indrawing and crepitation on auscultation
Significant bleeding	Recurrent or prolonged bleeding (from nose, gums, or venipuncture sites), hematemesis, or melena
Shock	Compensated shock: capillary refill ≥3 seconds or temperature gradient on leg (mid to proximal limb), but no hypotension Decompensated shock: SBP <70 mmHg in children or < 80 mmHg in adults, with evidence of impaired perfusion (cool peripheries or prolonged capillary refill)
Hyperparasitemia	*P. falciparum* parasitemia >10% (> 500,000/mcL)

Treating the Patient

1. Uncomplicated malaria
   - Oral antimalarial medications are the definitive treatment.
   - Antimalarial medications *should not be initiated* until diagnosis has been confirmed by laboratory investigations.
   - Adequate hydration is encouraged to hasten recovery.

2. Complicated malaria: considered a medical emergency
   • *A*irway, *B*reathing, *C*irculation, *D*isability, and *E*xposure approach should be followed to assess and manage the patient
   • Antimalarials
     – Intravenous therapy is preferred. The risk of death in severe malaria, especially in cerebral malaria, is the greatest in the first 24 hours after clinical presentation. Therefore, intravenous therapy should be commenced as soon as possible.
     – If there is a high suspicion for cerebral malaria with confirmed travel to endemic area, treatment can be started before getting the results of the malaria smear.
     – IV quinidine gluconate was previously the only IV drug available in the USA for severe malaria. As an antiarrhythmic with antimalarial effect, quinidine can cause QTc prolongation. Hence, an EKG must be obtained prior to commencing IV quinidine.
     – IV artesunate is available upon request from CDC and is provided to patients with severe malaria if registered under their protocol [26].
   • Antibiotic
     – Severe malaria constitutes a risk factor for bacterial infection such as bacteremia or pneumonia and in children, and concomitant bacterial infection can occur. Children with clinically diagnosed severe malaria have a higher prevalence of bacteremia than controls [27–30]. Bacteremia cannot be confidently identified or ruled out at bedside or immediate tests.
     – Hence, broad spectrum antibiotics should be commenced in all children with suspected severe malaria until negative bacterial culture results.
     – Acyclovir should also be considered until CSF-negative cultures for HSV.
   • Anti-epileptics
     – Seizures should be treated using intranasal or intravenous benzodiazepines.
     – Prophylactic anticonvulsants are not proven beneficial in uncomplicated malaria [18].
   • Exchange Transfusion
     – CDC previously recommended exchange transfusion as an adjunct to IV antimalarial agents for parasitemias >10% or complications such as cerebral malaria, acute respiratory distress syndrome (ARDS), or renal compromise [31, 32]. Exchange transfusion was thought to have beneficial effects by removing infected red cells, improving the rheological properties of blood, and reducing toxic factors such as parasite-derived toxins, harmful metabolites, and cytokines. Exchange transfusion has some theoretical advantages, but due to insufficient evidence, it is no longer recommended. A comprehensive review US National Malaria Surveillance System data and published literature regarding efficacy in severe malaria showed no effect on survival [30].

Case 1 Conclusion

- Received atovaquone/proguanil (Malarone) 250/100 mg PO daily for 3 days.
- Daily blood parasitemia was evaluated, see table below:

Day of hospitalization	1	2	3	4
Malaria parasitemia (%)	0.4	1.6	<0.1	0
Hemoglobin/hematocrit	8.5 g/dL	8.9 g/dL	8.2 g/dL	9.3 g/dL
Bilirubin	1.2 mg/dL	0.6 mg/dL		

- By day 3 of hospitalization, patient clinically improved with a documented decrease in HR to 108. She had improved oral intake and was noted to be playing actively in the playroom.
- She was discharged on day 4 with the diagnosis of uncomplicated malaria.

Case 2 Conclusion

A few hours after admission, patient's condition worsened with severe headache, lethargy, and confusion. Head CT was negative for any structural abnormalities.

Patient was continued on IV quinidine. By day 3 of hospitalization, malaria parasite density peaked at 43%. Based on the CDC expert opinion, the patient received exchange transfusion despite it being not the current recommendation.

By the end of the third day, patient's mental status improved, but the EKG showed prolonged QTc of 590 ms. Since he was able to tolerate PO at the time, patient was switched to oral quinine, which has less effect on the QT interval than the IV version. The patient also received broad spectrum antibiotics until negative culture results were obtained.

While inpatient, he developed acute kidney injury and pulmonary edema requiring fluid management and supplemental oxygen. The patient progressively recovered and was discharged on day 12 with all complications resolved. The final diagnosis was severe malaria.

Day of Hospitalization	1	2	3	6	Discharge
Parasitemia %	15%	32%	42%	<0.1	0
Creatinine	0.8 mg/dL	1 mg/dL	2.4 mg/dL	3.6 mg/dL	0.86 mg/dL
Platelets	43 K/uL	52 K/uL	24 K/uL	105 K/uL	248 K/uL
Hemoglobin	8.9 g/dL	10.3 g/dL	8.8 g/dL	7.9 g/dL	12.9 g/dL
WBC	3.3 K/uL	6.2 K/uL	6.5 K/uL	9.3 K/uL	8.8 K/uL
Total bilirubin/ direct bilirubin	6.7/3.8 mg/ dL	17.2/13.3 mg/ dL	15.3/12.1 mg/ dL	10.6/8.2 mg/ dL	7.8/5.4 mg/ dL

Discussion

Uncomplicated malaria is easy to treat but also easy to miss!

Perform malaria identification testing on all patients with symptoms suggestive of malaria with recent epidemiologic exposure. If an infant has symptoms suggestive of malaria, but has negative parasite smear, assess whether there is a recent travel history to malaria endemic regions or current case of malaria in the household. Consider hospitalizing the patient or recommend a close outpatient follow-up. Children with exposure to *Plasmodium* may manifest symptoms at undetectable parasite densities. Therefore, smears must be repeated every 12 hours until they are negative 3 times.

In cases of altered mental status, seizures, and fever, ED providers may be more familiar with infectious processes (e.g., meningitis) or toxic ingestions rather than cerebral malaria. This is especially true in nonendemic regions. Therefore, a recent travel history can make a difference in diagnosis. In suspected cases of cerebral malaria with altered mental status, perform a funduscopic exam to search for malarial retinopathy. This is best seen via indirect ophthalmoscopy.

Patients with seizure disorders pose a challenge in diagnosing cerebral malaria. However, because the mortality rate of cerebral malaria is high, patients with seizures and a positive falciparum smear should be treated as severe malaria until parasite density is quantified.

Pattern Recognition

- Periodic fever with recent travel history
- Altered mental status with recent travel to endemic location
- Positive parasite smear

Disclosure Statement The authors of this chapter report no significant disclosures.

References

1. World Malaria Report 2016. Geneva: World Health Organization; 2016. Licence: CC BY-NC-SA 3.0 IGO. Page 42
2. Mace KE, Arguin PM, Tan KR. Malaria surveillance—United States, 2015. MMWR Surveill Summ. 2018;67(7):1.
3. Isaacson M. Airport malaria- a review. Bull World Health Organ. 1989;67(6):737–43.
4. Velasco E, Gomez-Barroso D, Varela C, Diaz O, Cano R. Non-imported malaria in non-endemic countries: a review of cases in Spain. Malar J. 2017;16:260.
5. Zoller T, Naucke TJ, May J, et al. Malaria transmission in non-endemic areas: case report, review of the literature and implications for public health management. Malar J. 2009;8:71.
6. Kitchen AD, Chiodini PL. Malaria and blood transfusion. Vox Sang. 2006;90(2):77–84.

7. Fischer L, Sterneck M, Claus M, et al. Transmission of malaria tertiana by multi-organ donation. Clin Transpl. 1999;13(6):491–5.
8. Sotimehin SA, Runsewe-Abiodun TI, Oladapo OT, Njokanma OF, Olanrewaju DM. Possible risk factors for congenital malaria at a Tertiary Care Hospital in Sagamu, Ogun State, South-West Nigeria. J Trop Pediatr. 2008;54(5):313–20.
9. Trampuz A, Jereb M, Muzlovic I, Prabhu RM. Clinical review: severe malaria. Crit Care. 2003;7(4):315–23.
10. Brasil P, Costa AD, Pedro RS, et al. Unexpectedly long incubation period of Plasmodium vivax malaria, in the absence of chemoprophylaxis, in patients diagnosed outside the transmission area in Brazil. Malar J. 2011;10:122.
11. Beeson JG, Drew DR, Boyle MJ, Feng GQ, Fowkes FJ, Richards JS. Merozoite surface proteins in red blood cell invasion, immunity and vaccines against malaria. FEMS Microbiol Rev. 2016;40(3):343–72.
12. Kwiatkowski D, Nowak M. Periodic and chaotic host-parasite interactions in human malaria. Proc Natl Acad Sci U S A. 1991;88(12):5111–3.
13. Tjitra E, Anstey NM, Sugiarto P, et al. Multidrug-resistant Plasmodium vivax associated with severe and fatal malaria: a prospective study in Papua, Indonesia. PLoS Med. 2008;5(6):890–9.
14. Cox-Singh J, Davis TME, Lee KS, et al. Plasmodium knowlesi malaria in humans is widely distributed and potentially life threatening. Clin Infect Dis. 2008;46(2):165–71.
15. Flegel KM. Symptoms and signs of malaria. Can Med Assoc J. 1976;115(5):409–10.
16. Taylor TE, Fu WJJ, Carr RA, et al. Differentiating the pathologies of cerebral malaria by post-mortem parasite counts. Nat Med. 2004;10(2):143–5.
17. Román GC, S N. Neurological manifestations of malaria. Arq Neuropsiquiatr. 1992;50(1):03–9.
18. World Health Organization. Guidelines for the treatment of malaria. 3rd ed; 2015. http://apps.who.int/medicinedocs/documents/s21839en/s21839en.pdf. Accessed 7th Feb 2019
19. Tangpukdee N, Duangdee C, Wilairatana P, Krudsood S. Malaria diagnosis: a brief review. Korean J Parasitol. 2009;47(2):93–102.
20. World Health Organization. Severe malaria. Trop Med Int Health. 2014;19:7–131.
21. Center for Disease Control and Prevention. Guidelines for treatment of malaria in the United States. In: 2013. https://www.cdc.gov/malaria/resources/pdf/treatmenttable.pdf. Accessed 7th Feb 2019.
22. Misra UK, Kalita J, Prabhakar S, Chakravarty A, Kochar D, Nair PP. Cerebral malaria and bacterial meningitis. Ann Indian Acad Neurol. 2011;14:S35–9.
23. Beare NAV, Lewallen S, Taylor TE, Molyneux ME. Redefining cerebral malaria by including malaria retinopathy. Future Microbiol. 2011;6(3):349–55.
24. Hirneiss CKV, Wilke M, Kampik A, Taylor TE, Lewallen S. Ocular changes in tropical malaria with cerebral involvement--results from the Blantyre Malaria Project. Klin Monatsbl Augenheilkd. 2005;222(9):704–8.
25. Newton C, Peshu N, Kendall B, et al. Brain -swelling and Ischemia in Kenyans with Cererbal malaria. Arch Dis Child. 1994;70(4):281–7.
26. Center for Disease Control and Prevention. Artesunate is available to treat severe malaria in the United States. In: 2018.
27. Berkley J, Mwarumba S, Bramham K, Lowe B, Marsh K. Bacteraemia complicating severe malaria in children. Trans R Soc Trop Med Hyg. 1999;93(3):283–6.
28. Berkley JA, Lowe BS, Mwangi I, et al. Bacteraemia among children admitted to a rural hospital in Kenya. N Engl J Med. 2005;352(1):39–47.
29. Evans JA, Adusei A, Timmann C, et al. High mortality of infant bacteraemia clinically indistinguishable from severe malaria. QJM. 2004;97(9):591–7.
30. Tan KR, Wiegand RE, Arguin PM. Exchange transfusion for severe malaria: evidence base and literature review. Clin Infect Dis. 2013;57(7):923–8.
31. Griffith KS, Lewis LS, Mali S, Parise ME. Treatment of malaria in the United States - a systematic review. JAMA. 2007;297(20):2264–77.
32. Miller KD, Greenberg AE, Campbell CC. Treatment of malaria in the United States with a continous infusion of quindine gluconate and exchange transfusion. N Engl J Med. 1989;321(2):65–70.

Internal Hernias: *No Bulge, No Hernia?*

38

Andrew D. Chou and Colin G. Kaide

Case 1

Abdominal Pain after Roux-En-Y

Pertinent History A 47-year-old female presented to the emergency department (ED) complaining of abdominal pain, nausea, and vomiting. The pain is located in the epigastric area, and symptoms have been intermittent but have progressively worsened over the past 3 days to the point that she is now unable to tolerate any oral intake, even liquids. She has not had any fevers. She normally has bowel movements every day but thinks that she has not had one in 2 days. She is not passing flatus. She has not had any diarrhea and denies any sick contacts.

Pertinent Physical Exam

Except as noted below, the findings of the complete physical exam are within normal limits.

- Vitals: Temperature 98.7, HR 115, BP 143/86, RR 18, O2 saturation 99% on room air
- HEENT: Dry mucous membranes
- CV: Mild tachycardia
- Abdomen: Mild guarding with moderate associated tenderness in the epigastric area. No rebound tenderness

PMH Morbid obesity, hypertension, hyperlipidemia, type 2 diabetes, GERD. Roux-en-Y gastric bypass performed 8 years ago

A. D. Chou (✉) · C. G. Kaide
Department of Emergency Medicine, Wexner Medical Center at The Ohio State University, Columbus, OH, USA
e-mail: Andrew.Chou@osumc.edu

© Springer Nature Switzerland AG 2020
C. G. Kaide, C. E. San Miguel (eds.), *Case Studies in Emergency Medicine*,
https://doi.org/10.1007/978-3-030-22445-5_38

385

SH Ten pack-year previous smoker, social alcohol drinker, denies illicit drug use

FH Hypertension, diabetes, hyperlipidemia, coronary artery disease on both sides of the family

Pertinent Test Results

Test	Result	Units	Normal Range
WBC	13.7	K/uL	3.8–11.0 10^3/mm^3
Hgb	12	g/dL	(Male) 14–18 g/dL
			(Female) 11–16 g/dL
Platelets	286	K/uL	140–450 K/uL
Sodium	137	mEq/L	135–148 mEq/L
Potassium	3.6	mEq/L	3.5–5.5 mEq/L
Chloride	94	mEq/L	96–112 mEq/L
Bicarbonate	22	mEq/L	21–34 mEq/L
BUN	18	mg/dL	6–23 mg/dL
Creatinine	1.4	mg/dL	0.6–1.5 mg/dL
Glucose	146	mg/dL	65–99 mg/dL
Lipase	47	U/L	12–70
Troponin	<0.01	ng/dl	<0.04
Lactate	3.5	mmol/L	<2.0

ED Management

The patient was given intravenous morphine, ondansetron, and fluids for symptom control and hydration. Given her abnormal abdominal exam as well as her significant surgical history, a CT scan of the abdomen and pelvis with both intravenous and oral contrast was performed. Imaging revealed a "swirl" sign consistent with an internal hernia.

Updates on ED Course

The bariatrics team was consulted in the ED, and the patient was subsequently admitted to the surgical service with plans for urgent operative repair.

Learning Points

Priming Questions
1. What are common and uncommon complications of gastric bypass surgery?
2. Which patients should raise your suspicion for possibly having an internal hernia?
3. How much utility do labs and imaging have in diagnosing internal hernias?
4. What is the management of a patient with an internal hernia?

Introduction/Background

1. Internal hernias are a rare but very important cause of abdominal pain and small bowel obstruction in bariatric patients who have undergone Roux-en-Y gastric bypass. Aside from acute post-surgical problems such as perforation or a leaking anastamosis, internal hernias are one of the most serious acute complications. Additional more serious problems specific to this surgery can include marginal ulcers, malnutrition, and bowel obstructions from chronic adhesions.
2. Incidence has been estimated to vary between 1% and 5% after bypass [1–3].
3. Internal hernias are considered a late complication of Roux-en-Y surgery but can happen at any time.
4. Labs and even imaging can be deceptively unrevealing in patients with internal hernias, so a high index of suspicion must be maintained in patients with unexplained symptoms.

Roux-en-Y Gastric Bypass Surgery

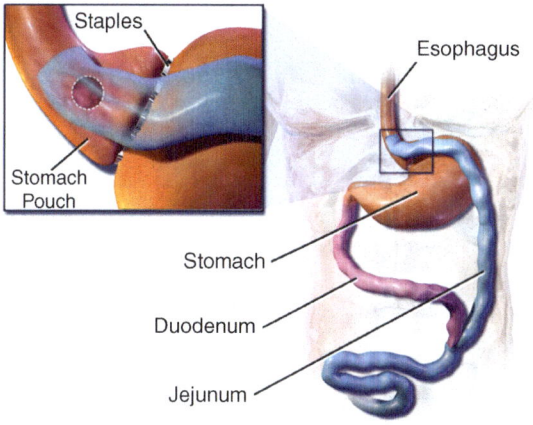

Blausen.com staff (2014). "Medical gallery of Blausen Medical 2014". WikiJournal of Medicine 1(2).   10.15347/wjm/2014.010.   ISSN   2002-4436.   (https://commons.wikimedia.org/wiki/File:Blausen_0776_Roux-En-Y_01.png), Blausen 0776 Roux-En-Y 01, https://creativecommons.org/licenses/by/3.0/legalcode. (Published with kind permission of © Colin G. Kaide 2019. All Rights Reserved)

Physiology/Pathophysiology

1. Roux-en-Y gastric bypass creates multiple mesenteric defects which can subsequently lead to internal hernias.
   - Petersen's defect refers to the space between the Roux-limb mesentery and the transverse mesentery.

- Patients with a retrocolic Roux limb are at risk for hernias through the transverse mesentery.
- A defect also occurs at the distal jejunojejunal anastomosis.
2. Bowel entrapment through any of these defects will result in an internal hernia.
3. Patients will often present with nonspecific symptoms which are not classic for obstruction, particularly if the hernia involves part of the bypassed small bowel, which is no longer in continuity with the remainder of the digestive tract.

"Petersen's Hernia" Resulting from the Intentional Creation of a Mesenteric Defect During a Roux-en-Y Gastric Bypass

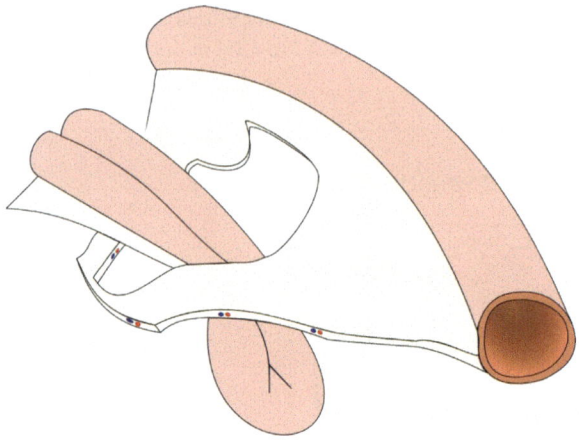

Image courtesy of Niels Olson via Wikicommons. (Published with kind permission of © Colin G. Kaide 2019. All Rights Reserved)

Making the Diagnosis

Differential Diagnosis
- Adhesive disease
- Incisional hernia
- Biliary disease
- Marginal ulcer
- Intussusception
- Anastomotic stricture
- Gastric remnant distention

1. Patients will typically be expected to have abdominal pain, which may be epigastric, and/or radiate to the back [4].
   - Symptoms are often intermittent, and the abdominal exam can appear benign unless the bowel has already become ischemic.

- Classic obstructive signs of nausea and vomiting may be absent, as the hernia may involve portions of bypassed small bowel.
2. Laboratory values can also be unrevealing.
   - A normal white blood cell count cannot rule out an internal hernia. Even patients with nonviable bowel can have a normal white blood cell count. Two studies showed that leukocytosis was only present in 20–30% of patients with internal hernias [5, 6].
   - Similarly, multiple patients with internal hernias were also found to have normal lactate levels [3].
3. Imaging studies can assist with the diagnosis but can be falsely reassuring.
   - Abdominal plain films, if obtained, may not show air-fluid levels classic for obstruction for the same reason that the patients do not have obstructive symptoms.
   - Computed tomography scans can reveal the classic "swirl" sign caused by twisting of the mesentery.
     - However, a significant percentage of patients may have negative CT scans, particularly given the intermittent nature of many of these hernias [5].

Swirl Sign Seen on Abdominal CT

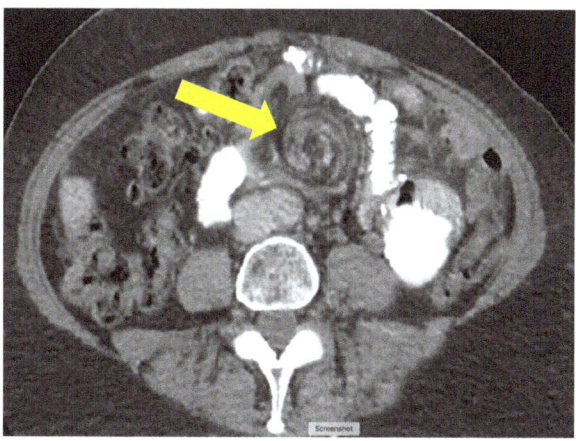

Published with kind permission of © Colin G. Kaide 2019. All Rights Reserved

Treating the Patient

1. The overall role of the emergency physician is to make the diagnosis, alert a surgeon familiar with this problem, and provide initial resuscitation.
2. Resuscitate the patient as needed, as patients with advanced pathology may have ischemic bowel, peritonitis, and/or sepsis.
   - This may include volume resuscitation with crystalloid. If the vomiting has been prolonged, significant dehydration can develop.

- Antibiotics may be indicated if the patient appears septic. Antimicrobial coverage should be directed against enteric pathogens.
3. Early consultation with bariatric surgery for consideration of operative exploration is mandatory. Some general surgeons may not be comfortable caring for patients who are post-op for bariatric procedures. If so, determine this early and arrange appropriate transfer.
4. The patient should remain NPO.
5. Symptom control should include medication for pain and nausea/vomiting.

Case Conclusion

Given her persistent symptoms, the patient was taken to the operating room for laparoscopic exploration. She was found to have an internal hernia through Petersen's defect with incarceration. Fortunately, the bowel was still viable, and the defect was closed with nonabsorbable suture after reduction of the bowel. The patient's abdominal pain resolved after the surgery, and her immediate postoperative course was uncomplicated.

Discussion

Internal hernias are an easily missed cause of abdominal pain in gastric bypass patients, and delays in diagnosis can lead to irreversible bowel ischemia. This pathology can present at any time after Roux-en-Y gastric bypass, so consider the diagnosis even in patients whose surgeries were performed years ago. Remember that labs and even CT imaging can be falsely reassuring. Early consultation with a bariatric surgeon is critical for good outcomes with these patients.

Pattern Recognition

Internal Hernia
- History of Roux-en-Y gastric bypass
- Nonspecific abdominal symptoms, usually with pain and or vomiting
- Possibly signs of obstruction (may be absent)

Disclosure Statement Andrew Chou: No disclosures

Colin Kaide: Callibra, Inc.-Discharge 123 medical software company. Medical Advisory Board Portola Pharmaceuticals. I have no relationship with a commercial company that has a direct financial interest in subject matter or materials discussed in article or with a company making a competing product.

References

1. Al Harakeh AB, et al. Bowel obstruction rates in antecolic/antegastric versus retrocolic/retro-gastric Roux limb gastric bypass: a meta-analysis. Surg Obes Relat Dis. 2016;12(1):194–8. Web. Jan 14, 2019.
2. Elms L, et al. Causes of small bowel obstruction after Roux-en-Y gastric bypass: a review of 2,395 cases at a single institution. Surg Endosc. 2014;28(5):1624–8. Web. Jan 14, 2019.
3. Garza E, et al. Internal hernias after laparoscopic Roux-en-Y gastric bypass. Am J Surg. 2004;188(6):796–800. Web. Jan 14, 2019.
4. Edwards ED, et al. Presentation and management of common post-weight loss surgery problems in the emergency department. Ann Emerg Med. 2006;47(2):160–6. Web. Feb 6, 2019.
5. Comeau E, et al. Symptomatic internal hernias after laparoscopic bariatric surgery. Surg Endosc. 2005;19(1):34–9. Web. Jan 14, 2019.
6. Srikanth MS, et al. Computed tomography patterns in small bowel obstruction after open distal gastric bypass. Obes Surg. 2004;14(6):811–22. Web. Feb 6, 2019.

Mesenteric Ischemia: *When a Benign Exam Means Danger Close*

39

Caleb J. Taylor and Christopher E. San Miguel

Case

Abdominal Pain

Pertinent History

The patient is a 79-year-old female with a past medical history of dementia, hypertension, paroxysmal atrial fibrillation, and gastroesophageal reflux disease who presented to the emergency department (ED) with acute abdominal pain. Her pain began 3 hours prior to her arrival in the ED. She describes her pain as diffuse and constant, with occasional radiation to her back. She denies urinary and vaginal symptoms. She notes associated nausea and has had two episodes of vomiting. Her emesis was nonbloody and nonbilious. Her nausea started at the same as her pain. She denied diarrhea, fevers, chills, trauma to her abdomen, or a history of GI bleeding.

Past Medical History The patient has a history of atrial fibrillation and is currently taking Coumadin. Her past INRs have indicated good compliance with her therapy.
- She had no allergies.

Pertinent Exam

Vitals: T: 97.6   P: 78   BP: 145/94   RR: 18   02: 100%

C. J. Taylor (✉) · C. E. San Miguel
Department of Emergency Medicine, Wexner Medical Center at The Ohio State University, Columbus, OH, USA
e-mail: CALEB.TAYLOR@OSUMC.EDU; christopher.sanmiguel@osumc.edu

© Springer Nature Switzerland AG 2020
C. G. Kaide, C. E. San Miguel (eds.), *Case Studies in Emergency Medicine*,
https://doi.org/10.1007/978-3-030-22445-5_39

Except as noted below, the findings of a complete physical examination were within normal limits.

- General: elderly female appeared stated age, NAD, appeared uncomfortable
- HEENT: no JVD
- Cardiovascular: RRR, normal S1 and S2, no S3, no m/g/r
- Lungs: no wheezes or rales
- Abdomen: Soft, normal bowel sounds, no distention, no masses, generalized tenderness, no rebound, no guarding
- Skin: no rashes or lesions

Plan Labs including a lactate, CT with contrast, pain management

Pertinent Diagnostic Testing

Test	Result in the ED	Result on the floor	Units	Normal Range
WBC	6.57	4.98	K/uL	3.8–11.0 $10^3/mm^3$
Hgb	14.2	7.6 ↓	g/dL	(Male) 14–18 g/dL
				(Female) 11–16 g/dL
Platelets	201	377	K/uL	140–450 K/uL
Creatinine	0.82	0.88	mg/dL	0.6–1.5 mg/dL
Lactate	4.14 ↑	1.1	mmol/L	<2.0 mmol/L

Abdominal XR No gross free air.

CT Aneurysm Study with Contrast No evidence of acute thoracic or abdominal aortic aneurysm or dissection. Multiple hypoattenuating foci within the hepatic parenchyma favored to represent cysts or hemangiomas. Left nonobstructing renal calculus is present without hydronephrosis.

Update 1 (2 Hours after Arrival to ED, 15 Minutes after Negative CT Aneurysms Study) The patient was given fluid resuscitation of 2 liters normal saline and treated for gastroenteritis and dehydration and her lactate normalized to 1.1. The diagnosis of mesenteric ischemia was considered; however, her symptoms were ultimately diagnosed as severe gastroenteritis and dehydration. She was admitted to a med/surg level of care for treatment of her gastroenteritis.

Learning Points: Acute mesenteric ischemia

Priming Questions
1. What are some risk factors for acute mesenteric ischemia that should be sought in a history and physical examination?
2. How is the diagnosis of mesenteric ischemia made?
3. What is the definitive treatment for mesenteric ischemia?

1. Acute mesenteric ischemia (AMI) is a rare vascular emergency that results in reduced blood flow to the stomach, small bowel, and/or to the colon.
2. AMI is a difficult diagnosis to make in the ED and a high index of suspicion is required to make the diagnosis.
3. The mortality for this condition is up to 60–80% in most studies even with early detection and intervention [2, 5, 6, 9]. Despite this, early diagnosis and treatment are the goals of therapy for AMI.
4. AMI is a clinical entity made up of multiple etiologies. Four main syndromes make up the vast majority of cases:
   - Mesenteric arterial embolus
   - Mesenteric arterial thrombosis
   - Nonocclusive mesenteric ischemia
   - Mesenteric venous thrombosis
5. Acute nonocclusive mesenteric ischemia is most commonly encountered in profoundly morbid ICU patients. Chronic nonocclusive mesenteric ischemia is a distinct clinical entity and will not be covered in this review.
6. The approximate case distribution is 50% arterial embolus, 20% arterial thrombus, 20% nonocclusive mesenteric ischemia, and 10% venous thrombus [2].

Physiology/Pathophysiology

1. Acute mesenteric ischemia results from an acute reduction in blood flow to a mesenteric vessel.
   - It can occur in the distribution of the celiac artery, superior mesenteric artery, inferior mesenteric artery, or the corresponding veins. It can occur anywhere along the course of the vessel.
   - The superior mesenteric artery is most likely to be involved especially if cardiac emboli are the cause (see Fig. 39.1).

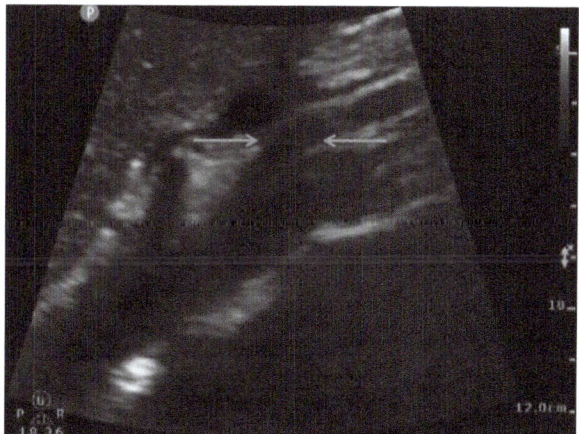

Fig. 39.1 The image above is a transabdominal sagittal ultrasound of a healthy aorta, celiac trunk, and superior mesenteric artery (SMA). Blue arrows highlight the takeoff of the SMA from the aorta. The narrow angle of this takeoff invites embolism from cardiac sources to lodge in the distal SMA and cause mesenteric ischemia. (Used with permission courtesy of Dr. Taylor and Dr. Van Sambeek)

- Embolism is more likely to occur distally in the vessel especially in the distal superior mesenteric artery due to is straight course and narrow take off angle from the aorta.
- The extent of bowel infarction depends most on the time since ischemia or initiation of ischemia reperfusion, the site of obstruction (proximal versus distal vessel involvement), and the adequacy of collateral flow. The amount of bowel involved and the duration of ischemia or ischemia reperfusion will determine the presenting symptoms.
- In situ thrombosis is more likely to occur at the origin of the vessel.

2. Acute mesenteric arterial embolus
   - An occlusion of the mesenteric artery is caused by an emboli, often a thrombus from the left atrium or septic emboli from endocarditis.
   - Risk factors include advanced age, malignancy, atrial fibrillation, digoxin, recent MI, and CHF, previous arterial emboli, hypercoagulable states, hypovolemia, shock, and vasopressors [2, 5, 8, 9].

3. Acute mesenteric arterial thrombus
   - An occlusion of the mesenteric artery is caused by progressive atherosclerosis of the mesenteric vasculature.
   - These patients may have a medical history of other vascular diseases including coronary artery disease, cerebrovascular disease, or peripheral vascular disease. Patients may have an acute mesenteric ischemia develop in a background of the chronic syndrome. Thus, the presence of a chronic mesenteric ischemia does not rule out an acute on chronic phenomenon and the astute physician should maintain a high index of suspicion that symptoms in such patients are due to acute mesenteric ischemia until proven otherwise [2, 5, 9].

4. Mesenteric venous thrombosis
   - A thrombus forms in the mesenteric venous system. This prevents venous return and can result in increased splanchnic vasculature pressures to the point which prevents perfusion.
   - Possible risk factors for this entity include malignancy, portal hypertension, nephrotic syndrome, exogenous estrogen supplementation, pancreatitis, or other causes of intra-abdominal inflammation, surgery, factor V Leiden mutation, protein C or protein S deficiency, anti-phospholipid antibody syndrome, polycythemia, and others. Up to 75% of these patients have an inherited or acquired coagulopathy identified [6].
   - The symptoms may be present for a longer duration than the arterial thrombus or embolus etiology and thus the presence of a subacute timeframe for symptoms should not distract the physician from suspecting acute mesenteric ischemia [2, 5, 6, 9].

5. Nonocclusive mesenteric ischemia
   - Hypoperfusion of the mesentery as a result of decreased cardiac output or mesenteric vasoconstriction, comparable to demand ischemia of the heart.
   - This often occurs in extremely morbid hospitalized patients. It occurs in absence of obstruction and is the result of vasospasm and/or low arterial flow.

Risk factors as the same as for acute mesenteric ischemia due to embolism and thrombosis. Additional risk factors include vasopressor use, cocaine use, and hypotension [2, 6, 9].

6. Once ischemia has been initiated, mucosal sloughing can occur in as little as 3 hours. Transmural necrosis and perforation can occur in as little as 6 hours [2, 9].

Making the Diagnosis

Think about mesenteric ischemia if diagnosing the following
- Abdominal aortic aneurysm
- Small bowel obstruction
- Gastroenteritis
- Appendicitis
- Nephrolithiasis
- Sepsis
- Cholecystitis

1. Physical exam
   - Pain is the most common symptom. It has many descriptors and the classically taught pain out of proportion to exam is not sensitive and is thought to be present <50% of the time [6]. These patients may experience intense pain but have a soft abdomen and no increase in pain on palpation. Pain, not pain out of proportion to exam, is the most sensitive finding [6]. Often the pain is acute in nature and patients may be able to recall exactly what they were doing when pain started. This should raise your index of suspicion especially if pain started less than 3–6 hours ago.
   - Signs of gastric emptying such as diarrhea or vomiting may accompany the pain. Similarly, occult of gross GI bleeding may be present. These are neither sensitive nor specific [2, 5, 6, 9].
   - Peritonitis indicating whole bowel wall infarction is present approximately 16% of the time [6]. If this has occurred it is more likely that the patient will have other signs of complications such as shock, sepsis, and perforation, but overall these signs are also insensitive and nonspecific.
2. Laboratory evaluation
   - There is currently no single sensitive laboratory test. The single most useful test is a serum lactate; however, it is not sensitive enough to rule out mesenteric ischemia if negative [9].
   - Other laboratory tests that should be considered include a basic chemistry, CBC, and a blood gas analysis. This may show an elevated hematocrit, leukocytosis, or a metabolic acidosis, but this is nonspecific and not sensitive [5, 9].

3. Imaging
   - Plain films are not sensitive or specific. Early in the course of illness, nothing may be seen. Late in the course of illness, mesenteric thumb printing (mesenteric edema), pneumatosis intestinalis, or perforation may be seen [5, 6, 9].
   - Standard abdominal CT scans have a specificity and sensitivity of 92% and 62%, respectively [5]. They are generally not useful unless late findings or complications such as perforation are present. Both vascular and intestinal abnormalities may be seen.
   - Mesenteric angiography is the gold standard; however, it is rarely performed [9]. Multidetector CT angiography has largely replaced standard angiography and has a specificity and sensitivity of 95% and 93%, respectively [3, 4, 7].
   - One way to enhance the sensitivity of both standard abdominal CT and CT angiography is to alert the reading emergency radiologist of the clinical suspicion for mesenteric ischemia. In one study, this resulted in increased reporting of critical findings for mesenteric ischemia from 81% of scans to 97% [7].

Treating the Patient

1. The different etiologies of acute mesenteric ischemia each have unique treatments. Regardless of the etiology treatment begins with aggressive resuscitation starting with the ABCs of emergency medicine. Intubate if airway protection is indicated. Use aggressive fluids and/or vasopressors if the patient is hypotensive. Regardless of the etiology of mesenteric ischemia, antibiotics effective against enteric pathogens are indicated. Common remines include piperacillin/tazobactam, ertapenem, or ciprofloxacin with metronidazole. Surgical consultation should occur as soon as acute mesenteric ischemia is suspected because mesenteric ischemia is a clinical diagnosis and does not need to wait until it has been confirmed via imaging. This is especially true if peritonitis, shock, or evidence of perforation or infarction is present.
2. The goals of treatment are to restore mesenteric blood flow quickly and treat any complications the patient may have.
3. Acute mesenteric embolus or thrombosis are essentially treated in the same manner. Definitive management is exploratory laparotomy (ex lap) [2, 5, 6, 9]. The decision to proceed with this therapy should be made in conjunction with a surgical consultant. The surgeon should be involved as soon as you suspect the diagnosis and they should be told that you suspect mesenteric ischemia.
4. Ex lap allows for surgical revascularization and a direct assessment of bowel viability and intervention if there is evidence of nonviability.
5. There are small, single-center studies that report improved mortality and reduced post-op complications when treating acute obstructive mesenteric ischemia with immediate revascularization via percutaneous techniques [1, 2, 6, 10]. This therapy is not available at all centers and has not replaced ex lap as definitive management at this time.
6. The treatment of acute nonocclusive mesenteric ischemia depends on the presence of complications. If complications are present, they should be addressed in

standard fashion as above. If complications are absent, care is mostly supportive. Interventions include aggressive fluid resuscitation and vasodilators [2, 6]. If angiography is performed papaverine, a vasodilator may be infused directly into the mesenteric vessel in question [6]. Patients who require pressors may require a therapeutic switch to an alternate agent with less vasoconstriction or a dose reduction if tolerated. If the patient does not improve or if evidence of complications becomes apparent, an emergent ex lap is indicated to rule out bowel infarction and facilitate intervention. A surgical consultant should still be involved in their care early even in absence of complications.

7. Treatment of acute mesenteric venous thrombosis differs from the other etiologies. In the absence of complications, heparin infusion alone may be sufficient treatment [2, 5, 6, 9]. In addition to treatment of the underlying venous clot, a work up for a hypercoagulable state should be performed on all patients with acute mesenteric venous thrombosis, if a cause is not already apparent [2, 5, 6, 9]. If the patient is not improving with conservative therapy, then an emergent ex lap is indicated. A surgical consultant should still be involved in their care early.

8. All patients with confirmed or suspect acute mesenteric ischemia should be admitted to the ICU level of care [6].

Case Conclusion

Approximately 3 hours after admission, the patient had frank hematochezia and hypotension on the floor requiring stat transfusion of 2 units of uncross-matched blood, and a transfer to the ICU for close monitoring. Her hemoglobin immediately prior to her ICU transfer was 7.6 and her lactate was 7.2. She remained diffusely tender to palpation and general surgery was consulted for evaluation for emergent laparotomy given the high index of suspicion for acute mesenteric ischemia. She was made NPO, ertapenem was started, and she was taken for laparotomy where she was definitively diagnosed with acute mesenteric ischemia likely from a cardiac source embolism. A small bowel resection of the nonviable bowel was performed. She survived to hospital discharge and is doing well postoperatively.

Type of Ischemia	Pathophysiology	Treatment	Other
Mesenteric arterial embolus	Emboli travels from elsewhere, usually the heart, and blocks the mesenteric artery	Antibiotics and Surgery, possible benefit of intravascular intervention	
Mesenteric arterial thrombosis	Atherosclerosis forms in the mesenteric artery	Antibiotics and Surgery, possible benefit of intravascular intervention	
Non-occlusive mesenteric ischemia	Poor cardiac output and vasoconstrictions decreases Perfusion of the ischemia	Antibiotics, treat underlying condition, weaning of vasopressors, intravascular treatment with papaverine	Usually found in very sick patients on vasopressors
Mesenteric venous thrombosis	A thrombus forms in the mesenteric vein	Antibiotics, systemic anticoagulation	Somewhat more indolent course, presents subacutetly

Discussion

1. Acute mesenteric ischemia is a difficult diagnosis to make in the ED. It is rare and often presents with vague symptoms. Acute mesenteric ischemia with obvious peritonitis or septic shock is striking and the presentation overwhelmingly suggests a grave diagnosis and the diagnosis in that circumstance may be easier to make.
2. Unfortunately, conventional teachings of intestinal angina and pain out or proportion to exam may not be present early in the disease [2, 5, 6, 9]. The only way to make the diagnosis and intervene is to have a high index of suspicion.
3. Conditions that raise the pretest probability are age greater than 50, comorbid cardiac conditions, and acute onset of pain. Similarly, unexplained elevated lactate with abdominal pain in an elderly patient is mesenteric ischemia until you prove it is not. Mesenteric ischemia is a clinical diagnosis, and imaging is not required to make the diagnosis. You should not rely on a standard CT scan to evaluate for this etiology. If you do require imaging, CT angiography is the most widely available and reliable modality.
4. When discussing the case with surgical consultants and radiologists, it is important to mention that you are suspicious for mesenteric ischemia and then divulge to them if your exam was positive for any complications that they may want to know about such as peritonitis [4].

Pattern Recognition

Acute mesenteric ischemia
- Advanced age
- Severe, sudden-onset abdominal pain
- Cardiac comorbidities (atrial fibrillation, CAD, CHF, MI, thrombus, vegetation)
- Symptoms of gastric emptying (nausea or diarrhea)

Disclosure Statement   The authors of this chapter report no significant disclosures.

References

1. Arthurs ZM, Titus J, Bannazedeh M, et al. A comparison of endovascular revascularization with traditional therapy for the treatment of acute mesenteric ischemia. J Vasc Surg. 2011;53:698–705.
2. Cudnik MT, Darbha S, Jones J, et al. The diagnosis of acute mesenteric ischemia: a systemic review and meta-analysis. Acad Emerg Med. 2013;20:1087–100.
3. Karkkainen JM, Acosta S. Acute mesenteric ischemia (part I) – incidence etiologies and how to improve early diagnosis. Best Pract Res Clin Gastroenterol. 2017;31(1):15–25.

4. Lehtimaki TT, Karkkainen JM, Saari P, Manninen H, Paajanen H, Vanninen R. Detecting acute mesenteric ischemia in CT of the acute abdomen is dependent on clinical suspicion: review of 95 consecutive patients. Eur J Radiol. 2015;84(12):2444–53.
5. Lo BM. Lower gastrointestinal bleeding. In: Tintinalli JE, et al., editors. Tintinalli's emergency medicine: a comprehensive study guide. 8th ed. New York: McGraw-Hill; 2016.
6. Long B, Koyfman A. The dangerous miss: recognizing acute mesenteric ischemia [internet]. 2016 May: [cited June 30th 2018] Available from http://epmonthly.com/article/the-dangerous-miss/.
7. Meke J. Diagnostic accuracy of multidetector CT in acute mesenteric ischemia: systematic review and meta-analysis. Radiology. 2010;256:93–101.
8. Menke J, Luthje L, Kastrup A, et al. Thromboembolism in atrial fibrillation. Am J Cardiol. 105:502–10.
9. Rosen P, Walls RM, Hockberger RS, Gausche-Hill M, Bakes KM. Rosen's emergency medicine: concepts and clinical practice. Philadelphia: Elsevier; 2018.
10. Resch TA, Acosta S, Sonesson B. Endovascular techniques in acute arterial mesenteric ischemia. Semin Vasc Surg. 2010;23:29–35.

Mucormycosis: *"There's a Fungus Among Us!"*

Tatiana Thema and Sorabh Khandelwal

Case

Persistent "Orbital Cellulitis"

Pertinent History

A 56-year-old woman with poorly controlled diabetes mellitis (DM) was transferred from an outside hospital due to concern for orbital cellulitis. She was seen at the outside hospital 5 days previously with left-sided ophthalmoplegia, facial numbness, and sinus symptoms. She was evaluated for a possible CVA. After a negative work up, she was discharged on levofloxacin (Levaquin®) with a diagnosis of sinusitis. She had a negative CT scan on the first visit. She returned to the hospital in diabetic ketoacidosis c/o fevers, headache, and loss of vision in her left eye. Following evaluation, she was transferred to the local tertiary care center for further care.

Pertinent Physical Exam

Except as noted below, the findings of the complete physical exam are within normal limits.

- HEENT: Complete ophthalmoplegia/vision loss of left eye, nonreactive to light, proptosis, erythema, and periorbital swelling. Decreased sensation of her left face, some weakness of facial muscles. Necrotic tissue present in the left nares, ecchymotic and partially necrotic palate, and midline uvula.

T. Thema · S. Khandelwal (✉)
Department of Emergency Medicine, Wexner Medical Center at The Ohio State University, Columbus, OH, USA
e-mail: Sorabh.khandelwal@osumc.edu

© Springer Nature Switzerland AG 2020
C. G. Kaide, C. E. San Miguel (eds.), *Case Studies in Emergency Medicine*,
https://doi.org/10.1007/978-3-030-22445-5_40

PMH
DM

Emergency Department Management

Patient's DKA was managed with insulin and fluids and she was started on Amphotericin. After evaluation by ENT and ophthalmology, she was taken directly to surgery.

Necrotic Tissue in Nostrils and Soft Palate

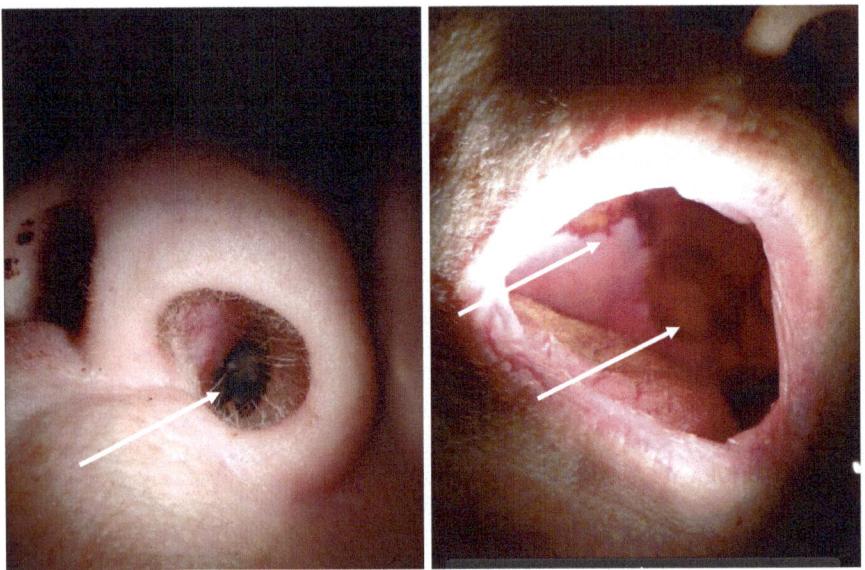

Used with permission, courtesy of Colin Kaide, MD

Orbital Infection

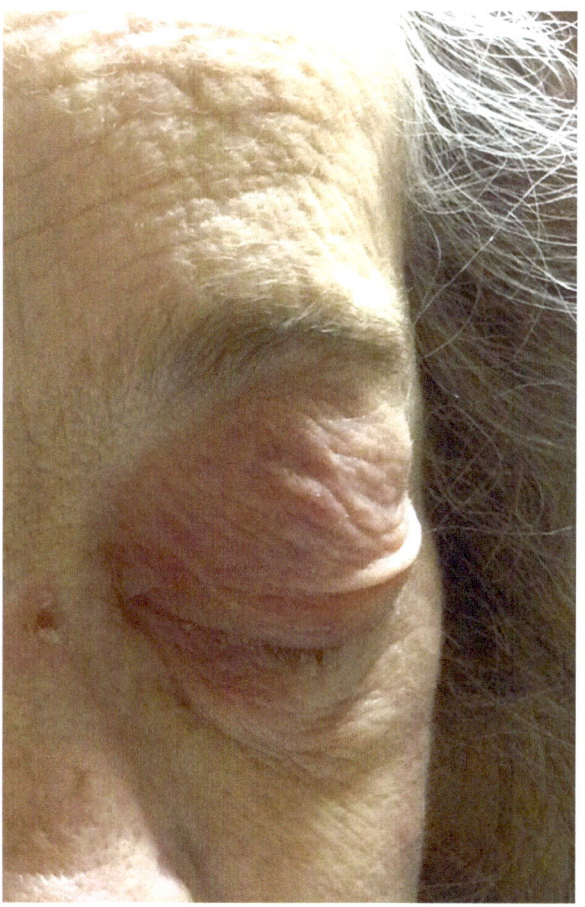

Used with permission, courtesy of Colin Kaide, MD

Learning Points

Priming Questions
1. What is particular about the pathophysiology of mucormycosis compared to other soft tissue infections?
2. How is mucormycosis diagnosed?
3. Are laboratory and imaging studies helpful in the diagnosis?
4. What is the role of the emergency physician in the treatment of mucormycosis?

Introduction/Background

1. Mucormycosis is a rare but rapid life-threatening infection with a high mortality rate. It is caused by fungal pathogens from the Mucorales order. The most common culprit identified is from *Rhizopus* species.
2. Overall mortality ranges from 25% to 62%, with the best prognosis in patients with infection confined to the sinuses. Mortality increases with pulmonary involvement and disseminated disease [1].
3. Common underlying conditions that can facilitate this infection [2]:
   - DM (particularly with ketoacidosis)
   - Organ or stem cell transplant
   - Hematologic malignancies
   - Metabolic acidosis
   - High dose glucocorticoid treatment
   - Chemotherapy treatments
   - Anti-rejection transplant medications
   - Penetrating trauma/burns
   - Iron overload states
   - AIDS
   - Injection drug use
   - Malnutrition
   - Treatment with deferoxamine
4. The host's immunity and underlying medical condition dictate the clinical presentation of mucormycosis types. From the most to least common: rhino-orbital-cerebral, pulmonary, cutaneous, gastrointestinal, disseminated, and atypical [3]. This review will focus on the rhino-orbital-cerebral presentation, which comprises between 20% and 34% of all cases [4]. The majority of rhino-orbital-cerebral involvement occurs in diabetic patients (about 70%) [5].

Physiology/Pathophysiology

1. Normal host: Phagocytes (mononuclear, polymorphonuclear) → oxidative metabolites + cationic peptides defensins → prevent germination and kill hyphal form.

2. Mucorales' ability to thrive in the host is multifactorial. Inhalation of fungi spores from environmental sources is the most common mode of acquisition [4]. This is followed by disruption of mucocutaneous barrier as well as percutaneous inoculation [4].
   - Via inhalation, ingestion, or cutaneous inoculation → mucorales kill mononuclear and polymorphonuclear phagocytes → germination into hyphae (angioinvasive form) → local angioinvasive growth → surrounding tissue infarction and necrosis [3, 4].
   - Blood vessel invasion → vessel wall necrosis → mycotic thrombi → tissue infarction → hematogenous dissemination → extensive necrosis.
3. Set up: Phagocytic activity disruption, either from insufficient recruitment (neutropenia) or functional impediment (hyperglycemia, glucocorticoids, acidosis) → unchallenged fungi growth [5].
   - Hyperglycemia: Rhizopus oryzae hyphal form adheres to the endothelial cell by GRP78, a glucose-related protein, which has increased expression in hyperglycemia [2].
     - Hyperglycemia also independently causes disruption of neutrophil and phagocyte recruitment, in addition to compromising their cell function.
   - Glucocorticoids cause compromised chemotaxis and lower fungicidal mechanisms [4].
   - Free iron: This boosts virulence by increasing proliferation. Several mechanisms of obtention of free iron by the fungus have been described.
     - Acidosis (pH < 7.4) (i.e., from DKA) decreases transferrin's ability to bind and sequester free iron, thereby leaving more free iron for the fungus.
     - Chelator deferoxamine for severe hemochromatosis or aluminum toxicity in dialysis patients (rarely seen today): Rhizopus oryzae plus the deferoxamine complex creates a ferrioxamine complex that frees iron via reductive process leading to free iron moving intracellularly [4]. Other iron chelating agents (i.e., deferasirox, deferiprone) do not act as siderophores and therefore do not increase risk of disease [2].
     - Multiple blood transfusions can lead to iron overload allowing for more free iron for the fungi [3].

Making the Diagnosis

Having a high index of suspicion remains crucial in making the diagnosis. Misdiagnosis or delayed diagnosis can be fatal. Absence of classic necrotic lesions does not rule out the disease. It is a late sign and occurs in <50% of patients in the early phase of the disease! [4] *Be on your guard for rapidly worsening or failed treatment of facial/oral cellulitis in suspect patients! Pause to look carefully for suspicious lesions and do a quick neurological exam.*

Differential Diagnosis
- Preseptal cellulitis
- Orbital cellulitis
- Dental abscess
- Acute sinusitis
- Migraine headache
- Orbital tumor
- Cavernous sinus thrombosis

1. The presentation can vary tremendously from sinus pain to the signature necrotic lesions. Consequently, maintaining a high index of suspicion is paramount in making the diagnosis.
   - In suspect patients, ostensibly mild-to-moderate symptoms include fever, congestion, headache, sinus or mouth or facial pain, hyposmia, anosmia, epistaxis, and black nasal discharge [4]. There might be associated tissue erythema or violaceous hue.
   - Presence of a painful necrotic eschar (ear canals, hard palate, nasal cavity, turbinates, face, eyelids) is often a late sign that indicates rapid evolution of infection [4, 6].
   - Other symptoms include periorbital edema, proptosis, orbital edema, preseptal edema, chemosis, monocular or binocular pain, blurry vision or vision loss, diplopia, ophthalmoplegia, infraorbital facial numbness, trigeminal nerve palsy, cranial nerve palsy, and any cranial neuropathy [3, 4, 6].
   - Extension of the disease tends to be to contiguous structures. Therefore, consider intracranial/central involvement: cavernous sinus thrombosis, internal carotid artery thrombosis, epidural and subdural abscesses, basilar artery aneurysm, meningitis (rare), and sagittal sinus thrombosis (rare) [4].
   - In patients with cough, consider pulmonary involvement [4].
2. Ultimately, the definitive diagnosis is made from biopsy of the necrotic lesion and histologic study of frozen sections [6]. However, upon encountering this disease, it falls on the astute clinician to recognize it quickly and start empiric antifungal treatment well before definitive diagnosis is established.
3. Adjunctive work up:
   - Labs include:
     – CBC to assess for neutropenia; however, leukocytosis is also possible.
     – ABG or VBG to assess for acidosis.
     – Chemistry panel with glucose.
4. Imaging with CT and MRI may be helpful in establishing the diagnosis or guaging the extent of disease.
   - CT findings of the head and face include extraorbital muscle thickening, air–fluid levels, bony erosions, mucosal thickening, and intracranial involvement [3–6].

- Extraorbital muscle thickening on CT or MRI should trigger empirical antifungal treatment [4, 6].
- MRI, more sensitive than CT, is useful in identifying the extent of tissue involvement and guide the need for surgery [7].

Treating the Patient

Due to the rarity of the disease, there is no comparative prospective study on the primary antifungal treatment for mucormycosis. Therefore, the best approach is still not established.

1. Currently, the multidisciplinary (e.g., internal medicine, infectious diseases, clinical microbiology, head and neck surgery, pathology, plastic surgery, ophthalmology) approach combines medical management and surgical debridement. Untreated, survival rates are about 3% [8]. Medical management alone is often inadequate.
2. Medical management.
   - Antifungal therapy:
     - Liposomal formulation of Amphotericin B (AmBisome): 5–10 mg/kg per day is most likely the drug to be used due to its safety profile and efficacy compared to Amphotericin B deoxycholate (nephrotoxic) [5, 7].
   - Optimization of other treatments as indicated: ketoacidosis reversal, hyperglycemia control, rapid glucocorticoid tapering, cessation of deferoxamine treatment, etc.
3. Surgery: Due to the aggressive nature of the mucormycosis, excision and debridement of infected tissue is important and should be expedited. Multiple surgeries might be needed to contain the infection [5]. In rhinocerebral involvement, debriding the retro-orbital space has been associated with preventing extension to the eye, avoiding enucleation [5].
4. Hyperbaric oxygen therapy (HBOT): It may be beneficial as an adjunct therapy. It has been used status postsurgical debridement. The Undersea and Hyperbaric Medical Society recommends its use early in the treatment given the success seen in numerous published case reports [9].

Case Conclusion

The patient was taken emergently to the operating room for surgical debridement. The procedures performed included:

- Left medial maxillectomy
- Bilateral sphenoidotomies
- Total left ethmoidectomy
- Septectomy
- Palatectomy
- Exenteration orbital contents

Pathology

Angioinvasive and tissue-invasive fungi consistent with mucormycosis, involving respiratory type tissue, extensive necrosis, and abscess. The microbiology: *Rhizopus* species.

Postdebridment, the patient received 3 HBO treatments but ultimately succumbed to the infection.

Discussion

Rhinocerebral mucormycosis can be swift and deadly and leave the patient with severe cosmetic or functional impairment even with optimal treatment. Therefore, the astute clinician should approach facial/mucosal cellulitis with caution in diabetic or immunocompromised patients.

Remember that this clinician should keep a high clinical suspicion for this disease, as it can be very vague in its presentation. The presence of a necrotic painful eschar is the hallmark finding, but it indicates advanced disease. It is much better to think of this diagnosis before the pathognomonic findings develop! It is important to start medical treatment and get surgery involved early in the management of mucormycosis.

Pattern Recognition

- Immunocompromised patients
- Mimics bacterial sinusitis
- Unilateral headache
- Retro-orbital Headache
- Facial pain
- Unilateral congestion to black discharge

Disclosure Statement The authors of this chapter report no significant disclosures.

References

1. Roden MM, Zaoutis TE, Buchanan WL, Knudsen TA, Sarkisova TA, Schaufele RL, Sein M, Sein T, Chiou CC, Chu JH, Kontoyiannis DP, Walsh TJ. Epidemiology and outcome of zygomycosis: a review of 929 reported cases. Clin Infect Dis. 2005;41(5):634.
2. Cox G. Mucormycosis (zygoycosis). In: Kauffman CA, Thorner AR, editors. UpToDate. Waltham: UpToDate Inc. https://www.uptodate.com (Accessed on 25 Feb 2019).
3. Ibrahim AS, Walsh TJ, Kontayiannis DP. Pathogenesis of mucormycosis. Clin Infect Dis. 2012;54(S1):S16–21.

4. Kontoyiannis DP, Lewis RE. In: Bennett JE, Dolin R, Blaser MJ, editors. Agents of mucormycosis and entomophthoramycosis. Mandell, Douglas, and Bennett's infectious disease essentials. 8th ed. Philadelphia. Chapter 260.: Elsevier; 2015. p. 2909–2919.e4.
5. Spellberg B, Edwards J Jr, Ibrahim A. Novel perspectives on mucormycosis: pathophysiology, presentation, and management. Clin Microbiol Rev. 2005;18(3):556–69.
6. Kontoyiannis DP. In: Goldman L, Schafer AI, editors. Mucormycosis. Goldman-Cecil medicine. 25th ed. Philadelphia: Elsevier Saunders; 2016. p. 2087–2091.e2, chapter 340.
7. Baugh WP. (2018). Rhinocerebral mucormycosis. Wallace MR (ed). [online] Emedicine.medscape.com. Available at https://emedicine.medscape.com/article/227586-differential. Accessed 25 Feb 2019.
8. Wali U, Balkhair A, Al-Mujaini A. Cerebro-rhino orbital mucormycosis: an update. J Infect Public Health. 2012;5(2):116–26.
9. Jacoby I. Necrotizing soft tissue infections. In: Hyperbaric oxygen therapy indications: Undersea and Hyperbaric Medical Society, Inc; 2014. p. 167–72. Chapter 11.

Radiology Case 8

41

Caitlin Hackett and Joshua K. Aalberg

Indication for Examination: 20-year-old male presents with right-sided chest pain and dyspnea. On exam, there are diminished breath sounds and hyperresonance on the right.

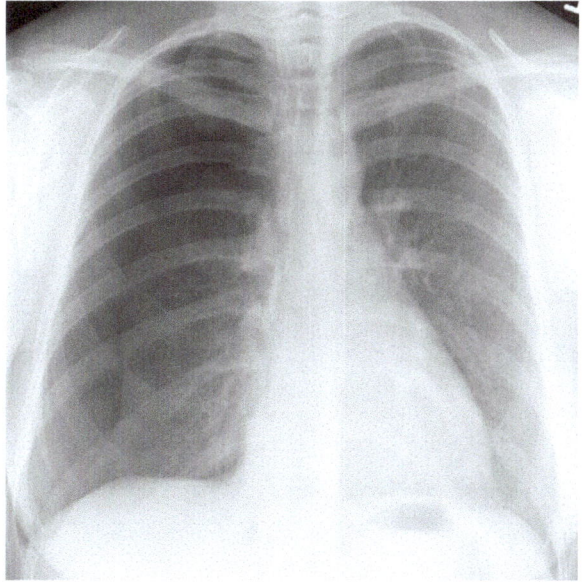

Radiographic Findings Lack of extension of the right lung to the edge of the chest cavity

C. Hackett · J. K. Aalberg (✉)
Department of Emergency Medicine, Wexner Medical Center at The Ohio State University, Columbus, OH, USA
e-mail: Caitlin.Hackett@osumc.edu; joshua.aalberg@osumc.edu

© Springer Nature Switzerland AG 2020
C. G. Kaide, C. E. San Miguel (eds.), *Case Studies in Emergency Medicine*,
https://doi.org/10.1007/978-3-030-22445-5_41

Diagnosis Large right pneumothorax

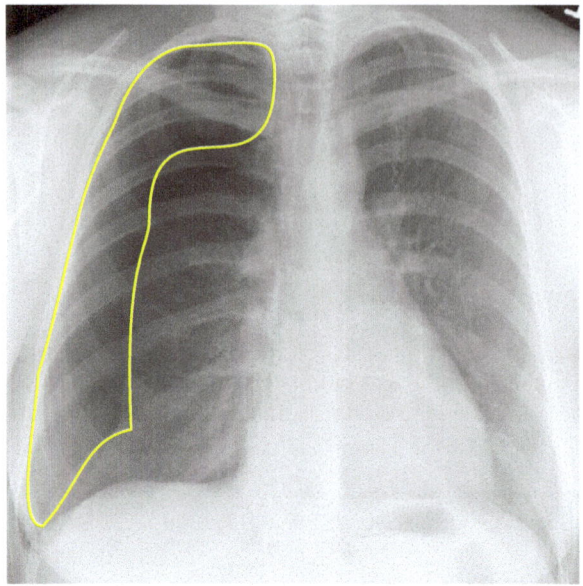

Learning Points

Priming questions
- What are the best patient positions to evaluate for pneumothorax on X-ray?
- What are some common mimics of pneumothorax?
- What are signs of tension pneumothorax?

Introduction

- Pneumothorax is an abnormal collection of air within the pleural space, which can cause mass effect on the adjacent lung.
- Tension pneumothorax occurs when air accumulates and causes pressure on the mediastinal structures eventually causing decreased venous return and cardiopulmonary collapse [1].

Pathophysiology/Mechanism

- There are many causes of pneumothorax.
  - Primary spontaneous pneumothorax is seen in patients with no underlying lung disease, most commonly thin young men.

- Blunt trauma, approximately 30–40% of patients with blunt chest trauma have an associated pneumothorax.
- Iatrogenic
  - Barotrauma from ventilation
  - Post bronchoscopy
  - Post thoracentesis or lung biopsy
  - Following central line placement.
- Infection including pneumocystis and necrotizing pneumonia
- Tumors
- More rare causes include
  - Cystic lung disease from Langerhans cell histiocytosis or lymphangioleiomyomatosis.
  - Smokers and patients with emphysema are at increased risk of developing a pneumothorax [2].

Making the Diagnosis

Chest radiograph is the initial test of choice to evaluate for pneumothorax.

- Ideally, the radiograph should be obtained in the upright position, as this allows air to rise to the apex, making the pneumothorax more apparent. The outer margin of visceral pleura and lung is separated from parietal pleura and chest wall, which appears as a thin white line on the radiograph. There is a lack of vessel markings beyond this line.
  - If an upright film cannot be obtained, there are several indirect signs of pneumothorax.
    - There may be relative lucency of the affected hemithorax or increased sharpness of the mediastinal margins.
    - The deep sulcus sign is a lucent costophrenic angle, which is deeper than the contralateral side. However, patients with hyperexpanded lungs may exhibit deepened costophrenic angles due to hyperaeration.
    - The double diaphragm sign refers to air outlining the anterior portions of the hemidiaphragm causing visualization of the anterior costophrenic sulcus. The ipsilateral hemidiaphragm may be depressed.
- Expiratory images may accentuate contrast between lung and gas.
- Lateral decubitus films may also be helpful if the patient is not able to stand for upright images. The hemithorax of interest should be placed in the nondecubitus position so that the air can rise. Decubitus films can detect as little as 5 ml of air.

Computed tomography (CT) can be used in patients when radiographs are equivocal. CT should also be considered in patients who have pneumothorax of uncertain etiology to assess for undiagnosed lung disease.

Bedsides, ultrasound is also being utilized more often to evaluate for pneumothorax. Absence of lung sliding is characteristic for pneumothorax, but can also be seen anytime the lung being examined is not being aerated, such as in mainstem intubations (if the contralateral mainstem is in fact the one with the endotracheal tube) and bronchial obstruction.

There are several entities that can mimic pneumothorax that clinicians should rule out prior to placing a chest tube.

- Skin folds, the scapular line, and external equipment can all cause pseudo-pneumothorax.
  - Unlike the pleural line seen with pneumothorax, the pseudo-pleural line will be thicker and more ill-defined.
  - The line will also be straighter. The pleural line should follow that natural curve of the chest cavity.
  - The scapular line can be identified if it connects with the rest of the bone.
  - Lung markings will extend to the periphery of the lung beyond a pseudo-pleural line.
  - Some of these findings are subtle and require aggressive windowing. As stated above, there are multiple different views that can help clinicians solve the problem [4].

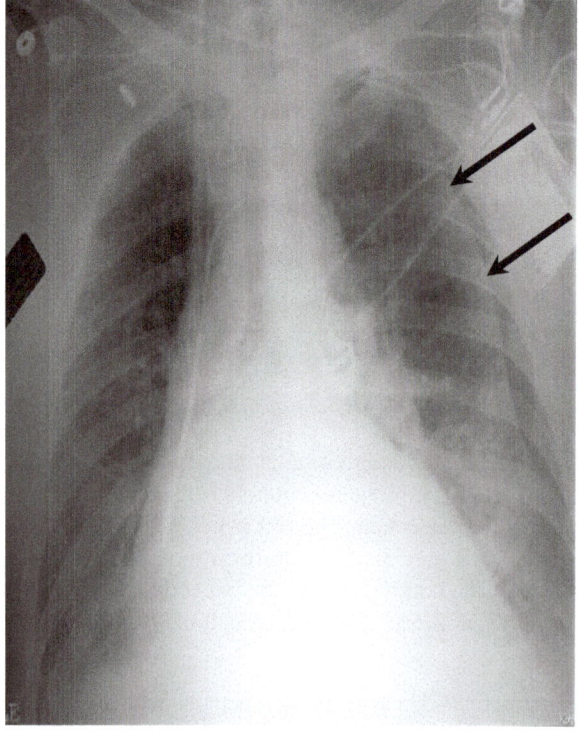

Skin fold mimicking a left pneumothorax

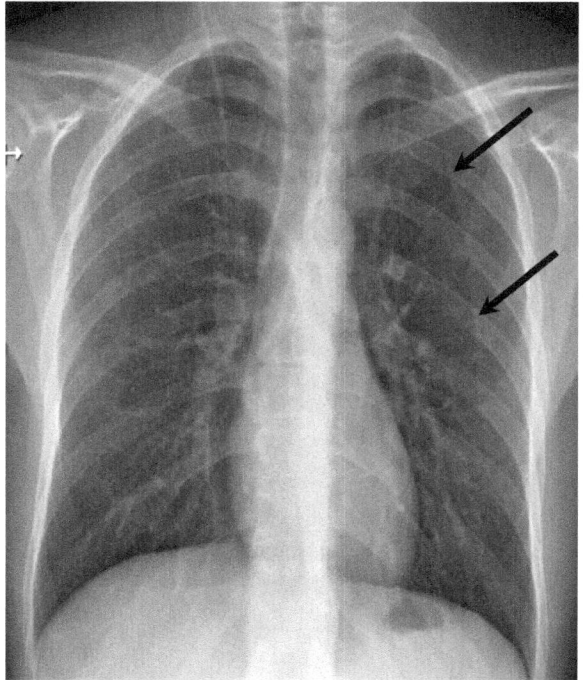

Scapular line mimicking pneumothorax

Radiographic findings of tension pneumothorax include contralateral shift of the mediastinum, depression of the hemidiaphragm, and ipsilateral increase in the intercostal spaces [3]. This however remains a clinical diagnosis and any hemodynamic instability in the setting of a pneumothorax should prompt emergent decompression without waiting for radiographic confirmation.

Treating the Patient

- Patients with tension pneumothorax, regardless of the cause require emergent decompression via needle depression, finger thoracostomy, or chest tube placement, whichever can be achieved fastest.
- There are myriad options for the treatment of a stable patient with a pneumothorax. These include high flow oxygen and reassessment, aspiration, placement of a small catheter, and placement of a traditional chest tube. Recurrent pneumothoraxes and those secondary to underlying pathology are more likely to benefit from traditional chest tube placement. Similarly, most experts agree that traumatic pneumothoraxes seen on chest X-ray require a traditional chest tube for treatment. However, small pneumothoraxes seen on CT only in an asymptomatic patient can be observed over time [5, 6].
- See the Pneumothorax chapter for more details.

Discussion

- Pneumothorax is a critical diagnosis to make, but can be deceptively difficult with false positives such as skin folds, scapular lines, and external equipment causing pseudopleural lines.
- Alternative imaging modalities include bedside ultrasound and CT of the chest.
- Treatment depends on the severity of the pathology, underlying cause (or lack thereof), and local practice patterns and resources. If a patient is hemodynamically unstable from their pneumothorax regardless of cause, they require immediate decompression.

Disclosure Statement   The authors of this chapter report no significant disclosures.

References

1. Weissleder R, et al. Primer of diagnostic imaging. 5th ed. Philadelphia: Elsevier; 2011.
2. Soto JA, Lucey BC. Emergency radiology requisites. 2nd ed. Philadelphia: Elsevier; 2017.
3. Goodman LR. Felson's principles of chest roentgenology. 4th ed. Philadelphia: Elsevier; 2015.
4. O'Connor AR, Morgan WE. Radiological review of pneumothorax. BMJ. 2005;330(7506): 1493–7.
5. Zarogoulidis P, et al. Pneumothorax: from definition to diagnosis and treatment. J Thorac Dis. 2014;6(Suppl 4):S372–6.
6. Mirvis SE, et al. Emergency radiology case review. 1st ed. Philadelphia: Elsevier; 2009.

Multiligament Knee Injuries: *The Knee Bone Is Connected to … Almost Nothing*

42

Mark J. Conroy and Ryan McGrath

Case

Knee Pain and Swelling Following Trauma

Pertinent History The patient presented to the emergency department (ED) after crashing his mountain bike while out on a ride. His front tire got caught and he went over the handlebars coming down awkwardly on his right leg. He cannot recall the exact position of his leg when he landed, but he felt a pop and immediate pain in his knee. Since the accident he has been unable to ambulate due to the pain and swelling. He has never injured this knee before and has noticed some numbness in his right foot since the accident.

Pertinent Physical Exam

- BP: 136/84, Pulse: 92, Temperature 98.4 °F (36.9 °C), RR 12, SpO2 99%.

Except as noted below, the findings of the complete physical exam are within normal limits.

- Extremity: 2+ femoral pulses bilaterally, 2+ left DP/PT pulses, 1+ right DP/PT pulses, no ecchymosis or abrasions noted.
- Musculoskeletal: Negative log roll of the bilateral lower extremities. Right knee exam reveals an effusion and diffuse tenderness with limited range of motion. There is laxity and pain with varus and valgus stress at 0 and 30°, especially when compared with the left. Lachman testing reveals increased translation compared with the left with no firm endpoint appreciated.

PMH None.

M. J. Conroy (✉) · R. McGrath
Department of Emergency Medicine, Wexner Medical Center at The Ohio State University, Columbus, OH, USA
e-mail: Mark.Conroy@osumc.edu; Ryan.McGrath@osumc.edu

© Springer Nature Switzerland AG 2020
C. G. Kaide, C. E. San Miguel (eds.), *Case Studies in Emergency Medicine*, https://doi.org/10.1007/978-3-030-22445-5_42

Pertinent Test Results

Right knee X-ray: Effusion with normal alignment and no signs of fracture.

ED Management

Knee immobilizer, crutches, pain control with urgent orthopedic referral.

Updates on Emergency Department Course

While waiting for his discharge, the patient reported increasing numbness to his right foot and lower leg. His knee pain was worsening despite pain medication. On re-examination, his right foot was dusky and cool and his distal pulses were no longer palpable. An ankle-brachial index (ABI) is obtained and a CT angiogram of his right lower extremity was ordered with emergent orthopedic surgery and vascular surgery consults. The CTA demonstrated an occlusion of the right popliteal artery. The patient was taken emergently to the OR for stabilization and revascularization.

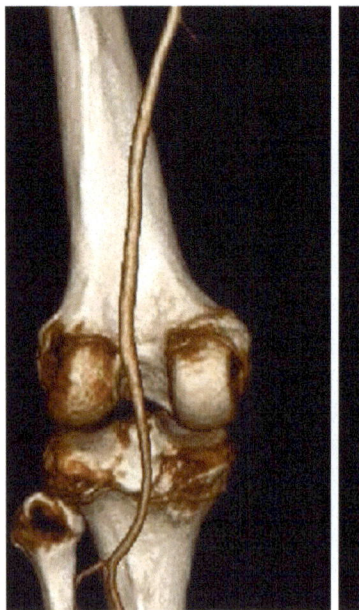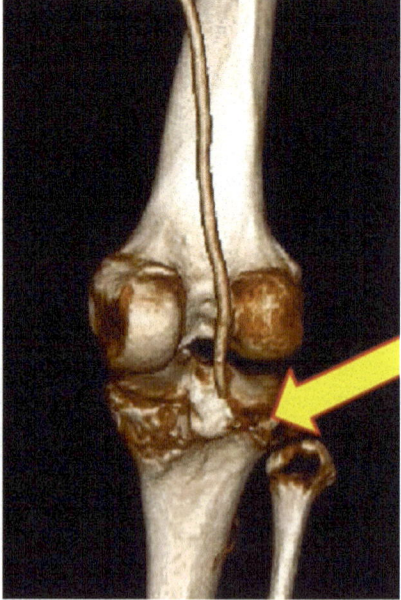

Anthony Dean Godfrey, Fadi Hindi, Callum Ettles, Mark Pemberton, and Perbinder Grewal (https://commons.wikimedia.org/wiki/File:CTAngioOcclusionRtPop.jpg), https://creativecommons.org/licenses/by/4.0/legalcode

Learning Points

Priming Questions
1. What injury mechanisms are most commonly associated with knee dislocations?
2. How is this diagnosis made and what role does advanced imaging play in its immediate evaluation?
3. What is the expected disposition for all patients with multiligament knee injuries?

Introduction/Background

1. Although uncommon, multiligament knee injuries with dislocation/relocation, or identifiable knee dislocations, represent a limb-threatening emergency due to compromise of the vascular supply to the limb and, thus, must be recognized and acted upon urgently. Although the estimated incidence of knee dislocation is less than 0.02% of orthopedic injuries annually [1] or 2–29 orthopedic injuries per million annually, it is imperative to act swiftly and appropriately to avoid significant patient morbidity [2, 3]. In particular, it is important to maintain a high index of suspicion, as nearly 50% of knee dislocations spontaneously reduce prior to arrival in the emergency department (ED) and reduction does not preclude vascular injury [4].

Physiology/Pathophysiology

1. Knee dislocations most commonly result from high-velocity mechanisms leading to blunt force against the knee and its many ligamentous attachments. Shearing of these stabilizing structures precedes translational movement of the tibia and fibula in reference to the femur and ultimately dislocation. Occasionally, low-energy mechanisms have resulted in dislocation injuries and typically involve an element of rotational force, particularly in obese patients. The translational displacement of the bones of the knee ultimately places significant stress on the limb's vascular supply.
   - The knee joint is stabilized primarily by four collateral ligaments that are susceptible to rotational and shearing forces including the anterior and posterior cruciate ligaments as well as the medial and lateral collateral ligaments. In knee dislocations, typically three of the four stabilizing ligaments of the knee are disrupted, leaving the tibia and fibula vulnerable to translational displacement in reference to the femur resulting in dislocation [1].
     - The Kennedy system classifies knee dislocation based on displacement of the tibia in reference to the femur. Anterior dislocations are the most common, accounting for 30–50% of cases and generally occur with forced hyperextension of the knee [5]. Posterior dislocations are the second most

common occurring in 25% of cases and are associated with the highest rate of complete tearing of the vascular supply of the lower leg [6]. Lateral dislocation occurs in approximately 13% of cases and result in the highest rate of peroneal nerve injury. Medial and rotational dislocation of the tibia occur infrequently [7].

- The femoral artery gives rise to the popliteal artery that provides collateral circulation to the knee via five geniculate arteries and the remainder of the lower extremity below the level of the knee. The popliteal artery is tethered at both ends of the knee joint within the popliteal fossa by the tendinous hiatus proximally and tendinous arch of the soleus distally. Due to this anatomy, the popliteal artery is susceptible to potential occlusion and tearing when shearing forces are applied to the knee as is the case with dislocation of the knee joint.
  - Although injury to the popliteal artery is most typically associated with knee dislocation, injury to both the popliteal veins and peroneal nerve (in 25% of dislocations) are also common and contribute to the emergent nature of this diagnosis [8].

Making the Diagnosis

Diagnosing a knee dislocation can either be quite simple or particularly tedious, as these dislocations have a tendency to self-reduce, making the appearance of gross deformity and instability on knee examination unreliable.

Differential Diagnosis
- *Isolated ligament/tendon injury*
- *Patellar dislocation*
- *Tibial plateau fracture*
- *Fracture of femur, tibia, fibula*
- *Cartilage tear*

1. Patients who present with significant deformities of the knee on visualization or striking instability on examination strongly suggest disruption of the joint and dislocation of the knee.
2. Recognition of more subtle presentations of knee dislocation requires greater focus on the physical examination particularly in evaluation of the integrity of the ligaments of the knee.
   - Knee dislocations typically occur with the disruption of at least three of the four stabilizing ligaments of the knee including the ACL, PCL, MCL, and LCL. *Thus, any knee examination with instability in multiple planes should be considered a dislocation of the knee until proven otherwise.*
     - Dislocation of the knee can still occur with disruption of only two knee ligaments, but there is approximately a 31% increased incidence of associated vascular injury when three of the four ligaments are injured [9].

3. Evaluation of the vascular patency of the limb is the most important aspect in evaluation of a potential knee dislocation.
    - The circulatory status of the limb should be assessed by palpating pulses distal to the popliteal artery, assessing for the presence of pulses with continuous wave form Doppler, or use of bedside ultrasound with color flow. Additionally, an ABI should be obtained. An ABI with a value less than 0.90 indicates compromised arterial supply to the extremity and has been found to have a nearly 100% positive predictive value in assessing a vascular injury needing repair [10]. Ultimately, if there are any hard signs of vascular compromise, an immediate vascular surgery consultation should be obtained. Hard signs of vascular compromise include:
        - Absence of pulses
        - External signs of limb ischemia (asymmetric pallor or duskiness)
        - Paresthesia or paralysis
        - Expanding hematoma
        - Bruit or thrill over the popliteal fossa
    - The presence of distal pulses or signs of increased perfusion after reduction of the dislocation does not exclude injury to popliteal vessels, and thus angiography is typically required for complete evaluation [6].
4. Imaging is required in the evaluation of a potentially dislocated knee but should not delay reduction with any signs of neurovascular compromise.
    - Plain films should be obtained in the initial evaluation for confirmation of the suspected diagnosis if there is uncertainty.
        - Evaluate for asymmetry of the joint and joint space as well as avulsion fractures, particularly of the lateral tibial plateau, which can be a secondary sign of ligament injury and dislocation [1].
    - Angiography remains the gold standard for evaluation of a potential vascular injury to the limb [7].
    - CT and MRI angiography have become increasingly accepted as noninvasive imaging studies for evaluation of the vasculature of the lower extremity following knee dislocation [7].

Treating the Patient

1. Immediate management
    - If obviously dislocated, steps should be taken to urgently reduce the dislocation even prior to obtaining confirmatory radiographs. This step is critical if there is any evidence of neurovascular compromise as a delay in reduction and reestablishing arterial flow greater than 8 hours is associated with amputation in as many as 85% of cases [9].
        - Special attention must be made to recognize a posterolateral dislocation, as these are considered irreducible at the bedside. Closed reduction of posterior dislocations can compromise the integrity of skin overlying the lateral femoral condyle leading to necrosis. A characteristic "dimple sign" at the anteromedial aspect of the knee due to excess skin folding is due to the anatomic distortion inherent to this injury. This dimple may become

more pronounced with longitudinal traction. If posterolateral dislocation is suspected emergent consultation to vascular surgery and orthopedic surgery should be performed [11].
- To perform a bedside reduction, typically the application of gentle longitudinal traction and counter-traction is all that is needed while the patient is adequately sedated. It is imperative to avoid excessive force, as the significant instability of a knee that has already been severely "stretched" places the patient at increased risk for additional injury. With anterior dislocations (the most common type) lifting of the femur may occasionally be required to achieve adequate reduction. Similarly, lifting of the tibia may be required for posterior dislocations [1].
- The patient should be placed in a long leg posterior splint or knee immobilizer with 15–20° of flexion following reduction [1]. *In all cases, knee dislocations require admission and observation for compartment and neurovascular checks due to potential delayed vascular injury and other complications.*

2. Postreduction management
- Neurovascular examination should be performed following reduction, although it is of limited accuracy. ABIs and advanced imaging to assess the integrity of the vascular supply should still be pursued [6].
- Emergent evaluation by vascular surgery should be completed with evidence of vascular injury on exam (hard signs) or imaging.
- Monitor for postreduction complications, which include:
  - Compartment Syndrome
  - Peroneal Nerve Injury (Foot drop)
  - DVT
  - Postreduction fractures and ligamentous injury
- An orthopedic specialist should be involved as soon as possible should the patient show evidence of a posterolateral knee dislocation or an irreducible dislocation. *Do not hesitate to involve specialists given the high risk of morbidity associated with this injury.*

Case Conclusion

The patient was taken urgently to the OR for revascularization and external fixation. His lower leg was preserved; however, he developed compartment syndrome requiring fasciotomy. Ultimately, he was discharged home with plans for a delayed reconstruction of his multiligament knee injury at a later date.

Discussion

These observations are made based on the writer's experience with multiligament knee injuries.

1. As many multi-ligament knee injuries with dislocation spontaneously reduce prior to formal evaluation, a high level of suspicion must be present whenever a

high-energy mechanism results in knee pain or evidence of injury even if visual inspection does not suggest gross abnormality. Failure to recognize a spontaneously reduced knee dislocation results from a failure to suspect and can result in significant morbidity.

2. Once a knee dislocation is recognized, it is imperitive to think quickly and act swiftly in mobilizing resources. Reduce the obviously dislocated knee then immediately divert attention to assessing the vascular supply of the limb. Presence of distal pulses and an ABI higher than 0.9 still requires admission or prolonged observation. Presence of distal pulses but an ABI less than 0.9 warrants imaging, likely CT angiography, of the limb to assess for vascular injury. Absent distal pulses or hard signs of ischemia warrant immediate vascular surgery consultation and emergent surgical repair. The patient should be admitted or observed for a prolonged time period in all cases, but determination of need for surgical repair is critical for preservation of the limb. In resource-limited settings, erring on the side of caution with immediate vascular imaging followed by emergent transfer for evaluation by vascular surgery is warranted given the potential morbidity associated with this injury.

Pattern Recognition

- High energy or low energy rotational mechanism
- Significant multiligament knee instability
- Signs of distal neurovascular compromise
- Spontaneous reduction in 50% of cases

Disclosure Statement   The authors of this chapter report no significant disclosures.

References

1. Rihn JA, Groff YJ, Harner CD, Cha PS. The acutely dislocated knee: evaluation and management. J Am Acad-Orthop Surg. 2004;12(5):334–46.
2. Peltola EK, Lindahl J, Hietaranta H, Koskinen SK. Knee dislocation in overweight patients. AJR Am J Roentgenol. 2009;192(1):101–6.
3. Sillanpää PJ, Kannus P, Niemi ST, Rolf C, Felländer-Tsai L, Mattila VM. Incidence of knee dislocation and concomitant vascular injury requiring surgery: a nationwide study. J Trauma Acute Care Surg. 2014;76(3):715–9.
4. Seroyer ST, Musahl V, Harner CD. Management of the acute knee dislocation: the Pittsburgh experience. Injury. 2008;39(7):710–8.
5. Henrichs A. A review of knee dislocations. J Athl Train. 2004;39(4):365–9.
6. Barnes CJ, Pietrobon R, Higgins LD. Does the pulse examination in patients with traumatic knee dislocation predict a surgical arterial injury? A meta-analysis. J Trauma. 2002;53:1109.
7. Medina O, Arom GA, Yeranosian MG, Petrigliano FA, McAllister DR. Vascular and nerve injury after knee dislocation: a systematic review. Clin Orthop Relat Res. 2014;472(9):2621–9. https://doi.org/10.1007/s11999-014-3511-3.

8. Niall DM, Nutton RW, Keating JF. Palsy of the common peroneal nerve after traumatic dislocation of the knee. J Bone Joint Surg Br. 2005;87(5):664–7.
9. Patterson BM, Agel J, Swiontkowski MF, Mackenzie EJ. Knee dislocations with vascular injury: outcomes in the Lower Extremity Assessment Project (LEAP) Study. J Trauma. 2007;63(4):855–8.
10. Mills WJ, Barrei DP, McNair P. The value of the ankle-brachial index for diagnosing arterial injury after knee dislocation: a prospective study. J Trauma. 2004;56(6):1261–5.
11. Wand JS. A physical sign denoting irreducibility of a dislocated knee. J Bone Joint Surg Br. 1989;71(5):862.

Acute Myocarditis: *"I Thought My Soul Was Weak, but My Heart??"*

43

Grace Rodriguez and Jennifer Yee

Case

"I'm having trouble catching my breath!"

Pertinent History

A previously healthy 19-year-old male presented to the emergency department with a chief complaint of progressive shortness of breath and fatigue. He was seen by his family doctor 3 weeks ago for an upper respiratory infection and was treated symptomatically with acetaminophen/diphenhydramine combination. He has had improvement of his rhinorrhea, congestion, and sore throat; yet, for the past 3 days, he has had progressive difficulty walking a flight of stairs due to shortness of breath, and he has noticed swelling in bilateral lower legs. He reports intermittent palpitations and "heaviness" in his chest.

He denies recent travel, productive cough, hemoptysis, unilateral extremity swelling, and syncope. He endorses intermittent low-grade fever (Tmax 100.6 °F/38.1 °C yesterday), and a 12 lb. weight gain over the past week with no change in his diet.

PMH

No significant medical history. No medications other than Tylenol PM as needed No vitamins or supplements.

G. Rodriguez (✉) · J. Yee
Department of Emergency Medicine, Wexner Medical Center at The Ohio State University, Columbus, OH, USA
e-mail: Grace.rodriguez@osumc.edu; Jennifer.yee@osumc.edu

© Springer Nature Switzerland AG 2020
C. G. Kaide, C. E. San Miguel (eds.), *Case Studies in Emergency Medicine*,
https://doi.org/10.1007/978-3-030-22445-5_43

Social History
- Drinks 2–3 alcoholic beverages per week
- Smokes marijuana occasionally. No tobacco products.

Family History
Noncontributory

Pertinent Physical Exam

- HR 122, RR 32, BP 120/65, Temperature 99.3 °F/37.4 °C, SpO2 95% on room air

Except as noted below, the findings of the physical exam are within normal limits.

- ENT: Thyroid has no palpable nodules and is normal in size. JVD present (11 cm H2O) with a positive hepatojugular reflex.
- Cardiovascular: Regular tachycardic rhythm, S3 gallop present.
- Pulmonary: Tachypnea with bibasilar crackles. Speaking in 5–6-word sentences at a time.
- Abdomen: No hepatosplenomegaly, abdomen soft and nontender in all quadrants with normal bowel sounds.
- Extremities: Bilateral 2+ pitting edema to mid-shin. Equal, symmetric pulses in all extremities.
- Skin: Diaphoretic and cool to the touch. No rashes, ecchymoses, or erythema.

Pertinent Test Results

- ECG showed sinus tachycardia with new LBBB, but did not meet Sgarbossa criteria.
- Chest X-ray showed bilateral interstitial edema and cardiomegaly.

Lab Results			
Test	Results	Units	Normal Range
Troponin	6.3	ng/ml	<0.04
BNP	800	pg/ml	<100

TSH/T4, Chemistry, CBC, and D-dimer were all within normal limits.

Emergency Department Management

He was placed on continuous telemetry. Bedside ultrasound was performed, which demonstrated a LV with thickened walls with global decrease in cardiac contractility and evidence of interstitial pulmonary edema bilaterally. The inferior vena cava was plethoric and showed <50% collapsibility. The patient was given 40 mg IV furosemide, 325 mg aspirin and started on CPAP for work of breathing and to decrease his preload and afterload. Nitroglycerin was held initially as patient was normotensive.

Updates on Emergency Department Course

Upon initial reassessment, it was noted that patient was tolerating CPAP well and was less tachypneic. He reported feeling that his dyspnea had subjectively improved. ECG and troponin were repeated without significant change from previous findings. He was admitted to the cardiology service for suspected myocarditis with acute decompensated heart failure.

Learning Points

Priming Questions
1. What are the important historical and clinical features of myocarditis?
2. What diagnostic studies should you order to evaluate a patient for myocarditis?
3. What are your first steps in treating a patient with acute myocarditis?

Introduction/Background

1. Myocarditis is defined as an inflammatory disease of the myocardium that is diagnosed by defined histological, immunological, and immunohistochemical criteria according to the current WHO classification [1].
2. Myocarditis has a wide spectrum of illness severity: it may be a mild and self-limiting condition, or it can be fulminant and life threatening [2].
3. There are multiple etiologies of myocarditis, the most common of these is viral infections. Adenovirus, parvovirus B-19, and human herpesvirus 6 are the most common viruses attributed to the development of myocarditis. Enteroviruses, notably Coxsackie B, were the most common etiology up until the 1990s [2].
   - Other notable etiologies of myocarditis include bacterial (associated with Lyme disease), autoimmune diseases such as Churg–Strauss syndrome or Crohn's Disease, hypersensitivity reactions to drugs (some examples include clozapine, penicillins, sulfonamides, and mesalamine), and toxic reaction to drugs (sympathomimetics, alcohol) [3].
4. While it is difficult to ascertain the natural history of myocarditis, as many cases may be subclinical, the US Myocarditis Treatment trial enrolled adults with biopsy proven myocarditis, the mortality in a group of 111 patients was 20% at 1 year and 56% at 4.3 years [4].
   - The composite rate of cardiomyopathy, transplantation, and death in North America, for those with biopsy-proven myocarditis, was found to be greater than 50% after 5 years [5].
   - Children diagnosed with acute myocarditis have only a 60% likelihood of transplantation-free survival at 10 years [6].

Physiology/Pathophysiology

1. The pathophysiology of acute myocarditis manifests in three distinct phases: the acute phase, the subacute phase, and the chronic phase [3].
   - The acute phase occurs in the first 1–3 days and consists of viral entry into the cardiac myocytes through a specific receptor: the coxsackie virus and adenovirus receptor [CAR]. Studies on explanted hearts with dilated cardiomyopathy have demonstrated higher CAR expression than in the myocardium of patients who do not have dilated cardiomyopathy [7]. Interestingly, when CAR is eliminated in rodent models, neither infection with coxsackievirus nor histologic evidence of myocarditis occurs [8].
     - During the acute phase, viral entry into myocytes induces cellular injury and eventual myocyte necrosis leading to exposure of intracellular antigens (myosin) and activation of the host's innate immune system [3].
   - The subacute phase can last a few weeks to several months, and it includes activated virus-specific T cells that target the host myocardium. This leads to T-cell-induced myocardial injury with subsequent myocardial necrosis. In addition, high levels of cytokines, particularly TNF, and antibodies are produced during this phase [9].
     - In most patients, the host immune response subsides following viral elimination, and LV function is able to recover without sequelae; however, in some patients, the cardiomyopathy enters a chronic and irreversible stage [1].
   - The chronic phase develops if there is a persistent inflammatory response—cytokines activate matrix metalloproteinases, which destroy the natural interstitial collagen and elastin framework of the heart [10].
2. There are three commonly recognized histological types of myocarditis: lymphocytic myocarditis, eosinophilic myocarditis, and giant cell myocarditis [2].
   - Lymphocytic myocarditis is the most common type and is most frequently caused by viruses, it is characterized by lymphocytic invasion, myocytolysis, and fibrosis and a heterogenous clinical presentation [2].
   - Eosinophilic myocarditis is a rare cause of myocarditis and is most frequently caused by autoimmune diseases, parasitic infections, hypersensitivity to drugs and substances, and vaccinations [11].
   - Giant cell myocarditis (GCM) is a rare cause of myocarditis, but it is rapidly progressive and is frequently fatal [12]. It is particularly aggressive in children, in a review of 15 pediatric GCM cases, all patients either died or required a heart transplant. The etiology of GCM is unknown, although it is often associated with autoimmune diseases and cancers involving immune cells, such as lymphoma. It is believed to occur secondary to autoimmune dysregulation [13].

Making the Diagnosis

> **Differential Diagnosis**
> - Pericarditis without myocarditis
> - ACS
> - Pneumonia
> - Primary dysrhythmia
> - Structural heart disease
> - Toxicologic: sympathomimetics
> - Thyrotoxicosis
> - Aortic dissection
> - Pericardial effusion
> - Pleural effusion
> - PE

1. Clinical presentation has a wide degree of variability. According to Sagar and colleagues [14] common presentations include:
   - Subclinical acute myocarditis—transient troponin elevations or ECG abnormalities following a viral illness or vaccination, patients have no symptoms of heart failure. The long-term risk of developing heart failure following transient elevations in cardiac biomarkers in the setting of a recent preceding viral infection or vaccination is unknown.
   - Acute heart failure with dilated cardiomyopathy—presents as acute heart failure with dyspnea, fatigue, poor exercise tolerance, and orthopnea; these patients are ill-appearing and often need endomyocardial biopsies to determine histologic diagnosis, treatment, and prognosis [15].
   - Myopericarditis resembling acute coronary syndrome—symptoms can mimic those of an acute MI, but without significant obstructive coronary artery disease on cardiac catheterization and with preserved LV function. There may be a component of coronary vasospasm [16].
   - Ventricular dysrhythmias or heart block presenting with presyncope or syncope—unexplained atrioventricular block and/or ventricular arrhythmias, may present with syncope or presyncope [17].
   - Heart failure with chronic or progressive dilated cardiomyopathy—up to 40% of patients with chronic dilated cardiomyopathy and subsequent heart failure have immunohistologic criteria consistent with myocarditis. These patients may present months to years following acute myocarditis (may have even had subclinical myocarditis) with symptoms of new-onset heart failure [18].

2. ECG—A variety of changes may be seen, including nonspecific T-wave changes, ST segment changes, pathologic Q waves, and a variety of dysrhythmias [19].
   - Although ECG is nonspecific, if suspicious for myocarditis, the ECG can be used as a risk-stratifying tool, as the presence of Q waves or a new left bundle branch block has been associated with higher rates of cardiac death or heart transplantation [20].
   - Other ECG findings that have been shown in studies to portend a poor prognosis include a QRS >120 ms, QTc >440 ms, an abnormal QRS axis, and ventricular ectopic beats [21].

The Most Common ECG Findings
- Sinus tachycardia
- Diffuse T-wave inversions
- ST-segment elevation without reciprocal depression.
- Low voltage of the QRS complexes
- Arrhythmias
  - Atrial and ventricular ectopic beats
  - Atrial and ventricular tachycardias
- Heart block is frequently observed in giant cell myocarditis and cardiac sarcoidosis.
- These EKG changes may persist for several months before they resolve spontaneously.

Feldman AM, McNamara D (2000). Myocarditis. N Engl J Med. 2000;343(19):1388–98.

---

3. Laboratory analysis—An elevated troponin level has been reported to have a sensitivity of 71% and a specificity of 83% in childhood myocarditis [22, 23].
   - Other nonspecific markers of inflammation may be elevated, including CRP, ESR, and leukocyte count, although their low specificity limits diagnostic value [7].
4. Chest X-ray may show interstitial infiltrates, pleural effusions, pulmonary vascular congestion, and cardiomegaly [19].
5. Echocardiogram findings are nonspecific. These may include new regional or global wall motion abnormalities that do not represent a normal coronary distribution. Fulminant cases often show thickened walls secondary to edema. Impaired right ventricular function is a strong predictor of death or need for transplant [24].
6. Cardiovascular magnetic resonance imaging (MRI) has become an incredibly powerful diagnostic imaging modality, as it can demonstrate myocardial inflammation, myocardial edema, fibrosis, and necrosis. Cardiac MRI has become the primary noninvasive tool of choice to diagnose myocardial inflammation in suspected acute myocarditis [25].

7. Coronary angiography is recommended to rule out coronary artery disease as an underlying etiology for myocardial damage [26].
8. Endomyocardial biopsy has long been the gold standard for diagnosing acute myocarditis. The 1987 Dallas Criteria for acute myocarditis requires confirmed lymphocytic invasion with myocyte injury without evidence of ischemia [27]. While these criteria are very specific for acute myocarditis, they are only 10–22% sensitive as myocardial inflammation is often patchy and thus predisposes to sampling error and a high false-negative rate [28, 29].

Treating the Patient

1. The treatment for acute myocarditis varies according to the spectrum of disease. For patients who present with symptoms of acute heart failure secondary to dilated cardiomyopathy, they typically respond well to standard heart failure treatment [7].
2. Initial treatment for patients who present with symptoms of acute decompensated heart failure in the ED is supportive. According to ACEP Guidelines, important recommendations include:
   • In patients who are acutely dyspneic secondary to acute heart failure and who are not hypotensive or who do not require emergent intubation, use CPAP at 5–10 mm Hg to reduce heart rate, respiratory rate, blood pressure, and the need for intubation (Level B Recommendation).
   • For patients who are not hypotensive with acute heart failure syndrome and associated dyspnea, use IV nitrates (Level B Recommendation).
   • Treat patients with moderate to severe pulmonary edema resulting from heart failure with IV Furosemide (Level B Recommendation) [30].
3. Patients with hemodynamically stable heart failure should be treated with: diuretics, an ACE inhibitor, and beta-blockers [1].
4. It is important to note that NSAIDs are the treatment of choice for pericarditis, yet they have been associated with increased mortality in experimental models of myocarditis [1].
5. Management of dysrhythmias is also an important step in emergent treatment. Patients should remain on continuous cardiac monitoring, and patients with complete AV block may require temporary pacing [1].
6. All patients diagnosed with myocarditis should be instructed to avoid exercise, as this may predispose to dysrhythmias [1].
7. Endomyocardial biopsy provides therapeutic guidance. Steroids and immunosuppressants have been shown to be beneficial in eosinophilic myocarditis, while immunosuppression and IVIG has been shown to be beneficial in giant cell myocarditis [31].
8. Patients presenting with fulminant myocarditis and cardiogenic shock whose condition worsens despite maximal medical therapy will likely need mechanical circulatory support, such as an intra-aortic balloon pump, a ventricular assist device or extracorporeal membrane oxygenation as a bridge to transplant [32].

Case Conclusion

The patient was admitted to the cardiology service where he had a cardiac MRI, which showed moderate–severe impairment of both his left and right ventricular function with gadolinium enhancement consistent with acute myocarditis. An echocardiogram showed an EF of 25–30% without valvular abnormalities. He underwent a left heart catheterization with coronary angiogram, which did not show any evidence of obstructive coronary artery disease. A right heart catheterization was performed to obtain endomyocardial biopsies, which were nondiagnostic. On hospital day 3, he clinically worsened with multiple runs of sustained ventricular tachycardia and acute pulmonary edema. He was intubated and underwent two rounds of synchronized cardioversion with an amiodarone bolus. Patient achieved return to sinus rhythm with persistent previous LBBB. He was taken emergently for ICD and intra-aortic balloon pump placement. He was placed on the cardiac transplantation list and received an LVAD and temporary RVAD while awaiting transplant.

Discussion

Acute myocarditis represents a wide spectrum of disease; it can range from asymptomatic presentations to fulminant heart failure. It is important to remember to keep a broad differential, as presentations are often nonspecific. Important diagnostic tools include: ECG, CXR, bedside ultrasound or echocardiogram, and measurement of a troponin level. Any patient you suspect of having acute myocarditis, with or without symptoms of heart failure, should be admitted to the hospital, as they are at high risk for clinical deterioration. Initial management should always include an airway evaluation, an assessment of cardiopulmonary status, and continuous cardiac monitoring with close monitoring of their hemodynamics. Management in the ED includes supportive care, including hemodynamic support, ventilatory support, and dysrhythmia management.

Pattern Recognition

- Recent Viral Illness
- New-onset heart failure in previously healthy individual
- Troponin elevation
- New Dysrhythmias: AV block, ventricular tachycardia, bundle branch blocks

Disclosure Statement The authors of this chapter report no significant disclosures.

References

1. Caforio AL, et al. Current state of knowledge on aetiology, diagnosis, management, and therapy of myocarditis: a position statement of the European Society of Cardiology Working Group on Myocardial and Pericardial Diseases. Eur Heart J. 2013;34:2636–48.
2. Ginsberg F, Parillo JE. Fulminant myocarditis. Crit Care Clin. 2013;29:465–83.
3. Kindermann I, et al. Update on myocarditis. J Amer Coll Cardiol. 2012;59:779–92. https://doi.org/10.1016/j.jacc.2011.09.074.
4. Mason JW, O'Connell JB, Herskowitz A, et al. A clinical trial of immunosuppressive therapy for myocarditis. N Engl J Med. 1995;333:269–75.
5. Cooper LT, et al. The global burden of myocarditis. Glob Heart. 2014;9:121–9.
6. Towbin JA, et al. Incidence, causes, and outcomes of dilated cardiomyopathy in children. JAMA. 2006;296:1867–76.
7. Noutsias M, Fechner H, de Jonge H, et al. Human coxsackie-adenovirus receptor is colocalized with integrins alpha(v)beta(3) and alpha(v)beta(5) on the cardiomyocyte sarcolemma and upregulated in dilated cardiomyopathy: implications for cardiotropic viral infections. Circulation. 2001;104:275–82.
8. Shi Y, et al. Cardiac deletion of the coxsackievirus-adenovirus receptor abolishes coxsackievirus B3 infection and prevents myocarditis in vivo. J Am Coll Cardiol. 2009;53:1219–26.
9. Pollack A, et al. Viral myocarditis—diagnosis, treatment options, and current controversies. Nat Rev Cardiol. 2015;12:670–8.
10. Lee JK, Zaidi SH, Liu P, et al. A serine elastase inhibitor reduces inflammation and fibrosis and preserves. Nat Med. 1998;4:1383–91.
11. Aslan I, et al. Eosinophilic myocarditis in an adolescent: a case report and review of the literature. Cardiol Young. 2013;23:277–83.
12. Xu J, Brooks EG. Giant cell myocarditis. Arch Pathol Lab Med. 2016;140:1429–34.
13. Das BB, Recto M, Johnsrude C. Cardiac transplantation for pediatric giant cell myocarditis. J Heart Lung Transplant. 2006;25(4):474–8.
14. Sagar S, et al. Myocarditis. Lancet. 2012;379(9817):738–47. https://doi.org/10.1016/S0140-6736(11)60648-X.
15. Cooper LT, Baughman KL, Feldman AM, et al. The role of endomyocardial biopsy in the management of cardiovascular disease: a scientific statement from the American Heart Association, the American College of Cardiology, and the European Society of Cardiology. Circulation. 2007;116:2216–33.
16. Yilmaz A, Mahrholdt H, Athanasiadis A, et al. Coronary vasospasm as the underlying cause for chest pain in patients with PVB19 myocarditis. Heart. 2008;94:1456–63.
17. Uemura A, Morimoto S, Hiramitsu S, Hishida H. Endomyocardial biopsy findings in 50 patients with idiopathic atrioventricular block: presence of myocarditis. Jpn Heart J. 2001;42:691–700.
18. Wojnicz R, Nowalany-Kozielska E, Wojciechowska C, et al. Randomized, placebo-controlled study for immunosuppressive treatment of inflammatory dilated cardiomyopathy: two-year follow-up results. Circulation. 2001;104:39–45.
19. Kühl U, Schultheiss HP. Myocarditis in children. Heart Fail Clin. 2019;6:483–96.
20. Nakashima H, et al. Q wave and non-Q wave myocarditis with special reference to clinical significance. Jpn Heart J. 1998;39:763–74.
21. Ukena C, et al. Prognostic electrocardiographic parameters in patients with suspected myocarditis. Eur J Heart Fail. 2011;13:398–405.
22. Smith SC, Ladenson JH, Mason JW, et al. Elevations of cardiac troponin I associated with myocarditis. Experimental and clinical correlates. Circulation. 1997;95:163–8.
23. Soongswang J, Durongpisitkul K, Nana A, et al. Cardiac troponin T: a marker in the diagnosis of acute myocarditis in children. Ped Cardiol. 2005;26:45–9.

24. Skouri HN, Dec GW, Friedrich MG, Cooper LT. Noninvasive imaging in myocarditis. J Am Coll Cardiol. 2006;48:2085–93.
25. Matthias G, et al. Cardiovascular magnetic resonance in myocarditis: a JACC white paper. J Amer Coll Cardiol. 2009;53 https://doi.org/10.1016/j.jacc.2009.02.007.
26. Jensen L, Marchant D. Emerging pharmacologic targets and treatment for myocarditis. Pharmacol Ther. 2016;161:40–51.
27. Aretz H, et al. Myocarditis. A histopathological definition and classification. Am J Cardiovasc Pathol. 1987;1:3–14.
28. Chow L, et al. Insensitivity of right ventricular endomyocardial biopsy in the diagnosis of myocarditis. J Am Coll Cardiol. 1989;14:915–20.
29. Hauck A, et al. Evaluation of postmortem endomyocardial biopsy specimens from 38 patients with lymphocytic myocarditis: implications for role of sampling error. Mayo Clin Proc. 1989;64:1235–45.
30. Silvers S, et al. Clinical policy: critical issues in the evaluation and management of adult patients presenting to the emergency department with acute heart failure syndromes. Ann Emer Med. 2007;49:627–38.
31. Rose NR. Viral myocarditis. Curr Opin Rheum. 2016;28:383–9.
32. Shauer A, et al. Acute viral myocarditis: current concepts in diagnosis and treatment. Isr Med Assoc J. 2013;15:180–5.

Necrotizing Fasciitis: *Flesh Eating Follies*

44

Colin G. Kaide

Case

Rapidly Progressing Cellulitis

Pertinent History

A patient presented to the emergency department (ED) at midnight with pain in the posterior aspect of her left calf and shin area with associated redness and warmth. The pain began at 9 PM, 3 hours prior to arrival. She denies any specific trauma and has been well up until last evening. She does have chronic lower extremity edema. She also has rheumatoid arthritis for which she takes immunosuppressant medications.

PMH Rheumatoid arthritis
   Meds: Anakrina, prednisone, denosumab and others

SH Nonsmoker, no drug use

Pertinent Physical Exam

- BP 152/103, Pulse 120, Temp 98.1 °F (36.7 °C), RR 17, SpO2 97%

Except as noted below, the findings of a complete physical exam are within normal limits.

C. G. Kaide (✉)
Department of Emergency Medicine, Wexner Medical Center at The Ohio State University, Columbus, OH, USA
e-mail: Colin.kaide@osumc.edu

© Springer Nature Switzerland AG 2020
C. G. Kaide, C. E. San Miguel (eds.), *Case Studies in Emergency Medicine*,
https://doi.org/10.1007/978-3-030-22445-5_44

- Cardiovascular: Tachycardia with regular rhythm, normal heart sounds, and intact distal pulses. Exam reveals no gallop and no friction rub or murmur heard.
- Extremity: She has 3+ pitting edema of the bilateral lower extremities, but on the left side there is spreading erythema and warmth on the anterior and posterior aspect. She also has associated tenderness generally in that area. The knee itself is not tender.

Pertinent Diagnostic Testing

Test	Results 02:03	Results 08:24	Results 10:54	Units	Normals
WBC	6.06	10.67	11.12	K/uL	$3.8–11.0 \times 10^3/mm^3$
Hgb	10.9	9.2	9.4	g/dL	Male: 14–18 g/dL
					Female: 11–16 g/dL
Na	139	139	141	mEq/L	135–148 mEq/L
pH	7.33	7.40	–	–	7.35–7.45
Lactate	1.8	3.9	4.8	mmol/L	< 2.0
CRP	5.7	24.5	–	Mg/L	< 8 mg/L
Cr	0.79	0.72	0.73	mg/dL	0.6–1.5 mg/dL
Glucose	149	115	120	mg/dL	65–99 mg/dL

Computed Tomography (CT) CT findings are suggestive of lower leg cellulitis without any evidence of subcutaneous air or organized fluid collections. Findings, however, do not exclude a necrotizing infection.

Emergency Department Course

The initial plan was to treat for cellulitis. A CT of the tibia/fibula (tib/fib) was obtained and did not show gas or fluid collections. The patient was started on piperacillin–tazobactam. Plan was for admission.

Update 1: (0300) Patient's cellulitis progressed rapidly and she continued to have pain out of proportion on examination. Vancomycin and clindamycin were added to her antibiotic regimen. She continued to be tachycardic and had minimal decrease in pain after getting hydromorphone. There became a mounting concern for necrotizing fasciitis as she was on chronic immunosuppressant drugs. The general surgery service was consulted and the resident who saw the patient believed this was not necrotizing fasciitis (NF). They would continue to follow. However, the ED team continued to keep NF on the differential and treat accordingly.

Update 2: (0730) As per recheck around 07:30, patient's area of cellulitis progressed rapidly, her pain is still out of proportion and she is still tachycardic. A phone call placed to the general surgery attending regarding our pressing concern for necrotizing fasciitis as the leading diagnosis.

- As of this moment, she has received IV vancomycin, piperacillin/tazobactam, and clindamycin.

- The general surgery attending came to re-evaluate the patient. The patient was scheduled to go to the operating room.
- Central line placed.

Update 3: (0845) Patient to OR

Learning Points: Necrotizing Soft Tissue Infections

Priming Questions
1. In terms of pathophysiology, what sets Necrotizing Fasciitis apart from other soft tissue infections?
2. How is this diagnosis made, and what roles do laboratory and imaging studies play?
3. What is the definitive treatment of Necrotizing Fasciitis and what treatment should be initiated in the Emergency Department?

Introduction/Background

1. Although uncommon, Necrotizing Fasciitis (NF) produces a life-threatening infection with a mortality rate from 25% to 35%, despite maximal therapy [1]. NF has been reported to occur in around 500–1500 patients annually in the United States [2, 3].
2. NF is soft tissue infection that rapidly progresses to cause necrosis of muscle fascia and subcutaneous tissues via endotoxins, exotoxins, and protease enzymes. They produce an expanding local tissue injury while also causing severe systemic toxicity [4].
   - The infection has been reported to spread at the rate of 1 inch (2.54 cm) per hour without manifesting overlying skin changes until the infection is in its advanced state.
   - Those who survive the initial infection frequently undergo multiple surgical debridements and sometimes amputations.
   - This is usually followed by surgical reconstruction of the original infection sites, leading to significant ongoing morbidity.

Physiology/Pathophysiology

1. NF tends to occur in two different but occasionally overlapping patterns. Some acknowledge it as Type III infection. Each one is characterized by different organisms and typically affects different populations of patients.
   - Type I NF (the most common form) is a polymicrobial infection and tends to develop in older and sicker patients who have a history of chronic systemic disease such as peripheral vascular disease, immunosuppression, or diabetes.

Although the inciting factor can include various forms of skin trauma such as decubitus ulcers, postoperative wounds, animal or insect bites, or insulin injection sites, often there is no obvious source of injury and the cause is unclear.

- The bacteria present in Type I NF include aerobic and anaerobic bacteria. Wound cultures frequently grow S. aureus, E. coli, B. fragilis, and various species of Enterococci, Peptostreptococcus, Prevotella, and Porphyromonas. Clostridium perfringens, the same organism that usually causes "gas gangrene" is often reported in Type I NF, though it is less frequently isolated [5–7]. Group A, Beta-Hemolytic Strep (Strep pyogenes) is usually also present.
- Fournier's gangrene, a form of NF that attacks the perineal region and abdominal wall, is also polymicrobial but enteric organisms predominate.
- Type II NF accounts for about 15–20% of cases [8–10].
  - It is the monomicrobial form and until recently, was caused almost exclusively by Group A Streptococcus (Streptococcus pyogenes). Recently, however, community-associated methicillin-resistant S aureus (MRSA) has been increasingly reported as the sole organism [11, 12].
  - Type II NF can develop spontaneously in apparently healthy people who have no known causative factor or portal of entry for bacteria [13]. In most patients, however, predisposing factors, such as minor skin trauma and blunt injury, can be identified. IV drug use has emerged as another significant cause of Type II NF [14].
- Type III NF: Although not universally accepted, some experts use the designation of a Type III to describe a rare, but virulent form of NF caused by Vibrio vulnificus. This is seen in coastal communities and is associated with exposure of an open wound to warm sea water [15, 16].
2. The damage created by infection with these organisms is multifactorial.
- *Clostridium* species produce alpha-toxin. Along with local tissue destruction, it causes significant systemic symptoms, often including cardiovascular collapse.
- *Staphylococcus aureus* and *Streptococci pyogenes* elaborate surface proteins M-1 and M-3, exotoxins A, B, C, streptolysin O, and superantigen.
  - These proteins have various effects including enhanced bacterial adherence, endothelial damage, tissue edema, and impaired microvascular tissue blood flow.
- Tumor necrosis factors and interleukins further stimulate the inflammatory response leading to additional microvascular injury and multisystem organ dysfunction.
- Activation of the clotting cascade produces small vessel thrombosis leading to increasing tissue ischemia [17]. The final common pathway is tissue ischemia causing interference with destruction of bacteria by polymorphonuclear leukocytes (PMNs) and blocking of the delivery of antibiotics to affected tissue [18].

Making the Diagnosis

The Differential – Think of NF Before Making These Diagnoses
- Cellulitis
- Deep Venous Thrombosis
- Abscess
- Hematoma
- Bullous Pemphigoid
- Chronic Venous Stasis

Wow…This can be either strikingly easy or a really complicated diagnosis to make, depending on how advanced the infection is on presentation and how quickly you recognize that this "particular cellulitis" doesn't look like the other 1000 cases you saw last year!

1. Just to make things more confusing, studies looking at the classic presentation consisting of rapidly progressing pain, diaphoresis, and anxiety in association with an injury or break in the skin, only seem to occur in 10–40% of the patients [19, 20]. Furthermore, most patients do not present with shock, fever, altered mental status, and impending cardiovascular collapse (that happens later!).
   - Most studies of presenting symptoms in NF look similar to cellulitis…erythema, swelling, and pain.
   - One striking feature that is frequently seen is tenderness beyond the margins of the overtly infected area. The pain seems to be frequently "out of proportion" to a garden-variety cellulitis. This may be the only clue that there is serious badness brewing just a centimeter or two deeper!

Cellulitis-looking Early Necrotizing Fasciitis

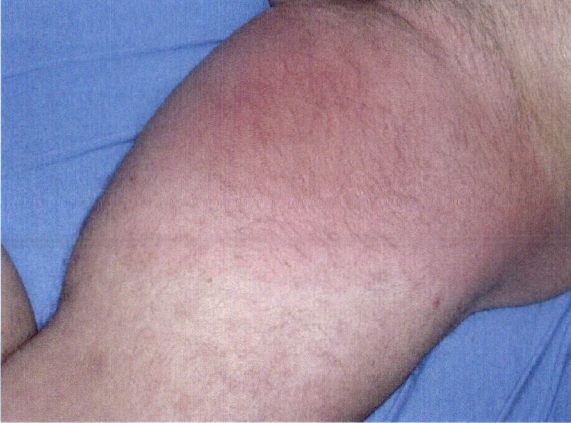

Published with kind permission of © Colin G. Kaide 2019. All Rights Reserved

Progression of Necrotizing Fasciitis Demonstrating Hemorrhagic Bullae

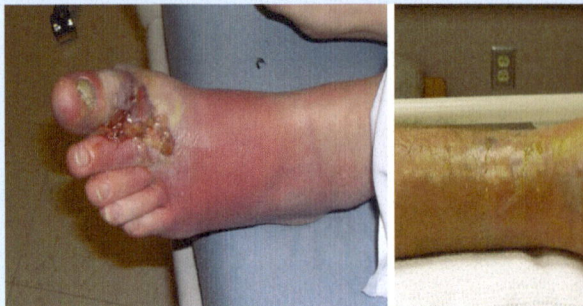

2. Certainly, if a patient does present with the characteristic findings along with fever and shock, NF should be strongly considered. The later skin findings include blistering and bullae formation. In the final stages, the bullae convert to hemorrhagic bullae and skin anesthesia and necrosis can quickly follow.
3. *The presence of crepitus and the issue of finding of gas on X-ray can be confusing.*
   - Various studies have reported crepitus in only 13–31% of patients presenting with NF.
   - Gas found on X-ray is very predictive of NF, but unfortunately, it is a rare finding. CT is more sensitive for gas than X-ray and can show gas in the deeper tissue planes.

Gas on X-ray of Patient with Necrotizing Fasciitis

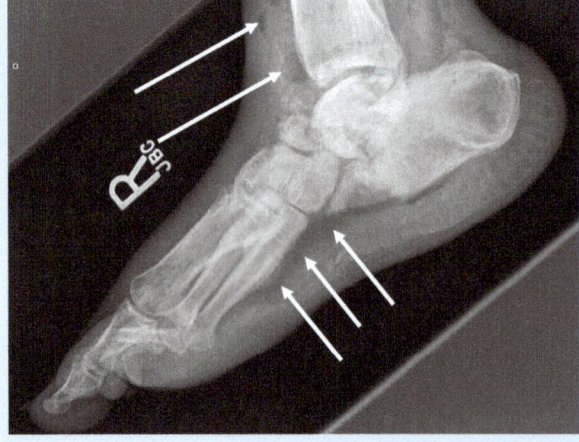

- Regardless of the imaging modality, gas is found in only 25% of NF. This seems to make sense since only a small number of the organisms involved in NF are gas formers. Clostridium perfringens is a classic gas former but is only a component of the mix in Type 1 NF. If, however, the patient does have crepitus on exam or gas is identified on imaging, the probability of NF is very high.
4. Lab Testing
   - Commonly abnormal lab values in NF include an elevated white count (>15,000), and a low sodium (<135). Other markers of inflammation are often elevated.
   - A scoring system was devised to help predict the presence of NF. This can help to appropriately risk stratify patients for whom you should strongly consider the diagnosis of NF. A total of less than six points confers a 96% negative predictive value for NF whereas a score of six or greater shows a positive

Laboratory Risk Indicator for Necrotizing Fasciitis (LRINEC) [23]

Test/variable	Points
C-reactive protein (mg/L)	
<15	0
≥15	4
White blood count (1000/mm³)	
<15 K	0
15–25 K	1
>25 K	2
Hemoglobin (g/dl)	
>13.5	0
11–13.5	1
<11	2
Sodium (mmol/L)	
≥135	0
<135	2
Creatinine (mg/dl)	
≤1.60 (≤141 μmol/L)	0
>1.60 (>141 μmol/L)	2
Glucose (mg/dl)	
≤180 (≤10 mmol/L)	0
>180 (>10 mmol/L)	1

A score <6 suggests a 96% negative predictive value for NF, and a score of 6 or greater suggests a 92% positive.

predictive value of 92%. Like all scoring systems, this one is not perfect. Subsequent, albeit less well-done, studies have challenged the degree of predictive value of the system. Regardless, this system is another tool to help make the case for rapid evaluation by a surgeon for definitive surgical diagnosis and definitive treatment [21–24].
5. Imaging: When NF is suspected but not yet clearly identified to such a degree as to convince a surgeon to take the patient to the OR, imaging can be helpful.

- Plain X-rays showing gas in the tissues is very convincing for NF. However, it is a big mistake to assume that the absence of gas rules out NF. Gas on X-ray or even on CT is found in only about 25% of cases. CT can demonstrate fluid collections and inflammatory changes consistent with possible NF and its sensitivity is quoted as high as 80% [25].
- Magnetic Resonance Imaging (MRI) remains the most definitive imaging modality with sensitivities of 90–100%. Specificities lag, however, and are only reported to be 50–85% [26, 27]. MRI can be problematic to do in a patient who is beginning to develop systemic symptoms of disease as it is a longer test and frequently located remotely from the ED.
- Overall, imaging studies are not perfect and are generally only indicated in cases in which the diagnosis is questionable. Obvious cases of NF do not need things to get between them and cold, hard surgical steel!
6. Direct Exploration: A very effective but seldom performed way to diagnose NF in clinically suspicious cases is to do a 2-cm bedside incision over the affected area, continued down to the muscle fascia. The ability to slide a finger easily along the disrupted fascia, along with the finding of gray-brown purulent fluid and necrotic tissue, pretty much clinches it! [27, 28]

Treating the Patient

1. Surgery: Definitive treatment for NF is surgical debridement. The mortality of NF is directly proportional to the duration of delay in getting the patient to the OR. Delays of 24 hours confer a nine-fold increase in mortality [20]. A recent Australian study described a clear correlation with survival and early surgical debridement [29].
2. Antibiotics: Antibiotic therapy is not curative, as antibiotics do not penetrate into the areas of active infection well, owing to ischemia. It is, however, very important in the treatment of sepsis and in helping to control the spread of the disease. Empiric therapy should include coverage for MRSA and methacillin-sensitive S aureus (MSSA) along with gram negative and anaerobic bacteria. Piperacillin/tazobactam plus vancomycin with the addition of clindamycin is a typical regimen. Clindamycin decreases the elaboration production of certain toxins specifically Clostridial alpha-toxin and M-proteins expressed by Strep and Staph [30, 31].
3. Hyperbaric Oxygen: Hyperbaric Oxygen Therapy (HBOT) creates a hyperoxic environment by subjecting the entire patient's body to 100% oxygen at pressures of 2.5–3 atmospheres absolute. Inhaled oxygen at these pressures generates a partial pressure of oxygen as high as 2200 mmHg. At this PaO_2, some physiologic and biochemical changes can have a significant antibacterial effect [32].
   - These include:
     - Suppression of clostridial alpha toxin production in gas gangrene.
     - Enhancement of leukocyte-killing activity.
     - Bacterial growth suppression in hyperoxic tissues.

- Improved antibiotic efficacy in a hyperoxic environment (Aminoglycosides, trimethoprim, sulfamethoxazole, and sulfisoxazole).
- Hypoxic environments decrease the effectiveness of fluoroquinolones and vancomycin. This can be reversed by HBO.
- Improvement in tissue repair.
- Suppression of the anaerobic bacteria.
- HBOT is an adjunctive treatment only. It should never delay definitive surgical therapy. It is best used after debridement. Studies to date have shown a decrease in mortality, number of surgical redebridements, and a decrease in amputations when HBO is added to aggressive surgery [32, 33]. In centers where HBOT is readily available, it should be considered.

Case Conclusion

The patient was taken emergently to the OR and underwent extensive debridement for the finding of purulent material and extensive necrotic tissue. The cultures grew predominantly Group A, beta-hemolytic streptococcus. She was taken to the OR three times for ongoing debridement. Supplemental hyperbaric oxygen was utilized for 20-, 90-minute treatments at 2.5 atmospheres absolute. She did not require an amputation, but remained on the ventilator and vasopressors for 7 days. She was extubated and transferred to stepdown with plans for skin grafting and rehabilitation. Final diagnosis was necrotizing fasciitis, Type II.

Case Discussion

These observations are made based on this writer's experience with acute necrotizing fasciitis.

This diagnosis can be a "no man's land." It can fall into the domain of many specialties including general surgery, orthopedics, urology, obstertics/gynecology (OB/Gyn), etc. Because of the wide variability of caregivers who might have a patient with necrotizing fasciitis, this patient may be owned by everybody, and nobody at the same time!

Even when the diagnosis is obvious… such as a patient with diabetes presenting with a rapidly progressive cellulitis, blebs and blisters on an extremity, elevated markers of infection, and abnormal vital signs…things may still progress at an average pace if the consultants are not made acutely aware of the degree of your concern. No one wants to believe the patient has NF, especially over the phone in the middle of the night. In highly suspicious cases, it is imperative that the physician who suspects NF be decisive and confident when explaining to the surgeon why they need to see the patients right now.

When the situation is less obvious and a person comes into the emergency department with a cellulitis that looks "different" then most of the cellulitis you have seen with in your expensive careers in emergency medicine (EM)…plus or minus abnormal labs and vital signs…the problem may stagnate to the point of disaster! This is where your training in EM is put to the test and where you and the patient win or lose at the end of the day. Ask yourself: "What is different about this and why should I be concerned…?" If something is not right…a large red flag should pop up in your visual field!

Pattern Recognition

- Rapidly progressing cellulitis
- Pain out of proportion to exam
- Signs of systemic illness
- If present, gas in the tissues on X-ray

Disclosure Statement Callibra, Inc.-Discharge 123 medical software company. Medical Advisory Board Portola Pharmaceuticals. I have no relationship with a commercial company that has a direct financial interest in subject matter or materials discussed in article or with a company making a competing product.

References

1. Shiroff AM HGN, Gracias VH. Necrotizing soft tissue infections. J Intensive Care Med. 2014;29(3):138–44.
2. Jallali WS, Butler PE. Hyperbaric oxygen as adjuvant therapy in the management of necrotizing fasciitis. Am J Surg. 2005;189(4):462–6.
3. Levine EG, Manders SM. Life-threatening necrotizing fasciitis. Clin Dermatol. 2005;23(2):144–7.
4. Mandell GL, et al. Mandell, Douglas, and Bennett's principles and practice of infectious diseases. New York: Churchill-Livingston; 2005.
5. Brook I, Frazier E. Clinical and microbiological features of necrotizing fasciitis. J Clin Microbiol. 1995;33(9):2382–7.
6. Hasham S, et al. Necrotising fasciitis. BMJ. 2005;330(7495):830–3.
7. Sarani B, Strong M, Pascual J, Schwab CW. Necrotizing fasciitis: current concepts and review of the literature. J Am Coll Surg. 2009;208(2):279–88.
8. VanUnnik A. Inhibition of toxin production in Clostridium perfringens in vitro by hyperbaric oxygen. Antonie Leeuwenhoek Microbiol. 1965;31:181–6.
9. Jonsson K, Hunt TK. Oxygen as an isolated variable influences resistance to infection. Ann Surg. 1988;208(6):783–7.
10. Wong CH, Chang HC, Pasupathy S, Khin LW, Tan JL, Low CO. Necrotizing fasciitis: clinical presentation, microbiology, and determinants of mortality. J Bone Joint Surg Am. 2003;85(8):1454–60.
11. Miller LG, et al. Necrotizing fasciitis caused by community-associated methicillin-resistant Staphylococcus aureus in Los Angeles. N Engl J Med. 2005;352(14):1445–53.
12. Lee TC, Carrick MM, Scott BG, Hodges JC, Pham HQ. Incidence and clinical characteristics of methicillin-resistant Staphylococcus aureus necrotizing fasciitis in a large urban hospital. Am J Surg. 2007;194(6):809–12.
13. Childers BJ, et al. Necrotizing fasciitis: a fourteen-year retrospective study of 163 consecutive patients. Am Surg. 2002;68(2):109–16.

14. Chen JL, Fullerton KE, Flynn NM. Necrotizing fasciitis associated with injection drug use. Clin Infect Dis. 2001;33(1):6–15.
15. Kuo Chou TN, Chao WN, Yang C, et al. Predictors of mortality in skin and soft-tissue infections caused by Vibrio vulnificus. World J Surg. 2010;34:1669–75.
16. Chen SC, Chan KS, Chao WN, et al. Clinical outcomes and prognostic factors for patients with Vibrio vulnificus infections requiring intensive care: a 10-yr retrospective study. Crit Care Med. 2010;38:1984–90.
17. Salcido RS. Necrotizing fasciitis: reviewing the causes and treatment strategies. Adv SkinWound Care. 2007;20:288–93.
18. Cainzos M, Gonzalez-Rodriguez FJ. Necrotizing soft tissue infections. Curr Opin Crit Care. 2007;13:433–9.
19. McHenry CR, Piotrowski JJ, Petrinic D, Malangoni MA. Determinants of mortality for necrotizing soft-tissue infections. Ann Surg. 1995;221:558–63; discussion 563–565.
20. Wong CH, Haw-Chong C, Shanker P, et al. Necrotizing fasciitis: clinical presentation, microbiology, and determinants of mortality. J Bone Joint Surg Am. 2003;85:1454–60.
21. Wall DB, Kleain SR, Black S, de Virgilio C. A simple model to help distinguish necrotizing from non-necrotizing soft tissue infection. J Am Coll Surg. 2000;191(3):227–31.
22. Wall DB, de Virgilio C, Black S, Klein SR. Objective criteria may assist in distinguishing necrotizing fasciitis from non-necrotizing soft tissue infection. Am J Surg. 2000;179(1):17–21.
23. Wong CH, Khin LW, Heng KS, Tan KC, Low CO. The LRINEC (Laboratory Risk Indicator for Necrotising Fasciitis) score: a tool for distinguishing necrotizing fasciitis from other soft tissue infections. Crit Care Med. 2004;32(7):1535–41.
24. Holland MJ. Application of the Laboratory Risk Indicator in Necrotising Fasciitis (LRINEC) score to patients in a tropical tertiary referral centre. Anaesth Intensive Care. 2009;37(4):588–92.
25. Wysoki MG, Santora TA, Shah RM, Friedman AC. Necrotizing fasciitis: CT characteristics. Radiology. 1997;203:859–63.
26. Seok JH, Jee WH, Chun KA, Kim JY, Jung CK, Kim YR, et al. Necrotizing fasciitis versus pyomyositis: discrimination with using MR imaging. Korean J Radiol. 2009;10(2):121–8.
27. Kim KT, Kim YJ, Won Lee J, Kim YJ, Park SW, Lim MK, et al. Can necrotizing infectious fasciitis be differentiated from nonnecrotizing infectious fasciitis with MR imaging? Radiology. 2011;259(3):816–24.
28. Andreasen TJ, Green SD, Childers BJ. Massive soft-tissue injury: diagnosis and management of necrotizing fasciitis and purpura fulminans. Plast Reconstr Surg. 2001;107(4):1025–35.
29. Kelly Bucca K, Spencer R, Orford N, Cattigan C, Athan E, McDonald A. Early diagnosis and treatment of necrotizing fasciitis can improve survival: an observational intensive care unit cohort study. ANZ J Surg. 2013;83:365–70.
30. Gemmell CG, Peterson PK, Schmeling D, et al. Potentiation of opsonization and phagocytosis of Streptococcus pyogenes following growth in the presence of clindamycin. J Clin Invest. 1981;67(5):1249–56. [Medline]. [Full Text].
31. Stevens DL, Bryant AE, Yan S. Invasive group a streptococcal infection: new concepts in antibiotic treatment. Int J Antimicrob Agent. 1994;4:297–301.
32. Kaide CG, Khandelwal S. Hyperbaric oxygen: applications in infectious disease. Emerg Med Clin North Am. 2008;26:571–95, xi. https://doi.org/10.1016/j.emc.2008.01.005.
33. Joshua J, Shaw JJ, Psoinos C, Emhoff TA, Shah SA, Santry HP. Not just full of hot air: hyperbaric oxygen therapy increases survival in cases of necrotizing soft tissue infections. Surg Infect. 2014;15(3):328–35.

Organophosphate Poisoning: *Of Mice and Men*

45

Betty Y. Yang and Nicholas Kman

Case 1

Farmer Dan: Found Down in a Field

Pertinent History

A 30-year-old man was brought, minimally responsive, to the emergency department by ambulance. He was found down with an empty bottle of hard liquor next to him and an empty gallon of pesticide. There was vomit next to him, and he had sweat through his clothing. He complained of difficulty breathing, nausea, blurred vision, weakness, and diarrhea. He was given naloxone in route, with no change in mental status.

Pertinent Physical Exam

Except as noted below, the findings of the complete physical exam are within normal limits.

- HR 50, BP 110/70, RR 30, Temp 98F, 87% on nonrebreather mask (NRB).
- General: Diaphoretic, smells like garlic.
- Head, eyes, ears, nose, throat: Pupils pinpoint, copious salivation, and lacrimation.
- Lungs: Shallow respirations with diffuse coarse breath sounds and rhonchi and wheezing.
- Heart: Bradycardia.
- Abdomen: Hyperactive bowel sounds, urinary incontinence, and fecal incontinence.

B. Y. Yang · N. Kman (✉)

Department of Emergency Medicine, Wexner Medical Center at The Ohio State University, Columbus, OH, USA

e-mail: Betty.Yang@osumc.edu; Nicholas.Kman@osumc.edu

© Springer Nature Switzerland AG 2020

C. G. Kaide, C. E. San Miguel (eds.), *Case Studies in Emergency Medicine*, https://doi.org/10.1007/978-3-030-22445-5_45

449

- Neuro: Diffuse weakness noted in upper and lower extremities bilaterally. Fasciculations were noted throughout.
- Bedside pulmonary function testing (PFTs): Negative Inspiratory Force (NIF) was −20.

Past medical history (PMH) Hypertension

Social history (SH) He works as a farmer, and his friend said he had been struggling to make ends meet.

ED Management

The nurse who triaged the patient started to feel dizzy and short of breath. An announcement was made for everyone encountering this patient to have full personal protective equipment (PPE). He was quickly decontaminated with soapy water and showered. He was then subsequently intubated for all the saliva and secretions. He was initially very difficult to ventilate, until he was loaded with atropine and pralidoxime (2-PAM).

Updates on ED Course

The patient required multiple escalating doses of atropine, until the wheezing and secretions improved. He received a total of 62 mg. He was admitted to the ICU.

Case 2: Colonel Boris Collapsed on a Bench

Pertinent History

A 66-year-old male Russian retired military intelligence colonel and his 33-year-old daughter were found collapsed on a bench outside a shopping mall. A witness observed him holding his palms up, shrugging, with his right hand twitching, out of his control. His eyes were open, but he appeared frozen and unable to move. His daughter was seen stiffening and shaking all her extremities and slumping over afterwards. She had lost control of her bowel movements. He had noisy, agonal breathing. The patient was in respiratory failure with poor effort, when he was found by the first responders, and intubated prior to transport to the ED.

Pertinent Physical Exam

Except as noted below, the findings of the complete physical exam are within normal limits.

- HR 50, BP 110/70, RR 30, Temp 98F, 88% intubated.
- HEENT: Intubated, endotracheal tube secretions.
- Lungs: Diffuse coarse breath sounds, rhonchi and wheezing.
- Heart: Bradycardia.
- Abdomen: Hyperactive bowel sounds.
- Neuro: Poor tone. Not following commands.

PMH None

SH Patient previously worked as a double agent. His daughter just traveled from Russia the day before.

ED Management

Both victims were decontaminated upon arrival to the ED. For Boris, Atropine and 2-PAM were given with some improvement in vital signs. Several doses of diazepam were given for the seizures. Patient was treated with supportive care.

Updates on ED Course

Patient was admitted to the ICU. Several of the first responders were initially hospitalized as well with itchy eyes and wheezing. Another 21 people in the area needed medical evaluation.

Learning Points: Pesticide Poisoning and Nerve Agent Toxicity

Priming Questions
1. What distinguishes organophosphate poisoning from other intoxications? What aspects of the history point toward organophosphate poisoning?
2. How does pesticide poisoning differ from nerve agents?
3. What are the elements of the cholinergic toxidrome? What will kill the patient first?
4. How is the diagnosis made? What role is there for laboratory studies?
5. What is the management of organophosphate poisoning?

Introduction/Background

1. Organophosphate (OP) and carbamate poisonings can lead to significant morbidity and mortality when recognition is delayed. These cholinesterase inhibitors

work by inhibiting the normal breakdown of the neurotransmitter acetylcholine, leading to an excess amount of acetylcholine at skeletal neuromuscular junctions and synapses. Thousands of structurally similar substances have been developed since their discovery.

2. Common pesticides used in agriculture are parathion, Malathion, Diazinon, Chlorpyrofos, and Dichlorvos. The use is primarily to protect livestock, crops, and communities from insects, but these compounds also pose a threat. Each year an estimated 500,000 deaths occur in rural Asia due to suicide, and an estimated 200,000 of these are due to intentional organophosphate poisoning [1].

3. Nerve agents are extremely potent organophosphates developed for chemical warfare and used in acts of terror. They were developed initially by German military scientists in the 1930s. The G-type nerve agents, [i.e., Tabun (GA), Sarin (GB), Soman (GD), and Cyclosarin (GF)] are clear, colorless, and tasteless liquids. The most recognizable use of Sarin (GB) in a terrorist attack was in the Tokyo Subway Attack in 1995 where 5500 civilians sought medical care [1–4]. The attack left 12 dead, 50 critically injured, and 1000 suffering temporary vision problems. More recently, Sarin was used as a weapon of mass destruction when it was deployed in Syria.

4. The next group developed by the British in the 1950's was the V-series, many times more powerful than the G-type nerve agents. VX is an amber-colored, oily liquid with low volatility until exposed to high temperatures. The adult VX LD_{50} is only 3 mg [2, 4–6]. VX was used in the assassination of the Kim Jong Nam December 2017. Beyond the V-series, the development of the Novichok series, Russian for "newcomer," were developed by the Soviets and had not been used in known attacks until the Sergei and Yulia Kripal were poisoned in the UK in March 2018. These newer agents are several times more potent than VX.

Physiology/Pathophysiology

1. Acetylcholine is a neurotransmitter that triggers stimulation of postsynaptic nerves, muscles, and exocrine glands. Acetylcholinesterase (AChE) breaks down acetylcholine, so there is no overstimulation. Organophosphates and carbamates are anticholinesterase inhibitors; blockade of AChE leads to the accumulation of excessive amounts of acetylcholine at muscarinic receptors and nicotinic receptors and in the CNS.

2. Maturation of the bond between AChE and AChE inhibitor is called "aging." Blockade of AChE may be reversible for a period, but once the bond ages, then the blockade becomes irreversible. For some agents, like Soman "aging" is only 2 minutes, whereas for Sarin "aging" takes 8.5 hours, and for Malathion, it is approximately 72 hours.

Acetylcholine, Acetylcholinesterase and Acetylcholinesterase Inhibitors

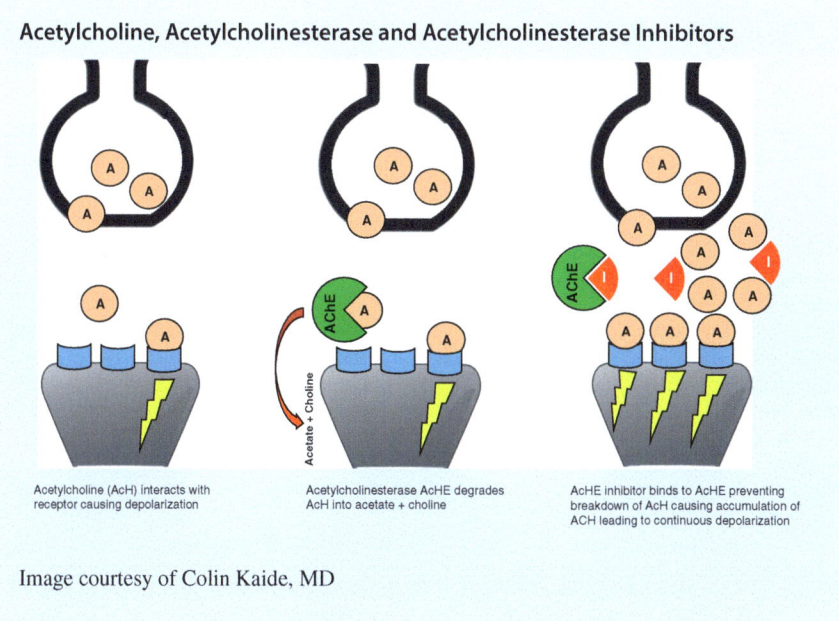

Acetylcholine (AcH) interacts with receptor causing depolarization

Acetylcholinesterase AcHE degrades AcH into acetate + choline

AcHE inhibitor binds to AcHE preventing breakdown of AcH causing accumulation of ACH leading to continuous depolarization

Image courtesy of Colin Kaide, MD

3. Carbamate poisoning has similar acute effects as OP poisoning, but toxicity is not as severe. Unlike OP, carbamates do not "age" the AChE enzyme; the bond between carbamate and AChE will spontaneously lyse, resulting in recovery of enzyme activity within several hours [3]. CNS effects are also less prominent, since they do not cross the blood-brain barrier as easily [3].

4. Onset of toxicity depends on the mode of delivery and the agent involved. The term "nerve gas" is a misnomer as these agents are liquids under temperate conditions. Depending how they are dispersed, they may present as a vapor, aerosol, or liquid. The tendency of vapor is to sink to the ground, as these agents are heavier than air. Dermal agents frequently have local fasciculations at the site of exposure before weakness. Inhalation can lead to death under a minute, with massive exposure. Very high doses of nerve agents can act quickly, even if dermal. Certain chemical compounds lead to more rapid onset.

Onset of action of organophosphate toxicity	
Mode of delivery	Onset
Inhalation	Fastest – seconds to minutes
Ingestion	30–90 minutes
Dermal	Slowest – up to 18 hours

5. Clinical presentation – Four types of clinical pathology related to the period of onset [2, 3]:

- *Cholinergic toxidrome* is the acute clinical findings due to excess acetylcholine affecting the nicotinic and muscarinic receptors. The most likely presentation seen in the ED will be the acute effects, which may be classified into three categories: the muscarinic, nicotinic, and CNS effects.
  - Muscarinic receptors are in the parasympathetic nervous system (cardiac conduction, exocrine glands, and smooth muscles), sympathetic nervous system (sweat glands), and the central nervous system.

Muscarinic effects mnemonics [3]	
I B SLUDGED	**DUMBELS**
MIosis	
Bronchorrhea, bronchospasm, bradycardia	Defecation/diaphoresis
Salivation	Urination
Lacrimation	Miosis
Urination	Bronchorrhea, bronchospasm, bradycardia
Defecation	Emesis
GI pain	Lacrimation
Emesis	Salivation
Diaphoresis	

  - Nicotinic receptors are located in the neuromuscular junctions of skeletal muscles and the sympathetic nervous system. The activation at the neuromuscular junction triggers muscle contraction rapidly when stimulated by acetylcholine. The cholinesterase inhibitor leads to hyperstimulation of the muscle, with continued contraction that leads to fasciculations and myoclonic jerks, followed by muscle fatigue, weakness, and paralysis. Beyond the skeletal system, nicotinic receptors also affect the sympathetic nervous system, due to ganglionic stimulation of the adrenal gland.

Nicotinic effects mnemonic [3]	
Monday	Mydriasis (pupillary dilatation)
Tuesday	Tachycardia, tachydysrhythmia
Wednesday	Weakness
Thursday	Hypertension
Friday	Fasciculation and myotonic jerks

  - CNS effects result from both muscarinic and nicotinic receptor activation. The main effects are:
    - Agitation, irritability, loss of consciousness
    - Seizure
    - Coma
    - Respiratory failure, apnea
  - Patients may die from bronchorrhea and bronchospasm, essentially drowning in secretions, but most frequently, they die from nicotinic effects and respiratory arrest. Cause of death is usually from respiratory compromise due to:
    - Bronchorrhea
    - Bronchospasm
    - Central respiratory depression
    - Weakness and paralysis

> *Nerve agents are exceedingly toxic and can cause convulsions in seconds and death from respiratory arrest within minutes.*

- Pediatric cases may present with different clinical findings from adults [2, 3].
  - ○ More nicotinic effects and CNS effects are notable, than muscarinic. Children frequently present with flaccid muscle weakness, lethargy, seizures, and coma. It is important to look for neuromuscular weakness, since tone may be overlooked, unless directly assessed. Less common are muscarinic effects, like bradycardia, fasciculations, and sweating.
  - ○ Generalized seizures are more common in pediatrics, while only appearing for severe organophosphate exposures in adults.
- *Intermediate syndrome* – Delayed neuromuscular dysfunction, occurring 24–96 hours after significant and severe poisoning, that usually resolves spontaneously after 1–2 weeks. Patients can suddenly develop peripheral respiratory failure, after having recovered from the acute cholinergic toxidrome. It is important to monitor neck flexion strength immediately after toxicity, since it appears to be a good indicator.
- *Organophosphate-Induced Delayed Neuropathy* – Delayed neuropathy with onset 1–5 weeks after acute cholinergic toxidrome with weakness, paralysis, pain, and paresthesia. Sensation recovers, but motor deficits may be permanent.
- *Organophosphorus Ester-Induced Chronic Neurotoxicity* – Chronic neurotoxicity with neuropsychiatric findings, lasting from weeks to years after acute cholinergic toxidrome.

Making the Diagnosis

Differential Diagnosis [2]
- Viral upper respiratory infection, influenza, pneumonia
- Mental illness
- Diabetic ketoacidosis
- Gastroenteritis
- Myasthenia crisis
- Guillain-Barre syndrome
- Nicotine poisoning
- Cholinergic intoxication (pilocarpine, carbachol, bethanechol, and methacholine)
- Opiate overdose
- Intoxication
- Hypertensive encephalopathy
- Asthma attack
- Hydrocarbon ingestion
- Coronary ischemia, myocardial infarction, congestive heart failure, cardiogenic shock
- Severe pyrethroid insecticide toxicity

A patient presenting with the full toxidrome would be straightforward, but patients may only present with a few of the clinical symptoms and signs. The presentation also differs in children.

1. Exposure history is fundamental to diagnosis. Occupational risks in pharmaceuticals, pesticides, chemical warfare agents, industrial materials, and traditional medical remedies. Multiple victims with a common exposure may be a key clue.
   - Beyond the muscarinic, nicotinic, and CNS effects, nerve agents have a specific toxidromes, in order of onset, described below [4]:
     - Primary: Mental status changes, fasciculations, muscle weakness, paralysis
     - Secondary: Increased secretions, miosis
     - Tertiary: Shallow breaths
   - Subsequent signs and symptoms are noted as convulsions, coma, and respiratory arrest.
2. Laboratory assessment: Cholinesterase levels are not especially useful in the emergent setting. There are two types of cholinesterase levels, which must be interpreted with caution: red blood cell acetylcholinesterase and plasma pseudocholinesterase aka butyrylcholinesterase [1–3].
3. Other laboratory testing: arterial blood gas, pulse oximetry, ECG, electrolytes, glucose, BUN, creatinine, lactic acid, creatinine kinase, lipase, liver function tests, and chest X-ray.
4. Other adjunct testing: Respiratory function tests – spirometry and negative inspiratory force (NIF) can be used to assess the severity of respiratory weakness. Electromyographic and nerve stimulation studies can determine patients at high risk for respiratory failure.

Treating the Patient

1. Emergency supportive care. ABCs first. Aggressive respiratory support is needed, since most fatalities from organophosphate poisoning is due to respiratory failure.

> **Pro Tip:**
> Remember! If intubation is needed, a nondepolarizing agent, like rocuronium, should be used. Depolarizing neuromuscular blockers, like succinylcholine, will have a prolonged paralytic effect, because it should be metabolized by AChE, which is blocked by the organophosphate poisoning. Due to the excessive acetylcholine in the neuromuscular junction, rocuronium onset may be delayed and large doses may be needed.

   - The patient should be closely monitored and reassessed, evaluating secretions, oxygen saturation, and respiratory rate every 5–10 minutes.
   - Supportive care should be provided for hydrocarbon pneumonitis, bradycardia, dysrhythmias, hypotension, seizure, and coma.

2. Atropine – Treatment of Muscarinic Effects
   - Atropine competitively inhibits AchE inhibitors to overcome the effects the cholinergic toxidrome. An atropine challenge is sometimes recommended to aid in diagnosis. If the patient does not have an anticholinergic response, the likely culprit is presumed to be organophosphate poisoning.
   - Atropine is given 2–5 mg IV initially, then double the dose every 5 minutes, until clinical improvement is evident. The most important indication for redosing is persistent wheezing, bronchorrhea, or bradyarrhythmia, as well as bradyarrhythmias and atrioventricular nodal (A–V) blocks.
   - Atropine is the undisputed cornerstone of treatment for acute cholinergic syndrome. Dosage requirements for pesticide toxicity can be orders of magnitude higher. Large cumulative doses (100+ mg in severe cases) are sometimes required [7–9].
   - Nerve agents typically target nicotinic receptors, so nerve agent poisoning does not require a significant amount of atropine.
   - Other antimuscarinics, like glycopyrrolate, have improved peripheral muscarinic toxicity, but do not penetrate CNS, like atropine.
3. Oximes – Treatment of the Nicotinic Effects.
   - Oximes (2-PAM aka Pralidoxime) can lyse the bond between AChE and the AChE inhibitor, as long as it is given before the bond matures. Oximes break the organophosphate-acetylcholinesterase bonds, reactivating the acetylcholinesterase to degrade excess acetylcholine. 2-PAM should be given with atropine, which has been noted to have a synergistic effect.
   - Pralidoxime is given as a loading dose (30–50 mg/kg, total 1–2 g in adults) over 30 minutes, followed by a continuous infusion of 8–20 mg/kg/h (up to 650 mg/h). Initial dose can be repeated in 1 hour if muscle weakness and fasciculations not improved.
   - Oximes are most effective if given early, before irreversible phosphorylation. However, they may still be effective after exposure, due to highly lipid-soluble compounds released into the blood from fat store over days to weeks.
   - The efficacy of oximes in OP poisoning remains controversial. There have been numerous studies worldwide, attempting to evaluate the efficacy of oximes as a treatment of OP poisoning. A recent Cochran review published in 2018 evaluated data from five randomized controlled trials, which showed no significant difference in treatment with 2-PAM with atropine and treatment with atropine alone [10]. Some countries do not utilize oximes, but 2-PAM remains part of the standard treatment regimen in the United States.
4. Benzodiazepine – Seizure Treatment and Prophylaxis.
   - Benzodiazepines are recommended to treat organophosphate poisoning whenever seizure or pronounced muscle fasciculations are present. It has been shown that the combination of atropine and diazepam is more effective in reducing mortality than atropine or oxime alone [9].
   - Diazepam (5–10 mg in adults and 0.2–0.5 mg/kg in children) should be used to control seizures. Lorazepam or other benzodiazepines may be used but barbiturates, phenytoin, and other anticonvulsants are not effective.

5. Autoinjectors – Scene and military treatment of Nerve Agent Poisoning.
   • If the military Mark I kits containing autoinjectors are available, they provide the best way to administer the antidotes. One autoinjector automatically delivers 2 mg atropine and the other automatically delivers 600 mg 2-PAM Cl.
   • Each prefilled DuoDote® Auto-Injector provides a single intramuscular dose of atropine and pralidoxime chloride in a self-contained unit, specifically designed for administration by emergency medical services personnel.
     – When activated, each DuoDote® Auto-Injector delivers 2.1 mg of atropine and 600 mg of pralidoxime chloride.
   • ANY severe symptoms immediately administer three (3) DuoDotes to the mid-outer thigh in rapid succession.

Minor and Severe Symptoms of Organophosphate Exposure, per Duodote [6]	
Minor symptoms	Severe symptoms
Blurred vision, miosis	Strange or confused behavior
Excessive, unexplained teary eyes	Severe difficulty breathing or copious secretions
Excessive, unexplained runny nose	from lungs/airway
Increased salivation such as sudden drooling	Severe muscle twitching and general weakness
Chest tightness or difficulty breathing	Involuntary urination or defecation
Tremors throughout the body or muscular	Convulsions
twitches	Unconsciousness
Nausea and/or vomiting	
Unexplained wheezing, coughing, or	
increased airway secretions	
Acute onset of stomach cramps	
Tachycardia or bradycardia	

6. Secondary exposure. Patients can expose others to and continue to be exposed to the poisons.
   • Rescuers and caregivers should wear appropriate personal protective equipment (PPE), and isolate and decontaminate patients.
   • The Occupational Safety and Health Administration (OSHA) recommendation for an incident with an unknown agent is to use Level A protective equipment. Level A suits include a self-contained breathing apparatus with positive pressure and totally encapsulating (head-to-toe and sealed), chemical protection. This is the highest degree of personal protective equipment available [4].
   • Decontamination. Delayed effects from skin exposure to nerve agents may not develop for 18 hours after exposure. Before transport, all exposures must be decontaminated. If liquid agent exposure is suspected, cut and remove all clothing. If showers or water are limited, 0.5% sodium hypochlorite solution, or absorbent powders, like flour, talcum powder can be used [5].
     – Skin and mucous membrane. Remove all contaminated clothing and wash exposed areas with water and soap. Irrigate eyes with copious water or saline. Decontamination of patient should not delay atropine administration or airway management, in severely poisoned patient.

- Inhalation. Ventilatory support is key. Antidotes, supplemental oxygen and suction may be sufficient. Resistance to ventilation may occur from bronchospasm and improve with atropine.
- Ingestion. Do no induce emesis, due to risks of aspiration. Gastric lavage or aspiration of liquid stomach contents may be appropriate within 30 minutes of ingestions, but lavage should be performed after airway secured. No significant evidence present for activated charcoal improving outcomes.
  - Dialysis is generally not indicated due to large volume of distribution. Studies are currently underway to evaluate the utility of plasmapheresis.

US Airforce Photo

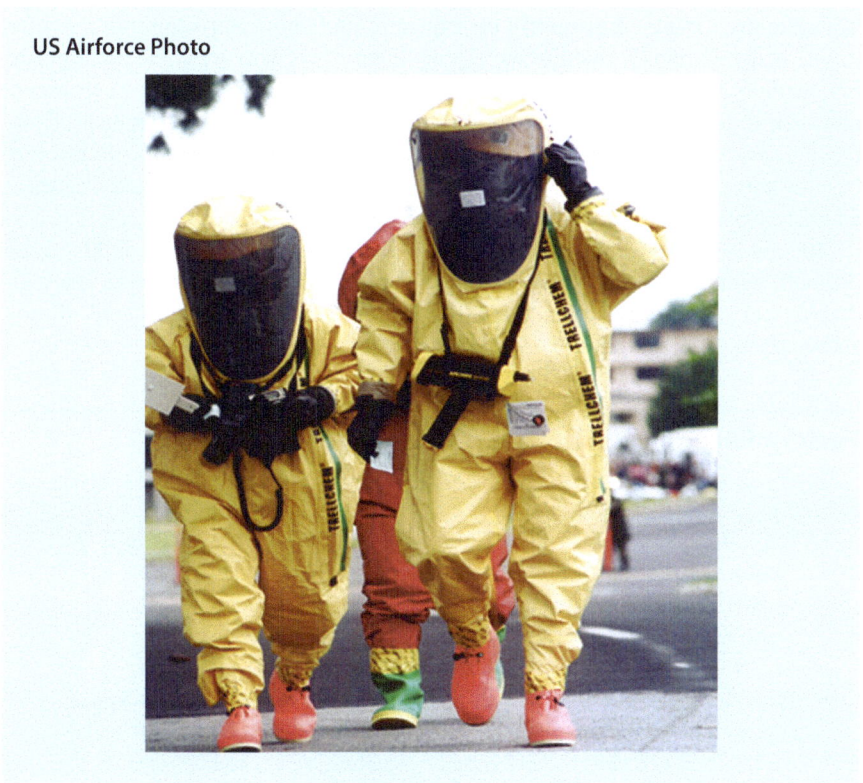

7. All exposures need to be observed closely for decompensation for at least 8–12 hours, even after mild exposures.

Case Conclusion

Case 1: The farmer found down had intentionally ingested a toxic amount of pesticide. He required more than 60 mg atropine administered for his life-threatening signs and symptoms to improve. He was extubated 2 days later and returned to baseline 1 week afterwards. He was evaluated by psychiatry for this suicide attempt.

Case 2: The use of a nerve agent was suspected, given the severity of the symptoms and the story. A full investigation was launched immediately, with the notification of emergency medical services. All potential sources of the chemical attack were isolated and examined. After suffering from a nerve agent attack, the patient stayed in the ICU for several months. Further testing and investigation revealed that the nerve agent was Novichok, a newer agent that was most prominently found on the front door handle and in the luggage of his daughter. He was last known to no longer be in critical condition, but his neurologic status remains to be seen.

Discussion

The diagnosis is based primarily on exposure and signs and symptoms. A high index of suspicion is needed to make this diagnosis. There are some distinguishing features that would make a cholinergic toxidrome more likely. Significant clues for diagnosis beyond history are multiple victims and the presence of fasciculations and weakness. In a mass casualty setting, a flowchart for toxidrome-based rapid identification of chemical warfare agents would facilitate treatment and safety planning [4].

The use of nerve agents in the civilian setting makes the diagnosis slightly more difficult, without the context clues of occupation and exposure. However, the toxidrome can be recognized and supportive care can be administered during stabilization.

Pattern Recognition: Organophosphate Poisoning

- Exposure history.
- Cholinergic toxidrome.
  - Nicotinic effects: Fasciculations, then weakness and paralysis.
  - Muscarinic effects: I B SLUDGED/DUMBELS.
  - CNS effects: Agitation, seizure, coma.
- What kills the patient: Bronchorrea, bronchospasm, central respiratory depression, weakness, and paralysis.

Disclosure Statement The authors of this chapter report no significant disclosures.

References

1. Eddleston M, Buckley NA, Eyer P, Dawson AH. Management of acute organophosphorus pesticide poisoning. Lancet. 2008;371(9612):597–607.
2. Auf der Heide E. Cholinesterase inhibitors: including pesticides & chemical warfare nerve agents section. Agency for toxic substances and disease registry; 2007. https://www.atsdr.cdc.gov/csem/csem.asp?csem=11&po. Accessed 15 May 2018.

3. Vohra R. Organophosphorus and carbamate insecticides. In: Olson K, editor. Poisoning & drug overdose. 7th ed: McGraw-Hill Education; Columbus, OH, USA. 2018. p. 353–60.
4. Ciottone GR. Toxidrome recognition in chemical-weapons attacks. N Engl J Med. 2018;378(17):1611–20.
5. CDC Medical Management Guidelines for Nerve Agents: Tabun (GA); Sarin (GB); Soman (GD); and VX. Agency for toxic substances and disease registry; 2014. https://www.atsdr.cdc.gov/mmg/mmg.asp?id=523&tid=93. Accessed 12 June 2018.
6. Duodote. https://www.meridianmeds.com/products/duodote. Accessed 12 June 2018.
7. Leibson T, Lifshitz M. Organophosphate and carbamate poisoning: review of the current literature and summary of clinical and laboratory experience in southern Israel. Isr Med Assoc J. 2008;10(11):767–70.
8. Aardema H, Meertens JHJM, Ligtenberg JJM, Peters-Polman OM, Tulleken JE, Zijlstra JG. Organophosphorus pesticide poisoning: cases and developments. Neth J Med. 2008;66(4):149–53.
9. Jokanović M, Kosanović M. Neurotoxic effects in patients poisoned with organophosphorus pesticides. Environ Toxicol Pharmacol. 2010;29(3):195–201.
10. Blumenberg A, Benabbas R, deSouza IS, Conigliaro A, Paladino L, Warman E, Sinert R, Wiener SW. Utility of 2-pyridine aldoxime methyl chloride (2-PAM) for acute organophosphate poisoning: a systematic review and meta-analysis. J Med Toxicol. 2018;14(1):91–8. https://doi.org/10.1007/s13181-017-0636-2. Epub 2017 Dec 11.

46

James Flannery and Joshua K. Aalberg

Indication for the Exam *33 y/o f with a past medical history of blood clots presents with 2 days of headache and generalized weakness.*

Diagnosis Sagittal venous sinus thrombosis

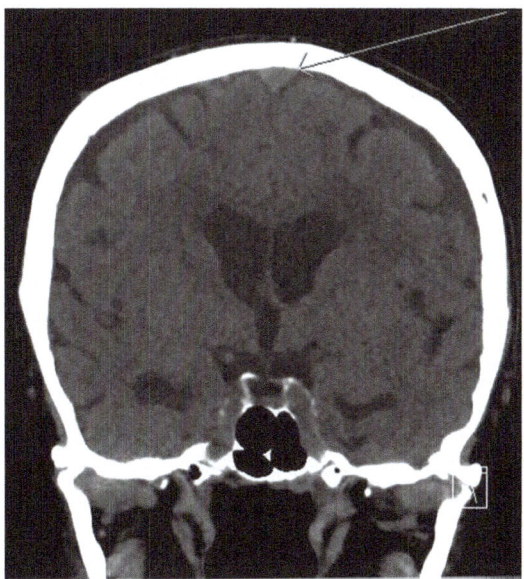

Hyperdense dural sinus indicating an acute thrombus in the superior sagittal sinus on a non-contrast head computed tomography (CT)

J. Flannery · J. K. Aalberg (✉)
Department of Emergency Medicine, Wexner Medical Center at The Ohio State University, Columbus, OH, USA
e-mail: James.flannery@osumc.edu; joshua.aalberg@osumc.edu

© Springer Nature Switzerland AG 2020
C. G. Kaide, C. E. San Miguel (eds.), *Case Studies in Emergency Medicine*,
https://doi.org/10.1007/978-3-030-22445-5_46

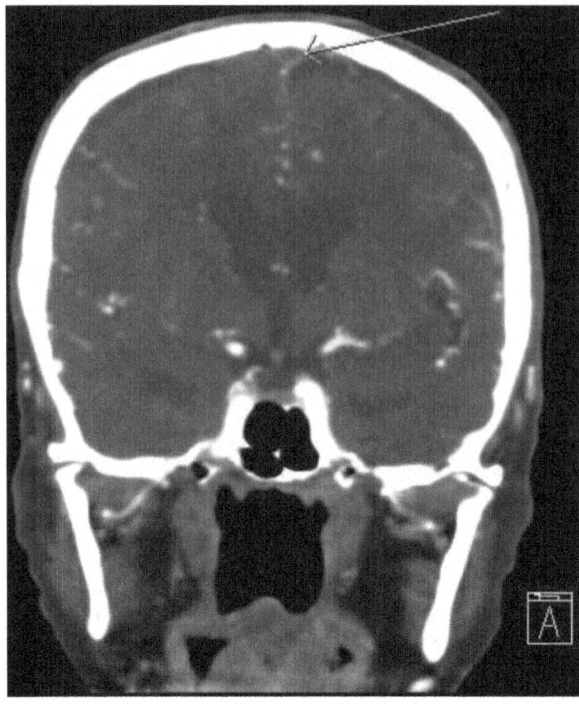

Thrombus surrounded by enhancing dura creates an "empty delta sign" on the venous phase contrast head CT (CTV)

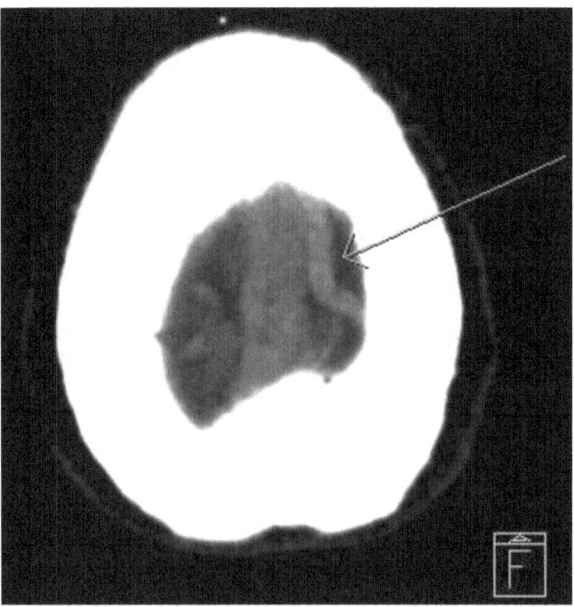

A hyperdense cortical vein causes a "cord sign," indicating an acute thrombosis involving a cortical vein on this non-contrast head CT

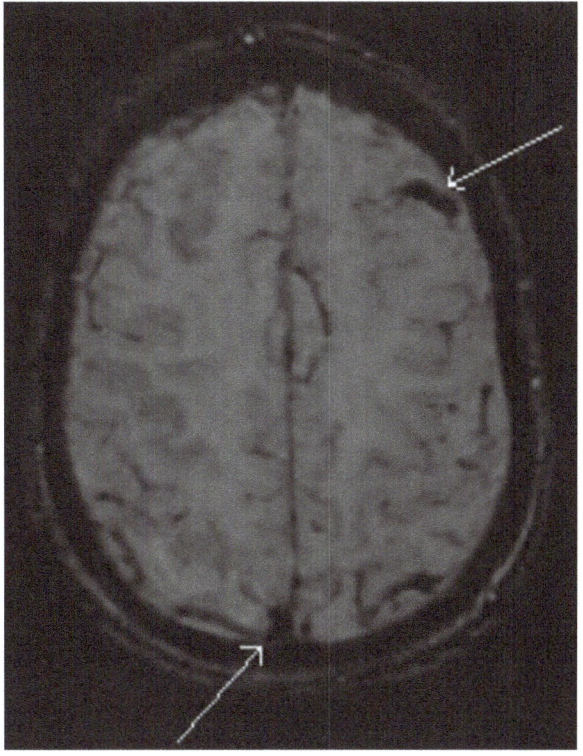

"Blooming artifact" indicates acute dural and cortical venous thrombosis on this Magnetic Resonance Imaging (MRI) Susceptibility weighted imaging (SWI) sequence

Learning Points

Priming Questions
- What will a dural venous thrombosis look like on non-contrasted versus contrasted head CTs?
- How do you distinguish true thrombus versus variant anatomy?
- What patients are at high risk for dural venous thrombosis?

Introduction/Background

Dural venous thrombosis (or cerebral venous thrombosis, CVT) is an occlusion of the intracranial dural sinuses, which function to drain intracranial venous blood and cerebrospinal fluid. The network of dural venous sinuses is extensive and eventually drains into the internal jugular veins. A CVT can cause a wide range of neurologic symptoms but the most common presentation is headache. Other potential symptoms include seizure, focal neurological deficits which may mimic typical stroke symptoms, papilledema, and encephalopathy.[8] Dural venous thrombosis accounts for 0.5–1% of all strokes [1].

Pathophysiology/Mechanism

Dural venous thrombus leads to occlusion of the venous drainage and eventually local edema and intracranial hypertension which can progress to ischemia and/or hemorrhage. The clinical course is highly variable, ranging from hours to upwards of 1 month [2]. A risk factor for venous thrombosis is identified in a majority of cases and should raise clinical suspicion if present. There are numerous risk factors, but some of the most commonly encountered include:

- pregnancy
- oral contraceptive use
- malignancy
- dehydration
- inflammation/infection
- trauma/fracture [3, 4].

Consider CVT in a young or middle-aged female with stroke-like symptoms. Another important consideration is genetic prothrombotic predisposition (such as lupus anticoagulant, antithrombin III, protein S or C deficiencies, factor V leiden) which is identified in 20–25% of CVT cases [5].

Making the Diagnosis

Non-contrasted head CT can show the thrombosed dural sinus as hyperdense attenuation, indicating acute thrombosis. Thrombosed cortical veins can also appear as tubular hyperdensities overlying the involved cerebral hemisphere. The most commonly involved sinuses are the superior sagittal and transverse sinuses, although multiple sinuses are often involved [4]. Cortical vein involvement will typically be adjacent to the dural sinus thrombus. These findings are insensitive though seen in only approximately 25–30% of cases [2, 6].

- Contrast-enhanced head CT in the venous phase increases diagnosis sensitivity by opacifing the dural venous sinuses. A thrombosed sinus will show a filling defect within the opacified sinus, referred to as the "empty delta sign" because of the triangular shape of the sinuses in cross section.
  - Common CT pitfalls:
    - False-positive cases of hyperdense dural sinuses can be seen in cases of high hematocrit such as polycythemia and dehydration, especially in children. In these cases, the cerebral arteries are frequently hyperdense as well

which can help distinguish a true thrombus [7]. Also, the density of a true acute thrombus will typically measure over 70 haunsfield units or have a haunsfield unit to hematocrit ratio > 2.0 [8].

- ○ Additional false-positive cases on non-contrasted CT are seen in the setting of acute subarachnoid or subdural hemorrhage adjacent to the sinus, which will also appear hyperdense and can typically be distinguished with a contrasted CT or MRI. It is important to remember that intracranial hemorrhage and dural venous thrombosis can be seen concurrently in 30–40% of patients [3].
- ○ False-positive cases on contrasted head CT include normal anatomic structures such as arachnoid granulations. These structures occupy the dural sinuses and can replicate a thrombus. However, arachnoid granulations will appear to be short and rounded in the long axis and have a density similar to cerebrospinal fluid [7]. A true clot is long and linear. Anatomic variations can also mimic a true thrombus, including sinus hypoplasia or intrasinus septa [3].

If there is a nondiagnostic or equivocal head CT for dural venous thrombosis with continued clinical suspicion, a contrasted brain MRI or MR venogram can be considered for more definitive diagnosis. Even with suspected dural venous thrombus on initial evaluation, CT or MR venogram is recommended to evaluate extent of the thrombus [3].

Treating the Patient

There are many proposed management guidelines for treatment of dural venous thrombosis, but in general terms:

- Anticoagulation with either intravenous heparin or subcutaneous low molecular weight heparin should be initiated immediately if no contraindication (e.g., intracranial hemorrhage), followed by transition to long-term oral anticoagulation after the acute episode.
- Endovascular therapy such as direct thrombolysis may be considered in patients who have a contraindication to anticoagulation or show worsening neurological symptoms despite anticoagulation.
- Decompressive hemicraniectomy is reserved for severe cases with significant mass effect.

Discussion

Dural venous thrombosis can be a difficult clinical diagnosis, but recognition of early signs on initial head CT can direct appropriate work up and therapy. It is imperative to exclude intracranial hemorrhage, as anticoagulation can propagate the bleed.

- Again, findings on CT include:
  - Hyperdense attenuation in a dural venous sinus on the non-contrasted head CT.
  - Hypodense filling defect in a contrast-enhanced sinus, known as the "empty delta" sign on contrasted head CT.
  - Be aware of possible false-positive imaging findings including high hematocrit or anatomic variants.

A first episode of dural sinus thrombus should warrant workup for a potential cause. This includes:

- Hypercoagulable states such as pregnancy, oral contraceptive use, or malignancy.
- Prothrombotic congenital conditions are also potential causes.
- Management of dural venous thrombosis is based on neurologic symptoms and imaging findings.
- Anticoagulation is first-line treatment; immediate initiation of heparin followed by long-term oral anticoagulation is the typical treatment course.
- Endovascular therapy such as direct thrombolysis is reserved for patients who have worsening neurological symptoms despite anticoagulation.
- Neurosurgical intervention may be indicated given significant intracranial findings such as severe mass effect or midline shift.

References

1. Bonneville F. Imaging of cerebral venous thrombosis. Diagn Interv Imaging. 2014;95(12):1145–50; Tomandl BF, et al. Comprehensive imaging of ischemic stroke with multisection CT. Radiographics. 2003;23(3):565–92.
2. Lee EJ. The empty delta sign. Radiology. 2002;224(3):788–9.
3. Saposnik G, et al. Diagnosis and management of cerebral venous thrombosis. Stroke. 2011;42:1158–92.
4. Stam J. Thrombosis of the cerebral veins and sinuses. N Engl J Med. 2005;352:1791–8.
5. Bousser MG, Ferro JM. Cerebral venous thrombosis: an update. Lancet Neurol. 2007;6:162–70.
6. Wasay M, Bakshi R, Bobustuc G, Kojan S, Sheikh Z, Dai A, Cheema Z. Cerebral venous thrombosis: analysis of a multicenter cohort from the United States. J Stroke Cerebrovasc Dis. 2008;17:49–54.
7. Provenzale JM, et al. Dural sinus thrombosis: sources of error in image interpretation. AJR Am J Roentgenol. 2011;196(1):23–31. Review. Erratum in: AJR Am J Roentgenol. 2011 May;196(5):1237. AJR Am J Roentgenol. 196(3):743, 2011ol. 2007;6:162–170.
8. Black DF, et al. Cerebral venous sinus density on noncontrast CT correlates with hematocrit. AJNR Am J Neuroradiol. 2011;32(7):1354–7.

Breakin' (Pacemakers): *Electric Boogaloo*

47

Matthew Malone and Ashish Panchal

Case

Syncope in a Patient with a Pacemaker

Pertinent History
This patient is a 76-year-old male who presented to a free-standing ED approximately 1 hour after a syncopal episode. He reports that he woke up this morning feeling well. This afternoon, the patient had an episode of syncope where he passed out and woke up on the floor. The episode was witnessed by his wife, who reports that he was only unconscious for a few seconds and had no seizure-like activity, confusion upon waking, tongue biting, or incontinence. Prior to his syncopal episode, he was painting the trim above a door at home. As he was painting, he became lightheaded. He had no CP, SOB, or other preceding symptoms. He did not hit his head and does not have any injuries. He is currently asymptomatic.

Past Medical History
Hypertension, Coronary Artery Disease, Complete Heart Block

Past Surgical History
Pacemaker implantation for complete heart block

Medications
Lisinopril, Atorvastatin

Social History
Remote tobacco use, no drug use, occasional alcohol use

M. Malone (✉) · A. Panchal
Department of Emergency Medicine, Wexner Medical Center at The Ohio State University, Columbus, OH, USA
e-mail: Matthew.malone@osumc.edu

© Springer Nature Switzerland AG 2020
C. G. Kaide, C. E. San Miguel (eds.), *Case Studies in Emergency Medicine*,
https://doi.org/10.1007/978-3-030-22445-5_47

469

Pertinent Physical Exam

- BP 128/77, Pulse 80, Temp 98.1 °F (36.7 °C), RR 14, SpO2 99%.
- HEENT: Normocephalic, atraumatic.
- Chest Wall: Right upper chest AICD battery without overlying erythema or tenderness to palpation.
- Neurological: Cranial nerves II-XII intact, Gross motor intact.

Except as noted above, the findings of a complete physical exam are within normal limits.

Pertinent Test Results

EKG
Paced rhythm with rate of 80 in LBBB pattern, complete capture of pacer spikes, unchanged from previous

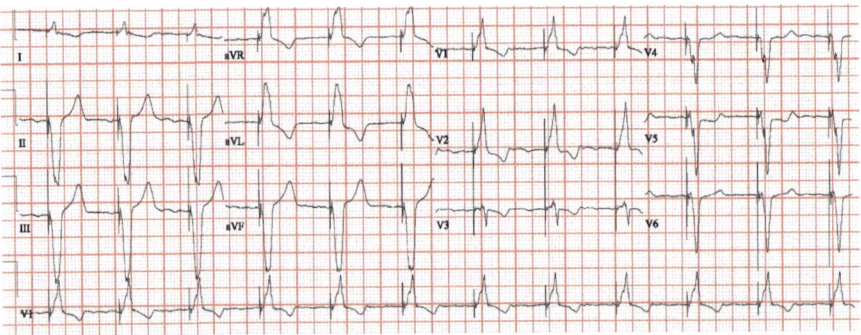

Courtesy of Matthew Malone, MD

Laboratory Evaluation:

Test	Result	Units	Normal range
WBC	6.01	K/uL	3.8–11.0 10^3 / mm³
Hgb	13.1 ↓	g/dL	(Male) 14–18 g/dL
			(Female) 11–16 g/dL
Platelets	300	K/uL	140–450 K /uL
Sodium	139	mEq/L	135–148 mEq/L
Potassium	4.0	mEq/L	3.5–5.5 mEq/L
Chloride	108	mEq/L	96–112 mEq/L
Bicarbonate	25	mEq/L	21–34 mEq/L
BUN	8	mg/dL	6–23 mg/dL
Creatinine	0.79	mg/dL	0.6–1.5 mg/dL
Glucose	92	mg/dL	65–99 mg/dL
Magnesium	2.1	mg/dL	1.6–2.6 mg/dL
Troponin	<0.01	ng/dl	< 0.11 ng/dl

CXR Single lead pacemaker in place without evidence of lead fracture or displacement, no other acute cardiopulmonary process.

Device Interrogation You do not have the ability to interrogate this patient's device in your clinical setting.

Updates on ED Course
Update 1: Cardiology is consulted and returns your page. They ask you to conduct an evaluation with the patient's assistance. The patient is asked to reproduce the movements he was performing prior to losing consciousness. While connected to a continuous cardiac monitor and with direct monitoring of the femoral pulse, he reproduces the actions of the painting above his head. The monitor demonstrates significant artifact due to movement, but it appears similar to a wide complex rhythm with a rate around 100. At this time, the patient's palpated pulse is between 30 and 40 bpm. He reports lightheadedness and feels like he will pass out. At this time, you have the patient lie back and stop the activity.

Cardiology believes the malfunction is oversensing of muscular activity. He recommends discharge with activity precautions and expedited cardiology follow-up for adjustment of device settings.

Learning Points: Pacemaker Malfunction

Priming Questions
1. What are the types of pacemaker malfunction and the common underlying causes of each?
2. What is the evaluation for a patient presumed to have a pacemaker malfunction?
3. What are other common complications associated with pacemaker implantation?

Introduction/Background

1. Indications for pacemakers are numerous, but all pacemakers are placed to maintain or restore a normal heartbeat. Common indications include pacing for sinus node dysfunction, acquired atrio-ventricular block, chronic bifascicular block, pacing for atrioventricular block associated with myocardial infarction, hypersensitive carotid sinus syndrome, and neurocardiogenic syncope. Often, the necessity of permanent pacemaker implantation is driven by a nonreversible conduction abnormality associated with symptomatic bradycardia [1, 2].
2. Pacemakers can be single or dual chamber, depending on the indication for placement. Single-chamber pacemakers have a single lead placed in either the right atrium or right ventricle. Dual-chamber pacemakers have 2 leads, one in the right atrium and the other in the right ventricle. The common terminology and settings for pacemakers are defined and describe the chamber paced and sensed,

the response to sensing, the programmability of the device, and the anti-tachycardia function of the device (e.g., pacing, shock) [3].

3. With the exception of a few specific examples which will be discussed, pacemaker malfunction usually leads to intermittent or complete return to the patient's underlying intrinsic cardiac rhythm.

Making the Diagnosis

Differential Diagnosis
- Failure to Pace (Output Failure)
  - Pacing stimulus is not generated as expected
  - No pacemaker spikes or pacer-induced QRS complexes
- Failure to Capture
  - Impulse given but does not depolarize myocardium
  - Pacer spikes on EKG
- Failure to Sense
  - Oversensing
  - Undersensing
- Pseudomalfunction
  - Crosstalk
  - Pacemaker-mediated tachycardia
  - Sensor-induced tachycardia
  - Runaway pacemaker
  - Lead-displacement dysrhythmia
  - Twiddler syndrome

1. The first goal for this patient is to determine hemodynamic stability. Place the patient on continuous cardiac monitoring and obtain a full set of vital signs.
2. If the patient is able to provide a history, ask about the indication for pacemaker placement, history of prior pacemaker malfunctions/complications and any current cardiac medications (especially antiarrhythmics).
3. Most patients with a pacemaker complication or malfunction related to their pacemaker will present symptomatically, often with similar symptoms to what required the pacemaker in the first place. For instance, a patient with a pacemaker for SA node dysfunction will present bradycardic and lightheaded, while a patient with a pacemaker for cardiac resynchronization therapy in severe CHF will likely present with acute heart failure.
4. Symptoms preceding and the circumstances surrounding the symptom onset may also identify the cause of the malfunction.
5. It is also important to maintain a wide differential diagnosis as many symptoms caused by pacemaker malfunction are vague and could be attributed to other causes, such as tachyarrhythmia, electrolyte imbalance, acute coronary symptom, congestive heart failure, sepsis, or dehydration.

6. Once a history has been obtained and the patient has been stabilized, a few additional tests may help to narrow the differential.
   - Chest radiography can identify lead fracture or displacement, as well as other issues such as twiddler syndrome.
   - Electrolyte abnormalities can contribute to various arrhythmias and should be evaluated and corrected as needed.
   - In the patient presenting with chest pain or SOB, cardiac biomarkers are important to evaluate for acute ischemia.
   - Device interrogation is helpful to identify specific causes of malfunction. Patients often carry a card to identify the make and model of their pacemaker. If not, the manufacturer code is visible on chest X-ray located on the pulse generator. Interrogations should include mode, rate, capture threshold, and sensitivity [4].
   - A 12-lead ECG should be obtained to identify the patient's current rhythm. This will likely also give important clues to if and why the pacemaker is malfunctioning.
     – Absence of pacer spikes indicates native depolarization, which might appropriate based on the current pacemaker settings or might represent a malfunction such as output failure.
     – Pacer spikes preceding myocardial depolarizations indicate successful pacing and capture.
     – Leads in RV apex produce LBBB pattern with appropriate discordance.
     – RBBB pattern may indicate the lead is in the LV [5].
7. The malfunctions can be categorized into the following general categories:
   - Failure to Pace (Output Failure):
     – In output failure, the EKG will be absent of pacing spikes or pacmaker-induced QRS complexes.
     – Output failure can be caused by lead malfunction, unstable connection, insufficient power/battery failure, cross-talk inhibition, and oversensing [6].
   - Failure to Capture:
     – The impulse is given by the device but fails to depolarize the myocardium.
     – Pacer spikes are seen on the EKG but no myocardial depolarizations are due to this impulse.
     – Failure to capture is usually due to some specific mechanical problem with wires and connectivity, but can also be seen in battery depletion, fibrosis at wire-myocardium interface, MI, electrolyte imbalance, or as the result of antiarrhythmic/rate control medications [6].
   - Failure to Sense: Oversensing and Undersensing
     – Oversensing occurs when any electrical signal with sufficient amplitude and frequency is inappropriately recognized as native cardiac activity, resulting in pacemaker output inhibition. These inappropriate signals may be large P or T waves, skeletal muscle activity, or lead contact problems. These abnormal signals may be transient and/or not be evident on ECG. Because of the lack of pacing spikes, oversensing can be difficult to distinguish from other types of output failure [6].

- Undersensing occurs when the pacemaker fails to detect spontaneous myocardial depolarization, which results in atrial or ventricular pacing spikes asynchronous to P waves or QRS complexes. Undersensing is most often caused by an improper sensing threshold, insufficient myocardial voltage signal, lead fracture, or fibrosis or electrolyte abnormalities [6].
- Pseudomalfunction:
  - Crosstalk: Crosstalk can occur in a dual chamber pacemaker when the atrial pacemaker spike is misinterpreted as a ventricular depolarization by the ventricular wire, which inhibits ventricular pacemaker wire output or vice versa. To correct crosstalk, reduce sensitivity and output in the atrial, or ventricular channel.
  - Pacemaker-mediated tachycardia: In pacemaker-mediated tachycardia, atrial sensing of a ventricular spike is interpreted as an atrial depolarization, which triggers another ventricular impulse. This is similar to a re-entrant tachycardia.
    ○ This is usually avoided by programming a long post-ventricular atrial refractory period.
    ○ Placing a magnet over the pacemaker will terminate the tachycardia by suspending the pacemaker's sensing function.
    ○ Adenosine can also be used to terminate the loop.
  - Sensor-induced tachycardia: Sensor-induced tachycardia occurs in newer generation pacemakers that increase heart rates in response to physiological stimuli such as exercise, tachypnea, hypercapnia, or acidemia. Vibrations, loud noises, fever, limb movements, hyperventilation, or electrocautery can be misinterpreted by the pacemaker sensors, resulting in pacing at an inappropriately fast rate. Magnet application will terminate the tachycardia [7].
  - Runaway pacemaker: A runaway pacemaker occurs in older-generation models in the setting of low battery voltage. The pacemaker delivers paroxysms of pacing spikes at 2000 bpm. This can provoke ventricular fibrillation or result in failure to capture. This is a true emergency and can be aborted by application of a magnet [8].
  - Lead-displacement arrhythmia: occurs when a dislodged pacing wire inside the right ventricle intermittently contacts the myocardium, resulting in ventricular ectopy. An EKG that has changed from an LBBB pattern to an RBBB pattern suggests that the electrode has eroded through the interventricular septum. This can be confirmed on chest X-ray [9].
  - Twiddler's syndrome: Twiddler's syndrome is when the patient rotates the pacemaker generator on its long axis, resulting in dislodgement of pacing leads or more rarely, diaphragmatic or brachial plexus pacing. Reel's syndrome has the same outcomes, except the generator is rotated on its transverse axis to cause lead dislodgement [10].

Treating the Patient

1. As there is significant overlap in the above causes of failure, the next steps in management are similar.
   - Check the power, battery, and connections by device interrogation and chest X-ray.
   - Identify and correct any potential underlying medical etiologies, including volume overload, dehydration, sepsis, electrolyte abnormality, ischemia, etc.
   - If you believe there is output failure secondary to oversensing, place a magnet on the pacemaker to switch it to an asynchronous mode. If oversensing was the problem, the patient should now be paced at the device's default rate [9].
   - In the setting of pacemaker-mediated, symptomatic tachycardia, a magnet can again be key to terminating the malfunctioning process [9].
   - If a pacemaker-dependent patient is symptomatically bradycardic, Advanced Cardiac Life Support (ACLS) protocols should be followed.
     - The patient may require external pacing. Transcutaneous pacing is less invasive and procedurally simply, however mechanical capture can be challenging. In contrast, temporary transvenous pacing is more successful but involves a more complicated invasive procedure [11, 12].
     - Mechanical capture can be confirmed on bedside echo by observing LV contractions that match the pacemaker spikes on the cardiac monitor [13].
   - Essentially all the above causes will eventually require adjustment of pacemaker settings by the device representative or the patient's electrophysiologist.

Case Conclusion

The patient was comfortable with the plan to be discharged home. He had no additional events. He met with his cardiologist the following morning. Device interrogation was performed and oversensing was confirmed. His cardiologist subsequently increased the absolute value of device sensitivity, making it harder for muscle contraction to inhibit output.

Discussion

1. It is rare for a pacemaker to change its functionality unless there is a component malfunction. Given the complexity of contemporary pacemakers, evaluation of the entire system through device interrogation and imaging, often in consultation with a specialist, should be performed to ensure normal functionality of the device if malfunction is suspected by the clinical scenario.

2. Transcutaneous or transcutaneous pacing may be required if the patient is hemo-dynamically unstable in the setting of permanent pacemaker malfunction. Transcutaneous pacemaker should be trialed first in the hemodynamically unstable patient, as it is much faster to apply than placing a transvenous pacemaker.

3. If transcutaneous pacing fails at maximum settings, emergent placement of a transvenous pacemaker should be attempted. If transcutaneous pacing is successful at correcting hemodynamics, the patient may still need placement of a temporary transvenous pacemaker as the patient may not tolerate transcutaneous pacing while awake and sedation for the discomfort may worsen hemodynamics.

Pattern Recognition

- Presence of a pacemaker
- Syncope
- Symptomatic bradycardia or tachycardia

Disclosure Statement The authors of this chapter report no significant disclosures.

References

1. Epstein AE, DiMarco JP, Ellenbogen KA, Estes NA 3rd, Freedman RA, Gettes LS, et al. ACC/AHA/HRS 2008 Guidelines for Device-Based Therapy of Cardiac Rhythm Abnormalities: a report of the American College of Cardiology/American Heart Association Task Force on Practice Guidelines (Writing Committee to Revise the ACC/AHA/NASPE 2002 Guideline Update for Implantation of Cardiac Pacemakers and Antiarrhythmia Devices): developed in collaboration with the American Association for Thoracic Surgery and Society of Thoracic Surgeons. Circulation. 2008;117(21):e350–408. https://doi.org/10.1161/CIRCUALTIONAHA.108.189742.
2. Epstein AE, DiMarco JP, Ellenbogen KA, Estes NA 3rd, Freedman RA, Gettes LS, et al. 2012 ACCF/AHA/HRS focused update incorporated into the ACCF/AHA/HRS 2008 guidelines for device-based therapy of cardiac rhythm abnormalities: a report of the American College of Cardiology Foundation/American Heart Association Task Force on Practice Guidelines and the Heart Rhythm Society. J Am Coll Cardiol. 2013;61(3):e6–75. https://doi.org/10.1016/j.jacc.2012.11.007.
3. Bernstein AD, Daubert JC, Fletcher RD, Hayes DL, Luderitz B, Reynolds DW, et al. The revised NASPE/BPEG generic code for antibradycardia, adaptive-rate, and multi-site pacing. North American Society of Pacing and Electrophysiology/British Pacing and Electrophysiology Group Pacing. Clin Electrophysiol. 2002;25(2):260–4.
4. Neuenschwander JF, Hiestand BC, Peacock WF, Billings JM, Sondrup C, Hummel JD, et al. A pilot study of implantable cardiac device interrogation by emergency department personnel. Crit Pathw Cardiol. 2014;13(1):6–8. https://doi.org/10.1097/HPC.0000000000000000.
5. Jain R, Mohanan S, Haridasan V, Rajesh GN, Mangalath Narayanan K, Sajeer K. A change in QRS morphology in right ventricular apical pacing: is it a red flag sign? Heart Asia. 2014;6(1):152–4. https://doi.org/10.1136/heartasia-2014-010556.

6. Safavi-Naeini P, Saeed M. Pacemaker troubleshooting: common clinical scenarios. Tex Heart Inst J. 2016;43(5):415–8. https://doi.org/10.14503/THIJ-16-5918.

7. Ip JE, Markowitz SM, Liu CF, Cheung JW, Thomas G, Lerman BB. Differentiating pacemaker-mediated tachycardia from tachycardia due to atrial tracking: utility of V-A-A-V versus V-A-V response after postventricular atrial refractory period extension. Heart Rhythm. 2011;8(8):1185–91. https://doi.org/10.1016/j.hrthm.2011.02.036.

8. Ortega DF, Sammartino MV, Pellegrino GM, Barja LD, Albina G, Segura EV, et al. Runaway pacemaker: a forgotten phenomenon? Europace. 2005;7(6):592–7. https://doi.org/10.1016/j.eupc.2005.06.004.

9. Burns E. Pacemaker malfunction. 2019. https://litfl.com/pacemaker-malfunction-ecg-library/. Accessed 6 Feb 2019.

10. Nicholson WJ, Tuohy KA, Tilkemeier P. Twiddler's syndrome. N Engl J Med. 2003;348(17):1726–7. https://doi.org/10.1056/NEJM200304243481722.

11. Vukmir RB. Emergency cardiac pacing. Am J Emerg Med. 1993;11(2):166–76.

12. Allison MG, Mallemat HA. Emergency care of patients with pacemakers and defibrillators. Emerg Med Clin North Am. 2015;33(3):653–67. https://doi.org/10.1016/j.emc.2015.05.001.

13. Tam MM. Ultrasound for primary confirmation of mechanical capture in emergency transcutaneous pacing. Emerg Med (Fremantle). 2003;15(2):192–4.

Pediatric Drowning: *The Cold Water Blues*

48

Colleen J. Bressler and Maegan Reynolds

Case

Pertinent History

This 8-year-old male presented to the Emergency Department (ED) in full cardiac arrest. The patient had been waiting to be picked up for school and fell through an iced retaining pond. Time from fall to retrieval from the water was estimated at about 25 minutes. Cardiopulmonary resuscitation (CPR) was initiated and he arrived at the ED about 25 minutes after retrieval. He was intubated and had received 4 doses of epinephrine by Emergency Medical Services (EMS) en route to the ED.

Pertinent Physical Exam

- Active CPR, Temperature 31.6 °C (88.9 °F)

Except as noted below, the findings of a complete physician exam are within normal limits.

Primary Survey
- Airway – Intubated with 5.0 cuffed endotracheal tube (ETT) at 22 cm at the teeth.
- Breathing – Breath sounds bilaterally with bagging, positive color change noted on colorimeter. Circulation – no palpable pulses, CPR ongoing.

Secondary Survey.
- Head – abrasion to the right forehead. Bilateral pupils fixed and dilated.
- Neck – in c-collar.

C. J. Bressler (✉) · M. Reynolds
Department of Emergency Medicine, Nationwide Children's Hospital, Columbus, OH, USA
e-mail: colleen.bressler@nationwidechildrens.org

© Springer Nature Switzerland AG 2020
C. G. Kaide, C. E. San Miguel (eds.), *Case Studies in Emergency Medicine*,
https://doi.org/10.1007/978-3-030-22445-5_48

- Chest – Right with clear breath sounds, Left diminished breath sounds – ETT pulled back to 18 cm at the teeth with improved breath sounds bilaterally.
- Abdomen – soft, distended.
- Pelvis – stable, normal rectal tone, no rectal blood.
- Extremities – no pulses, no deformities.

Pertinent Diagnostic Testing

Test	Result	Units	Normal range
pH (arterial)	6.7 ↓	–	7.35–7.45
pCO$_2$ (arterial)	113 ↑	mmHg	35–45 mmHg
Base excess	−22 ↓	mmol/L	−3.0–3.0 mmol/L
Bicarbonate	15 ↓	mEq/L	21–34 mEq/L
Hgb	10.9 ↓	g/dL	(Male) 14–18 g/dL
			(Female) 11–16 g/dL
Hematocrit	32 ↓	%	34.9–44.3%

Plan
Continue Pediatric Advanced Life Support (PALS) and rewarming

Update 1/Resuscitation Efforts Resuscitation efforts continued following PALS algorithms. Two intraosseous (IO) catheters were placed in the patient's bilateral tibias. The patient received a total of 6 doses of epinephrine and was then started on an epinephrine drip. As noted above, the ET tube was pulled back with improved breath sounds. The patient received 40 ml/kg of *warmed* IV fluids and 10 mL/kg of pRBCs. Return of spontaneous circulation (ROSC) was achieved about 15 minutes after his arrival to the ED. His temperature at the time of ROSC was 28.8 °C (83.8 °F), which was lower than his initial presenting temperature.

Update 2/Rewarming Efforts In addition to the resuscitation listed above, active rewarming was initiated in the ED. This included the following:

- Removal of wet clothing
- Application of warm blankets
- Ceiling warmers (convection heating)
- Forced-air blanket placed on the patient
- Warmed saline via IV boluses
- Foley catheter placed with bladder lavage with *warmed* fluid (10 mL NS/kg ×3)
- Chest tubes were placed. 2 chest tubes were placed on the right side, a lower argyle chest tube and an upper pigtail. 3 L of *warmed* saline, in 1 L increments, were placed via the pigtail and drained through the argyle chest tube. One chest tube was placed on the left and approximately 150 mL of *warmed* fluid was instilled via the left chest tube.

Update 3

The patient was transferred to the Pediatric Intensive Care Unit (PICU). In the PICU, a femoral central line was placed. The patient was placed on temperature-regulating equipment through his femoral line which can allow for controlled rewarming. The patient's temperature gradually improved.

Learning Points: Pediatric Drowning

Priming Questions
1. What are some of the complications of drowning that you have to worry about in the ED?
2. How is this diagnosis made, and what roles do laboratory and imaging studies play (blood gas, CXR, decision to admit/transfer)?
3. What variables have shown to affect patient outcomes in drowning?
4. What are some of the treatments for hypothermia that can be initiated in the Emergency Department?

Introduction/Background

1. There has been a national campaign in part through the CDC and American Academy of Pediatrics to increase awareness of pediatric drowning. Much has been publicized on drowning prevention strategies such as increased supervision, CPR teaching to parents, installing pool fences, and wearing life jackets around lakes or the ocean even for experienced swimmers [1, 2].
2. Across the United States approximately 3 children die every day from unintentional drowning, and drownings are a leading cause of death for children age 1–14. For every death, 5 more children are treated in EDs for non-fatal drowning injuries [1].
3. Drowning is defined as "a process resulting in primary respiratory impairment from submersion/immersion in a liquid medium." This is the term that should be used regardless of outcome and regardless of chronicity of symptoms. "Drowning" should be broadly applied and should replace other terms such as "near drowning," "wet drowning," "dry drowning," and "secondary drowning." [3]

Physiology/Pathophysiology

1. Drowning is first and foremost a hypoxic event. This can be secondary to a few processes such as laryngospasm, apnea, and/or aspiration. Those who suffer cardiac arrest at the primary event of drowning likely have suffered a fatal arrhythmia as a result of the hypoxia, hypercarbia, and acidosis.

2. Many of the complications from drowning are due to both the initial hypoxic-ischemic insult and reperfusion injuries after rescue [3].
   - Lung injury – often caused by abnormal surfactant function and increased capillary endothelial permeability [3].
     - This can lead to pulmonary edema, ventilation/perfusion mismatch, atelectasis, poor compliance, and acute respiratory distress syndrome (ARDS) [3].
     - Aspiration of fresh water vs salt water was classically taught to result in varying electrolyte abnormalities; however, this has recently been questioned and the salinity of the water is now thought to be of little to any clinical significance [3].
   - Shock – This can be caused by a combination of decreased oxygenation of the blood and severe myocardial dysfunction [4]. Hypothermia can also contribute to this state of poor tissue perfusion.
   - Hypoxic brain injury – irreversible central nervous system (CNS) damage begins after 4–6 minutes of hypoxia [4].
3. Patients should also be evaluated for traumatic injuries, as these can be the inciting event which caused the drowning to occur.

Making the Diagnosis

Differential Diagnosis
- Pneumonia
- ARDS
- Asthma Attack
- Heart Failure
- Flash Pulmonary Edema

1. This diagnosis is generally readily apparent from the history, but identifying the degree of injury from a drowning relies heavily on the physical exam.
   - Respiratory rate, respiratory effort, oxygen saturation, pulmonary exam, and mental status are going to provide key information about whether or not the patient has suffered injury from an aspiration event. Vital sign values and mental status should be analyzed in the context of age-appropriate parameters.
   - Lung injury from drowning typically occurs relatively quickly, within 6 to 8 hours of the event [3].
     - Patients without vital sign or physical exam abnormalities can typically be observed for 6–12 hours. If no vital sign abnormalities or significant respiratory distress occurs, they do not always require admission to the hospital and can be discharged from the Emergency Department following their observation period [3, 4].

- As some of the processes which lead to pulmonary dysfunction can take a few hours to fully manifest, it is certainly possible to have a patient with mild to moderate symptoms who then decompensates, which is why it is generally recommended that moderately symptomatic patients be admitted for prolonged observation. This process is what some in the lay community may refer to as "secondary drowning." As above, however, it is exceedingly rare for patients to decompensate after being completely asymptomatic with a normal exam, work up, and brief observation period.
- Common tests to help assist with the identification of a lung injury is a chest radiograph and a blood gas. However, radiographic changes may not be apparent until 6–8 hours after the injury.
- Cardiac and pulse oximetry monitoring should be provided for all patients while being evaluated.

Treating the Patient

1. Initial resuscitative efforts should focus on correcting hypoxia. This is one circumstance where the previously recommended ABC approach to resuscitation remains valid in both pediatrics and adults. This is not to say that drowning victims should not receive chest compressions or be assessed for arrhythmias, but rather that the priority should be on airway management, even in the setting of cardiac arrest. Of note, the Heimlich maneuver and other procedures to remove fluid from the lungs are not recommended. Not only are they ineffective, but they delay time to definitive treatment and they can cause vomiting and subsequent aspiration of gastric contents [3].
2. Treatment for symptomatic patients not in cardiac arrest is largely supportive to ensure they continue to be able to oxygenate and ventilate. These therapies can include supplemental oxygen, noninvasive positive pressure ventilation (NIPPV), invasive ventilator support, extracorporeal membrane oxygenation (ECMO), and/or inotropic support as needed.
3. Antibiotics can be used if there is a concern that pneumonia is worsening the patient's ARDS. Fresh water and salt water aspirations are at risk for developing a pneumonia. However, routine antibiotic administration in the emergency department is not advised [3].
4. Steroids and/or aerosol treatments such as albuterol are not typically indicated acutely for drowning-induced lung disease [3].
5. Prognostic factors
   - Patient outcomes typically depend on a number of factors – age, EMS response time, duration of immersion, type of water, water temperature, witnessed drowning, resuscitation, and degree of pulmonary involvement [3, 5, 6].
   - Favorable outcomes have been seen in shorter EMS response times and in salt water, when compared to fresh water [5, 7–13].

- In regards to hypothermic drownings, those with severe hypothermia often do better. Children also have better outcomes in hypothermic drownings when compared to adults.
- Effective and immediate CPR was the single most important factor in survival and positive neurologic outcomes in hypothermic drownings [11, 14, 15].
- The most common instances of a miraculous survival with good neurologic recovery following a submersion injury occurred in small children who were submerged in icy water with rapid hypothermia prior to hypoxia. Researchers hypothesize that these favorable outcomes are due to the larger body surface area in small children inducing more rapid cooling [12, 16–24].

6. Treatment of Hypothermic Drownings
   - It is important to clarify that hypothermia can be a complication of drowning in any water temperature below the normal body temperature. Victims who drown in warmer temperatures that become hypothermic often have worse outcomes because hypothermia is often associated with longer submersion times [3, 4].
   - There are many different treatment options for rewarming a drowning victim who has hypothermia. The degree of hypothermia and a patient's overall prognosis should be considered when choosing which warming modality to implement.

Type of rewarming	Definition	Rewarming rate (°C/F per hour)	Notes/complications
Passive rewarming	Allowing the patient's body to rewarm itself Mitigating causes of hypothermia, i.e., removal of the patient's wet clothing	0.5–4°C (0.9–7.2°F)	Best for mildly hypothermic patients
Passive rewarming with activity	Using movement of the patient's body to increase temperature	1–5°C (1.8–9°F)	May increase afterdrop
Active external rewarming	External surface rewarming by forced air assistive heating devices, warm blankets, bags of warm fluids to axilla and groin	0.5–4°C (0.9–7.2°F)	Only rewarms patient's surface May increase afterdrop
Bladder lavage	Warmed fluid flushes into the patient's bladder	Variable 0.5–1°C (0.9–1.8°F)	Small surface area, catheterization may be difficult in some patients
Gastric lavage	Warmed fluid flushes into the patient's stomach via NG/OG	0.5–1°C (0.9–1.8°F)	Potential for aspiration and electrolyte or fluid imbalance
Thoracic or peritoneal lavage	Warmed fluid via chest tubes or catheters into patient's thoracic or peritoneal cavities	1–2°C (1.8–3.6°F)	Potential hemorrhage, trauma to organs, electrolyte or fluid imbalance. – thoracic may impair CPR quality
Intravascular catheter rewarming	Central venous catheter that has temperature probe that warms blood as it is pumped passed probe	Device specific: 0.5–2.5°C (0.9–4.5°F)	Potential for hemorrhage, thrombus, or may worsen hypotension
ECMO	Circulatory and/or ventilator support	4–10°C (7.2–18°F)	Most invasive with possible complications of hemorrhage, thrombosis, hemolysis

Adapted from *Accidental hypothermia- an update* [25]

- Afterdrop is the process of heat redistribution within the body that leads to further decrease in core body temperatures following rewarming attempts. That is, despite active rewarming attempts as cold blood is redistributed from the extremities to the core, measured body temperature may initially decline, then increase as above. Afterdrop may lead to increased complications including a higher risk for cardiac arrest as cold blood is shunted to vital organs [25–28].
- The risk of cardiac arrest increases as a patient's core temperature decreases to below 32 °C (89.6°F). However, cardiac arrest is unlikely to be due solely to hypothermia until the temperature is <28 °C (82.4°F) and alternative causes, such as hypoxia or hypovolemia, should be considered [25, 29, 30]. Some patients can still have vital signs at <24 °C (75.2°F) [25, 29, 30]. At 18°C (64.4°F) the brain tolerates cardiac arrest for up to 10 times longer than at 37 °C (98.6°F) [25].
- The American Heart Association guidelines allow additional defibrillation attempts concurrent with rewarming strategies and state that it may be reasonable to consider epinephrine administration during cardiac arrest according to the standard ALS algorithm [31].
- ECMO can be considered as a therapy for hypothermic cardiac arrest or signs of imminent cardiac arrest.
- Risk factors for imminent cardiac arrest include temperature < 28 °C (82.4°F), ventricular arrhythmia, systolic blood pressure < 90 mmHg, and those who have already arrested [25].

Case Conclusion

The patient was placed on veno-arterial (VA) ECMO on hospital day (HOD) 2 for 9 days. He was bridged from ECMO to continuous renal replacement therapies (CRRT) for 3 days. He ended up with 5 different chest tubes due to a multitude of reasons (including resuscitation and pneumothoraces). He had a bronchoscopy on HOD 4 that showed copious thin secretions, concerning for alveolar hemorrhage. He was extubated on HOD 21 and weaned to room air on HOD 30. He was then sent to inpatient rehab on HOD 37. He was discharged home on HOD 74. He has some minor deficits requiring wrist splints and is still receiving physical, occupational, and speech therapy, but the patient can speak in full sentences and ambulate without assistance.

Case Discussion

Although many pediatric patients may be evaluated in the ED for possible drowning, severe disease is rare. When assessing a drowning patient the most important diagnostic and prognostic factors are vital signs and exam changes. While a chest X-ray or ABG may be helpful, these are preceded by exam changes and abnormalities on diagnostic testing may not be apparent for 6–8 hours following the initial event. While hypothermia is often a protective factor, a drowning patient's rewarming should be initiated in the ED. Care must be taken to lessen the afterdrop phenomenon, and the type of rewarming should be based on the patient's severity of illness and overall prognosis. For patients with minimal symptoms, if there are no exam changes or testing abnormalities after an observation period of at least 6–8 hours they may be discharged from the ED. The primary treatment in the ED of a drowning patient is supportive care. The overall primary treatment for drowning is prevention through pool and water safety education, including encouraging early bystander CPR and rapid mobilization of EMS.

Pattern Recognition

Drowning
- Progressively worsening respiratory symptoms after a drowning event
- Hypothermia
- Hypoxia and impaired ventilation
- Pulmonary edema on chest X-ray

Disclosure Statement The authors of this chapter report no significant disclosures.

References

1. Centers for Disease Control and Prevention, National Center for Injury Prevention and Control, Division of Unintentional Injury Prevention. Drowning Prevention. 2016; https://www.cdc.gov/safechild/drowning/index.html.
2. American Academy of Pediatrics, Committee on Injury, Violence, and Poison Prevention. Policy Statement- Prevention of Drowning. Pediatrics. 2010;126:1: 1–8.
3. Meyer RJ, Theodorou AA, Berg RA. Childhood drowning. Pediatr Rev. 2006;27:163–9. https://doi.org/10.1542/pir.27-5-163.
4. Seeyave DM, Brown KN. Environmental emergencies, radiological emergencies, bites and stings. In: Shaw K, Bachur R, editors. Fleisher & Ludwig's textbook of pediatric emergency medicine. 7th ed. Philadelphia: Wolters Kluwer; 2016. p. 718–60.
5. Quan L, et al. Predicting outcome of drowning at the scene: a systematic review and meta-analyses. Resuscitation. 2016;104:63–75.
6. Claesson A, Lindqvist J, Ortenwall P, Herlitz J. Characteristics of lifesaving from drowning as reported by the Swedish Fire and Rescue Services 1996–2010. Resuscitation. 2012;83:1072–7.
7. Dyson K, Morgans A, Bray J, Matthews B, Smith K. Drowning related out-of-hospital cardiac arrests: characteristics and outcomes. Resuscitation. 2013;84:1114–8.
8. Blasco Alonso J, Moreno Perez D, Milano Manso G, Calvo Marcias C, Jurado Ortiz A. Drowning in pediatric patients. An Pediatr (Barc). 2005;62:20–4.
9. Mizuta R, Fujita H, Osamura T, Kidowaki T, Kiyosawa N. Childhood drownings and near-drownings in Japan. Acta Paediatr Jpn. 1993;35:186–92.
10. Orlowski JP. Prognostic factors in pediatric cases of drowning and neardrowning. JACEP. 1979;8:176–9.

11. Quan L, Mack CD, Schiff MA. Association of water temperature and submersion duration and drowning outcome. Resuscitation. 2014;85:790–4.
12. Bierens J, van der Velde EA, van Berkel M, zan Zanten JJ. Submersion cases in the Netherlands: prognostic indicators and results of resuscitations. Ann Emerg Med. 1990;19:1390–5.
13. Forler J, Carsin A, Arlaud K, et al. Respiratory complications of accidental drownings in children. Arch Pediatr. 2010;17:14–8.
14. Suominen PK, Korpela RE, Silfvast TGO, Olkkola KT. Does water temperature affect outcome of nearly drowned children. Resuscitation. 1997;35:111–5.
15. Cummings P. Methods for estimating adjusted risk ratios. Stata J. 2009;9:175–96.
16. Avramidis S, Butterly R. Drowning survival in icy water: a review. Int J Aquatic Res Educ. 2008;2(4):Article 8. https://doi.org/10.25035/ijare.02.04.08.
17. Antretter H, Muller LC, Cottogni M, Dapunt OE. Successful resuscitation in severe hypothermia following near-drowning. Dtsch Med Wochenschr. 1994;119:837–40.
18. Biggart MJ, Bohn DJ. Effect of hypothermia and cardiac arrest on outcome of near-drowning accidents in children. J Pediatr. 1990;117(2 Pt 1):179–83.
19. Fretschner R, Kloss T, Borowczak C, Berkel H. First aid and prognosis following drowning accidents: results of a retrospective study of 115 cases. Anasthesiologie, Intensivmedizin, Notfallmedizin, Schmerztherapie. 1993;28:363–8.
20. Kemp AM, Sibert JR. Outcome in children who nearly drown: a British Isles study. Br Med J. 1991;302:931–3.
21. Kyriacou DN, Arcinue EL, Peek C, Kraus JF. Effect of immediate resuscitation on children with submersion injury. Pediatrics. 1994;94(2 Pt 1):137–42.
22. Estebe JP, Kabura L, Miorcec de Kerdanet M, Betremieux P, Malledant Y. Hypothermia helps in the drowned child: report of a case. Annales de Pediatrie. 1991;38:476–8.
23. Fritz KW, Kasperczyk W, Galaske R. Successful resuscitation in accidental hypothermia following drowning. Anaesthesist. 1988;37:331–4.
24. Leitz KH, Tsilimingas N, Guse HG, Meier P, Bachmann HJ. Accidental drowning with extreme hypothermia- rewarming with extracorporeal circulation. Der Chirurg Zeitschrift fur alle Gebiete der Operativen Medizen. 1989;60:352–5.
25. Paal P, et al. Accidental hypothermia–an update: the content of this review is endorsed by the International Commission for Mountain Emergency Medicine (ICAR MEDCOM). Scand J Trauma Resusc Emerg Med. 2016;24:111. https://doi.org/10.1186/s13049-016-0303-7.
26. Hayward JS, Eckerson JD, Kemna D. Thermal and cardiovascular changes during three methods of resuscitation from mild hypothermia. Resuscitation. 1984;11(1–2):21–33.
27. Giesbrecht GG, Bristow GK. The convective afterdrop component during hypothermic exercise decreases with delayed exercise onset. Aviat Space Environ Med. 1998;69(1):17–22. 108.
28. Giesbrecht GG, Bristow GK. A second postcooling afterdrop: more evidence for a convective mechanism. J Appl Physiol. 1992;73(4):1253–8.
29. Pasquier M, Zurron N, Weith B, Turini P, Dami F, Carron PN, et al. Deep accidental hypothermia with core temperature below 24° c presenting with vital signs. High Alt Med Biol. 2014;15(1):58–63. https://doi.org/10.1089/ham.2013.1085.
30. Anderson S, Herbring BG, Widman B. Accidental profound hypothermia. Br J Anaesth. 1970;42(7):653–5. 233.
31. AHA, Vanden Hoek TL, Morrison LJ, Shuster M, Donnino M, Sinz E, Lavonas EJ, et al. Part 12: cardiac arrest in special situations: 2010 American Heart Association Guidelines for Cardiopulmonary Resuscitation and Emergency Cardiovascular Care. Circulation. 2010;122(18 Suppl 3):S829–61. https://doi.org/10.1161/CIRCULATIONAHA.110.971069.

Pneumothorax: *"Hmmm, I Guess Dr. Heimlich Had More Than One Maneuver!"*

49

Christine Luo and Andrew King

Case 1

Pertinent History

The patient is an 18-year-old male who presents to the emergency department with right-sided chest pain. He states that he was simply watching a soccer game when he developed acute onset right-sided chest pain. The pain radiates into his back and is worse with breathing and coughing. It is not exacerbated by movement, and he has no recollection of any muscular injury. The pain was accompanied by dyspnea. He has had no preceding illnesses or similar symptoms in the past.

Pertinent Physical Exam

Except as noted below, the findings of the complete physical exam are within normal limits.

- Vitals: Blood pressure 156/71, pulse 82, temperature 98.1 °F (36.7 °C), respiratory rate 22, SpO_2 100%. SpO_2 desaturates to 90% while speaking.
- Constitutional: Appears uncomfortable while seated. Tall, thin body habitus.
- HEENT: No stridor.
- Cardiovascular: Normal rate and regular rhythm. 2+ radial and dorsalis pedis pulses bilaterally.

C. Luo · A. King (✉)
Department of Emergency Medicine, Wexner Medical Center at The Ohio State University, Columbus, OH, USA
e-mail: Andrew.king3@osumc.edu

© Springer Nature Switzerland AG 2020
C. G. Kaide, C. E. San Miguel (eds.), *Case Studies in Emergency Medicine*,
https://doi.org/10.1007/978-3-030-22445-5_49

- Pulmonary/Chest: No significant respiratory distress. No use of accessory muscles during respiration. Mildly diminished breath sounds on right. No wheezes, rhonchi, rales. No chest wall tenderness or crepitus on palpation.
- Extremities: No peripheral edema noted.

Past Medical and Surgical History

Unremarkable and non-contributory aside from a penicillin allergy.

Social History

The patient recently started college and has been training daily with the college water polo team. He has been exposed to tobacco smoke since a young age, but he denies tobacco, alcohol, and illicit drug use.

Family History

Both the patient's father and cousin have previously required hospitalizations for "tubes in the chest."

Pertinent Test Results

An ECG showed normal sinus rhythm with no evidence of ischemic changes.

The chest X-ray demonstrates a right-sided pneumothorax.

ED Management

The emergency department physician placed an 8 French catheter-style chest tube complete with Heimlich valve. The patient remained in the emergency department for further observation following the placement of the catheter.

Case 2

Pertinent History

A 63-year-old male presents to the emergency department after a motor vehicle accident. The patient was an unrestrained driver in a head-on collision at moderate speed. On presentation, the patient complained of sharp, unrelenting left-sided chest pain. EMS reports that the patient's breathing became much more labored since their initial evaluation. The patient had no loss of consciousness and reports no additional complaints or injuries.

Pertinent Physical Exam

Except as noted below, the findings of the complete physical exam are within normal limits.

- Vitals: Blood pressure 82/50, pulse 115, temperature 99.3 °F (37.4 °C), respiratory rate 42, SpO2 92% on non-rebreather mask.
- Constitutional: Appears in significant respiratory distress.
- HEENT: No stridor. There was evidence of jugular venous distension and tracheal deviation on examination.
- Cardiovascular: Tachycardic and regular rhythm. 2+ radial and dorsalis pedis pulses bilaterally.
- Pulmonary/Chest: Severe respiratory distress. Diminished breath sounds on the left with obvious signs of chest trauma.

Past Medical and Surgical History

The patient has a history of COPD, and type 2 diabetes mellitus for which he takes metformin and multiple inhaled medications. The patient continues to smoke and uses alcohol socially. The remainder of his history is non-contributory.

Pertinent Test Results

An ECG revealed sinus tachycardia with no acute ischemic changes. The treatment team performed a bedside ultrasound to assess for pneumothorax. The first ultrasound image of the right lung shows normal lung sliding with the normal appearance of the "seashore" sign on M-mode. The second ultrasound image shows the left lung and the presence of a pneumothorax. There is absent lung sliding as evidenced by the "bar-code" sign on M-mode.

ED Management

The team of emergency physicians quickly identified tension pneumothorax pathology, and a 14-gauge angiocatheter was placed in the left second to third intercostal space in the mid-clavicular line for immediate decompression. Upon completion of the initial trauma survey, a 36 French chest tube was placed in the fifth intercostal space in the mid-axillary line. The chest tube was placed to water seal and vacuum.

Learning Points

Priming Questions
1. What is a pneumothorax?
2. How are pneumothoraces classified?
3. What conditions predispose patients to develop pneumothoraces?
4. What management options are present for pneumothoraces?
5. Are there outpatient options available for pneumothorax treatment?

Introduction/Background

1. What is a pneumothorax?
   - A pneumothorax occurs when air becomes trapped between the visceral and parietal pleura. This may occur due to compromise of either pleural membrane.
2. Pneumothorax Classification:
   - A pneumothorax can be spontaneous, traumatic or iatrogenic in etiology. Spontaneous pneumothoraces are further categorized as primary or secondary.
     - Primary spontaneous pneumothoraces occur in patients without clinically apparent lung disease (often young, tall men, aged 20–40 years, who usually smoke). Of note, the onset of a primary pneumothorax has not been correlated with physical activity and muscle effort [1].
     - Secondary pneumothoraxes are a complication of preexisting underlying pulmonary disease, trauma or medical treatment.
       Underlying pulmonary diseases such as COPD, pneumonia particularly *Pneumocystis jiroveci* pneumonia, cystic fibrosis, asthma, and tuberculosis can be predisposing factors.
     - Traumatic pneumothorax can be due to either blunt or penetrating chest trauma.
     - Iatrogenic pneumothorax may occur during subclavian or internal jugular line placement, thoracentesis, or following lung or pleural biopsy. A pneumothorax may also result from barotrauma during positive pressure ventilation.
   - Pneumothorax Size Classification:
     - By the British Medical Society definition, a large pneumothorax is differentiated from a small pneumothorax by measuring greater than 2cm from the lung margin to the chest wall at the level of the hilum. Although subject to multiple limitations including pneumothorax localization and lung shape, the 2cm guideline is thought to estimate a 50% pneumothorax by volume [2].

3. Incidence:
   - Primary spontaneous pneumothorax has been estimated to have an incidence of 7.4 and 1.2 per 100,000 per annum for males and females, respectively. Likewise, the incidence of secondary spontaneous pneumothorax has been estimated to be 6.3/100,000 per annum for males and 2.0/1000,000 per annum for females [3]. In a United Kingdom study, emergency hospital admissions for pneumothorax were 16.7 and 5.8 per 100,000 per year for men and women, respectively [4].

Physiology/Pathophysiology

1. Lung Anatomy
   - A membranous lining, the visceral pleura, encases the lung parenchyma and continues on to line the chest wall, as the parietal pleura. The potential space between the visceral and parietal pleura is the pleural space.
   - Under homeostatic conditions, a small amount (5-15mL) of fluid is secreted between visceral and parietal pleura into the pleural space and no air or gas is present [5]. This pleural fluid lubricates and facilitates the sliding of the visceral and parietal pleura against each other during respiration.
2. Development of the pneumothorax
   - Air enters the pleural space when either the visceral or parietal pleura are compromised or when gas-producing organisms invade [6].
   - The pathogenesis of spontaneous pneumothorax is unclear at this time. Rupture of an underlying subpleural bleb or bulla has been considered. Taller individuals may be predisposed to apical subpleural bleb development due to a larger increasing gradient of negative pleural pressure from the lung base to apices and subsequent increased apical alveolar distension. However, other lesions of "pleural porosity," such as a more porous inflammatory fibroelastic layer replacing the visceral pleural mesothelium, may contribute to the development of the spontaneous pneumothorax [6].
3. Tension pneumothorax
   - When increasing amounts of air become trapped in the pleural space, increasing pressure is exerted on the lung parenchyma and mediastinal structures, leading to hemodynamic instability. This is known as a tension pneumothorax. Lung compression leads to increasing lung atelectasis and vascular shunting. Deviation of mediastinal structures can cause decreased vena caval filling and decreased cardiac output [7].
   - Positive pressure ventilation can worsen any pneumothorax.
     - During positive pressure ventilation, intrapleural pressure continuously increases during all phases of respiration as positive pressure forces air through a given defect and into the pleural space [8].

Making the Diagnosis

Differential Diagnosis
- Cardiac tamponade
- Acute coronary syndrome
- Aortic dissection
- Pericarditis
- Pneumonia
- Hemothorax
- Diaphragm rupture

1. Clinical Symptoms
   - Sudden onset dyspnea and chest pain are common symptoms associated with the development of a pneumothorax. The larger the pneumothorax, the more likely the patient is symptomatic.
   - Physical exam:
     In a systematic review of clinical symptoms for tension pneumothorax, over 20% of patients with unassisted breathing presented with [8]:
     - Respiratory distress
     - Tachypnea (Respiratory rate ≥20)
     - SpO2 <92%
     - Hyperresonance upon percussion
     - Decreased air movement on auscultation
     - Tachycardia
     In the same study, over 20% of patients on assisted ventilation presented with [8]:
     - Subcutaneous emphysema
     - Decreased air entry on auscultation
     - Tachycardia
     - Hypotension
     - Cardiac arrest
   - Tension pneumothorax is a clinical diagnosis and treatment should not be delayed for imaging confirmation.
2. Imaging
   - Computed tomography (CT) is considered the reference or gold standard for pneumothorax identification [9, 10]. However, patients may not be stable enough to transport for CT scanning. Alternative options include chest X-ray and bedside ultrasound (US). Many studies comparing chest X-ray and ultrasound for pneumothorax detection have generally noted ultrasound to be more sensitive than chest X-ray [9].
   - Chest X-ray
     - A pneumothorax can be identified on a chest X-ray by the displacement of the visceral pleural margin away from the chest wall and a lack of

pulmonary markings between the margin and the chest wall. The lateral decubitus view is the most sensitive followed by a chest X-ray in the erect position; the supine view is least sensitive [9].

- Ultrasound
  - The patient is usually moved into a supine or semi-upright position. Air is expected to rise to the anterior chest. The linear ultrasound probe is then placed over the intercostal space and perpendicular to the rib margins [10].
  - On ultrasound, normal lung sliding, which occurs when the visceral pleura moves against the parietal pleura, will form a shimmering pleural line as noted in Fig 49.2. When viewed under M-mode, the nonmoving chest wall in the near field forms horizontal lines and the far field deep to the sliding pleura will form a grained image, also known as the **seashore sign**. Lung sliding rules out a pneumothorax at the scanned area with 100% sensitivity [9].
  - If a pneumothorax is present, the air between the parietal and visceral pleura scatters the sound waves. Thus, no shimmering pleural line will be seen and on M-mode horizontal lines representing the nonmoving chest wall structure in the near fields will again be seen; however, the far field deep to the parietal pleura will also appear nonmoving and will be represented also by horizontal lines on M-mode. This forms the **barcode sign** as seen in Figure 49.3. It should be noted that any pathology which prevents aeration of the lung, such as airway obstruction or mainstem intubation of the contralateral bronchus, can preclude lung sliding and will resemble a pneumothorax on ultrasound [10, 12].

Fig. 49.1 Chest X-ray indicating a right sided pneumothorax

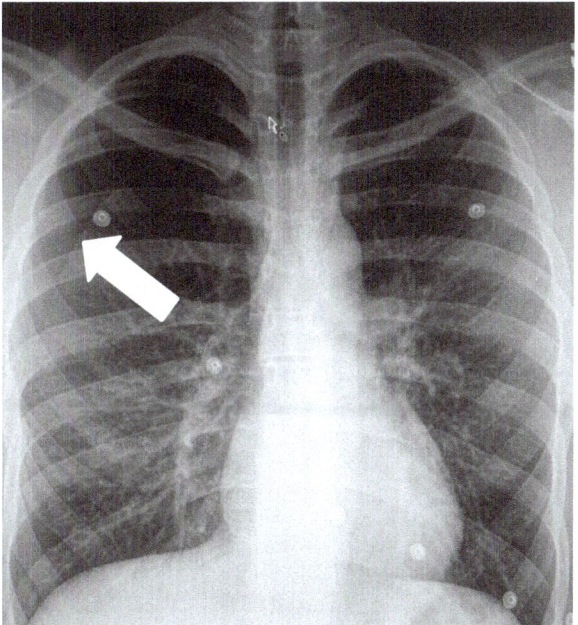

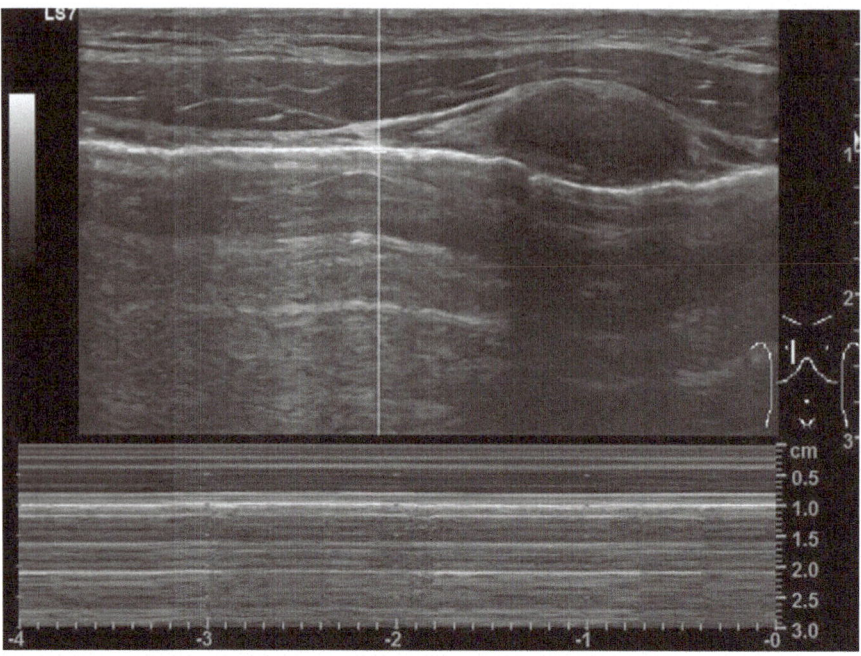

Fig. 49.2 Normal lung ultrasound - seashore sign

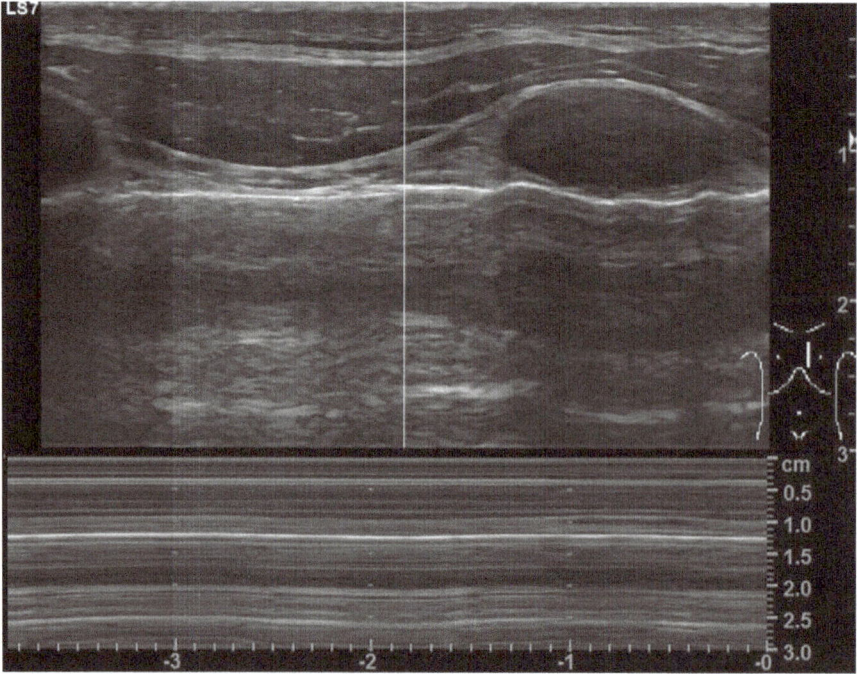

Fig. 49.3 Pneumothorax on lung ultrasound - barcode sign

- The **lung point sign** occurs at the interface between the pneumothorax and normal lung sliding. When the lung point is viewed under M-mode, juxtaposition of the barcode and seashore signs will be seen [10, 12].

Treating the Patient

1. Tension Pneumothorax
   - Patients who are exhibiting signs of tension pneumothorax, most notably hypotension and tachycardia, require immediate decompression. Traditionally, it was taught that an angiocatheter should be inserted into the 2nd or 3rd rib space on the mid-clavicular line. However, some experts are now recommending that the decompression take place along the anterior or mid axillary lines at the 4th or 5th intercostal spaces, arguing that body habitus limits access to the chest cavity from the mid-clavicular line. Others advocate for a finger thoracostomy procedure whereby a scalpel is used to access the intercostal space and either a finger or another blunt instrument is used to puncture through the pleura. There are pro's and con's to each technique, but in the moment you need to evacuate air from the chest cavity as quickly as you can, any way that you can.
2. Traumatic Pneumothorax
   - Many traumatic pneumothoraces need standard chest tube drainage. Among other reasons is the risk of concurrent hemothorax and the need to drain that as well. There is considerable debate however on how best to treat "occult pneumothoraces," those seen on CT scan of the chest, but not xray. A recent retrospective study found that 91% of pneumothoraces less than 35 mm in size which were originally treated conservatively without drainage, did not require any subsequent drainage [11].
3. Small Primary Pneumothorax
   - A small primary pneumothorax will usually resolve without treatment. Supplemental oxygen increases the rate of reabsorption slightly and is appropriate during a short period of observation in the emergency department.
   - Patients may also be treated with a small-bore catheter attached to a Heimlich valve. Normal respiration and coughing are often sufficient to create the pressure needed to remove the excess air from the pleural space, and the lung will then expand. The Heimlich valve does not require suction and has been used for outpatient therapy. You can place a catheter thoracostomy in the 4th or 5th intercostal space, in the anterior or mid axillary line, like a standard chest tube. The 5th intercostal space roughly corresponds with the same height as the nipple. This is an alternative location to the placement in the second intercostal space and it is equally effective. The end of the catheter is then attached to the Heimlich valve. Be sure it is oriented to allow air out of the chest but not back in. The direction of the air is usually indicated by an arrow.
     - Indications for outpatient management
       A stable primary spontaneous pneumothorax
       Close apposition of the lung to the lateral chest wall with initial thoracentesis and aspiration and drainage procedures

 Physician satisfaction with the position of the catheter
 An air leak that is manageable with one thoracentesis
- Contraindications for outpatient management
 Traumatic pneumothoraxes
 Secondary pneumothoraxes
 A patient with poor residual function
 A large air leak requiring tube thoracostomy
 A hemothorax
 Unacceptable residual collapse defined as poor apposition of the lateral lung to the lateral chest wall
 If the patient is not reliable
- Bring the patient back to the ED to have a follow-up X-ray in 2–3 days. If the lung is up, pull the tube.
- Sometimes the process does not fix the pneumothorax…but most often it does! Any chance to NOT have a huge tube in your chest with a 3-day hospitalization is a good thing!
- If the lung fails to re-expand after 24–48 hours then a 24F–28F standard chest tube attached to the water seal will be required.
- Simple aspiration of the pneumothorax is another option. A Cochrane review comparing it to large chest tube insertion found that aspiration had a higher fail rate but led to shorter hospital stays and possibly fewer adverse events [12].
4. Large, Secondary, or Symptomatic Pneumothorax
- Patients with secondary pneumothorax in general, will require standard chest tube drainage with a water seal device and admission to the hospital. The underlying illness often requires additional intervention such as antibiotics, surgery, or additional diagnostic evaluation.

NOTE: Many patients will experience pain as the lung begins to re-expand. Sometimes they feel like they have to cough excessively. This is commonly seen as the lung expands.

Case Conclusion

The patient in Case 1 was observed in the emergency department for 6 hours. A repeat chest X-ray revealed complete re-inflation of the lung. The patient was discharged with the Heimlich valve in place, and upon follow-up with thoracic surgery in 48 hours, the catheter was removed without complication. The patient in Case 2 was admitted to the surgical intensive care for a 24-hour period due to his tension pneumothorax. Aside from rib fractures, the patient had no additional injury. The chest tube was pulled when breathing status improved and the lung achieved adequate re-inflation.

Discussion

1. Tension pneumothorax with hemodynamic instability, jugular venous distension, and tracheal deviation is a medical emergency. This must be both recognized and treated with either an anterior needle decompression, axillary decompression, or finger thoracostomy without waiting for imaging.
2. Many treatment options exist for the management of simple, non-traumatic pneumothoraces. The appropriate treatment is typically dictated by the patient, size of the pneumothorax, and the degree of pain and distress.
3. Patients presenting to the emergency department with a pneumothorax CAN be safely discharged from the ED after a successful aspiration or with a Heimlich valve in place.

Pattern Recognition

Pneumothorax
- Chest pain
- Shortness of breath
- Decreased breath sounds
- Hypoxia
- Hypotension
- Jugular venous distension

Disclosure Statement   The authors of this chapter report no significant disclosures.

References

1. Bense L, et al. Onset of symptoms in spontaneous pneumothorax: correlations to physical activity. Eur J Respir Dis. 1987;71(3):181–6.
2. MacDuff A, et al. Management of spontaneous pneumothorax: British Thoracic Society pleural disease guideline 2010. Thorax. 2010;65(Suppl 2):ii18–31.
3. Melton LJ, et al. Incidence of spontaneous pneumothorax in Olmsted County. Minnesota. p. 1950 to 1974.
4. Gupta D, et al. Epidemiology of pneumothorax in England. Thorax. 2000;55:666–71.
5. Cafarotti S, Condoluci A, Inderbitzi R. Physiology and pathophysiology of the pleura In: Kiefer T, editor. Chest drains in daily clinical practice. Cham: Springer; 2017.
6. Noppen M. Spontaneous pneumothorax: epidemiology, pathophysiology and cause. Eur Respir Rev. 2010;19(117):217–9.
7. Walls RM, et al. Rosens emergency medicine: concepts and clinical practice. Philadelphia, PA: Elsevier; 2018.
8. Roberts DJ, et al. Clinical presentation of patients with tension pneumothorax. Ann Surg. 2015;261(6):1068–78.

9. Jalli R, et al. Value of ultrasound in diagnosis of pneumothorax: a prospective study. Emerg Radiol. 2013;20:131–4.
10. Husain LF, et al. Sonographic diagnosis of pneumothorax. J Emerg Trauma Shock. 2012;5(1):76–81.
11. Eddine SBZ, Boyle KA, Dodgion CM, et al. Observing pneumothoraces. J Trauma Acute Care Surg. 2019;1
12. Carson-Chahhoud KV, Wakai A, van Agteren JEM, Smith BJ, McCabe G, Brinn MP, O'Sullivan R. Simple aspiration versus intercostal tube drainage for primary spontaneous pneumothorax in adults. Cochrane Database Syst Rev 2017, Issue 9. Art. No.: CD004479. DOI: https://doi.org/10.1002/14651858.CD004479.pub3.

Peripartum Cardiomyopathy. *"Babies Are Breaking My Heart!"*

50

Meenal Sharkey and Natasha Boydstun

Case

Postpartum Shortness of Breath

Pertinent History

A 32-year-old female presents to the Emergency Department (ED) via ambulance after feeling short of breath and lightheaded. She did not feel comfortable driving. She reports she has had shortness of breath for the last 2 weeks with a dry cough. She is 3 weeks status post an uncomplicated vaginal delivery. She has had lower extremity edema for the past 2 months, but it has worsened in the past 2 weeks. She denies chest pain but has had some lightheadedness. She has not had any syncope, fevers, chills, or leg pain. Her pregnancy was overall uneventful; however, she did have worsening of her chronic hypertension that required hydralazine. She was induced at 40 weeks gestation and successfully delivered a healthy baby girl.

The original version of this chapter was revised. An correction to this chapter can be found at https://doi.org/10.1007/978-3-030-22445-5_68

M. Sharkey (✉)
USACS, Canton, OH, USA

Doctors Hospital Emergency Department, Columbus, OH, USA
e-mail: msharkey@usacs.com

N. Boydstun
Doctors Hospital Emergency Department, Columbus, OH, USA

PGY4, Emergency Medicine Resident, Columbus, OH, USA
e-mail: natasha.boydstun@ohiohealth.com

© Springer Nature Switzerland AG 2020
C. G. Kaide, C. E. San Miguel (eds.), *Case Studies in Emergency Medicine*,
https://doi.org/10.1007/978-3-030-22445-5_50

Past Medical History

1. Hypertension.
2. Three weeks post-partum

Past Surgical History
None

Medications
Hydralazine

Allergies
No known drug allergies (NKDA)

Family History
Noncontributory

Social History
She denies drinking alcohol and using tobacco products.

Physical Exam

- Vitals: HR 118, RR 22, BP 99/40, SpO2 88% on RA, corrected to 92% on 2 L NC
- General: Sitting in the gurney, looks anxious, tachypneic.
- HEENT: normal
- Cardiovascular: tachycardic. Normal S1, S2 sounds, + S3
- Pulmonary: moderate respiratory distress, tachypneic, conversational dyspnea, bibasilar crackles
- Abdomen: Soft, nontender, nondistended
- Extremities: no acute deformities, 2+ pitting edema up to the knees bilaterally. Cool extremities.
- Neurological: normal
- Psychiatric: normal

Pertinent Diagnostic Testing

| Test | Result | | | Units | Normal range |
	Day 1 Time 1400	Day 1 Time 2000	Day 3 Time 0200		
WBC	13 ↑	14 ↑	14 ↑	K/uL	3.8–11.0 10^3/mm^3
Hgb	11.3	11.1	10.9 ↓	g/dL	(Male) 14–18 g/dL (Female) 11–16 g/dL
Na	123 ↓	127 ↓	130 ↓	mEq/L	135–148 mEq/L
K	4.3	4.5	4.7	mEq/L	3.5–5.5 mEq/L
CO2	18 ↓	18 ↓	19 ↓	mEq/L	21–34 mEq/L
BUN	45 ↑	47 ↑	48 ↑	mg/dL	6–23 mg/dL
Cr	1.7 ↑	1.9 ↑	1.9 ↑	mg/dL	0.6–1.5 mg/dL

Test	Result Day 1 Time 1400	Day 1 Time 2000	Day 3 Time 0200	Units	Normal range
AST (U/L)	43 ↑	–	–	IU/L	8–32 IU/L
ALT (U/L)	55 ↑	–	–	IU/L	6–21 IU/L
TSH	2	–	–	uIU/mL	0.550–4.780 uIU/mL
BNP	8483 ↑	8512 ↑	–	pg/ml	<100 pg/ml
Troponin (ng/mL)	0.092	0.103	0.099	ng/mL	< 0.11 ng/mL
UA	2+ ketones ↑	–	–	–	Negative

Electrocardiogram (EKG)

- Sinus tachycardia at 123 bpm
- Left axis deviation
- Minimal criteria for left ventricular hypertrophy (LVH)
- Otherwise unremarkable

CXR

Mikael Häggström (https://commons.wikimedia.org/wiki/File:Chest_radiograph_with_signs_of_congestive_heart_failure_-_annotated.jpg), "Chest radiograph with signs of congestive heart failure – annotated", https://creativecommons.org/publicdomain/zero/1.0/legalcode

Emergency Department Course

The patient presented with concern for hypoxia, tachycardia, and volume overload. Due to recent delivery, with the hypoxia, there was concern for pulmonary embolism (PE). However, the patient's chest X-ray was most consistent with congestive heart failure and bilateral pleural effusions. The physical examination was concerning for significant bilateral lower extremity edema with associated S3 and tachycardia. Physical findings, X-rays, and the EKG, raised concern for PPCM versus (PE). There was a lower concern for preeclampsia given her relative hypotension, despite her prior history of hypertension and lower extremity edema. She was started on three doses of sublingual nitroglycerin, followed by the initiation of a nitroglycerin drip. The patient was started on BiPAP.

Update 1 (1600)

- Improved hemodynamics on Bilevel Positive Airway Pressure (BiPAP).
- CT-PE study negative, but shows concern for dilated cardiomyopathy, bibasilar effusions.
- Obstetrics and Gynecology (OB/GYN) consulted.
- Patient admitted to the intensive care unit (ICU) for diuresis, BiPAP management.
- Cardiology consulted for inpatient echo and further cardiac monitoring.

Learning Points: Peripartum Cardiomyopathy (PPCM)

Priming Questions

1. What risk factors put a pregnant patient at higher risk for developing PPCM?
2. What exam, lab, and radiographic findings would you expect in a patient with PPCM?
3. What is the treatment for PPCM? What is the prognosis for PPCM?

Introduction/Background

1. Peripartum cardiomyopathy (PPCM) affects approximately 1 in 3000–4000 postpartum women in the USA. In other parts of the world, such as Nigeria, the number can be as high as 1 in 100 [2, 13].
2. Risk factors for developing PPCM include multiparity, multiple gestations, obesity, chronic hypertension, pregnancy-related hypertension, age > 25 years old, African descent, and prolonged use of tocolytics [13].
3. Onset of PCCM can occur at any time during pregnancy, but it typically occurs in the last month of pregnancy up to 5 months postpartum. In a retrospective analysis, the later that PPCM is diagnosed, the higher the morbidity and mortality [12].

4. Prognosis
   - Reported mortality varies depending on the study from 0% to 9% [6].
   - One study of 182 PPCM patients found that 25% of patients suffered at least one of the following major adverse events: death, heart transplant, or other significant morbid events that were either life-threatening or had an important and long-lasting effect on quality of life. [6]
     - Delay in diagnosis was an independent risk factor for development of a major adverse event [6].
   - Sources also vary in their reported rates of recovery of cardiac function. Cardiac function recovery ranges from 20% to 82% of patients. Most experts agree that the majority of cardiac recovery occurs in the first 6 months after initiating optimal medical management, but a longer span of recovery over the years has also been reported [2].

Physiology/Pathophysiology

1. Although many experts have postulated different etiologies of PPCM, the exact cause remains unclear. In fact, if another typical cause for cardiomyopathy has been identified even in the context of pregnancy, PPCM is ruled out!
2. Some of the etiologies that have been discussed throughout the literature include:
   - Genetics
     - There are two case studies that support a genetic link; however, it was suggested that the patients may have had dilated cardiomyopathy that was unmasked by the physiological changes of pregnancy [10].
   - Hormonal changes: Elevated prolactin levels in pregnancy [7, 8].
     - Prolactin is a hormone that is released to allow women to produce milk to provide nutrition to their newborn baby.
     - Prolactin also plays a role in apoptosis of endothelial cells and interferes with the metabolism and contractility of cardiac myocytes.
     - There have even been case reports of women with PPCM who have been treated with bromocriptine (a prolactin inhibitor).
   - Chimerism [7].
     - Immune response develops due to fetal cells in the mother's bloodstream.
   - Sequelae from a viral infection [7].
     - An inappropriate immune response occurs that attacks the myocardium.
     - Viruses that have been implicated include: parvovirus B19, Epstein-Barr virus (EBV), cytomegalovirus (CMV), and human herpes virus 6.
   - Inappropriate apoptosis of cardiac myocytes [7].
   - Inability to compensate for the normal physiological changes in pregnancy [7].
   - Malnutrition (i.e., low selenium levels) [5].
     - Low selenium levels have been suggested as a possible contributor to the development of PPCM as the number of cases of PPCM continue to rise in lesser developed areas of the world (such as in Haiti and parts of Africa).
     - However, no epidemiologic studies have validated reported correlation between low selenium levels and PPCM.

Making the Diagnosis

The Differential: Other Diagnoses to Think About
- Normal pregnancy
- Anemia
- Thromboembolic disease (deep venous thrombosis (DVT) / pulmonary embolism (PE))
- Malignant hypertension (including secondary causes of this, i.e., preeclampsia)
- Coronary artery disease
- Acute renal failure
- Cardiomyopathy secondary to another identifiable cause
- Thyroid dysfunction
- Sequeale from infectious mycarditis

1. History and Physical Exam [10].
   - PPCM requires a high index of suspicion, so a thorough history and physical exam is crucial!
   - Patient identifier: female in last month of pregnancy or up to 5 months postpartum
   - Look for any signs of heart failure. Symptoms may include any of the following:
     - Fatigue
     - Shortness of breath at rest or exertional
     - Orthopnea
     - Jugular venous distension (JVD)
     - Leg edema
     - Palpitations
     - Hypotension
2. Workup
   - Laboratory studies [13]: There is no definitive laboratory study to "make" the diagnosis, but they are important to rule out other potential causes of the patient's symptoms
     - Complete Blood Count (CBC)
       ◦ Rule out anemia
       ◦ A significant leukocytosis may suggest an infectious process
     - Complete Metabolic Panel (CMP): Rule out evidence of acute renal failure, liver dysfunction, and acute electrolyte derangements
     - Brain Natriuretic Peptide (BNP): Usually elevated in PPCM
     - Thyroid Stimulating Hormone (TSH): Rule out hypo/hyperthryoidism
     - Troponin: Often elevated in the acute phase of PPCM

- Electrocardiogram. [3]
  - Remember to always compare to a prior EKG if able. The following can be seen in PPCM:
    - Sinus tachycardia (most common)
    - Left atrial/biatrial enlargement
    - Left ventricular hypertrophy
    - Left axis deviation
    - Widened QRS (>120 ms)
    - Ventricular ectopy [seen in severe cardiomyopathy]
    - Ventricular dysrhythmias
- Chest X-ray [13].
  - Cardiomegaly: Often seen in normal pregnancy as the heart is pushed upward and laterally, making the heart appear enlarged [9].
  - Cephalization of the pulmonary vessels
  - Bilateral pleural effusions
  - Pulmonary edema
- Echocardiogram [13].
  - Ejection fraction <45%
  - No evidence of valvular dysfunction
- Magnetic Resonance Imaging [9].
  - Can measure cardiac contraction
  - Helps rule out inflammatory processes
- Cardiac Catheterization [13]: Helps rule out ischemic etiology of the cardiomyopathy.
- Endocardial biopsy [13].

Treating the Patient

1. OB/GYN consultation
   - This should occur early in the patient's course, particularly if the patient is not yet postpartum, as there is a high morbidity and mortality for both mom and fetus if the diagnosis is not made.
   - Many therapies are teratogenic and can cause harm to the fetus.
2. Goals of treatment: optimize volume status without decreasing blood to the placenta if the patient is not yet postpartum.
   - Restrict fluids
   - Medications [11].
     - SAFE in pregnancy AND breastfeeding
       - Hydrochlorothiazide
       - Furosemide
       - Digoxin

- SAFE in pregnancy, CONTRAINDICATED in breastfeeding
    - Nitroglycerin: Some sources say that nitroglycerin (NTG) can cause fetal decelerations and bradycardia in the IV formulation; however, if benefits outweigh the risk, NTG is acceptable
    - Beta-blockers
- CONTRAINDICATED in pregnancy, SAFE in breastfeeding: Hydralazine (particularly unsafe when used in the third trimester)
- CONTRAINDICATED in pregnancy and breastfeeding
    - Angiotensin-converting enzyme inhibitor (ACEi)
    - Angiotensin II receptor blockers (ARBs)
    - Nitroglycerin: In pregnancy, nitroglycerin can cause fetal decelerations and bradycardia with the IV formulation. Breastfeeding woman are advised to avoid nitroglycerin for the first 6 months of the infact's life.
- BiPAP [4].
    - Respiratory physiology is changed in the pregnant woman as demonstrated by a higher minute ventilation. Minute ventilation increases due to the increase in tidal volume with relatively unchanged respiratory rate. Blood gas will show a normal pH with decreased CO_2 levels with compensatory decrease in bicarbonate levels.
    - If BiPAP is needed, use it! Be aware that BiPAP does carry an increased risk of vomiting when used in a pregnant woman as pregnancy causes weakening of the lower esophageal sphincter, increasing risk of aspiration.
- Anticoagulation [13].
    - Controversial: Current recommendations state that if atrial fibrillation is present or a left ventricular thrombus has been identified, anticoagulation should be started.

Case Conclusion

The patient spent 5 days in the ICU before she was transferred to step down and subsequently to telemetry with a total hospital stay of 10 days. The initial echocardiogram (Echo) showed decreased left ventricular (LV) function with an ejection fraction of 33%. During her hospitalization, she underwent aggressive diuresis, which complicated her initial acute kidney injury (AKI) on presentation; however, her creatinine started to trend down as her volume status improved. She required BiPAP for 3 days before she was transitioned to high flow nasal cannula (HFNC), nasal cannula (NC), and finally room air (RA). She did not require ventilator support. She was eventually discharged home on Lasix 20 mg daily with hopes that she will wean off all medication. A repeat Echo done 6 months later showed full recovery of LV function with an ejection fraction (EF) of 65%.

Discussion

This diagnosis is definitely easy to miss as a lot of the symptoms that are characteristic of PPCM are also characteristic of normal pregnancy, particularly early in the disease course. This diagnosis requires a very high index of suspicion as missing this diagnosis can be lethal if not treated. If the patient is not a first time mother, she can often be your greatest resource! She can tell you if this is her "normal" fatigue/dyspnea or if this is something different. The key is to listen to your patient!

If the patient is still pregnant, one of the main things to keep in mind is that the mortality of the fetus is 100% dependent on the mortality of the mother. There is no such thing as a category A medication when it comes to pregnancy and it is hit or miss if the medication is safe in breastfeeding. The best way to ensure survival for both of your patients, is to remember that saving the mother means saving the baby. Do what you think is best for mom and you are doing the best thing for baby!

After being diagnosed and treated for PPCM, a lot of women may wonder if it is safe to conceive again. The answer to this question is really dependent on how much cardiac recovery has been made. Even if full recovery of cardiac function has been made, she has a higher risk of developing PPCM during the next pregnancy than someone who has never had PPCM. If full cardiac recovery has not been made, future pregnancies are generally not recommended. [10]

Pattern Recognition

- Last month of pregnancy through the first 5 months postpartum
- Fatigue, dyspnea, leg edema, and orthopnea
- Echo with an EF <45%
- No other cause of cardiomyopathy

Disclosure Statement The authors of this chapter report no significant disclosures.

References

1. Al-Jobur D. HELLP!!! Pregnancy complications in the postpartum period. In: emDOCs.net – emergency medicine education; 2015. http://www.emdocs.net/hellp-pregnancy-complications-postpartum-period/.
2. Asad ZUA, Farah F, Dasari TW. Peripartum cardiomyopathy: a systematic review of the literature. Clin Cardiol. 2018. https://onlinelibrary.wiley.com/doi/abs/10.1002/clc.22932.

3. Burns E, Burns EBE. Prehospital & retrieval medicine. 2017 Dilated cardiomyopathy – life in the fast lane ECG library: LITFL • life in the fast lane medical blog. https://lifeinthefastlane.com/ecg-library/dilated-cardiomyopathy/.
4. Calicut A. Changes in respiratory system in pregnancy. In: LinkedIn SlideShare; 2013. https://www.slideshare.net/draslam1/changes-in-respiratory-system-in-pregnancy. Accessed 27 Jul 2018.
5. Fett JD, Ansari AA, Sundstrom JB, Combs GF. Peripartum cardiomyopathy: a selenium disconnection and an autoimmune connection. Egyptian J Med Human Genet. 2002. https://www.sciencedirect.com/science/article/pii/S0167527302003595.
6. Goland S, Modi K, Bitar F, Janmohamed M, Mirocha JM, Czer LS, et al. Clinical profile and predictors of complications in peripartum cardiomyopathy. J Card Fail. 2009;15(8):645–50. https://doi.org/10.1016/j.cardfail.2009.03.008.
7. Espinosa J, Caravello A, Wagner A, Norinsky AB. Dyspnea after delivery: a case of post-partum cardiomyopathy. In: OMICS international; 2016. https://www.omicsonline.org/open-access/dyspnea-after-delivery-a-case-of-postpartum-cardiomyopathy-mrcs-1000109.php?aid=71888.
8. J Jahns BG, Stein W, Hilfiker-Kleiner D, Pieske B, Emons G. Peripartum cardiomyopathy—a new treatment option by inhibition of prolactin secretion. Am J Obs Gynecol. 2008. https://www.ajog.org/article/S0002-9378(08)00682-0/fulltext.
9. Johnson-Coyle L, Jensen L, Sobey A. Peripartum cardiomyopathy: review and practice guidelines. 2012. http://ajcc.aacnjournals.org/content/21/2/89.full.
10. Peripartum Cardiomyopathy (PPCM). In: Peripartum cardiomyopathy. http://www.heart.org/HEARTORG/Conditions/More/Cardiomyopathy/Peripartum-Cardiomyopathy-PPCM_UCM_476261_Article.jsp#.W1s8kNhKgk9.
11. The #1 medical reference app. In: Point of care medical applications | Epocrates. http://www.epocrates.com/.
12. VC-C W, Chen T-H, Yeh J-K, et al. Clinical outcomes of peripartum cardiomyopathy: a 15-year nationwide population-based study in Asia. In: Advances in pediatrics; 2017. https://www.ncbi.nlm.nih.gov/pmc/articles/PMC5671863/.
13. Zaccardi MR, Bhimji SS. Cardiomyopathy, peripartum: StatPearls [Internet]; 2018.

Radiology Case 10

51

James Flannery and Joshua K. Aalberg

Indication for the Exam *73 y/o m presents with right hip pain after a fall. On exam there is significant pain with even passive range of motion (rom).*

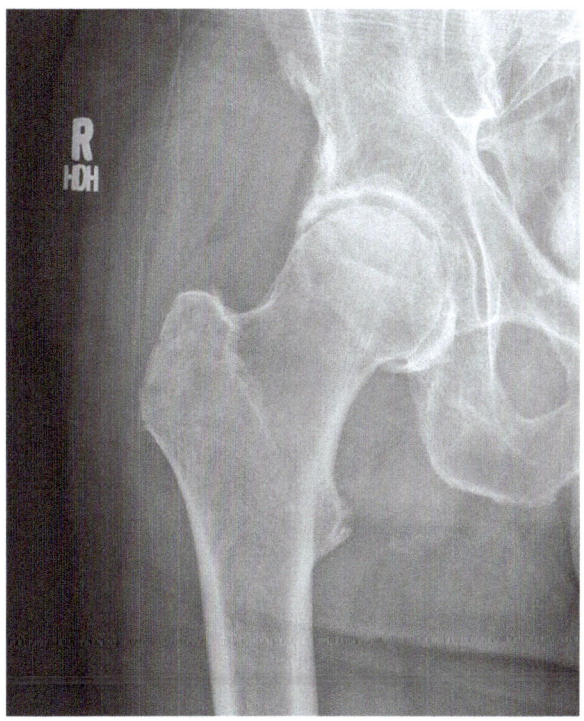

J. Flannery · J. K. Aalberg (✉)
Department of Emergency Medicine, Wexner Medical Center at The Ohio State University, Columbus, OH, USA
e-mail: James.flannery@osumc.edu; joshua.aalberg@osumc.edu

© Springer Nature Switzerland AG 2020
C. G. Kaide, C. E. San Miguel (eds.), *Case Studies in Emergency Medicine*,
https://doi.org/10.1007/978-3-030-22445-5_51

Radiologic Findings Anteroposterior (AP) view of the right hip – No apparent fracture.

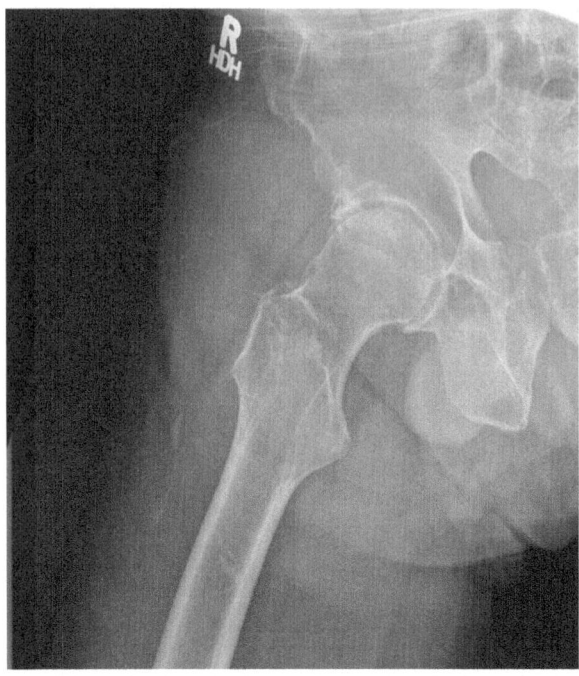

Radiologic Findings "Frog-leg" lateral view of the right hip – No apparent fracture.

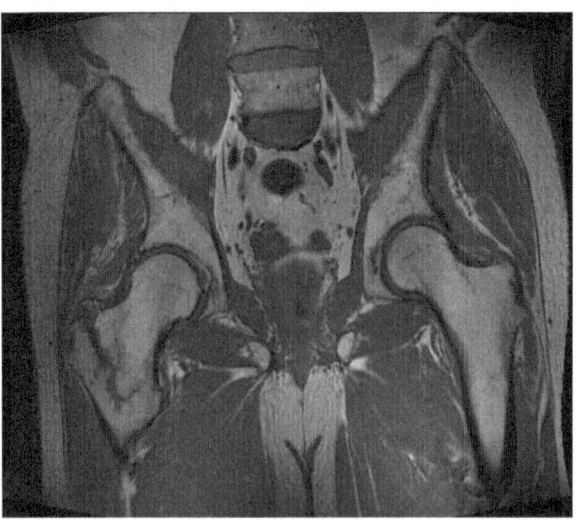

Radiologic Findings T1-weighted coronal magnetic resonance imaging (MRI) sequence – dark linear signal through the intertrochanteric region of the right femur

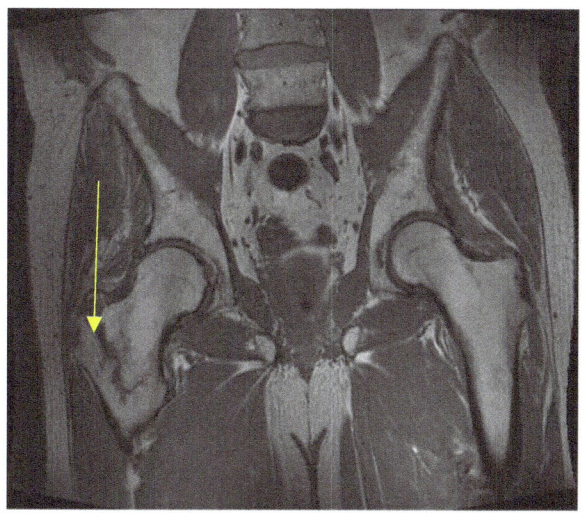

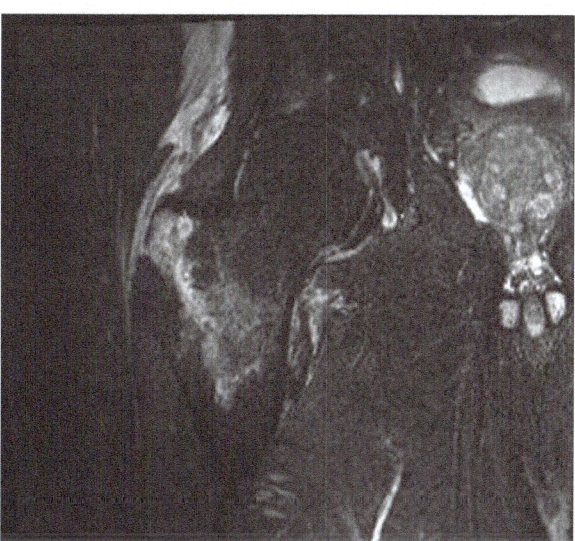

Short T1 inversion recovery "STIR" coronal MRI sequence – bright linear signal (edema) through the intertrochanteric region of the right femur.

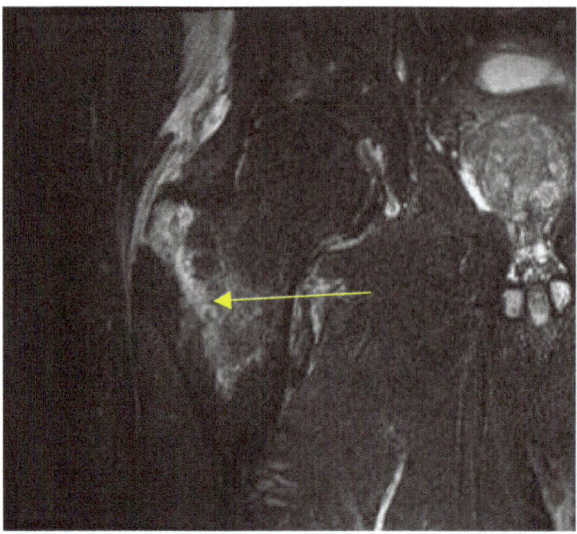

Diagnosis Nondisplaced intertrochanteric femur fracture

Learning Points

Priming Questions
- What are the different types of hip fractures?
- What are possible complications?
- What population is at the greatest risk?

Introduction/Background

The term "hip fracture" typically refers to a fracture of the proximal femur. Proximal femur fractures can be categorized broadly into intracapsular or extracapsular in relation to the hip joint.

- Intracapsular fractures include femoral head and femoral neck fractures.
- Extracapsular fractures include intertrochanteric and subtrochanteric fractures.

The elderly population is most at risk for these fractures, which lead to significant morbidity and mortality [1]. Approximately 320,000 hip fractures are diagnosed in the United States each year [2]. The prevalence of hip fractures is higher in women largely due to a higher risk of osteoporosis versus men.

Pathophysiology/Mechanism

The hip joint is a major weight bearing, ball-and-socket joint comprised of the acetabulum and proximal femur. Fracture mechanism depends on the segment of the femur involved but generally can occur with a hip dislocation, high-energy axial load such as a motor vehicle accident, repetitive stress fracture in athletes or fall in the case of an elderly patient [5]. With loss of bone density and trabecular bone, such as in the case of osteoporosis, the supportive tensile and compressive forces of the femoral neck are compromised and are susceptible to fractures [3].

Fractures of the femoral head-neck junction are of particular clinical concern due to the risk of avascular necrosis. The femoral artery branches into the lateral and medial circumflex femoral arteries, supplying the femoral neck. Small branches of these circumflex arteries course back proximally across the femoral neck towards the joint and anastomose with other branches at the femoral head. If these arteries are injured, then delayed healing and necrosis can ensue [4]. This complication is seen most commonly in subcapital (most proximal portion of the head-neck junction) neck fractures.

Isolated fractures of the lesser trochanter in adults are nearly always secondary to a tumor [6]. This finding should warrant workup for malignancy.

Making the Diagnosis

- Two view radiographs of the hip are usually obtained during the initial evaluation. Signs of fractures include cortical discontinuities or contour irregularities, disruption of the trabeculae, and head-neck angulations. Sensitivity of radiographs ranges between 90–98% and varies with bone density [7, 8].
- In the setting of a negative hip radiograph with high clinical suspicion for occult fracture in the emergency setting, computed tomography (CT) and magnetic resonance imaging (MRI) are the next imaging modalities of choice. MRI is more sensitive than CT in the setting of osteopenia or low-energy trauma and can pick up soft tissue injuries, such as muscle strains/tears, nerve injuries, synovitis, bursitis or infection. The downside to MRI is the time to acquire the sequences, cost and availability [9].
  - CT findings will be similar to the radiographic findings as described above. The diagnostic advantage lies in the three view or 3-dimensional perspective that CT provides.
  - MRI findings will show linear signal abnormalities on all sequences representing the fracture plane, along with bone marrow edema on fluid-sensitive sequences such as T2 or Short-TI Inversion Recovery (STIR).

Treating the Patient

Mostly all treatment options of hip fractures are surgical. The severity and location of the fracture along with the functioning status of the patient will determine the surgical approach.

- Nondisplaced femoral neck fractures are typically corrected by internal fixation.
- Displaced fractures may be internally fixated in younger patients and treated with total hip arthroplasty in the elderly.
- Fixation is typically indicated in all fractures to avoid risk of nonunion, malunion or avascular necrosis in the case of intracapsular fractures.

Discussion

- Hip fractures are highly prevalent, especially in the elderly population, and carry high morbidity and mortality.
- Radiographs are highly sensitive for a fracture, but the chances of missing an occult fracture increase in the setting of osteoporosis and low-energy mechanisms.
- If clinical suspicion is high after negative radiographs, consider further imaging with a CT or MRI. If available, MRI is the most sensitive modality.
- Surgical intervention is typically the preferred management of hip fractures in all patients.

References

1. Brauer CA, Coca-Perraillon M, Cutler DM, Rosen AB. Incidence and mortality of hip fractures in the United States. JAMA. 2009;302(14):1573–9.
2. Brown CA, Starr AZ, Nunley JA. Analysis of past secular trends of hip fractures and predicted number in the future 2010–2050. J Orthop Trauma. 2012;26(2):117–22.
3. Lotz JC, Cheal EJ, Hayes WC. Stress distributions within the proximal femur during gait and falls: implications for osteoporotic fracture. Osteoporos Int. 1995;5(4):252–61.
4. Ehlinger M, Moser T, Adam P, et al. Early prediction of femoral head avascular necrosis following neck fracture. Orthop Traumatol Surg Res. 2011;97(1):79–88.
5. Sheehan SE, et al. Proximal femoral fractures: what the orthopedic surgeon wants to know. Radiographics. 2015;35(5):1563–84.
6. James SL, Davies AM. Atraumatic avulsion of the lesser trochanter as an indicator of tumour infiltration. Eur Radiol. 2006;16(2):512–4.
7. Lubovsky O, Liebergall M, Mattan Y, et al. Early diagnosis of occult hip fractures MRI versus CT scan. Injury. 2005;36:788–92.
8. Cannon J, Salvatore Silvestri S, Mark Munro M. Imaging choices in occult hip fracture. J Emerg Med. 2009;37(2):144–52.
9. Kirby MW, Spritzer C. Radiographic detection of hip and pelvic fractures in the emergency department. AJR Am J Roentgenol. 2010;194(4):1054–60.

Pott's Puffy Tumor: *"I'm Not a Klingon, It's an Abscess!"*

52

Christopher Lee and David Bahner

Case

Pertinent History

An 18-year-old male presented with his roommate with 1 week of progressive forehead swelling and sleepiness. Patient had an upper respiratory infection starting 3 weeks ago with rhinorrhea, sore throat, and headache that progressed to sinus pain and fever. He saw his primary physician and was prescribed a 10-day course of amoxicillin. He had improvement of his symptoms but he did not feel completely back to baseline. For the past week, his headache has gotten worse and he noticed a tender bump on his forehead that had progressively gotten larger in addition to having low-grade fevers. This morning his roommate noticed that he was sleepier than usual and had an episode of vomiting, prompting him to bring the patient to the Emergency Department (ED). The roommate denied any knowledge of trauma and said that the patient was acting normally yesterday evening.

Pertinent Physical Exam

Except as noted below, the findings of the complete physical exam are within normal limits.

C. Lee (✉) · D. Bahner
Department of Emergency Medicine, Wexner Medical Center at The Ohio State University, Columbus, OH, USA
e-mail: christopher.lee@osumc.edu; david.bahner@osumc.edu

© Springer Nature Switzerland AG 2020
C. G. Kaide, C. E. San Miguel (eds.), *Case Studies in Emergency Medicine*,
https://doi.org/10.1007/978-3-030-22445-5_52

- Vitals: Temperature 101.8, Heart Rate 100, Respiratory Rate 14, Blood Pressure 100/50, Saturation 99% on room air
- Head, Ears, Eyes, Nose, and Throat (HEENT): Atraumatic, normocephalic, 3-cm diameter area of induration on the right forehead, tender to palpation, no overlying redness, drainage, nasal turbinates erythematous without drainage, bilateral tympanic membranes with intact light reflex.
- Eyes: Pupils Equal, Round, Reactive to Light and Accommodation (PERRLA); Extraocular Movements Intact (EOMI); no injection
- Cardiovascular (CV): Tachycardic, regular rhythm, no murmurs/rub/gallop, normal S1 and S2
- Neuro: Somnolent, GCS 14 (E3, V5, M6), CNII-XII intact, Strength 5/5 bilaterally in upper and lower extremities bilaterally, intact sensation, no dysmetria.

Past Medical History/Social History/Family History

Noncontributory

Pertinent lab work					
Test	Results 0700	Results 1200	Results 1500	Units	Normal range
WBC	12.3	15.5	17.9	K/uL	$3.8–11.0 \cdot 10^3/mm^3$
Hgb	13.3	12.9	13.0	g/dL	(Male) 14–18 g/dL (Female) 11–16 g/dL
Lactate	2.1	2.7	3.1	mmol/L	<2.0
pH	7.32	7.29	7.23	–	7.35–7.45
ESR	70	86	90	mm/h	(Male) 0–22 mm/h (Female) 0–29 mm/h
CRP	132	139	145	mg/L	<3 mg/L
Creatinine	0.75	0.79	0.77	mg/dL	0.6–1.5 mg/dL

WBC white blood cell, *Hgb* Hemoglobin, *ESR* Erythrocyte sedimentation rate, *CRP* C-reactive protein

CT Head 2 cm × 2 cm periosteal abscess in the right frontal bone anteriorly. Bilateral frontal sinuses completely opacified. Adjacent to this abscess, there is a complex subdural fluid collection with 2 mm of right-to-left midline shift.

ED Management

IN the ED the following were obtained: CT head, Chem-7, Complete Blood Count. The patient received an intravenous (IV) fluid bolus and IV antibiotics.

Update 1 (0800) Computed Tomography of the head resulted showing an abscess of the frontal bone with intracranial spread. Neurosurgery was consulted and their recommendations are pending. Patient remains somnolent but arousable and conversant.

Update 2 (1300)   Patient became more somnolent with a declining Glasgow Coma Scale (GCS). On repeat exam, he was found to have a dilated pupil, right eye (OD). Given declining mental exam and neurologic deficit, there was concern for herniation. Patient was intubated and a right femoral central venous catheter (CVC) was placed. The patient was treated with hypertonic saline boluses and a temporary course of hyperventilation. Neurosurgery was updated.

Update 3 (1330)   The patient was taken to the operating room.

Learning Points

Priming Questions
1. Through what avenues does Pott's Puffy Tumor spread intracranially?
2. Although rare, what are the common causes of Pott's Puffy Tumor?
3. How is Pott's Puffy Tumor managed?

Introduction/Background

1. Pott's Puffy Tumor (PPT) is a subperiosteal abscess with underlying osteomyelitis of the frontal bone. First described in 1760 by Sir Percivall Pott [1], the already uncommon incidence of PPT has declined dramatically with the advent of antibiotics [2]. The literature describing the disease has largely been confined to case reports and reviews thereof. Thirty-seven cases have been noted in the pediatric literature since 2006 [3] and 32 cases in adults since 2012 [4].
2. PPT is characterized by swelling and pain on the forehead which can lead to intracranial and orbital involvement. PPT has a male predominance with estimates ranging from 3:1 [4] to 5:1 [5]. It primarily affects teenagers although cases in patients as young as 2 years old have been reported [6].
3. PPT is commonly described as a complication of frontal bacterial sinusitis although head trauma is also prevalent. Rarer etiologies include odontogenic infections, iatrogenic causes from neurosurgical procedures, and chronic intranasal cocaine abuse [7, 8].

Physiology/Pathophysiology

1. Pott's Puffy Tumor is a complicated infection arising from bacterial sinusitis, thus bacteria such as *S. pneumoniae*, *H. influenzae*, *M. catarrhalis* are the predominant agents [9]. However, the low oxygen concentration that develops from the occluded sinuses can foster development of anaerobic species such as *Bacteroides* spp., and *Fusobacterium* [10–14].
2. The frontal sinuses begin as an anterosuperior aspect of the ethmoid air cells that become pneumatized at 2 years of age and become adult-sized in the late teens

[15, 16]. Intracranial communication to the dural venous plexus from the scalp and calvarium are accomplished from the emissary and diploic veins, respectively. These feeder veins lack valves. It is hypothesized that the diploic system is larger and more active in young adults, leading to the higher incidence of PPT in this population [10, 12, 13].

Making the Diagnosis

Differential Diagnosis
1. Hematoma
2. Subcutaneous abscess
3. Cellulitis
4. Contusion
5. Angioedema

1. Time course for diagnosis can be acute to chronic and is dependent on the etiology and presence of neurological or ophthalmological complications.
   - The most common cause is a preceding upper respiratory infection (URI). Mean time to diagnosis after onset of fever was 7 days [5]. Case reviews have not identified risk factors leading to the development of complications and poor outcome [4, 17]. Rate of complications is approximately 4% [18].
   - Time to diagnosis was found to be the most important aspect in reducing the incidence of intracranial complications [4].
2. The hallmark finding is forehead swelling. Infectious symptoms such as fever and headache (70%) are common. Neurological symptoms such as nausea and vomiting (23%), mental status changes (23%), focal neurological signs (12%), seizures (6%), and meningismus (6%) are rarer [19].
3. Lab work commonly demonstrates leukocytosis with elevations of C-reactive protein (CRP) and erythrocyte sedimentation rate (ESR). There are no clinical scoring tools to aid in diagnosis.
4. Imaging is invaluable for detecting the presence and extent of intracranial and/or orbital complications.
   - CT with contrast is the first line modality but magnetic resonance imaging (MRI) with and without contrast is more sensitive for intracranial complications.
   - Complications include: Meningitis, subdural empyema, intracerebral abscess, epidural abscess, cavernous sinus thrombosis, and orbital cellulitis.

T1 Sagittal brain MRI demonstrating intracranial involvement

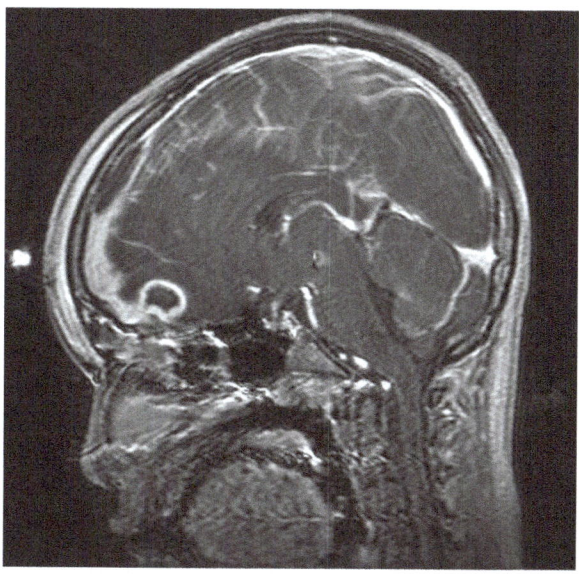

Radswiki   (https://commons.wikimedia.org/wiki/File:Potts-puffy-tumor-004.jpg),   "Potts-puffy-tumor-004", https://creativecommons.org/licenses/by-sa/3.0/legalcode

Treating the Patient

1. Surgical management ranges from minimally invasive endoscopic sinus surgery to craniectomy depending on the extent of disease. Specimen sampling is also vital for guiding antibiotic therapy. The morbidity and mortality of intracranial abscess is high with estimates of 30% in the modern antibiotic era in addition to chronic seizure disorders in 80% for patient with subdural abscesses [13].
2. Antibiotic therapy should be adjunctive to surgical debridement and drainage. While there are no established protocols in place, duration of therapy is typically 4–8 weeks given the presence of osteomyelitis.
3. Careful attention should be paid to the patient's neurological status and level of consciousness. Encephalopathy may be secondary to sepsis or neurological from herniation and midline shift. Consider intubation and emergent consultation if the patient is obtunded or has a declining Glasgow Coma Scale (GCS) and is exhibiting focal neurologic deficits.

Case Conclusion

Patient was taken emergently to the operating room where he underwent a craniotomy, drainage of subdural empyema, and washout without complication. Patient remained intubated in the neurocritical care unit with eventual recovery of his neurological status after 2 weeks. Intraoperative cultures resulted in *Peptostreptococcus spp* and *H. influenzae*. MRI confirmed osteomyelitis of the frontal bone. A peripherally inserted central catheter (PICC) line was placed, and the patient was discharged back home with home healthcare for continued IV antibiotics for osteomyelitis.

Discussion

The low incidence of PPT and the significant potential for morbidity and mortality begs the need for a high index of suspicion in any patient with signs of infection and frontal swelling. Thankfully, the differential for forehead swelling is narrow. Overt signs of infection can be absent on exam given the subperiosteal location of the abscess. Many of the subacute cases initially present to an ENT or neurosurgery clinic with undifferentiated symptoms [4]. Consider this diagnosis in the same realm as epiglottitis – a deadly disease that is now rare due to advances in medicine but is always on the differential diagnosis if the right conditions arise!

Usage of point-of-care ultrasound to aid in the diagnosis of abscess versus cellulitis is commonplace in emergency departments [20] and could have a role in diagnosis given concerns for the use of ionizing radiation in pediatric patients.

Pattern Recognition

- Forehead swelling after a sinus infection
- "Bruising" that persists after an episode of head trauma

References

1. Tattersall R. Pott's puffy tumor. Lancet. 2002;359:1060–3.
2. Babu BP, Todor R, Kasoff KS. Pott's puffy tumor: the forgotten entity. J Neurosurg. 1996;84:110–2.
3. Kombogiorgias D, Solanki GA. The Pott puffy tumor revisited: neurosurgical implications of this unforgotten entity. J Neurosurg. 2006;105(2 Suppl Pediatrics):143–9.
4. Akiyama K, Masayuki K, Mori N. Evaluation of adult Pott's puffy tumor: our five cases and 27 literature cases. Laryngoscope. 2012;122:2383–8.
5. Tsai BY, et al. Pott's puffy tumor in children. Childs Nerv Syst. 2010;26:53–60.
6. Rao M. A "hickey". Epidural brain abscess, osteomyelitis of the frontal bone, and subcutaneous abscess (Pott puffy tumor). Clin Pediatr. 2003;42:657–60.

7. Karaman E, Hacizade Y, Isildak H, Kaytaz A. Pott's puffy tumor. J Craniofac Surg. 2008;19:1694–7.
8. Noskin GA, Kalish SB. Pott's puffy tumor: a complication of intranasal cocaine abuse. Rev Infect Dis. 1991;13(4):606–8.
9. Kaliner KA, et al. Sinusitis: bench to bedside. J Allergy Clin Immunol. 1997;99(6):S829–48.
10. Bambakidis NC, Cohen AR. Intracranial complications of frontal sinusitis in children: Pott's puffy tumor revisited. Pediatr Neurosurg. 2001;35(2):82–9.
11. Clayman GL, Adams GL, Paugh DR, Koopmann CF. Intracranial complications of paranasal sinusitis: a combined institutional review. Laryngoscope. 1991;101(3):234–9.
12. Feder HM, Cates KL, Cementina AM. Pott puffy tumor: a serious occult infection. Pediatrics. 1987;79(4):625–9.
13. Remmler D, Boles R. Intracranial complications of frontal sinusitis. Laryngoscope. 1980;90(11):1814–24.
14. Uren RF, Howman-Giles RO. Pott's puffy tumor. Scintigraphic findings. Clin Nucl Med. 1992;17(9):724–7.
15. Tomas SJ. Developmental anatomy and physiology of the nose and sinuses. Clinical pediatric otolaryngology. St Louis, MO: Mosby; 1986. p. 269–79.
16. Rontal M, Anon JB, Zinreich SJ. Embryology and anatomy of the paranasal sinuses. Pediatr Otolaryngol. 2003;2:861.
17. Guillen A, Brell M, Cardona E, Claramunt E, Costa J. Pott's puffy tumour: still not an eradicated entity. Childs Nerv Syst. 2001;17(6):359–62.
18. Brook I. Microbiology and antimicrobial treatment of orbital and intracranial complications of sinusitis in children and their management. Int J Pediatr Otorhinolaryngol. 2009;73:1183–6.
19. Nisa L, Landis BN, Giger R. Orbital involvement in Pott's puffy tumor: a systematic review of published cases. Am J Rhinol Allergy. 2012;26(2):63–70.
20. Subramaniam S, Bober J, Chao J, Zehtabchi S. Point-of-care ultrasound for diagnosis of abscess in skin and soft tissue infections. Acad Emerg Med. 2016;23(11):1298–306.

Pulmonary Hypertension: *"You Take My Breath Away"*

53

Jennifer Cotton and Eric Adkins

Case

Flight med calls your department. "We have a 41-year-old cardiac patient of yours with a catheter coming from his chest that has broken off. Blood was coming from it, so we clamped it off. He's in respiratory distress and we'll be landing in 5 minutes."

Pertinent History

The patient is a 41-year-old male with a history of pulmonary hypertension who presents in respiratory distress. The broken line is used for a continuous infusion epoprostenol pump. The patient reports having non-bloody diarrhea for the last 3 days. He endorses nausea but has been tolerating fluids. He had mild SOB starting earlier today. However, just prior to calling EMS he fell due to lightheadedness while attempting to stand up quickly. His epoprostenol line caught on some furniture, causing it to tear. The broken off remainder is still in his chest. He did not lose consciousness or sustain any other injuries. Immediately following his line malfunction, he reports worsening shortness of breath, lightheadedness, and chest pressure.

J. Cotton (✉)
Division of Emergency Medicine, Department of Surgery, University of Utah Hospital, Salt Lake City, UT, USA
e-mail: Jennifer.Cotton@utah.edu

E. Adkins
Department of Emergency Medicine, Wexner Medical Center at The Ohio State University, Columbus, OH, USA
e-mail: Eric.Adkins@osumc.edu

© Springer Nature Switzerland AG 2020
C. G. Kaide, C. E. San Miguel (eds.), *Case Studies in Emergency Medicine*,
https://doi.org/10.1007/978-3-030-22445-5_53

Pertinent Physical Exam

- Vitals: HR 125, RR 28, O_2 sat 92% on 15 L/min, BP 102/74.

Except as noted below, the findings of a complete physical exam are within normal limits.

- General: The patient is in acute distress.
- Pulmonary: He is in respiratory distress and is speaking in 4–5-word sentences. Lungs are clear. Tachypneic with mild retractions.
- Cardiovascular: 2/6 systolic murmur, JVD to angle of mandible, and a regular rhythm, Extremities with 1+ pitting edema.
- Abdominal: Exam is benign except for mildly increased bowel sounds.
- Skin: Pale, cool, and diaphoretic.

PMH History of pulmonary hypertension and right heart failure. No other significant medical history. No surgical history.

SH Patient does not drink alcohol, use illicit drugs, or smoke. Patient worked as a school teacher prior to developing pulmonary hypertension. He is currently on disability.

Pertinent Test Result

Test	Result	Units	Normal range
WBC	10.7	K/uL	$3.8–11.0 \cdot 10^3/mm^3$
Hgb	16.3	g/dL	(Male) 14–18 g/dL
			(Female) 11–16 g/dL
Hematocrit	43	%	34.9%–44.3%
Platelets	264	K/uL	140–450 K/uL
Sodium	143	mEq/L	135–148 mEq/L
Potassium	3.3 ↓	mEq/L	3.5–5.5 mEq/L
Chloride	110	mEq/L	96–112 mEq/L
Bicarbonate	22	mEq/L	21–34 mEq/L
BUN	30 ↑	mg/dL	6–23 mg/dL
Creatinine	1.5 ↑	mg/dL	0.6–1.5 mg/dL
Glucose	86 ↑	mg/dL	65–99 mg/dL
pH (venous)	7.2 ↓	–	7.320–7.420
pCO_2 (venous)	25 ↓	mmHg	36.1–52.1 mmHg
pO_2 (venous)	36 ↓	mmHg	46.1–71.1 mmHg
Lactate	3 ↑	mmol/L	<2.0 mmol/L
Troponin	0.07	ng/dl	<0.11 ng/dl
BNP	510 ↑	pg/ml	<100 pg/ml

ECG – right axis deviation, tall P waves in inferior leads, prominent R wave in V1
Chest X-ray – mild cardiomegaly consistent with previous imaging, no evidence of pulmonary edema
POCUS – RV dilation and poor systolic function (Fig. 53.1), septal bowing into left ventricle, enlarged IVC with minimal respiratory variation

Learning Points

Priming Questions
1. What symptoms do patients with pulmonary HTN present with during acute episodes?
2. What objective findings can be present in decompensated pulmonary HTN?
3. What are the management goals for treating patient with acute episode of decompensated pulmonary hypertension?
4. What are the treatment options for the management of both an acute-episode and long-term pulmonary HTN?

Introduction/Background

1. Pulmonary hypertension is a high morbidity and mortality disease process caused by increased pulmonary vascular pressures and the resulting right ventricle (RV) failure.
2. There are several types of pulmonary hypertension that all increase pulmonary vascular resistance and meet the diagnostic criteria of elevated pulmonary artery pressures ≥25 mmHg (Table 53.1). Type 1 is due to hypertension of the pulmonary arteries. Type 2 is caused by left heart disease increasing pressure within the pulmonary vasculature. Type 3 is caused by chronic lung disease or hypoxia. Type 4 is due to chronic thromboemboli. Lastly, type 5 is a collection of unknown or multifactorial causes [1].
3. Initial symptoms are related to an inability to increase cardiac output; exertional chest pain due to subendocardial hypoperfusion, exertional syncope due to inability to increase output to meet demand, and extremity swelling due to fluid

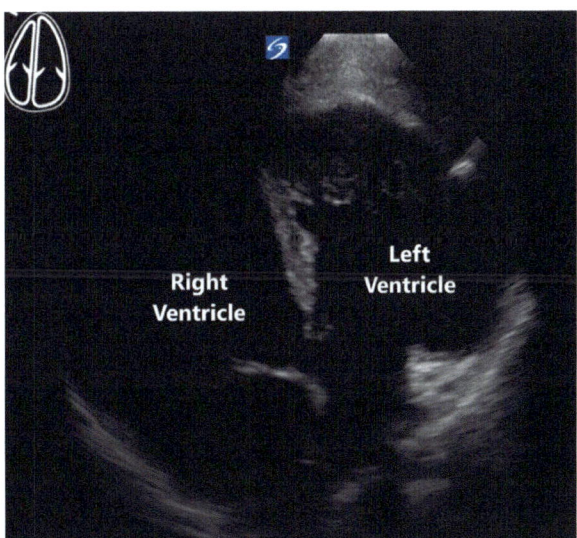

Fig. 53.1 Dilated right ventricle that is significantly larger than the left ventricle

Table 53.1 Different types of pulmonary hypertension

Type	Description
1	Primary hypertension of pulmonary arteries
2	Left heart failure causing increased pressure within pulmonary vasculature
3	Chronic lung disease or hypoxia (i.e., COPD)
4	Chronic thromboemboli
5	Everything else that does not fit into a category above

build-up from increased right heart pressures. Because initial symptoms are often subtle the average time to diagnosis is 2 years [1].

4. Outpatient treatments target reduction of RV afterload through vasodilation. Prostacyclin agonists, such as epoprostenol, are a common treatment delivered via permanent central line or subcutaneously infusion pump. Oral endothelin receptor antagonists, such as bosentan or ambrisentan, and PDE-5 inhibitors, such as sildenafil or tadalafil, can also be used.

5. Acute episodes of decompensation are typically due to medication delivery failure, fluid overload, dehydration, or progression of disease, which cause decreased RV output for different reasons.

6. There is a direct relationship between the RV function and renal perfusion. Any conditions that affect renal function or impair urine output will worsen RV function.

Physiology/Pathophysiology

1. Normally the pulmonary vasculature is a high flow, low resistance system. However, with pulmonary hypertension the resistance of the pulmonary vasculature rises and leads to RV failure.
   - Initially the RV hypertrophies in response to increased afterload, which over time progresses to RV dilation and systolic failure.
   - RV failure results in a state of preload-dependent right heart filling and output. RV dilation also leads to decreased contractility. Fluid overload only worsens this, causing the already dilated myocardium to further stretch, fall down the Starling curve, and reduce cardiac contractility even more.

2. Right coronary artery perfusion typically occurs during both systole and diastole. Perfusion is dependent on the pressure gradient between the aorta and the RV. However, as RV pressure rises perfusion during systole decreased until the RV is primarily perfused during diastole, further worsening RV function.

3. Hypercapnea and hypoxia are dangerous in pulmonary hypertension. They increase pulmonary vasoconstriction, increasing pulmonary artery pressures and worsening already tenuous cardiac output.

4. Volume overload causes decompensation by further increasing pressure within the RV and leading to reduced overall cardiac output.
   - Increased RV pressures lead to increased RV dilation and decreased contractility, reducing RV output.
   - Increased RV pressures cause the pressure gradient between aorta and RV to decrease, reducing RV perfusion and RV output

- Increased RV pressures, if high enough, can also cause septal bowing into the left ventricle (LV). This reduces LV preload by reducing its volume, leading to decreased LV function.
5. Dehydration or relative hypovolemia can also cause decompensation in these patients due to their preload-dependent cardiac output. Even mild volume losses can cause noticeable changes in RV function and decrease cardiac output.
6. Medication delivery failure is another important cause of acute decompensation. For the patient receiving continuous delivery of prostacyclin agonists medication failures will precipitate serious decompensation quickly.
   - Because the half-life of such medications is a few minutes its abrupt withdrawal will lead to a rapid increase in pulmonary vascular resistance [1].
   - The already failing RV cannot compensate for this abrupt change in afterload, leading to decreased RV and overall cardiac output.

Summary of Pathophysiology
- RV hypertrophy & ↑ pulmonary artery pressure → RV dilation → ↓ contractility
- ↑ RV pressures → septal bowing & ↓ LV filling → ↓ cardiac output
- ↑ RV pressures → ↓ aorta-RV pressure gradient → ↓ RCA perfusion → ↑ RV ischemia

Making the Diagnosis

Differential Diagnosis
- Decompensated pulmonary HTN
- Pulmonary embolism
- Acute coronary syndrome
- Pericardial effusion with tamponade

1. For the initial diagnosis of pulmonary hypertension, the history is key and should lead to further testing. Patients often describe exertional shortness of breath due to their inability to increase their cardiac output. They may also experience fatigue and exertional chest pain, lightheadedness, and syncope for similar reasons.
   - Echo is the initial diagnostic test of choice because it can estimate pulmonary artery pressures noninvasively. It can also detect evidence of more severe disease such as reduced RV function, RV dilation, right atrial dilation, and septal bowing.
   - A right heart cath remains the gold standard for diagnosis and quantification of disease. Pulmonary artery pressures ≥25 mmHg are diagnostic [2].
2. Diagnosing the acute cause of decompensation of the patient with established diagnoses is trickier. Patients live within a narrow margin of fluid balance and small changes in either direction can have significant effects. Clinical

decompensation is often due to fluid overload, too little fluid, arrhythmia, or abrupt withdrawal of medication.

3. Blood tests may be helpful, but are often nonspecific.
   - BNP is often elevated at baseline, so a single value is not very helpful. It is primarily helpful at the extremes and in comparison to previous values.
   - Lactate can indicate the degree of hypoperfusion.
   - Troponin elevations are associated with worse outcomes [1].

4. ECG can have right axis deviation and signs of right heart strain or right atrial enlargement. However, it typically does not change management significantly for acute decompensation due to pulmonary hypertension alone. It is important, however, for assessing for arrhythmias, which may occur with dilation of cardiac structures.

5. Chest X-rays may be normal. However, depending on the type of pulmonary hypertension, other findings such as cardiomegaly, pulmonary edema, or pulmonary vascular pruning may be present. It is additionally useful to assess for other causes of their symptoms [3].

6. Bedside ultrasound can be useful for guiding treatment in the initial evaluation of decompensated pulmonary hypertension.
   - The RV will often be dilated relative to the LV. Normal ratios of RV:LV are 0.6:1. As the RV dilates this ratio becomes 1:1 or worse. This can suggest worsening disease severity.
   - RV systolic function can easily be assessed to guide treatment plan and response to treatment. A tricuspid annular plane systolic excursion (TAPSE) measure is obtained with M-mode through the lateral annulus of the tricuspid valve of an apical four chamber view. Upward movement of this area <16 mm indicates significant systolic dysfunction and is associated with a worse prognosis.
   - Septal bowing into the LV indicates significant RV pressures and severe disease.
   - Due to baseline elevated RV pressures, IVC ultrasound is largely not helpful [4].

7. Physical exam can support your diagnosis of decompensated pulmonary hypertension and help guide treatment.
   - Every exam should include examination of the patient's epoprostenol pump. Pump failure is a reversible and common cause of decompensation. Examine the entire system: pump, reservoir, tubing, connection to the patient. Ask when it was last filled, if there has been leakage, when the battery was last changed.
   - Other physical exam findings include edema, JVD, pale or cool skin, diaphoresis, or systolic murmur. Lung sounds can be normal or abnormal [1].

8. Assessing fluid status is difficult in acute decompensation.
   - History of recent illness causing volume losses or noncompliance with treatment can support your diagnosis.
   - JVD and worsening edema potentially support fluid overload and definitely should make you question administering fluids.
   - Significant RV dilation or septal bowing into LV supports the patient not being volume down and potentially being fluid overloaded.

Treating the Patient

1. Check the pump. Check the pump. Check the pump. It cannot be emphasized enough. If there is a malfunction in prostacyclin agonist delivery, restart it immediately and at their home dose.
   - If there is any doubt that the prostacyclin agonist is not being delivered, administer peripherally. This can be done with patient's own pump until pharmacy brings up the fresh mixed medication. Often, patients will have a backup pump and extra supply of medication in case of any malfunction.
   - The half-life is typically minutes, so do not discontinue delivery under any circumstances. Hemodynamic collapse will occur from acute pulmonary artery vasoconstriction.
   - Expect side effects with restarting prostacyclin agonists; flushing, nausea, vomiting, diarrhea, and possibly hypotension. This is ok. Treat them as needed.
2. Support right heart contractility with dobutamine.
   - Start at 2 mcg/kg/min and titrate to a maximum of 10 mcg/kg/min. Avoid doses >10 mcg/kg/min as this actually increases pulmonary vascular resistance.
   - Anticipate the side effect of vasodilation causing hypotension. Have pressors at the bedside and ready use.
   - Dobutamine may cause arrhythmias.
   - Milrinone or calcium sensitizers, such as levosimendan, can be used as an alternative to dobutamine [1].
3. Support right coronary artery and RV perfusion with norepinephrine [5].
   - Increasing systemic vascular resistance will increase the pressure gradient between the aorta and RV, increasing flow to RCA and perfusion of RV.
   - Norepinephrine is the least vasoconstrictive of available pressors.
   - MAP >65 mmHg is a good goal, but perfusion of organs should be the ultimate guide of pressor therapy in these patients.
   - Dopamine and phenylephrine have significant pulmonary vasoconstriction and should be avoided [1].
4. Reduce RV afterload
   - As mentioned above, if prostacyclin agonist delivery has been interrupted, restart it immediately. However, this and other vasodilating medications are rarely initiated in the ED even for acute episodes.
   - Maintain oxygen saturation above 90%, as hypoxia will contribute to further pulmonary vasoconstriction. Give as much oxygen as needed for this, but avoid noninvasive positive pressure ventilation as this will decrease preload.
   - Hypercapnea also causes pulmonary vasoconstriction, so avoid if possible [6].
5. Do your best to assess the fluid status and make corrections as needed.
   - Use history, exam, and ultrasound to support your decision as much as possible. Small changes in fluid status can tip patients over the edge.
   - Give 250–500 ml boluses at a time and reassess frequently, if you decide to give fluids. Better yet try a passive leg raise to provide an auto-bolus that is reversible.

6. Sepsis requires a change from traditional management strategies.
   - Careful history is required to determine fluid status. If the patient history corresponds with dehydration from overdiuresis, poor oral intake, or losses from GI tract, then IV fluids may be appropriate.
   - A fluids first approach to resuscitation is dangerous. Consider early pressors and inotropic support, in some cases even before fluids.
   - Be sure to factor the volume of antibiotics into your calculation of fluids given.
   - The IVC will almost always appear enlarged on ultrasound when checking the collapsibility index. This is often unreliable in patients with pulmonary hypertension. A highly collapsible IVC may be an indicator of a patient that will respond to fluids.
7. Treat arrhythmias aggressively via cardioversion.
   - Atrial arrhythmias are common due to atrial stretch, but should be treated with electrical or chemical cardioversion.
   - Do not use calcium channel blockers or beta blockers because this will affect cardiac contractility and output.
8. Do not increase intrathoracic pressure, if at all possible.
   - Increasing intrathoracic pressure decreases preload, which will hurt cardiac output in the preload dependent RV of pulmonary hypertension.
   - Intubation should be a last resort. If performed, use the minimum amount of PEEP necessary to maintain oxygen saturation above 90%.
9. ECMO can be used as a bridge if other treatments fail to stabilize the patient.
   - Bridge patient to definitive treatment such as heart transplant or initiating pulmonary vasodilator medications.
10. Pulmonary HTN patients on ventilators
    - Minimize PEEP. Increases in PEEP will impair RV function.
    - Avoid hypercapnia which will cause acidosis and impair RV function [7].

Case Conclusion

The respiratory therapist brings bipap to the bedside to help with work of breathing and oxygenation, but the physician insists this should not be used and keeps the patient on non-rebreather. The patient's epoprostenol is re-initiated peripherally at his home dose. Dobutamine and norepinephrine are also prepared and hung, but not initiated yet. While the nurses are preparing these medications, a bedside cardiac ultrasound is performed. The right heart is enlarged with some septal bowing into the left ventricle. A TAPSE measurement is performed and shows decreased systolic function of the right heart (Fig. 53.2). Based on these findings, fluids are held until RV function is restored, despite a history that could suggest some dehydration. The patient's blood pressure drops to 88/56 shortly after initiating the epoprostenol and the patient's skin is flushed. Norepinephrine and dobutamine are initiated with

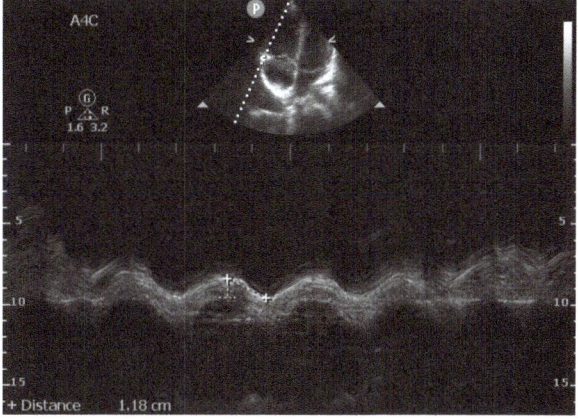

Fig. 53.2 TAPSE evaluation of right heart systolic function. Measurement taken from peak to trough of movement. Abnormal measurement of 11.8 mm present here

improvement in blood pressure to 104/70. The patient's shortness of breath improves and his extremities become warmer. The patient is admitted to the ICU for further care and appears significantly improved from his initial presentation.

Discussion

Pulmonary hypertension is a terrible disease process that causes right ventricular failure due to increased pulmonary afterload. Patients with this disease are on a number of medications to address the physiologic derangements in the pulmonary vasculature and right heart that occur. Medication delivery failures alone can precipitate serious decompensation. The tenuous fluid balance these patients live in also put them at risk for decompensation from small changes in volume status. Other events, such as arrhythmias, that can affect cardiac output will also lead to acute decompensations. This patient highlights how ill patients can become with abrupt discontinuation of prostacyclin agonist delivery. In addition, the case also highlights the importance of using ultrasound to help assess the RVs ability to respond to the fluid. This patient had a recent diarrheal illness but reported drinking fluids. One might consider giving a fluid bolus in a patient with this history, but bedside ultrasound found septal bowing into the LV. This supported the decision to not give fluids and prevented the administration of fluids that clearly would have harmed this patient. This case also highlights the mainstays of treatment for decompensation – supporting RV contractility, supporting RV perfusion, restarting prostacyclin agonists (and anticipating hypotension side effect), preventing hypoxia, and being thoughtful about fluid administration. The high mortality rate associated with this disease and ability of decompensated patients to quickly worsen or die with inappropriate treatment underscores the importance of emergency physicians being knowledgeable about this disease process and how to treat it.

Pattern Recognition

Decompensated Pulmonary HTN
- Shortness of breath
- Hypotension
- Right heart dilation with a thickened free wall on ultrasound
- Abrupt interruption in epoprostenol delivery

Disclosure Statement The authors of this chapter report no significant disclosures.

References

1. Winters ME. Pulmonary hypertension. In: Tintinalli J, editor. Tintinalli's emergency medicine. 8th ed. New York: McGraw-Hill Medical; 2016.
2. Badesch DB, Champion HC, Sanchez MA, et al. Diagnosis and assessment of pulmonary arterial hypertension. J Am Coll Cardiol. 2009;54:S55.
3. Galiè N, Humbert M, Vachiery JL, et al. 2015 ESC/ERS guidelines for the diagnosis and treatment of pulmonary hypertension: The Joint Task Force for the Diagnosis and Treatment of Pulmonary Hypertension of the European Society of Cardiology (ESC) and the European Respiratory Society (ERS). Eur Heart J. 2016;37:67.
4. Ghio S, Pica S, Klersy C, et al. Prognostic value of TAPSE after therapy optimisation in patients with pulmonary arterial hypertension is independent of the haemodynamic effects of therapy. Open Heart. 2016;3:e000408.
5. Taichman DB, Ornelas J, Chung L, et al. Pharmacologic therapy for pulmonary arterial hypertension in adults: CHEST guideline and expert panel report. Chest. 2014;146:449.
6. Nauser TD, Stites SW. Diagnosis and treatment of pulmonary hypertension. Am Fam Physician. 2001;63(9):1789–98.
7. Gayat E, Mebazaa A. Pulmonary hypertension in critical care. Curr Opin Crit Care. 2011;17:439–44; Galiè N, Corris PA, Frost A, et al. Updated treatment algorithm of pulmonary arterial hypertension. J Am Coll Cardiol. 2013; 62:D60.

Serotonin Syndrome: *When the Happy Hormone Gets Angry*

Greg Eisinger, Mena Botros, and Lauren Branditz

Case

Unexplained fever, tachycardia, and hypertension in the ICU.

Pertinent History

A 42-year-old male with a history of subglottic stenosis presented to the emergency department with dyspnea and stridor. He was evaluated by otolaryngology and taken to the operating room urgently for tracheal dilation. After intubation with a 4.0 endotracheal tube in the operating room, he was unable to be oxygenated or ventilated so emergent tracheotomy was performed. However, due to significant subglottic narrowing, a tracheostomy tube could not be placed. Instead, a 6.0 endotracheal tube was placed through the tracheotomy incision and left sutured in place with a plan for sedation and chemical paralysis to prevent dislodgement until revision could be performed in a few days. On arrival to the intensive care unit, the

G. Eisinger (✉) · L. Branditz
Department of Emergency Medicine, Wexner Medical Center at The Ohio State University, Columbus, OH, USA
e-mail: Gregory.Eisinger@osumc.edu; Lauren.Branditz@osumc.edu

M. Botros
Department of Emergency Medicine, Wexner Medical Center at The Ohio State University, Columbus, OH, USA

Department of Pediatrics – Nationwide Children's Hospital, Columbus, OH, USA
e-mail: Mena.Botros@osumc.edu

© Springer Nature Switzerland AG 2020
C. G. Kaide, C. E. San Miguel (eds.), *Case Studies in Emergency Medicine*,
https://doi.org/10.1007/978-3-030-22445-5_54

patient was agitated, tachycardic, and hypertensive with high requirements for sedation. Shortly later he developed fevers.

PMH Depression, PTSD, subglottic stenosis, factor V Leiden, obesity

Home Meds Oxycodone, clonazepam, paroxetine

Current Meds Midazolam 4 mg/hour, fentanyl 100 mcg/hour, propofol 50 mcg/kg/min, cisatracurium 2.5 mcg/kg/min

SH 5 pack-year smoking history, no EtOH or illicit drugs

Pertinent Physical Exam

- BP 179/73, Pulse 105, Temp 99.5 °F/37.5 °C, RR 26, SpO2 93% (on ventilator)

  Except as noted below, the findings of the complete physical exam are within normal limits

- *General:* Intubated, restless, and agitated
- *HEENT:* Bilateral mydriasis, metal-lined endotracheal tube with sutures intact per tracheotomy incision
- *CV:* Regular, tachycardic without murmurs
- *Pulm:* Clear mechanical breath sounds bilaterally
- *Abd:* Soft without obvious tenderness
- *Neuro:* Agitated, no facial asymmetry, moving all extremities equally with full strength
- *Ext:* Warm, well-perfused, no edema

Plan (2200)
Maintain deep sedation and chemical paralysis to avoid dislodgement of the endotracheal tube

Update 1 (0900) Patient with ongoing agitation, hypertension, and tachycardia despite heavy sedation regimen. Concern for anxiety due to inadequate sedation during neuromuscular blockade. Midazolam titrated up to 10 mg/hour and fentanyl to 300 mcg/hour. Cisatracurium rebolused. Dexmetetomidine added at 0.6 mcg/kg/hour.

Update 2 (1200) Called to bedside for BP 231/85, HR 133, and temperature 102.2. Septic workup initiated but concern raised for serotonin syndrome after paroxetine was noted on medication review. Repeat exam notable for ongoing agitation, bilateral mydriasis, ocular clonus, increased muscle tone, and sustained ankle clonus.

Fentanyl infusion stopped and cyproheptadine initiated at 4 mg per NG tube every 4 hours.

Update 3 (1600) Significant improvement in agitation. BP now 124/60, HR 60, Temp 99.7.

Learning Points

Priming Questions
1. What is the serotonin syndrome (SS)?
2. What are some of the most common and most overlooked medications that can precipitate SS?
3. How is SS diagnosed?
4. What are the most important features of the management of SS?

Introduction/Background

1. SS is a potentially life-threatening toxidrome caused by pharmacologic overactivation of 5-hydroxytryptamine (5HT) 1a and 2a receptors. It is characterized by the triad of altered mental status, neuromuscular abnormalities, and autonomic hyperactivity [1].
2. Incidence of SS has been increasing over the past several decades, partially owing to increased use of SSRIs in clinical practice [2], as well as likely increased symptom recognition by physicians.
3. Extrapolating from national poison center data [3], more than half of the cases are attributed to intentional ingestion, likely reflecting the frequent use of SSRIs in patients prone to suicidal and parasuicidal behaviors. The majority of other cases are likely due to drug-drug interactions and polypharmacy.
4. Though data on mortality rates are difficult to come by, death and major adverse outcomes are likely uncommon, though acute illness can be severe with multiorgan system failure.
5. Remember the Libby Zion case? Well you should! The headline-topping 1984 death of this young female patient due to the missed diagnosis of SS by allegedly overworked and under-supervised residents led to the Bell Commission that ultimately resulted in the ACGME duty hour regulations that we all know and love [4].

Libby Zion
Libby Zion, a college freshman, died on March 5, 1984. She was admitted to the hospital for rehydration and observation with "flu-like" symptoms. She was taking the antidepressant phenelzine daily. She was seen inpatient by an

intern and a second-year resident. She was noted to have unusual jerking movements and was given meperidine (Demerol®) to help control the symptoms. After becoming progressively more agitated, a phone order was given for haloperidol. The patient fell asleep, but early the next morning she was found to have a temperature of 107 °F (41.7 °C). When this was recognized, the team mobilized to begin cooling but before they were able to start the process, she suffered a fatal cardiac arrest. The cause of death was determined to be serotonin syndrome resulting from the combination of medications, all of which have effects on serotonin levels.

Physiology/Pathophysiology

1. 5HT is synthesized endogenously from the amino acid L-tryptophan and metabolized primarily in the liver by monoamine oxidase (MAO) to 5-hydroxyindoleacetic acid (5-HIAA) which is then excreted by the kidneys [5].
2. Approximately 90% of the body's 5HT is synthesized in the enterochromaffin cells of the gut with the remainder coming from serotonergic neurons in the CNS, particularly the brain's raphe nuclei, and in platelets [5].
3. The physiologic effects of 5HT are diverse and include systemic vasoconstriction, vasodilation in skeletal and cardiac muscle, bronchoconstriction, platelet aggregation, activation of gut peristalsis, modulation of mood, sleep, temperature, attention, and appetite, and stimulation of the vomiting reflex as well as both pain and itch sensation [5].
   - 5HT is involved in the pathophysiology of migraine, mood disorders, and carcinoid syndrome.
4. The list medications that have been described as precipitants of SS is long and spans multiple therapeutic classes including antidepressants, analgesics, anti-emetics, muscle relaxers, antibiotics, anti-Parkinsonian drugs, cough suppressants, and herbal supplements (see Table 54.1).
   - Illicit drugs such as cocaine and MDMA as well as over-the-counter drugs like dextromethorphan and St. John's Wart have been implicated.
   - SS associated with MAOI ingestion has been associated with more severe presentation and may portend worse outcomes [6, 7].
5. Opiates and SS:
   - SS related to opioid analgesics has been well-described, though the class as a whole remains an underrecognized cause of SS.
   - Most reports identify co-administration of opiates and several serotonergic agents, most commonly SSRIs and anti-emetics.
   - Postulated mechanisms for opioid-induced SS include weak serotonin reuptake inhibition and suppression of GABA-mediated inhibition of serotonergic neurons [9, 10].
     - Synthetic opioids also seem to inhibit the 5-HT transporter (SERT) in in-vitro studies [11].

Table 54.1 Drugs implicated in the development of serotonin syndrome by mechanism and class

Psychiatric medications	Non-psychiatric medications
Inhibitors of serotonin reuptake	
Selective serotonin reuptake inhibitors (e.g., sertraline, fluoxetine, citalopram)	Tricyclic skeletal muscle relaxants (e.g., cyclobenzaprine)
Serotonin norepinephrine reuptake inhibitors (e.g., duloxetine, venlafaxine)	Phenylpiperidine opioids (e.g., fentanyl, dextromethorphan)
Tricyclic antidepressants (e.g., amitriptyline, nortriptyline, clomipramine)	5HT3 receptor antagonists (e.g., ondansetron)
Dopamine-norephinephrine reuptake inhibitors (e.g., buproprion)	Local anesthetics (e.g., cocaine)
Serotonin modulators (e.g., trazodone)	Herbal supplements (e.g., St. John's Wort)
Tetracyclic antidepressants (e.g., mirtazapine)	Tramadol
	Meperidine
	Methadone
	MDMA
Inhibitors of serotonin metabolism	
Monoamine oxidase inhibitors (e.g., phenelzine, selegiline)	Other drugs which inhibit MAO (e.g., linezolid, methylene blue)
Drugs which increase serotonin synthesis or release	
Lithium	*L*-tryptophan
	Amphetamines
	Dopamine agonists (e.g., *L*-dopa, bromocriptine)
	MDMA
	Ethanol
	Lorcaserin
	Valerian root
	Cocaine
Serotonin receptor agonists	
Buspirone	Triptans
Vortioxetine	Anticonvulsants (e.g., valproate, carbamazepine)
Vilazodone	Ergot alkaloids
Atypical antipsychotics (e.g., quetiapine, aripiprazole, clozapine)	Fentanyl
	Metoclopramide
	LSD
Postsynaptic receptor sensitizers	
Lithium	

Adapted from Beakley et al. [8]

- Structural differences between opiate classes likely determine their propensity for 5HT agonism. Non-phenanthrenes (e.g., meperidine, tramadol, fentanyl, methadone) and the phenanthrenes lacking an oxygen bridge (e.g., dextromethorphan) exhibit serotonergic activity. Phenanthrenes containing an oxygen bridge (e.g., buprenorphine, codeine, oxycodone, hydrocodone, hydromorphone, morphine, naloxone, and naltrexone) do not [9, 12].
  - However, case reports involving several of the phenanthrenes with an oxygen bridge do call this hypothesis into question [13].

6. Possible triggers of SS include:
   - Introduction of a new serotonergic medication.
   - Deliberate or accidental overdose on a serotonergic medication.
   - Co-administration of several medications with serotonergic properties.
   - Altered metabolism of serotonergic drugs via inhibition of cyp450 enzymes.
   - Altered 5HT metabolism via inhibition of monoamine oxidase.
   - Discontinuation of a drug with 5HT antagonist properties (e.g., Clozapine) in patients taking a selective serotonin reuptake inhibitor (SSRI) [14].
   - Rarely, appropriate therapeutic dosing of a single serotonergic agent [15].

Making the Diagnosis

Differential Diagnosis of Serotonin Syndrome
- Neuroleptic malignant syndrome
- Malignant hyperthermia
- Sepsis
- Thyroid storm
- Alcohol/benzodiazepine withdrawal
- Anticholinergic toxidrome
- Sympathomimetic toxidrome

1. SS is diagnosed by recognition of its clinical features in the setting of serotonergic medication administration. No specific laboratory or radiographic findings are diagnostic.
2. The Hunter serotonin toxicity criteria [16] have demonstrated excellent diagnostic performance and are considered the standard tool for the diagnosis of SS (see Table 54.2 below).
   - In its retrospective derivation trial, the Hunter criteria performed significantly better than the older Sternbach criteria, with 84% sensitivity and 97% specificity relative to the gold standard of diagnosis by a certified medical toxicologist among 2222 patients admitted with an overdose of a serotonergic agent [16].
   - However, the Hunter criteria have yet to be prospectively validated.

Table 54.2 The Hunter serotonin toxicity criteria

1. Treatment with a serotonergic agent
and
2. At least one of the following:
   Spontaneous clonus
   Inducible clonus PLUS agitation or diaphoresis
   Ocular clonus PLUS agitation or diaphoresis
   Tremor PLUS hyperreflexia
   Hypertonia PLUS temperature > 38 °C PLUS ocular clonus or inducible clonus

Table 54.3 Differential diagnosis for conditions mimicking serotonin syndrome [1]

Disorder	Context	Distinguishing features
Serotonin Syndrome	Exposure to serotonergic agents; onset over a period of hours and resolution within 24 hours of treatment	Hyperreflexia, clonus (especially ocular), rigidity with lower extremity predominance, mydriasis, diarrhea/hyperactive bowel sounds
Neuroleptic Malignant Syndrome	Exposure to dopamine antagonists; onset over a period of days to weeks, resolution in ~9 days with treatment	Acute Parkinsonism, lead-pipe rigidity, bradyreflexia, normal to hypoactive bowel sounds
Malignant Hyperthermia	Exposure to inhalation anesthetics or depolarizing neuromuscular blockers; onset over minutes to hours, resolution within 24–48 hours with treatment	Normal mental status, rigidity (especially in masseter muscle), hypercarbia
Thyroid Storm	Elevated free T4 with suppressed or elevated TSH; history of hyperthyroidism	Goiter, exophthalmos, high-output heart failure, no neuromuscular findings
Sympathomimetic Toxicity	Exposure to stimulant agents	No neuromuscular findings, typically normothermic
Anticholinergic Toxicity	Exposure to anticholinergic agents	Dry skin, urinary retention, hypoactive bowel sounds, no neuromuscular findings, typically normothermic
Sepsis/meningitis	Localizing signs & symptoms and/or laboratory or radiographic evidence of infection	No neuromuscular findings, normal pupils, not typically hypertensive
Alcohol or Benzodiazepine Withdrawal	Known recent intoxication, laboratory evidence of ingestion, or known history of abuse/withdrawal	No neuromuscular findings, typically normothermic

3. Though not included in the Hunter criteria, differentiation from other conditions that present with similar clinical features is crucial in the diagnosis of SS (see Table 54.3 below).
   - Any time a febrile tachycardic patient presents with *HYPER*tension, you should pause and consider this differential before closing on the diagnosis of sepsis!
4. Onset of symptoms in SS is typically within 24 hours of the inciting event and resolution most often occurs within 24 hours of stopping the offending agent, though more protracted presentations may occur in the setting of longer-acting agents such as fluoxetine or the irreversible MAOIs [17].
5. Mild cases present similarly to the sympathomimetic toxidrome with agitation, mydriasis, diaphoresis, tremor, tachycardia, and hypertension. As severity increases, patients develop hyperpyrexia, muscular rigidity with hyperreflexia, myoclonus especially in the lower extremities, along with more pronounced mental status abnormalities. The most severe cases may result in rhabdomyolysis, acute renal failure, seizures, respiratory failure, coma, and cardiac arrest.

- Ocular clonus is a unique feature characterized by rapid, involuntary, spontaneous spastic eye movements in multiple directions and is essentially pathognomonic. If you've seen this once, you'll never miss it!
6. Labs and imaging:
    - Although this diagnosis is made solely based on clinical features, several studies should be ordered to screen for alternate diagnoses and identify complications of SS:
        - Urine and serum toxicology panels to confirm the presence of serotonergic agents and rule out other ingestions such as sympathomimetics, anticholinergics, and antidopaminergic agents.
        - CBC to assess for leukocytosis or anemia.
        - Blood cultures, urinalysis, and chest x-ray to identify possible sources of sepsis.
        - Consider lumbar puncture to rule out meningoencephalitis.
        - Complete metabolic panel and lactate to identify electrolyte abnormalities and assess for end-organ injury.
        - Creatine phosphokinase to assess for rhabdomyolysis.
        - Thyroid-stimulating hormone and free T4 levels to rule out thyroid storm.
        - EKG to assess for arrhythmia.
        - Blood gases to assess the adequacy of oxygenation and ventilation.

Treating the Patient

1. The definitive treatment for SS is discontinuation of all serotonergic drugs which typically leads to resolution of symptoms within 24 hours [1].
2. Supportive care includes benzodiazepines for agitation and seizures, IV fluids for rhabdomyolysis, and supplemental oxygen as needed.
    - Consider adding short-acting IV beta blockers or calcium channel blockers if hypertension remains uncontrolled despite treating agitation.
    - Tylenol and NSAIDs *will not* work for hyperthermia here because the heat is generated by increased neuromuscular activity rather than a typical hypothalamic fever.
3. Serotonin antagonist therapy is indicated for moderate to severe cases or when symptoms do not remit with the cessation of the offending agent.
    - Cyproheptadine is a first-generation antihistamine with 5-HT1A and 5-HT2A antagonist properties.
        - It is considered the gold-standard first-line therapy despite a dearth of evidence for its safety and efficacy.
        - The usual starting dose is 12 mg, followed by 2 mg every 2 hours as long as symptoms persist. A maintenance dose of 8 mg every 6 hours has been recommended, though the appropriate duration has not been established [1].
        - Therapy can be monitored via the assessment of pupils. In active SS, cyproheptadine will cause miosis due to 5HT antagonism but when SS has resolved it will cause mydriasis due to its anticholinergic effects [18].

- There is no parenteral formulation of cyproheptadine, limiting its use in patients without enteral access.
- Side-effects may include sedation and hypotension, which may be desirable in this setting. Anticholinergic properties may worsen hyperthermia by inhibition of diaphoresis [19].
- Also beware of exacerbating anticholinergic toxicity from co-ingestion in patients with suicide attempts.
4. Other agents have also been used to treat SS including chlorpromazine.
   • Chlorpromazine confers the benefit of a parental formulation. However, there is also a significant risk of hypotension, hyperthermia, and a theoretical risk of lowering seizure threshold which limits its use in this setting [19].
   - It is also not the best choice if NMS remains on the differential!
   - Based on reported cases, a reasonable starting dose is 50-100 mg IM with repeat dosing every 6 hours until symptoms resolve [19].
5. For the most severe cases involving profound encephalopathy, hemodynamic instability, or end-organ injury, the patient should be intubated, sedated, and started on continuous neuromuscular blockade.

Case Conclusion

Although the patient had a dramatic improvement in his symptoms with stopping the fentanyl infusion and administration of cyproheptadine, his symptoms did intermittently resurface over the next 48 hours requiring repeat doses of cyproheptadine, each time with improvement. He was eventually taken back to the operating room for completion of a formal tracheostomy and discharged from the hospital without any obvious sequelae of his SS.

Discussion

SS is an uncommon but likely underrecognized cause of altered mental status, autonomic instability, and neuromuscular abnormalities. Clinicians should be vigilant for this diagnosis in patients who are prescribed serotonergic medications, especially if taking multiple offenders or if a new agent was recently added or increased in dosage, and in patients with depression and suicidality. Always review the patient's current medication list including over-the-counter meds, herbal supplements, and illicit substances when prescribing a serotonergic agent. Use caution and provide counseling regarding SS if multiple serotonergic agents are to be used. You DO NOT want to be named in the next Libby Zion case! Do not forget about opioids as potential triggers of SS. Apply the Hunter criteria when suspecting SS. Always at least consider this diagnosis when you see a patient who is tachycardic and HYPERtensive with a fever. Obtain targeted laboratory and imaging studies to rule out other diagnoses and look for evidence of end-organ injury.

The mainstay of treatment is to stop the offending agent and provide supportive care. Consider serotonin antagonist therapy with cyproheptadine for moderate to severe cases. If the patient is truly unstable or has a severe end-organ injury, intubate and start continuous neuromuscular blockade.

Pattern Recognition

- Exposure to serotonergic agents
- Agitated delirium
- Hyperthermia, tachycardia, hypertension
- Myoclonus/hyperreflexia (LE > UE)
- Mydriasis
- Tremors
- Ocular clonus is essentially pathognomonic

Disclosure Statement The authors of this chapter report no significant disclosures.

References

1. Volpi-abadie J, Kaye AM, Kaye AD. Serotonin syndrome. The Ochsner Journal. 2013;13(4):533–40.
2. Boyer EW, Shannon M. Current concepts: the serotonin syndrome. N Engl J Med. 2005;352(11):1112–20.
3. Gummin D, Mowry J, Spyker D, Brooks D, Fraser M, Banner W. 2016 Annual Report of the American Association of Poison Control Centers' National Poison Data System (NPDS): 34th Annual Report. Clin Toxicol. 2017;55(10):1072–254.
4. Asch DA, Parker RM. The Libby Zion case. One step forward or two steps backward? N Engl J Med. 1988;318(12):771–5.
5. Trevor AJ, Katzung BG, Kruidering-Hall M, Trevor AJ, Katzung BG, Kruidering-Hall M. Antidepressants. In: Trevor AJ, et al., editors. Katzung & trevor's pharmacology: examination & board review. 11th ed. New York, NY: McGraw-Hill; 2015. http://accesspharmacy.mhmedical.com/content.aspx?bookid=1568&sectionid=95702844. Accessed 17 Sep 2019.
6. Isbister GK, N a B. The pathophysiology of serotonin toxicity in animals and humans: implications for diagnosis and treatment. Clin Neuropharmacol. 2005;28(5):205–14.
7. Ramsay RR, Dunford C, Gillman PK. Methylene blue and serotonin toxicity: inhibition of monoamine oxidase A (MAO A) confirms a theoretical prediction. Br J Pharmacol. 2007;152(6):946–51.
8. Beakley BD, Kaye AM, Kaye AD. Tramadol, pharmacology, side effects, and serotonin syndrome: a review. Pain Physician. 2015;18(10):395–400.
9. Gillman PK. Monoamine oxidase inhibitors, opioid analgesics and serotonin toxicity. Br J Anaesth. 2005;95(4):434–41.
10. Tao R, Auerbach SB. GABAergic and glutamatergic afferents in the dorsal raphe nucleus mediate morphine-induced increases in serotonin efflux in the rat central nervous system. J Pharmacol Exp Ther. 2002;303(2):704–10.

11. Rickli A, Liakoni E, Hoener MCLM. Opioid-induced inhibition of the human 5-HT and nor-adrenaline transporters in vitro: link to clinical reports of serotonin syndrome. Br J Pharmacol. 2018;175(3):532–43.

12. Codd EE, Shank RP, Schupsky JJ, Raffa RB. Serotonin and norepinephrine uptake inhibiting activity of centrally acting analgesics: structural determinants and role in antinociception. J Pharmacol Exp Ther. 1995;274(3):1263–70.

13. Jhun P, Bright A, Herbert M. Serotonin syndrome and opioids--what's the deal? Ann Emerg Med. 2015;65(4):434–5.

14. S. S, C.O. H, S. W, W. W. Serotonin syndrome precipitated by sertraline and discontinuation of clozapine. Clin Toxicol. 2015;53(8):840–1.

15. Robles L. Serotonin syndrome induced by fentanyl in a child: case report. Clin Neuropharmacol. 2015;38(5):206–8.

16. Dunkley EJC, Isbister GK, Sibbritt D, Dawson AH, Whyte IM. The hunter serotonin toxicity criteria: simple and accurate diagnostic decision rules for serotonin toxicity. QJM – Mon J Assoc Physicians. 2003;96(9):635–42.

17. Kolecki P. Venlafaxine induced serotonin syndrome occurring after abstinence from phenel-zine for more than two weeks. Toxicol Clin Toxicol. 1997;35:211–2.

18. McDaniel WW. Serotonin syndrome: early management with cyproheptadine. Ann Pharmacother. 2001;35(7–8):870–3.

19. Graudins A, Stearman A, Chan B, Kulig K. Treatment of the serotonin syndrome with cypro-heptadine. J Emerg Med. 1998;16(4):615–9.

Stevens Johnson Syndrome – *"Steven Who? And Why I Should Care About His Johnson?"*

55

Zachary E. Cardon, Colin G. Kaide, and Jason J. Bischof

Case

Sick Patient with a Rash

Pertinent History

A 22-year-old female presents with a diffuse rash including desquamation of mucous membranes and lips. She was recently started on lamotrigine (Lamictal®) at an initial dose of 100 mg, Clonazepam 0.5 mg, and Doxycycline approximately 2 weeks ago. She reports that the rash began 3 days prior to presentation. She was seen at an outside hospital and was diagnosed with hand, foot, and mouth disease and treated with supportive care. Her rash continued to worsen, spreading to her trunk, groin, and mouth. She is unable to tolerate drinking liquids due to severe pain. She describes the rash on her body as pruritic. She has no past medical history of skin disorders.

Z. E. Cardon
The University of North Carolina School of Medicine, Department of Emergency Medicine, Columbus, OH, USA

C. G. Kaide
Department of Emergency Medicine, Wexner Medical Center at The Ohio State University, Columbus, OH, USA

J. J. Bischof (✉)
The University of North Carolina School of Medicine, Department of Emergency Medicine, Columbus, OH, USA

Department of Emergency Medicine, Wexner Medical Center at The Ohio State University, Columbus, OH, USA
e-mail: jason.bischof@osumc.edu

© Springer Nature Switzerland AG 2020
C. G. Kaide, C. E. San Miguel (eds.), *Case Studies in Emergency Medicine*, https://doi.org/10.1007/978-3-030-22445-5_55

PMH Seizures, Anxiety Disorder

Meds Lamotrigine, Clonazepam, Doxycycline

Pertinent Physical Exam
- Blood pressure 130/70, pulse 116, temperature 99.9 °F (37.7 °C), RR 16, SpO2 99%.

Except as noted below, the findings of a complete physical exam are within normal limits.

- Mouth: Multiple lesions in mouth, yellow crusting and desquamation of mucous membranes of lips, tongue, and buccal mucosa.
- Eyes: Conjunctival injection present bilaterally.
- Cardiovascular: Tachycardia present, regular rhythms, no murmurs.
- GU: Vaginal mucosal lesions noted.
- Skin: Skin is warm and dry. No erythema. Diffuse maculo papular rash with pink papules coalescing into plaques with superimposed vesicles and bullae.

ED Management

The most likely diagnoses considered at the time of presentation were Erythema Multiforme Major and Stevens-Johnson Syndrome. Dermatology was consulted and evaluated the patient at the bedside. Based on the patient's clinical history and physical exam they felt the patient was more likely exhibiting Erythema Multiforme Major. The patient was admitted for further management and workup.

Learning Points

Priming Questions
1. What is the difference between Erythema Multiforme, Stevens-Johnson Syndrome, and Toxic Epidermal Necrolysis?
2. What are specific causes and risk factors of Stevens-Johnson Syndrome/Toxic Epidermal Necrolysis that I can look for in a patient's history?
3. What is the treatment and disposition of Stevens-Johnson/Toxic Epidermal Necrolysis?

Introduction/Background

1. Erythema Multiforme (EM) versus Stevens-Johnson Syndrome (SJS) versus Toxic Epidermal Necrolysis (TEN) is a confusing set of definitions. The definition has undergone revision over the years such that the final consensus definition divides the entities into two spectra [1].
   - Erythema Multiforme
     - Erythema Multiforme Minor: Typically presents with target lesions, however early on initial lesions may be raised erythematous papules. Typical target lesions contain three concentric zones. Lesions are most commonly on extensor surfaces of acral extremities (finger, hands, toes, feet) (Image 1) and spread centripetal [2, 3].
     - Erythema Multiforme Major: Combines the findings of EM minor with the involvement of one or more mucosal membranes. In one study, 63% of patients with EM had mucosal involvement [4]. Also by definition EM cannot have the detachment of skin greater than 10% of total body surface area (TBSA) [5].

Erythema Multiforme Minor of the Hand

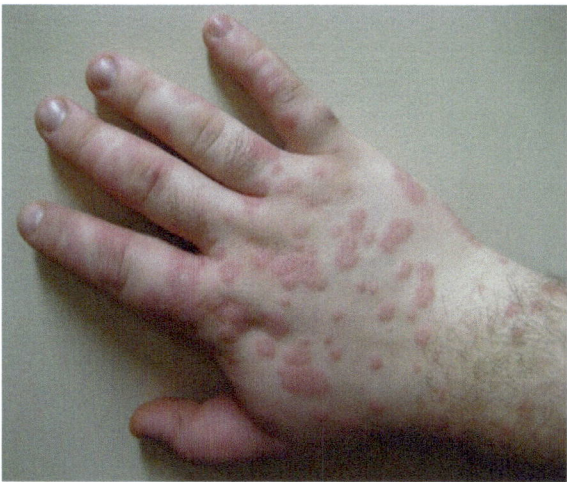

James Heilman, MD (https://commons.wikimedia.org/wiki/File: Erythema_multiforme_minor_of_the_hand.jpg), "Erythema multiforme minor of the hand", https://creativecommons.org/licenses/by-sa/3.0/legalcode

- SJS/TEN.
  - SJS/TEN are considered to be a single entity, just along different ends of the severity spectrum: When <10% of TBSA is involved, the disease is labeled as SJS. If >30% of TBSA is involved, it is called TEN. Between 10 and 30%, there is overlap between the two labels [6, 7].
  - Lesions predominate on the trunk and face and spread symmetrically to other areas of the body and the extremities (Image 2). This spectrum typically presents with diffuse erythema or purpuric macules and blistering. Ninety percent of the time one or more mucous membrane is affected with erosions (Image 3) [8, 9]. As the disease progresses, bullae form and coalesce, forming flaccid blisters with full thickness epidermal necrosis.

Stevens-Johnson Syndrome

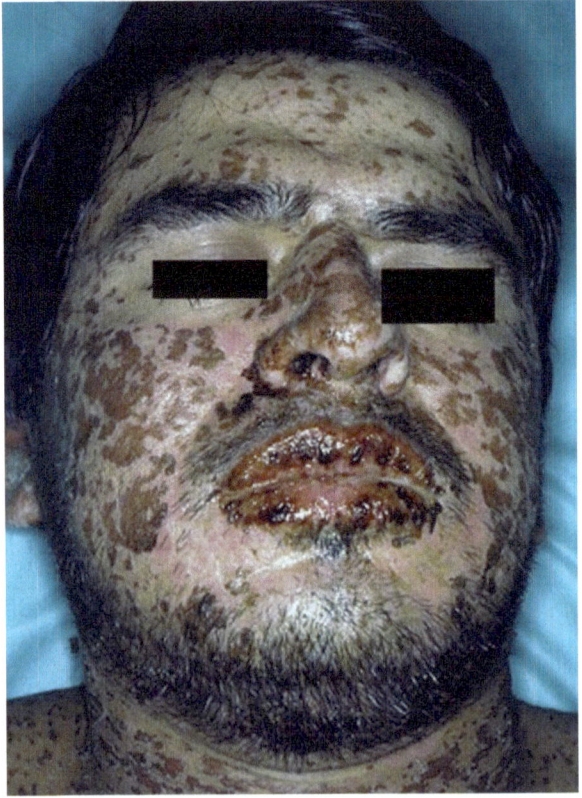

Dr. Thomas Habif (https://commons.wikimedia .org/wiki/File:Stevens-johnson syndrome.jpg), "Stevens-johnson-syndrome", https://creativecommons.org/licenses/by-sa/3.0/legalcode

Stevens-Johnson Syndrome

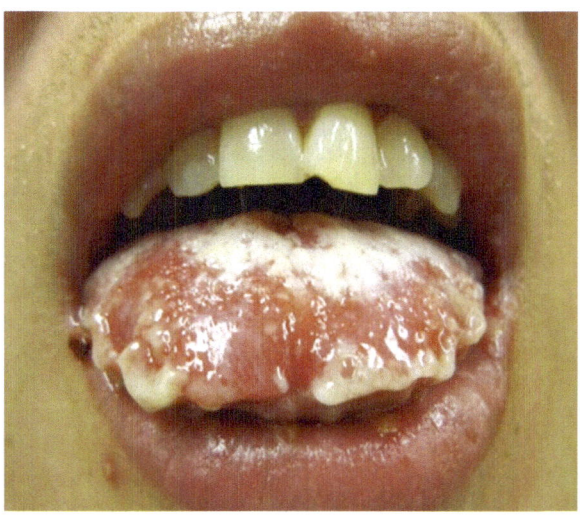

James Heilman, MD (https://commons.wikimedia. org/wiki/File: Mucosal_desquamation_in_a_ person_with_Stevens–Johnson_ syndrome.jpg), "Mucosal desquamation in a person with Stevens–Johnson syndrome", https://creativecommons.org/licenses/by-sa/3.0/legalcode

2. Ninety percent of cases of EM are thought to be triggered by infection with Herpes Simplex Virus (HSV) being the most commonly identified pathogen [2, 10]. Certain classes of medication, particularly barbiturates, hydantoins, nonsteroidal anti-inflammatory drugs, penicillin's, phenothiazines, and sulfonamides, can also trigger EM [11].

3. The incidence of SJS/TEN is roughly 4–6 cases per million person/year [12, 13]. Mortality is approximately 5% for Stevens-Johnson syndrome, and anywhere from 30–50% for toxic epidermal necrolysis [7]. Approximately 50% of cases of SJS and 80–90% of cases of TEN are drug induced [14]. Mycoplasma pneumonia is likely the second most common cause, particularly in children, though this is somewhat controversial as it also can be the cause of EM [15].

Physiology/Pathophysiology

1. The pathogenesis of SJS/TEN is not completely understood. It appears that through an unknown mechanism, cytotoxic T cells and natural killer cells begin to attack keratinocytes and cause massive apoptosis [16].

2. By and large, when suspecting possible SJS/TEN in patients and hunting for causes, it is all about the drug history. Certain drugs are more likely to cause SJS/TEN.

- Short-Term Drug Use vs Long-Term Drug Use.
  - The risk of SJS/TEN appears to be largely limited to the first 8 weeks of taking an at-risk medication. While it is possible to develop SJS/TEN after taking an at-risk drug for a longer period of time, it is unlikely [17, 18].
- Lamotrigine (Lamictal®) and SJS/TEN.
  - The patient in this case had been started on Lamotrigine around 2 weeks prior to her presentation to the ED. Seven to ten percent of patients started on Lamotrigine will develop a rash, but only 3 in 1000 will require hospitalization [19]. Rash and other skin conditions are more common in children, so this medication is often reserved for adults [20].
  - Appropriate dosing and dosing adjustment can prevent or decrease the risk of lamotrigine-associated rashes. In adults, the recommended initial dose of lamotrigine alone (in the absence of cytochrome P-450 inhibitors or enhancers) is 25 mg po daily for the first 2 weeks, 50 mg daily during weeks 3 and 4, and then weekly increases of 50–100 mg per day as clinically indicated. The patient in this case was started at 100 mg from day 1.

Drug	Relative risk
TMP/sulfa and other sulfonamide abx	172
Carbamazepine	90
Oxicam-NSAIDS	72
Corticosteroids	54
Phenytoin	53
Allopurinol	52
Phenobarbital	45
Valproic acid	25
Nevirapine	22
Cephalosporins	14
Pantoprazole	18
Tramadol	20
Lamotrigine	14
Sertraline	11
Quinolones	10
Aminopenicillins	6.7

3. There are certain patient risk factors that also make one more prone to develop SJS/TEN.
   - Patients with HIV are reported to have around 100-fold higher risk to develop SJS/TEN [21]. Active malignancy also increases the incidence, particularly hematologic cancers, at an estimate of at least two-fold [12]. High dose and rapid introduction of medications, systemic lupus, and radiation therapy also appear to increase the risk of SJS/TEN as well [22–24].

Making the Diagnosis

The Differential – Whoa! That Person Is Sick…and Look at that Rash!!
- Acute Generalized Exanthemtous Pustolosis
- Drug Eruption
- Erythema Multiforme
- Erythroderma
- Kawasaki Disease (kids)
- Pemphigus Vulgaris
- Bullous Pemphigoid
- Staph Scalded Skin Syndrome (kids)
- Toxic Shock Syndrome

1. The diagnosis of SJS/TEN in the emergency department will always be a clinical diagnosis. The are no specific labs or imaging that will clinch the diagnosis. The patient's history, particularly drug history, symptoms leading up to the start of a developing a rash, and identifying the rash itself will make up your three components.
   - Typically a prodrome of an influenza-like illness (fever, malaise, headache, cough, and conjunctivitis) develops 1–3 weeks after initiation of drug [25].
   - Skin lesions appear 1–3 days after the prodrome [14]. As discussed above in the introduction, lesions start out as ill-defined coalescing macules with purpuric centers on the face and trunk and spread to extremities and mature into large confluent blisters that undergo epidermal detachment [26].
     - Blistering and epidermal detachment lead to a positive Nikolsky sign (light lateral pressure at what appears to be unaffected skin leads to sloughing) as well as a positive Asboe-Hansen sign (lateral extension of bullae with downward pressure).

Nikolsky Sign

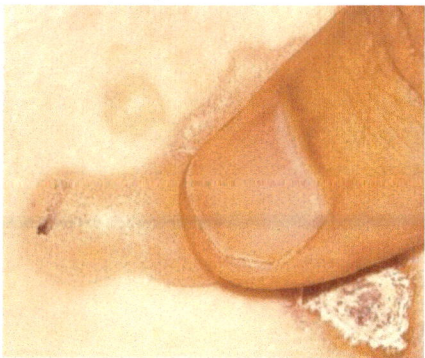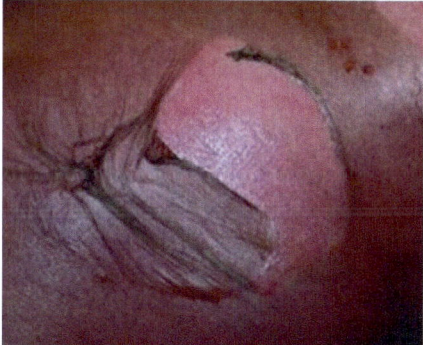

Source unknown—Public domain images

- Three to five days of sloughing lead to denuded or exposed underlying skin causing extreme pain, massive loss of fluid and protein, bleeding, evaporative heat loss with subsequent hypothermia, and infection.
- There is also simultaneous mucosal involvement with cutaneous presentation.
  - Oral mucosa and the vermillion border are involved with painful hemorrhagic erosions.
  - Eighty percent of patients also have ocular involvement including pain, photophobia, severe conjunctivitis with discharge, corneal ulceration, and uveitis [27].
2. Particular lab findings are often present though nonspecific, and while seeing these abnormalities can bolster your confidence in your diagnosis of SJS/TEN, there are no labs to hang your hat on.
   - Anemia and lymphopenia are often seen, and neutropenia can be seen as well in a third of patients. Neutropenia in particular is indicative of a worse prognosis. Thrombocytopenia is seen as well but only in 10–20% of patients. Elevated erythrocyte sedimentation rate, mildly elevated serum transaminases, and elevated BUN are also often noted [7].
3. As with many skin-related disorders, a biopsy can be very helpful and often definitively provide a diagnosis. Due to some skin diseases mimicking SJS/TEN, biopsy can be the only way to confirm the diagnosis. However, in the acute setting of the emergency department, skin biopsies are not going to happen, so the patient must be treated based on clinical judgment.

Treating the Patient

1. Stop the offending drug! Review medications that are frequently associated with SJS and stop them. While not generally used in the acute phase of illness, there is an algorithm, ALDEN, that has been developed to help define drug causality [28]. However in the ED setting you can stop all medications that seem possible culprits, particularly looking at medications started in the last 8 weeks.
2. Employ anti-shear handling and try to avoid breaking large bullae if you can. Denuded skin leaks serum and becomes coated with necrotic debris. This combined with hemorrhagic crusting acts as an excellent substrate for bacteria leading to infection and possible sepsis, the leading cause of death in SJS/TEN [8].
   - Hold on antibiotics unless you actually think there is a wound infection. Most of these patients will have fevers due to the associated inflammatory response. Pull the trigger if other signs of possible infection including confusion, hypotension, reduced urine output or oxygen saturation, or if an obvious wound infection is present. Be sure to cover for *Staphyloccocus* and *Pseudomonas* species with your antibiotic choice [8].
3. Remember that SJS/TEN can involve the mucosa and even the GI tract! Complications of pneumonias, ARDS, small bowel ulcers and colonic perforations have been reported [29–31].
4. The wounds from SJS/TEN can be thought of as similar to extensive burns. Treatment in a burn-unit setting is indicated and reduces mortality, particularly

with TEN [32–34]. There are some important differences between SJS/TEN and burns!

- In SJS/TEN, the extent of skin damage is limited to the superficial dermal layers of the skin.
- SJS/TEN has less fluid, electrolyte and energy requirements. 2 ml/kg × % affected TBSA of fluid is usually adequate to maintain urine output and blood pressure in the normal range [35]. Burns usually require more fluid recusitation [36].
- TEN often involves the GI tract, respiratory system, and the ocular system in addition to the skin. Significant sequelae in these organ systems are possible.

5. As there is frequent involvement of ocular surfaces and genital areas, often multiple specialties are involved in the inpatient management including ophthalmology and gynecology.
6. IVIG, steroids, and cyclosporin have all been used in the treatment of SJS/TEN with mixed results [37]. These may be started in consultation with other services or the admitting team. In the ED, initial treatment is mostly supportive care.
7. Prognosis.
   - SCORTEN scoring system (SCORe of Toxic Epidermal Necrosis) has been developed that predicts the probability of hospital mortality [38]. There are seven parameters including age, malignancy, heart rate, TBSA, serum urea, glucose, and bicarbonate. Each positive is 1 point for a total of 7 points. The higher the score the greater mortality.

Scorten		
Risk factor	0 Points	1 Point
Age	<40 years	>40 years
Associated malignancy	No	Yes
Heart rate	<120	>120
Serum BUN (mg/dL)	<28	>28
Detached or compromised body surface	<10%	>10%
Serum bicarbonate (mEq/L)	>20	<20
Serum glucose (mg/dL)	<252	>252

Risk factors and mortality rate: 0–1 (3.2%), 2 (12.1%), 3 (35.3%), 4 (58.3%), 5 or more (>90%)

Case Conclusion

A punch biopsy was performed that was inconclusive: Erythema Multiforme Major versus Stevens-Johnson Syndrome. The patient was treated with one dose of IVIG which was not continued due to poor patient tolerance. The patient gradually improved with supportive care.

Discussion

These observations are made based on this writer's experience with SJS/TEN.

As with all emergency department presentations, these patients can be sick or not sick. There are so many skin conditions and diseases out there, you are not going to diagnosis everyone. But look at the whole picture to determine whether you need a more thorough workup or need to get consultants involved. What are the vitals? How does the patient look? Are they septic? The fundamentals of emergency medicine will help guide your management.

For any patient with a rash that gives you a concern for SJS/TEN, get that good drug history. Luckily, the data show that there are certain drugs to look out for, and they were likely started in the last few weeks to a month. If they have one of the "likely suspects," then start becoming more concerned.

When in doubt, ask for help and ask for it early. If you see a rash on a patient that makes your skin hurt, lots of scattered bullae/open wounds, get those burn and/or dermatology consults in early. These patients experience a great deal of insensible water loss; they need early fluids, wound care, and admission.

And one more thing, when starting a new medication on a patient, follow the directions!

Pattern Recognition

Steven-Johnson Syndrome/Toxic Epidermal Necrolysis
- Prodrome of flu-like illness
- Painful rapidly progressing targetoid rash
- Nikolsky Sign
- Mucosal involvement
- Drug of notoriety recently started

Disclosure Statement Zachary Cardone and Jason Bischoff have no disclosures.
Colin Kaide: Callibra, Inc.-Discharge 123 medical software company. Medical Advisory Board Portola Pharmaceuticals. I have no relationship with a commercial company that has a direct financial interest in subject matter or materials discussed in article or with a company making a competing product.

References

1. Assier H, Bastuji-Garin S, Revuz J, et al. Erythema multiforme with mucous membrane involvement and Stevens-Johnson syndrome are clinically different disorders with distinct causes. Arch Dermatol. 1995;131:539–43.
2. Bastuji-Garin S, Rzany B, Stern RS, Shear NH, Naldi L, Roujeau JC. Clinical classification of cases of toxic epidermal necrolysis, Stevens-Johnson syndrome, and erythema multiforme. Arch Dermatol. 1993;129(1):92–6.
3. Huff JC, Weston WL, Tonnesen MG. Erythema multiforme: a critical review of characteristics, diagnostic criteria, and causes. J Am Acad Dermatol. 1983;8:763.
4. Wetter DA, Davis MD. Recurrent erythema multiforme: clinical characteristics, etiologic associations, and treatment in a series of 48 patients at Mayo Clinic, 2000 to 2007. J Am Acad Dermatol. 2010;62(1):45–53.
5. Lerch M, Mainetti C, Beretta-Piccoli B, Harr T. Current perspectives on erythema multiforme. Clin Rev Allergy Immunol. 2018;54:177–84.

6. Roujeau J-C. Stevens-Johnson syndrome and toxic epidermal necrolysis are severity variants of the same disease which differs from erythema multiforme. J Dermatol. 1997;24:726–9.
7. Fromowitz JS, Ramos-Caro FA, Flowers FP. Practical guidelines for the management of toxic epidermal necrolysis and Stevens-Johnson syndrome. Int J Dermatol. 2007;46(10):1092–4.
8. Roujeau JC, Hosidow O, Saiag P, Guillaume JC. Toxic epidermal necrolysis (Lyell syndrome). J Am Acad Dermatol. 1990;23:1039–58.
9. Bircher A. Symptoms and danger signs in acute drug hypersensitivity. Toxicology. 2005;209:201–7.
10. Weston WL. Herpes-associated erythema multiforme. J Investig Dermatol. 2005;124:xv–xvi.
11. Volcheck GW. Clinical evaluation and management of drug hypersensitivity. Immunol Allergy Clin N Am. 2004;24:357–71.
12. Frey N, Jossi J, Bodmer M, Bircher A, Jick SS, Meier CR, Spoendlin J. The epidemiology of Stevens-Johnson syndrome and toxic epidermal necrolysis in the UK. J Invest Dermatol. 2017;137(6):1240.
13. Chan HL, Stern RS, Arndt KA, Langlois J, Jick SS, Jick H, Walker AM. The incidence of erythema multiforme, Stevens-Johnson syndrome, and toxic epidermal necrolysis. A population-based study with particular reference to reactions caused by drugs among outpatients. Arch Dermatol. 1990;126(1):43.
14. Parrillo SJ. Stevens-Johnson syndrome and toxic epidermal necrolysis. Curr Allergy Asthma Rep. 2007;7(4):243–7.
15. Wetter DA, Camilleri MJ. Clinical, etiologic, and histopathologic features of Stevens-Johnson syndrome during an 8-year period at Mayo Clinic. Mayo Clin Proc. 2010;85(2):131.
16. Correia O, Delgado L, Ramos JP, Resende C, Torrinha JA. Arch Dermatol. 1993;129(4):466–8.
17. Roujeau JC, Kelly JP, Naldi L, et al. Medication use and the risk of Stevens-Johnson syndrome or toxic epidermal necrolysis. N Engl J Med. 1995;333:1600–7.
18. Mockenhaupt M, Viboud C, Dunant A, et al. Stevens-Johnson syndrome and toxic epidermal necrolysis: assessment of medication risks with emphasis on recently marketed drugs. The EuroSCAR-study. J Invest Dermatol. 2008;128:35–44.
19. Wang X-q, et al. Risk of a lamotrigine-related skin rash: current meta-analysis and postmarketing cohort analysis. Seizure. 2015;25:52–61.
20. Guberman AH, Besag FM, Brodie MJ, Dooley JM, Duchowny MS, Pellock JM, Richens A, Stern RS, Trevathan E. Lamotrigine-associated rash: risk/benefit considerations in adults and children. Epilepsia. 1999;40:985–91.
21. Mittmann N, Knowles SR, Koo M, Shear NH, Rachlis A, Rourke SB. Incidence of toxic epidermal necrolysis and Stevens-Johnson syndrome in an HIV cohort: an observational, retrospective case series study. Am J Clin Dermatol. 2012;13(1):49–54.
22. Horne NS, Narayan AR, Young RM, Frieri M. Toxic epidermal necrolysis in systemic lupus erythematosus. Autoimmun Rev. 2006;5(2):160.
23. Halevy S, Ghislain PD, Mockenhaupt M, Fagot JP, Bouwes Bavinck JN, Sidoroff A, Naldi L, Dunant A, Viboud C, Roujeau JC, EuroSCAR Study Group. Allopurinol is the most common cause of Stevens-Johnson syndrome and toxic epidermal necrolysis in Europe and Israel. J Am Acad Dermatol. 2008;58(1):25.
24. Sommers KR, Kong KM, Bui DT, Fruehauf JP, Holcombe RF. Stevens-Johnson syndrome/toxic epidermal necrolysis in a patient receiving concurrent radiation and gemcitabine. Anti-Cancer Drugs. 2003;14(8):659.
25. Roujeau JC. Immune mechanisms in drug allergy. Allergol Int. 2006;55(1):27.
26. Roujeau JC, Stern RS. Severe adverse cutaneous reactions to drugs. N Engl J Med. 1994;331(19):1272.
27. Kohanim S, Palioura S, Saeed HN, et al. Acute and chronic ophthalmic involvement in Stevens-Johnson syndrome/toxic epidermal necrolysis – a comprehensive review and guide to therapy. II. Ophthalmic disease. Ocul Surf. 2016;14:168–88.
28. Sassolas B, Haddad C, Mockenhaupt M, et al. ALDEN, an algorithm for assessment of drug causality in Stevens-Johnson syndrome and toxic epidermal necrolysis: comparison with case–control analysis. Clin Pharmacol Ther. 2010;88:60–8.

29. de Prost N, Mekontso-Dessap A, Valeyrie-Allanore L, Van Nhieu JT, Duong TA, Chosidow O, Wolkenstein P, Brun-Buisson C, Maître B. Acute respiratory failure in patients with toxic epidermal necrolysis: clinical features and factors associated with mechanical ventilation. Crit Care Med. 2014;42(1):118.

30. Sakai N, Yoshizawa Y, Amano A, Higashi N, Aoki M, Seo T, Suzuki K, Tanaka S, Tsukui T, Sakamoto C, Arai M, Yamamoto Y, Kawana S. Toxic epidermal necrolysis complicated by multiple intestinal ulcers. Int J Dermatol. 2008;47(2):180–2.

31. Carter FM, Mitchell CK. Toxic epidermal necrolysis–an unusual cause of colonic perforation. Report of a case. Dis Colon Rectum. 1993;36(8):773–7.

32. McGee T, Munster A. Toxic epidermal necrolysis syndrome: mortality rate reduced with early referral to regional burn center. Plast Reconstr Surg. 1998;102:1018–22.

33. Palmieri TL, Greenhalgh DG, Saffle JR, et al. A multicenter review of toxic epidermal necrolysis treated in U.S. burn centers at the end of the twentieth century. J Burn Care Rehabil. 2002;23:87–96.

34. Mahar PD, Wasiak J, Hii B, et al. A systematic review of the management and outcome of toxic epidermal necrolysis treated in burns centers. Burns. 2014;40:1245–54.

35. Shiga S, Cartotto R. What are the fluid requirements in toxic epidermal necrolysis? J Burn Care Res. 2010;31:100–4.

36. Cancio LC, et al. Protocolized resuscitation of burn patients. Crit Care Clin. 2016;32(4):599–610.

37. Creamer D, Walsh S, Dziewulski P, Exton L, Lee H, Dart J, Setterfield J, Bunker C, Ardern-Jones M, Watson K, Wong G, Philippidou M, Vercueil A, Martin R, Williams G, Shah M, Brown D, Williams P, Mohd Mustapa M, Smith C. U.K. guidelines for the management of Stevens–Johnson syndrome/toxic epidermal necrolysis in adults. Br J Dermatol. 2016;174:1194–227.

38. Bastuji-Garin S, Fouchard N, Bertocchi M, et al. SCORTEN: a severity-of-illness score for toxic epidermal necrolysis. J Invest Dermatol. 2000;115:149–53.

Radiology Case 11

56

James Flannery and Joshua K. Aalberg

Indications for the Exam *This patient, a 33-year-old female, with a past medical history of intravenous drug abuse presents with fever, left lower leg pain, and drainage from an ulcer on her lower left leg.*

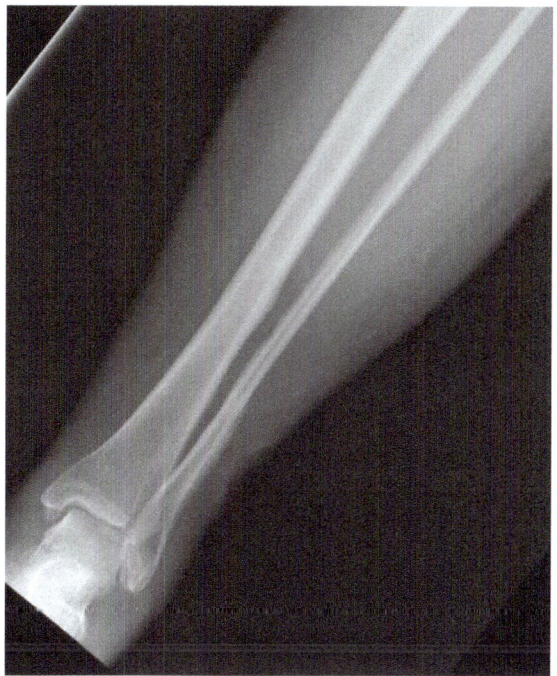

J. Flannery · J. K. Aalberg (✉)
Department of Emergency Medicine, Wexner Medical Center at The Ohio State University, Columbus, OH, USA
e-mail: James.flannery@osumc.edu; joshua.aalberg@osumc.edu

© Springer Nature Switzerland AG 2020
C. G. Kaide, C. E. San Miguel (eds.), *Case Studies in Emergency Medicine*,
https://doi.org/10.1007/978-3-030-22445-5_56

Radiologic Findings Anteroposterior (AP) radiograph of left tibia and fibula – diffuse soft tissue swelling with cutaneous ulceration of the distal lateral leg and periosteal reaction of distal tibia and fibula.

Diagnosis Osteomyelitis

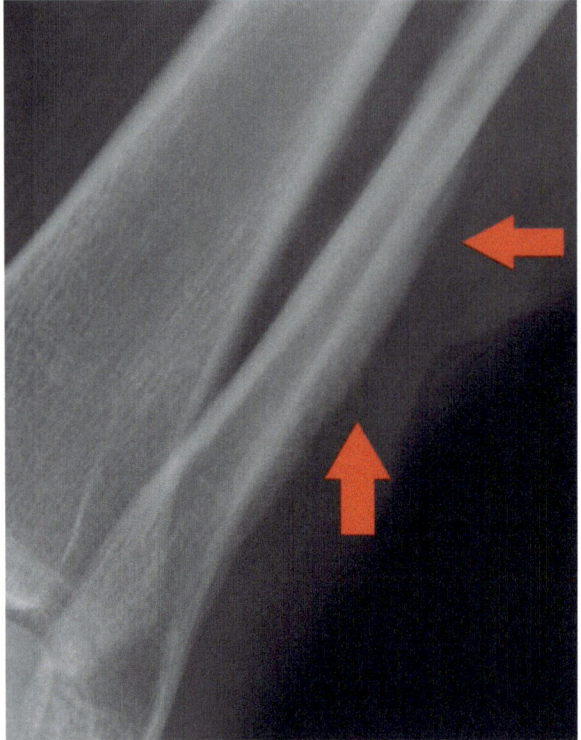

Learning Points

Priming Questions
- What is the normal evolution of imaging findings on radiographs in osteomyelitis?
- What are common pathogens for various patient populations?
- How is osteomyelitis different in the adult versus pediatric patient?

Introduction/Background

Osteomyelitis is an infection of the bone typically from a bacterial source. Acute cases progress over days to weeks which can evolve to a relapsing, chronic form after months to years. A majority of cases occur in children and the elderly, although it can be seen at any age, with a 3:1 male predominance [2]. Specific risk factors include diabetes, intravenous drug abuse, trauma or surgery, and sickle cell anemia.

Pathophysiology/Mechanism

There are two main origins for developing osteomyelitis: hematogenous spread and direct inoculation. Microorganisms such as bacteria embed into the bone and initiate an inflammatory response that leads to osteoclast activation and subsequent bone destruction. Osteoblasts counteract the bone loss with intense bone production which gives the periosteal reaction demonstrated in the above case. As the inflammatory response evolves, intraosseous vascular pathways are destroyed resulting in ischemia and osseous necrosis. Necrotic fragments then can be sequestered and serve as an infection nidus for chronic episodes of infection that are difficult to target medically. Sinus tracts can develop from the infected medullary cavity beyond the periosteum and drain pustulous material through the defect.

The most frequently encountered pathogen in all cases is *Staphylococcus aureus* [1, 2]. Particular pathogens have a higher propensity in specific populations, such as *Streptococci spp* and anaerobic bacteria in patients with diabetes, gram-negative species in IV drug abusers, and *Salmonella spp* in patients with sickle cell anemia [1].

Children are susceptible to osteomyelitis via the hematogenous route due to abundant vascularity with slow flow at the metaphyses of long bones, especially involving rapidly growing joints such as the knee [3, 5].

Making the Diagnosis

- Many radiographic findings in osteomyelitis are in fact secondary signs that are insensitive and typically appear days to weeks after infection has actually started to affect the bone. The earliest radiographic signs of developing infection are soft tissue edema and loss of the fat planes adjacent to the bone, which evolve over the period of days [5]. Apparent radiographic changes to the bone itself occur 10 days to weeks later and include cortical blurring or loss, trabeculae lysis, and periosteal reaction. [4, 5] Clinical history and physical exam findings such as cutaneous ulceration and recurring cellulitis and/or osteomyelitis episodes should warrant closer inspection for subtle imaging findings.
- The gold standard for diagnosis of osteomyelitis is bone biopsy but this is of course invasive. The other available imaging modality is Magnetic Resonance Imaging (MRI), which can detect early and subtle changes to the bone marrow that cannot be detected on radiographs [6].

Treating the Patient

Treatment for osteomyelitis is going to include antimicrobial therapy such as oral or intravenous antibiotics and/or surgical management.

- Isolation of the microbe via bone biopsy would give definitive antimicrobial sensitivities but again is often not practical due to the invasive nature of the procedure. Positive blood cultures may also provide a suspected source of infection and can guide therapy. Otherwise, broad antibiotic coverage can be utilized with special consideration given to patient population with unique organisms.
- Intravenous antibiotics are typically given over a period of weeks with eventually transition to oral agents.
- Chronic cases of osteomyelitis will generally need surgical management such as debridement in order to re-establish viable blood supply and eradicate dead bone.

Discussion

- Osteomyelitis can be a difficult entity to diagnose and treat. Recognizing subtle imaging clues on radiographs will help guide further work-up and treatment:
  - Soft tissue edema and loss of fat planes first.
  - Followed by changes to the bone including cortical destruction and periosteal reaction.
  - Changes from osteomyelitis are seen earlier and more reliably on MRI.
- It is important to understand that particular patient populations will have a propensity to be infected by specific organisms. But with that said, the most common organism in all populations is *Staphylococcus aureus*.
- Treatment involves extended antimicrobial therapy, surgical management, or both. This depends on the patient, severity, and nature of the disease and chronicity.

References

1. Lew DP, Waldvogel FA. Osteomyelitis. Lancet. 2004;364(9431):369–79.
2. Kremers HM, Nwojo ME, Ransom JE, Wood-Wentz CM, Joseph Melton L III, Huddleston PM III. Trends in the epidemiology of osteomyelitis: a population-based study, 1969 to 2009. J Bone Joint Surg Am. 2015;97(10):837–45.
3. Jaramillo D. Infection: musculoskeletal. Pediatr Radiol. 2011;41(Suppl 1):127.
4. Gold RH, Hawkins RA, Katz RD. Bacterial osteomyelitis: findings on plain radiography, CT, MR, and scintigraphy. Am J Roentgenol. 1991;157:365–70.
5. Miller TT, Schweitzer ME. Imaging of musculoskeletal infections. In: Hodler J, Zollikofer CL, Von Schulthess GK, editors. Musculoskeletal diseases. Milano: Springer; 2009–2012.
6. Kothari NA, Pelchovitz DJ, Meyer JS. Imaging of musculoskeletal infections. Radiol Clin N Am. 2001;39:653–71.

Thyroid Storm: *Glands Gone Wild!*

57

Natalie Ferretti and Jennifer Yee

Case

Palpitations and Diaphoresis

Pertinent History Patient is a 53-year-old female who presents to the Emergency Department accompanied by her husband. She states she has felt like her heart was racing all day today, and she feels hot and sweaty. She denies any upper respiratory symptoms, chest pain, shortness of breath, abdominal pain, vomiting, or diarrhea. She feels slightly nauseated. Her husband also adds that she has been mildly confused over the past few days and seems to get lost in familiar areas or intermittently forgets what she is doing, but she seems more agitated today. They deny any hallucinations or substance abuse. She does not have a history of dysrhythmias or coronary artery disease. She has never had a stress test or undergone cardiac catheterization. Her husband brought the patient's medication bottles with him. He denies that she has started any new medications, vitamins, or supplements recently.

Past Medical History Gastroesophageal reflux disease (GERD), hyperthyroidism, arthritis.

Family History Mother – hypertension, diabetes; Father – hypertension, Coronary Artery Disease, hyperlipidemia.

Surgical History Cesarean section.

Social History Nonsmoker, Consumes Alcohol Socially, Denies Intravenous Drug Use (IVDU)

N. Ferretti (✉) · J. Yee
Department of Emergency Medicine, Wexner Medical Center at The Ohio State University, Columbus, OH, USA
e-mail: natalie.ferretti@osumc.edu

© Springer Nature Switzerland AG 2020
C. G. Kaide, C. E. San Miguel (eds.), *Case Studies in Emergency Medicine*, https://doi.org/10.1007/978-3-030-22445-5_57

Pertinent Physical Exam

- Vitals: Heart Rate 160, Blood Pressure 130/74, Oxygen saturation (O2 sat) 98% on room air, Respiratory rate 24, Temperature 102.2 °F/39 °C.

Except as noted below, the findings of the complete physical exam are within normal limits.

- Head, Ears, Eyes, Nose, and Throat: Normocephalic, atraumatic. Exophthalmos present bilaterally. Ears and nose unremarkable. Neck supple. Enlarged thyroid palpated with nodules.

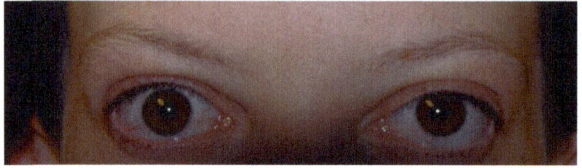

Exophthalmos. (Image courtesy of Colin Kaide, MD)

- Cardiovascular: Tachycardic, irregular rhythm. No murmurs. Intact symmetric distal pulses.
- Pulmonary: Lungs clear to auscultation bilaterally (CTAB), appropriate chest wall excursion. Speaking in slightly shortened sentences secondary to tachypnea at rest.
- Abdomen: Soft, Nontender/Nondistended, Positive bowel sounds.
- Extremities: No clubbing, cyanosis, or edema.
- Neuro: Hyperreflexia noted throughout all extremities. Generally tremulous at rest. No clonus or rigidity. No focal weakness or deficits. Appears anxious and delirious, occasionally staring off during questioning.
- Skin: Diaphoretic. Thin hair.

Pertinent Diagnostic testing

Lab results			
Test	Results	Units	Normal range
WBC	13.3	K/uL	3.8–11.0 10^3 / mm^3
Hgb	11	g/dL	(male) 14–18 g/dL
			(female) 11–16 g/dL
Platelets	212	K/uL	140–450 K /uL
Creatinine	0.8	Mg/dL	0.6–1.5 mg/dL
Potassium	4.3	mEq/L	3.5–5.5 mEq/L
Glucose	146	Mg/dL	65–99 mg/dL
Lactate	1.0	Mmol/L	< 2.0
Uric acid	11.6	Mg/dL	(3.5–7.7 mg/dL)
Troponin	<0.01	Ng/ml	< 0.04

Lab results			
Test	Results	Units	Normal range
BNP	170	Pg/ml	<100
TSH	0.0003	µU/mL	Less than 9 µU/mL
Free T4	6	µU/mL	5–13 µg/dL

WBC white blood cells, *Hgb* hemoglobin, *BNP* brain natriuretic peptide, *TSH* thyroid stimulating hormone

Chest X-Ray No acute cardiopulmonary findings.

Computed Tomography Angiogram Chest No pulmonary embolism identified. No focal consolidation or effusion bilaterally.

Urinalysis and Urine Drug Screen Negative.

Electrocardiogram Irregularly irregular rhythm rate of 160 bpm, narrow QRS, unable to identify P waves, nonspecific ST or T wave changes. Consistent with atrial fibrillation with rapid ventricular response.

Emergency Department (ED) Course

Patient's home medications were brought to the ED by husband and include chondroitin, aspirin, omeprazole, and methimazole. On further discussion with the patient's husband, he states they were recently traveling out of the country and she forgot to pack her medications, so she had not taken her methimazole for the past 5 days. Due to recent travel and new onset atrial fibrillation (a-fib), computer tomography angiography (CTA) of the chest was obtained to evaluate for pulmonary embolism, which was negative. Vitals were significant for tachycardia and hyperthermia. Labs were relatively unremarkable other than a mild leukocytosis, but she did not have overt signs of infection evident on her physical exam, chest X-ray, or urinalysis. Urine drug screen negative for tested substances. Electrocardiogram (EKG) showed atrial fibrillation with rapid ventricular response (RVR), which was new-onset atrial fibrillation as patient had no history of previous dysrhythmia. Given her history of hyperthyroidism and recent medication noncompliance, a clinical diagnosis of thyroid storm was suspected.

Update 1

Patient was given 1 mg IV propranolol every 15 minutes for heart rate control and 600 mg of oral propylthiouracil (PTU). 1 hour after PTU, 8 drops of Lugol's solution iodine was administered. She was also given hydrocortisone 300 mg IV and acetaminophen for hyperpyrexia. Blood and urine cultures were drawn. As her medication noncompliance was a reasonable cause of thyroid storm without identified infectious etiologies, broad-spectrum antibiotics were held. On reassessment, patient's heart rate improved to 138 from 160, her temperature was 98.6 °F/37 °C, she was more alert, oriented times 3, and answering questions appropriately. An admission to ICU was requested.

Learning Points: Thyroid Storm

Priming Questions
1. How do you differentiate between hyperthyroidism and thyroid storm? What is used to make the diagnosis of thyroid storm?
2. If so many people have thyroid dysfunction and hyperthyroidism, which subset of these people develop thyroid storm and who is predisposed?
3. When treating thyroid storm, does the order in which you give the medications make a difference?

Introduction/Background

1. Hyperthyroidism progresses to thyroid storm in approximately 12% of patients [1].
2. Thyroid storm is a life-threatening condition that can lead to end-organ damage and cardiovascular collapse if not treated emergently [2].
3. The cause of progression from hyperthyroidism to thyroid storm is not well defined but is thought to be due to altered peripheral response to thyroid hormone and resulting adrenergic hyperactivity [3].
4. The most common precipitating event of thyroid storm is infection, however, there are other physiologic triggers including burns, diabetic ketoacidosis (DKA), pulmonary embolism (PE), stroke, surgery, trauma, and parturition [4].
5. Thyroid storm has a nonspecific presentation that mimics many other more common ED presentations, thus the physician must maintain a high index of suspicion for the diagnosis.
6. The most common clinical features of thyroid storm are hyperpyrexia, tachycardia, central nervous system (CNS) dysfunction, and gastrointestinal (GI) manifestations [4–6].
7. Mortality of thyroid storm is currently reported at 10% [7].

Physiology/Pathophysiology

1. Hyperthyroidism is classically defined as low TSH and elevated free T3 and T4 hormone.
   - The hypothalamus secretes thyroid releasing hormone (TRH), which stimulates release of thyroid stimulating hormone (TSH) from the pituitary. TSH binds receptors on the thyroid cells to stimulate release of thyroid hormone [7].

- The T4 form of the hormone, thyroxine, is the most prevalent type in circulation; however, triiodothyronine (T3) is the active form that binds nuclear receptors [8].
- The ratio of T4 to T3 circulating in the blood stream is 20:1 [3].
- The majority of circulating thyroid hormone is bound to proteins including thyroid binding globulin (TBG), albumin, and transthyretin [7]. The percentage of free hormone determines thyroid activity.
- T4 undergoes conversion to T3 by 5′ deiodinase. T3 then enters the cells and binds to receptors, which affect gene regulation and transcription [7].

2. Excess thyroid hormone has effects including elevated metabolic rate, increased temperature and heart rate, increased cardiac contractility, as well as muscle and CNS excitability.
3. There is no clinical feature or single lab test that distinguishes hyperthyroidism from its more severe form, thyroid storm.
    - Thyroid storm occurs most commonly in patients with underlying Graves' disease, but may also be seen in patients with toxic multinodular goiter and other causes of elevated thyroid levels [9].
4. Thyroid storm is not well understood. It is currently believed that thyroid storm develops when there is upregulation of peripheral thyroid hormone receptors and increased sensitivity to catecholamines.
    - There is no evidence of increased production of T3/T4 in thyroid storm.
    - Typically some preceding stressor occurs which causes increased catecholamines and increased responsiveness peripherally, thus leading to excessive adrenergic response [9].
    - Increased levels of free hormone in circulation (unbound to proteins) contributes to increased adrenergic activity.
    - Multiple factors can interfere with hormone binding and may increase levels of free hormone including burns, trauma, surgery, ketoacidosis, infections, etc. [4]
    - Excess free T3 leads to enhanced beta-adrenergic receptor activity [8].
    - Multiple organ systems are sensitive to the adrenergic response, explaining the most common cause of death from thyroid storm: cardiovascular collapse and multiorgan failure [6, 7].
5. Complications of excessive thyroid stimulation most often include cardiovascular pathology such as heart failure or atrial fibrillation.
    - EKG findings typically show sinus tachycardia in 40% of patients and atrial fibrillation in 10% to 35% of patients [9].
    - Clinicians must be aware of an abnormal presentation of thyroid storm in the elderly known as apathetic thyrotoxicosis. Elderly patients may not develop the agitation or CNS excitability, but rather display depressed mental status, anorexia, or lethargy. Their presentation may only be new onset atrial fibrillation or heart failure, thus complicating the diagnosis of thyroid storm even further [10].
    - Thyrotoxic periodic paralysis is a serious and feared complication, but its incidence is only 0.2% in North America. The paralysis is caused by a shift of potassium into the cells, which inhibits muscle function. Treatment with potassium can restore muscle function [8, 11].

6. One of the predictors of mortality is total bilirubin level. It has been shown that level >3 mg/dL was associated with significantly higher mortality compared to people with bilirubin <3 mg/dL [2]. This is more specific than just the presence or absence of jaundice.

Making the Diagnosis

Understanding the pathophysiology of thyroid function and excess hormone effects in thyroid storm is the most important factor for making the diagnosis. There is no defining lab test or classic presentation of thyroid storm, so the key is to keep it on the differential in any patient that has a significant past medical history and presents with symptoms of increased sympathetic tone.

The diagnosis of thyroid storm may be challenging and is frequently overlooked. Clinical presentation of these patients is nonspecific and can mimic many other more common ED presentations. The diagnosis is clinical, and there are no routinely reliable lab tests to make the diagnosis [1].

1. The most common signs and symptoms are fever, tachycardia, CNS dysfunction, and GI manifestations [4]. These are not specific for any one condition! We see these presenting symptoms every day in the Emergency Department, and the cause is rarely thyroid storm.
2. The differential for these nonspecific symptoms is broad, including sepsis, heat stroke, meningitis, encephalitis, serotonin syndrome, neuroleptic malignant syndrome, stimulant toxidrome, adrenal insufficiency, pheochromocytoma, and many more.
3. The most important part of making the diagnosis is keeping thyroid storm on the differential and remaining mindful of a patient's past medical history and current medication list.
   - If the patient has a history of thyroid disorder and presents with the aforementioned symptoms, thyroid storm should always be considered. If suspected, it should be treated in an expeditious fashion, as delay or failure to treat may lead to poor outcomes and death.
   - Be aware that some people may take exogenous thyroid hormone for weight loss purposes; therefore, it is important to consider this during evaluation of patients with hyperthyroid presentations.
4. TSH and free T3/T4 levels are not always helpful in the diagnosis of acute phase thyroid storm.
   - T3 and T4 levels may be elevated in thyroid storm, but not always. Therefore, these labs cannot be used to make the diagnosis. Most important out of the thyroid tests is the free concentration of thyroid hormone [4].
   - It has also been proposed that maybe the rapidity of the rise in thyroid hormone, rather than a one-time level, may be a determinant for development of thyroid storm [7, 12].
5. Burch and Wartofsky developed a scoring system in 1993 to aid in the diagnosis of thyroid storm. It has been said that the scoring system leads to many false-positive diagnoses due to low specificity [2]. Patients with severe nonthyroidal illness will test positive on this scoring system.

Burch – Wartofsky's diagnostic criteria	
Thermoregulatory dysfunction	Scoring points
37.2–37.7	5
37.8–38.2	10
38.3–38.8	15
38.9–39.4	20
39.4–39.9	25
>40.0	30
Effects on CNS	
Mild (agitation)	10
Moderate (delirium, psychosis)	20
Severe (seizures, coma)	30
Gastrointestinal and liver dysfunction	
Moderate (diarrhea, N/V, abdominal pain)	10
Severe (unexplained jaundice)	20
Cardiovascular dysfunction (heart rate)	
99–109	5
110–119	10
120–129	15
130–139	20
≥140	25
Atrial fibrillation	10
Heart failure	
Mild (peripheral edema)	5
Moderate (bibasilar rales)	10
Severe (pulmonary edema)	15
History of triggering factor	
Negative	0
Positive	10

A score of 45 or greater is highly suggestive of thyroid storm, 25–44 suggestive of impending crisis, and below 25 unlikely to be thyroid storm [6, 13].

6. If thyroid storm is suspected based on history and clinical findings, the provider should begin empiric treatment immediately. This diagnosis is clinical and one should not rely on lab results [14].
7. These patients will always require admission and likely be admitted to the ICU due to the high mortality of the disease process and the propensity for hemodynamic instability and cardiovascular collapse [14].
8. Remember to investigate for any underlying triggers of thyroid storm and begin treatment for these as well. Currently, the most common precipitant is infection [7].

Treating the Patient

Once thyroid storm is recognized, treatment consists of several steps aimed at multiple points of the pathway. The keys to successful treatment include blocking additional thyroid hormone synthesis, inhibiting release of thyroid hormone, antagonizing peripheral effects of catecholamines, inhibiting peripheral conversion of T4 to active T3, and other supportive care directed at hemodynamic status and the inciting event that precipitated the storm. The American Thyroid Association recommends this multimodal approach to all patients in thyroid storm [1, 14, 15].

1. Decrease synthesis of new thyroid hormone.
   - Thionamides, most commonly propylthiouracil (PTU) or methimazole, are used.
   - Typically for hyperthyroidism, methimazole is used because it has less serious side effects compared to PTU, however in the case of thyroid storm, the American Thyroid Association recommends PTU as the first line thionamide [5, 15]. This is because PTU has an added benefit of also inhibiting peripheral conversion of T4 to T3. Dosing includes a 600 mg oral loading dose followed by 250 mg q4 h [7].
   - These medications are given orally; no intravenous form currently exists. If the patient is unable to take the medication orally, they can both be given via nasogastric (NG) tube or rectally via enema.
   - It is appropriate to give thionamides to pregnant patients in thyroid storm. PTU is typically the drug of choice in the first trimester, with methimazole preferred in the second and third trimesters [8, 11, 15]. Methimazole has been associated with teratogenic effects early on in pregnancy, but it is the preferred agent after the first trimester due to the risk of hepatotoxicity from PTU [8, 11].
2. Block release of preformed hormone from the thyroid gland.
   - Iodine prevents additional release.
   - It is important to wait 1 hour after administration of a thionamide before giving iodine, as iodine is a substrate for thyroid hormone production. Without blockade of the synthesis of new hormone, iodine administration would contribute to further synthesis of new hormone [9, 12].
   - Once the synthesis pathway is blocked, increases in iodine prevent release of hormone from the gland by the Wolff-Chaikoff effect. The principle states that increasing levels of iodine leads to decreased organification and hormone synthesis [3, 7].
   - Iodine is given in the form of Lugol's solution or SSKI. Dose is 8 drops of Lugol's every 6 hours or 5 drops of supersaturated potassium iodide (SSKI) every 6 hours [4, 7]. If the patient has a severe allergy to iodine, lithium can be used instead and has the same effect of decreasing release of hormone [4].
   - Lithium is a second-line agent. The mechanism of action is not clear; however lithium is also known to inhibit the coupling of iodotyrosine during thyroid hormone synthesis. Dosing is 300 mg every 6–8 hours with very close monitoring. The narrow therapeutic index of lithium makes it a less desirable option [4, 7].
3. Address the excess thyroid hormone already in circulation.
   - Thyroid hormone in circulation has a half-life of approximately 3–6 days in a thyrotoxic patient [4].
   - Beta-blockade is used to treat the symptoms of increased sympathetic tone. Propranolol is the most commonly used beta-blocker for thyroid storm because it has the additional benefit of inhibiting peripheral conversion of T4 to T3. Dose is either 1–2 mg IV q15 minutes or 60–120 mg PO q6 hours [4, 7].

- The downside of propranolol is that it has a relatively long half-life and suppresses cardiac contractility, which can worsen heart failure.
- Alternatives include esmolol, which has the benefit of a shorter half-life and more selective beta blockade, thus less bronchospasm. It can be used as a constant infusion and titrated easily making it an attractive option for the ED setting [7].
- Beta-blockers are the mainstay of treatment, but patients must be closely monitored for worsening heart failure. Some patients are already in high output heart failure due to their increased cardiac activity and decreased peripheral vascular resistance from thyroid storm. When beta-blockers are added and cardiac contractility is decreased, heart failure can worsen and fluid overload or pulmonary edema can develop rapidly. Echocardiography is recommended when using rate control in patients with thyroid storm [16].
- Cholestyramine is not a mainstay of treatment, but can be used to bind thyroid hormone and interrupt enterohepatic circulation thus facilitating elimination via the GI tract [4, 7].
- In severe situations where the patient is not responding to usual treatment within 24–48 hours of initiation, thyroid hormone can be removed from circulation via plasma exchange or dialysis [4, 7, 14, 18]. Plasma exchange removes thyroid binding globulin (TBG) with bound thyroid hormone and replaces it with free albumin, which contains unsaturated binding sites for remaining free thyroid hormone in circulation [7].

4. Block peripheral conversion of T4 to T3.
   - Propranolol and PTU both may block peripheral T4 to T3 conversion, however, the most potent blockade of peripheral conversion is from glucocorticoids [7].
   - Stress dose steroids are given; 300 mg hydrocortisone IV loading dose, followed by 100 mg q8 hours [7].
   - Steroids are often part of the treatment algorithm for this reason, as well as helping to counteract adrenal insufficiency in the shock state [4, 6].

5. Treat the underlying precipitant of the thyroid storm if one can be identified.
   - The most common precipitant is infection, so obtaining cultures, urinalysis, and chest X-ray are important diagnostics [4].
   - Often these patients will be started on broad spectrum antibiotics until underlying infection is either identified or excluded.
   - Other precipitating causes such as myocardial infarction (MI), pulmonary edema (PE), and diabetic ketoacidosis (DKA) should concurrently be treated using their respective typical standard of care measures.

6. Supportive Care
   - Volume resuscitation from fluid losses due to sweating, diarrhea, or vomiting.
   - Normal saline containing dextrose may help combat glycogen depletion from increased metabolic rate [3, 4].
   - Sometimes vasopressors may be needed to maintain an appropriate mean arterial pressure (MAP) in the acute phase.

- Hyperpyrexia is treated with acetaminophen. Avoid aspirin as it can disrupt binding of thyroid hormone to TBG, leading to increased free hormone levels and worsening of disease! [5, 12]
- External cooling measures: cool mist, cooling blanket, ice packs, etc.
7. Clinicians should keep in mind the pathophysiology of this condition when considering other medication use.
- Avoid medications that increase sympathetic tone such as ketamine, albuterol, or pseudoephedrine during acute thyroid storm for fear of worsening the adrenergic response [9].

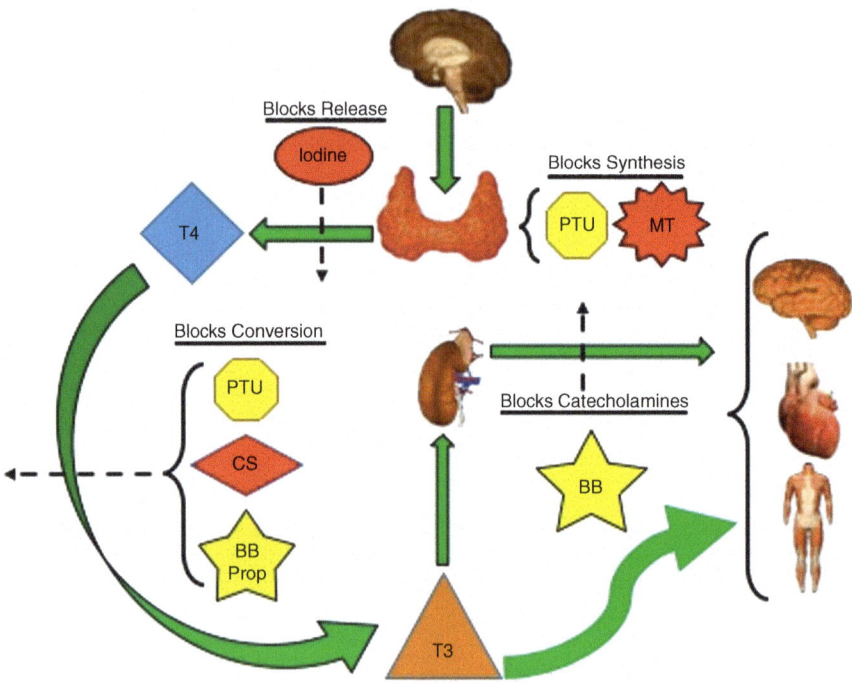

Thyroid Storm Treatment. (Graphic Courtesy of Colin Kaide, MD)

Treating thyroid storm		
Drug	Initial dose	Ongoing dosing
Propothiouracil	600 mg PO	250 mg q4 h
Methimazole	20–25 mg PO	20–25 mg PO q4 h
Propranolol	1–2 mg IV q15 min	60–120 mg PO q6 h
Iodine Lugol's solution	8 drops	8 drops q 6 h
Or	6 drops	6 drops q 6 h
SSKI (potassium iodide)		
Hydrocortisone	300 mg IV	100 mg q 8 h

Common Pitfalls

1. Failure to recognize and treat the underlying cause, which leads to persistent thyrotoxicosis [17].
2. Failure to recognize thyroid storm in a patient with history of hyperthyroidism [17].
3. Failure to treat in an expedited fashion [17].
4. Inducing cardiogenic shock from overaggressive beta-blockade treatment to lower heart rate too quickly [17].

Case Conclusion

The patient was treated with PTU, iodine, propranolol, and steroids in the ED and was subsequently admitted to the ICU. Once in the ICU, her blood and urine cultures were monitored and were negative for growth. She remained in the ICU for 3 days and her PTU, steroid, and propranolol were weaned. She was restarted on her methimazole and transferred to the floor.

Discussion

Maintain a high clinical suspicion for this can't miss diagnosis! For the patient who presents to the ED with hyperthermia, tachycardia, tachypnea, and altered mental status, the differential will be broad. More common causes such as sepsis and heat stroke should always be considered, but beware of anchoring and premature closure.

Review the patient's past medical history and medication list for diagnostic clues. Strongly consider the diagnosis in patients with hyperthyroidism on baseline PTU or methimazole, but also in patients with hypothyroidism who take thyroid hormone replacement. They can overdose on exogenous thyroid hormone and induce a hyperthyroid state or thyroid storm.

If you suspect thyroid storm, start treating it! This is a clinical diagnosis. If your treatment for sepsis is not working and you find yourself thinking 'something is not right', this should be a red flag prompting reconsideration of the diagnosis. Thyroid storm can be rapidly fatal so early and empiric treatment is important. Once it is suspected, begin treatment with thionamides, iodine, beta-blockers, and steroids right away.

Remember the correct order of treatment in order to prevent additional thyroid hormone synthesis. Remember supportive care such as intravenous fluids and antipyretics to maintain blood pressure and normothermia.

Pattern Recognition

- History of Hyperthyroidism or newly diagnosed hyperthyroidism
- Tachycardia
- Tachypnea
- Hyperthermia
- Altered mental status

Disclosure Statement The authors of this chapter report no significant disclosures.

References

1. Ross DS, Burch HB, Cooper DS, et al. 2016 American Thyroid Association guidelines for diagnosis and management of hyperthyroidism and other causes of thyrotoxicosis. Thyroid. 2016;26:1343–421.
2. Akamizu T, Satoh T, Isozaki O, et al. Diagnostic criteria, clinical features, and incidence of thyroid storm based on nationwide surveys. Thyroid. 2012;22:661–79.
3. Tintinalli JE, Stapczynski JS, Ma OJ, Cline D, Meckler GD, Yealy DM. Tintinallis emergency medicine: a comprehensive study guide. New York: McGraw-Hill Education; 2016.
4. Stathatos N, Wartofsky L. Thyrotoxic storm. J Intensive Care Med. 2002;17:1–7.
5. Bacuzzi A, Dionigi G, Guzzetti L, Martino AID, Severgnini P, Cuffari S. Predictive features associated with thyrotoxic storm and management. Gland Surg. 2017;6:546–51.
6. Wang H-I, Yiang G-T, Hsu C-W, Wang J-C, Lee C-H, Chen Y-L. Thyroid storm in a patient with trauma – a challenging diagnosis for the emergency physician: case report and literature review. J Emerg Med. 2017;52:292–8.
7. Chiha M, Samarasinghe S, Kabaker AS. Thyroid storm. J Intensive Care. 2013;30(3):131–40.
8. Franklyn JA, Boelaert K. Thyrotoxicosis. Lancet. 2012;379:1155–66.
9. Marx JA, Hockberger RS, Walls RM. Rosens emergency medicine: concepts and clinical practice. Vol 1 & 2. St Louis: Mosby; 2010.
10. Bhattacharyya A, Wiles PG. Thyrotoxic crisis presenting as acute abdomen. J R Soc Med. 1997;90:681–2.
11. Leo SD, Lee SY, Braverman LE. Hyperthyroidism. Lancet. 2016;388:906–18.
12. Yoshida D. Thyroid storm precipitated by trauma. J Emerg Med. 1996;14:697–701.
13. Sabir AA, Sada K, Yusuf BO, Aliyu I. Normothermic thyroid storm: an unusual presentation. Ther Adv Endocrinol Metab. 2016;7:200–1.
14. Satoh T, Isozaki O, Suzuki A, et al. 2016 guidelines for the management of thyroid storm from the Japan Thyroid Association and Japan Endocrine Society (first edition). Endocr J. 2016;63:1025–64.
15. Bahn RS, Burch HB, Cooper DS, et al. Hyperthyroidism and other causes of thyrotoxicosis: management guidelines of the American Thyroid Association and American Association of Clinical Endocrinologists. Thyroid. 2011;21:593–646.
16. Ngo SYA, Chew HC. When the storm passes unnoticed—a case series of thyroid storm. Resuscitation. 2007;73:485–90.
17. Wolfson AB, Cloutier RL, Hendey GW, Ling L, Rosen CL, Schaider J. Harwood- Nuss clinical practice of emergency medicine. Philadelphia: Wolters Kluwer; 2015.
18. Deng Y, Zheng W, Zhu J. Successful treatment of thyroid crisis accompanied by hypoglycemia, lactic acidosis, and multiple organ failure. Am J Emerg Med. 2012; https://doi.org/10.1016/j.ajem.2012.01.003.

Thrombotic Thrombocytopenia Purpura (TTP): *"Who Are You Calling a FAT RN?"*

58

Joshua Faucher and Colin G. Kaide

Case

Shortness of Breath and Irregular Heartbeat.

Pertinent History

The patient is a 48-year-old female with complex history including heart failure with reduced ejection fraction, chronic relapsing thrombotic thrombocytopenia purpura (TTP), paroxysmal atrial fibrillation, chronic obstruction pulmonary disease (COPD), and hyperthyroidism who presents for evaluation of shortness of breath. The patient had these symptoms for approximately 2 days. She has also noticed some bruising on her arms and legs and has felt fatigued. She stated this is what her previous TTP relapses have felt like. She denied any chest pain or cough. She endorsed subjective fevers without measured temperatures. She had no lower extremity swelling. Reportedly, she called EMS, and when they hooked her up to the monitor, they were concerned for atrial fibrillation with rapid ventricular response, and she was given 20 mg of Cardizem prior to arrival. She said this did not help.

J. Faucher
Rush Oak Park Hospital, Oak Park, Illinois, USA
e-mail: joshua.foucher@osumc.edu

C. G. Kaide (✉)
Department of Emergency Medicine, Wexner Medical Center at The Ohio State University, Columbus, OH, USA
e-mail: Colin.kaide@osumc.edu

© Springer Nature Switzerland AG 2020
C. G. Kaide, C. E. San Miguel (eds.), *Case Studies in Emergency Medicine*,
https://doi.org/10.1007/978-3-030-22445-5_58

Pertinent Physical Exam

Except as noted below, the findings of the complete physical exam are within normal limits.

- Blood pressure 119/77, pulse 117, temperature 97.8 °F (36.6 °C), temperature source Oral, respiratory rate 26, SpO2 95.00%.
- Constitutional: She is oriented to person, place, and time. She appears well-developed and well-nourished. She appears in distress.
- Cardiovascular: Increased rate, regular rhythm, normal heart sounds, and intact distal pulses. No murmur heard.
- Pulmonary/chest: Breath sounds normal. She is in respiratory distress. She has no wheezes. She has no rales. Dyspnea and tachypnea are present. She is unable to speak in full sentences.
- Abdominal: Soft. She exhibits no distension. There is no tenderness.
- Neurological: She is alert and oriented to person, place, and time. She exhibits normal muscle tone. Coordination normal. Exam changes during the course of the ED stay.
- Skin: Skin is warm and dry. Petechiae noted. She is not diaphoretic. There is pallor and mild jaundice present. Ecchymosis to left arm under BP cuff and bilateral ankles.

PMH

Heart failure with reduced ejection fraction (EF = 15%)
Previous thrombotic thrombocytopenic purpura with relapse several years prior
Paroxysmal atrial fibrillation

Pertinent Test Results

ECG: Sinus tachycardia

Test	Result	Units	Normal range
WBC	16.4	K/uL	3.8–11.0 10^3/mm^3
Hgb	12.3	g/dL	(Male) 14–18 g/dL
			(Female) 11–16 g/dL
Platelets	41	K/uL	140–450 K/uL
BUN	33	mg/dL	6–23 mg/dL
Creatinine	1.48	mg/dL	0.6–1.5 mg/dL
Glucose	231 ↑	mg/dL	65–99 mg/dL
Troponin	24.89	ng/ml	<0.04 ng/dl
BNP	2283	pg/ml	<100 pg/ml
Total bili	2.8	mg/dL	0.2–1.4 mg/dL

ED Management

On arrival, she was significantly tachycardic but otherwise hemodynamically stable. Her respiratory effort was increased, with her unable to speak complete sentences, but her oxygenation was within normal limits on a nasal cannula. We had initial concerns for repeat TTP exacerbation with a differential diagnosis including CHF exacerbation, acute coronary syndrome, or pulmonary pathology such as pneumonia or pneumothorax.

Initial chest X-ray showed cardiomegaly and a pleural effusion consistent with volume overload in the setting of CHF with poor ejection fraction. Chemistry revealed an acute kidney injury with a creatinine of 1.48. Hemoglobin was normal at 12. Platelets returned with thrombocytopenia at 41, with most recent previous values of 150–170. The clinical picture was consistent with an acute TTP. This was confirmed over the phone with the lab as they reported schistocytes on her smear. To complicate matters, her troponin came back significantly elevated at 24, consistent with cardiac ischemia. BNP was also elevated above 2000. At this point, there was concern that TTP was causing acute platelet plugging and an acute myocardial infarction; however serial EKGs did not show ST elevation.

We consulted hematology, who recommended plasmapheresis after bedside evaluation of the patient. The patient also had runs of ventricular tachycardia and continued to be tachycardic and symptomatic. Cardiology was consulted and recommended an amiodarone bolus followed by a drip.

Updates on ED Course

During the patient's ED course, she became hypoxic with oxygen saturations in the low 80s on nonrebreather and had declining mental status, with subsequent intubation in the ED. An apheresis catheter was placed, and the procedure was complicated by the lateral port clotting at the time of line placement. Per recommendations of hematology, the line was unclogged using tissue plasminogen activator (tPA). Hematology also recommended corticosteroids, which were administered. The patient also became secondarily hypotensive after intubation and remained hypotensive in the 80s over 50s throughout the rest of her ED stay. She was treated with multiple liters of IV fluids after intubation, with admission to the medical intensive care unit in critical condition.

Learning Points

Priming Questions

1. What signs and symptoms should prompt consideration of and evaluation for TTP, and what are the most reliable clinical indicators of its presence?
2. How can TTP be distinguished from other forms of microangiopathic hemolytic anemia, and what differential diagnoses can present with similar symptoms?
3. What are the critical actions that can be performed in the emergency department to increase the chance of patients with TTP surviving their disease?

Introduction/Background

1. TTP is a form of microangiopathic hemolytic anemia (MAHA) [1], and like other forms of MAHA such as hemolytic uremic syndrome (HUS) or disseminated intravascular coagulation (DIC), it is characterized by the destruction of erythrocytes associated with thrombosis in the small blood vessels of multiple organs.
2. TTP is a rare disorder, with an annual incidence of between 2 and 4 patients per million per year [1, 2]. Mortality for TTP was originally over 90%, but contemporary advances in care have decreased the mortality to as low as 10% with conventional treatments [1].
   - There is demographic variation in the incidence of TTP, with women and patients of African descent experiencing disproportionately higher rates of the disease [2, 3]. Large cohorts have demonstrated women making up over 70% of cases of idiopathic TTP and patients of African descent making up over a quarter of the patient population.
   - The majority of cases are idiopathic, but precursors associated with the development of TTP include preceding infections, HIV, pregnancy, autoimmune diseases (such as systemic lupus erythematosus), malignancy, and certain medications (e.g., quinine, ticlopidine, and clopidogrel) [1, 4].
3. Patients with idiopathic TTP have a 40% risk of recurrence, which usually manifests as a single episode within the first year after initial diagnosis, and may have a less severe presentation [5].

Pathophysiology

1. In normal physiology, a metalloproteinase referred to as ADAMTS13 circulates at functional levels in the bloodstream. As shear stress on the endothelial cells of the blood vessel walls exposes von Willebrand factor (vWF) multimers, ADAMTS13 cleaves these multimers inactivating their pro-thrombotic effect [6].
   - For the nerds, ADAMTS13 is "a disintegrin and metalloproteinase with a thrombospondin type 1 motif, member 13."

Normal Function of vonWillebrand's Factor

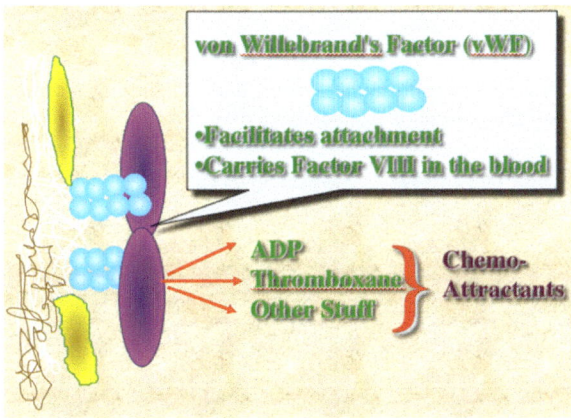

Courtesy of Colin Kaide, MD (Published with kind permission of © Colin G. Kaide 2019. All Rights Reserved

2. Patients with TTP have a deficiency of ADAMTS13, either due to a genetic defect leading to decreased production or an inhibiting antibody deactivating the enzyme [6, 7]. vWF thereby accumulate, promoting platelet adhesion and the deposition of microthrombi platelets in small blood vessels, with resulting organ damage. Because platelet activation typically does not happen in this process, the clotting cascade likewise remains mostly unactivated leading to very little fibrin in these predominantly platelet-vWF plugs. Consumption of platelets accounts for the notable thrombocytopenia ($<50 \times 10^9$/L, often as low as 10–15×10^9/L).

   - Those born with a hereditary ADAMTS13 deficiency have homozygous or double-heterozygous autosomal recessive mutation of the ADAMTS13 gene and manifest with symptoms in childhood [6]. These patients are treated with scheduled plasma transfusions to supplement levels of ADAMTS13.
   - Patients with acquired TTP have both deficiency levels of ADAMTS13 and a detectable inhibiting antibody causing autoimmune destruction of the functional enzyme [6].

vWF Multimers and Antibodies to ADAMTS13

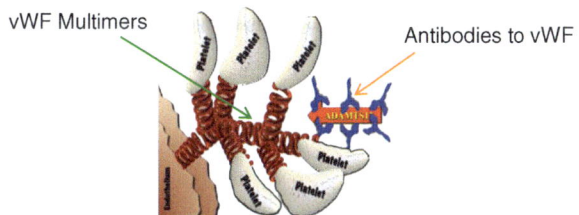

Courtesy of Colin Kaide, MD. (Published with kind permission of © Colin G. Kaide 2019. All Rights Reserved)

Virtually any organ system can be affected by ischemic damage caused by the microthrombi (e.g., central nervous system involvement with neurologic deficits, acute kidney injury, myocardial infarction) [1]. Notably, pulmonary compromise secondary to microthrombi without another identifiable cause is rare, possible due to lower shear stress in the pulmonary vasculature or the high compliance and collateral circulation of pulmonary vessels [8].

Micro Angiopathic Hemolytic Anemia—MAHA

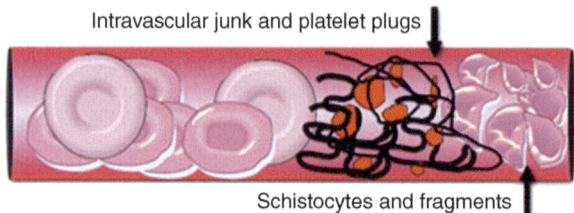

Courtesy of Colin Kaide, MD. (Published with kind permission of © Colin G. Kaide 2019. All Rights Reserved)

3. MAHA: As red blood cells (RBCs) pass through the network of long, tangles of thick, nearly occlusive vWF multimers and entangled platelets in microvascular, shearing of the red cells causes fracturing of their structure and the formation of RBC fragments called schictocytes [9]. Along with fragmented RBCs, this hemolysis spills lactate dehydrogenase (LDH) bilirubin and other intracellular contents including free hemoglobin into the blood. Free hemoglobin is then bound by haptoglobin leading to low haptoglobin levels.
4. Acquired TTP is most often idiopathic; however acquired cases with an identifiable trigger may occur due to autoimmune activation of the ADAMTS13 inhibitor via molecular mimicry [1].
   • Drugs associated with TTP include quinine [1] and ticlopidine [10]. The latter, an antiplatelet agent, carries an FDA black box warning describing a risk of TTP, which has been estimated to occur in approximately 1 in 5000 patients, usually during the first 3 months of treatment.
   • Clopidogrel has also been associated with the development of MHA; however the resulting syndrome is more reminiscent of HUS due to normal levels of ADAMTS13 activity and more severe renal failure, with thought that the drug may cause direct endothelial damage rather than production of an antibody [10].

Making the Diagnosis

While TTP is associated with the mnemonic FAT RN, that tool has both questionable taste and utility. TTP can present with highly nonspecific symptoms with no slam-dunk features to suggest the diagnosis on initial history and physical. Initial presentations require high clinical suspicion for successful diagnosis.

Differential Diagnosis: TTP Can Be Mistaken for Various More Common Disorders
- Other MHAs (HUS, DIC, HELLP syndrome)
- Immune thrombocytopenic purpura
- Ischemic stroke
- Acute coronary syndrome
- Sepsis
- Hematologic malignancy

1. TTP is traditionally described by the five-point mnemonic FAT RN, denoting the presence of fever, anemia, thrombocytopenia, renal dysfunction, and neurologic deficits, which were originally thought to be the hallmarks of the disease [11]. In reality, however, this pentad may be present in as low as 4% of patients [1] and in retrospect may have been more characteristic of extreme presentations of the natural history of the disease when it was still terminal.
   - Review of a database of cases over a 20-year period has demonstrated that nearly half of patients had no major neurologic deficits, 95% were without acute renal failure, and only 10% presented with fever [12]. The vast majority did, however, have platelet counts below 20,000 and a hematocrit less than 30%.
   - Further retrospective reviews have shown the most common presenting symptoms to include neurologic deficits ranging from mild headache to seizures or focal deficits (44% of patients) and typically isolated abdominal pain (23.5%), with significant bleeding in less than 10% of patients [12]. If there is an infection, malignancy, or other inciting illness, symptoms may in fact stem from that rather than the TTP itself.
2. The initial clues to the presence of TTP will likely be found on a CBC demonstrating mild anemia and platelets under 50,000 [1]. These results should trigger suspicion of MHA, which can be confirmed via a peripheral smear demonstrating schistocytes (fragment red blood cells).

Classic Clinical Presentation for TTP: FAT RN‡
F   *Fever*: Not as common in either disease and not required for the diagnosis (10%)∗.
A   *Anemia-microangiopathic hemolytic anemia (MAHA)*: *Schistocytes* occur when RBCs become trapped in the microthrombi and are forced through the clog, causing shearing of their membranes. LDH is *always* elevated when RBCs are broken. Haptoglobin will be low (another marker of hemolysis) (100%)∗.
T   *Thrombocytopenia*: Platelet counts can range from 5 to 100 × 10⁹/L (100%)∗. More severe thrombocytopenia is seen in TTP.

R   *Renal abnormalities*: This finding, seen in both forms, is more prominent with more severe complications in HUS. Renal insufficiency, azotemia, proteinuria, hematuria, and even renal failure occur (5%)∗.

N   *Neurologic abnormalities*: This feature is the hallmark of TTP (nearly a half of patients have this in TTP). It is found to a lesser degree in about 1/3 of patients with HUS. Findings include headache, confusion, cranial nerve palsies, seizures, and coma. These symptoms can wax and wane and be subtle in presentation, requiring the clinician to spend time getting the full neuro history (50%)∗.

Thrombocytopenia and MAHA are the only two things required for the diagnosis of TTP.

‡ *Never say FAT RN out loud in the ED or you might suffer bodily harm!*
∗Percent of patients having this finding according to Page et al. 2017 [12].
Created by Colin G. Kaide, MD

Image 2: Schistocytes on Peripheral Smear

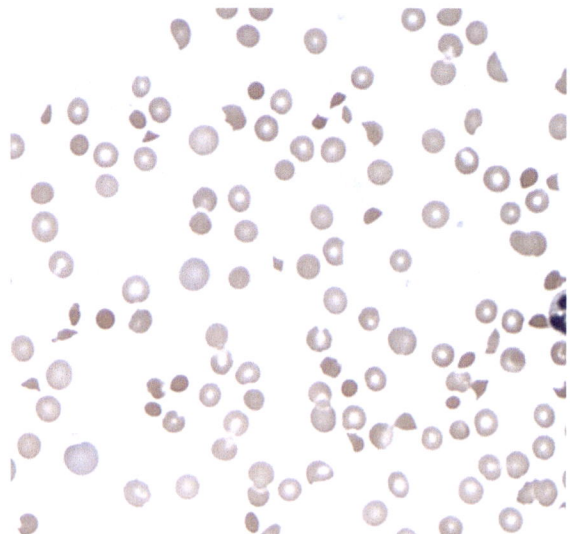

Image courtesy of Nicholas Nowacki, MD. (Published with kind permission of © Colin G. Kaide 2019. All Rights Reserved)

3. Since the presenting symptoms of TTP can be vague and nonspecific and other signs of organ dysfunction can be present, additional lab work should be aimed at detecting affected organs and excluding other causes of symtpoms [1]. These tests may include:
   - Additional confirmation of hemolytic anemia (LDH, haptoglobin, bilirubin)
   - Coagulation studies

- Type and cross
- Renal function tests
- Cardiac enzymes
- Blood/urine cultures and chest radiographs if there is suspicion for infection
- HIV screening
- Toxicology tests (as needed)
- CNS imaging if there are signs of neurologic deficits

4. Support for the diagnosis of TTP is obtained by demonstrating deficient serum levels of ADAMTS13 and in acquired TTP the presence of an inhibitor antibody [7]. Measurement of ADAMTS13 is likely best deferred by emergency providers, however, due to the fact that the lab is a sendout at most institutions and will not return before decisions for treatment must be made. ADAMTS13 levels are also highly variable depending on the assay used, can be low in other diseases, and are not considered specific or sensitive for diagnosis of TTP [13].

5. DIC is another form of MAHA that may present with multi-organ dysfunction and schistocytes on peripheral smear and must be differentiated from TTP. While TTP affects platelet aggregation mediated by vWF, DIC is a more complex consumptive coagulopathy affecting all clotting factors and as a result will have elevated INR, elevated PTT, decreased fibrinogen, and elevated D-dimer (in contrast to TTP, which will have only thrombocytopenia) [4].

Abnormal findings in HUS, atypical HUS, TTP, and DIC

Lab/findings	HUS	Atypical HUS	TTP	DIC
INR/PTT	Normal	Normal	Normal	Elevated
Platelets	Low	Low	Low	Low
Schistocytes	Present	Present	Present	Present
Renal abnormalities	+++	+++	+	NA[a]
Hemoglobin	Decreased	Decreased	Decreased	Decreased
LDH	Increased	Increased	Increased	Increased
Haptoglobin	Decreased	Decreased	Decreased	Decreased
ADAMTS 13	Normal	Normal	Low	Normal
Increased D-dimers	No	No	No	Yes
Decreased fibrinogen	No	No	No	Yes
Platelet plugs	Yes	Yes	Yes	No
Fibrin plugs	No	No	No	Yes

Created by Colin G. Kaide, MD
[a]Not unless the DIC specifically clots either renal or cerebral vessels or causes bleeding intrarenally or intracranially

6. The PLASMIC Score (named for the components of the score: **P**latelets, **L**ysis, **A**ctive cancer, **S**tem cell or solid organ transplant, **M**CV, **I**NR, and **C**reatinine) was described for use to generate a probability of the patient having TTP when testing for ADAMTS13 levels or inhibitor screens was delayed due to the "sendout" status of these tests in nonacademic settings [14]. A high score (6, 7) was found to both predict TTP with a 90% sensitivity and also to indicate a positive response to plasma exchange transfusion (PLEX). Similarly, a lower score of 0–5 predicted the absence of TTP with a 90% sensitivity and also indicated a low

response rate to PLEX. A score of 0–4 was 100% sensitive for predicting the absence of TTP [15].

- Although this score looks promising, the emergency physician should remember that it was derived and validated in an inpatient population that was admitted for suspicion of TTP. It has never been validated as a screening tool in emergency department patients.

The PLASMIC Score

Criteria	Points
Platelet count <30 × 10⁹/L	1
One or more indicators of hemolysis:	1
Reticulocyte count (percentage) >2.5% or	
haptoglobin undetectable or	
indirect bilirubin >2.0 mg/dL [>34 mcmol/L]	
No active cancer in the preceding year	1
No history of solid organ or hematopoietic stem cell transplant	1
Mean corpuscular volume (MCV) <90 femtoliters	1
International normalized ratio (INR) <1.5	1
Creatinine <2.0 mg/dL [<177 mcmol/L]	1

Created by Colin G. Kaide, MD Adapted from Li et al. 2017 [15]
0–4 Low probability
5 Intermediate probability
6–7 High probability

Treating the Patient

1. The mainstay of treatment for TTP is plasma exchange, which serves to replenish the plasma level of ADAMTS13 reversing its deficiency and also to remove the inhibitor antibody causing enzyme dysfunction in acquired TTP [1, 6, 16]. Plasma exchange requires central access via placement of an apheresis (or hemodialysis) catheter, which can be expediently performed in the emergency department. A Cochran review found no superiority of cryoprecipitate compared to fresh frozen plasma when utilized for plasma exchange, and sourcing of blood products should begin immediately upon suspicion of TTP [17].

   - Expert consultation with hematology should be made for facilitation of plasma exchange, and they may recommend additional adjunctive treatments commonly employed such as glucocorticoids and rituximab [1, 18].
   - PLEX is an invasive procedure with complications in up to 30 percent of patients [5, 19], the majority of which are catheter related (placement-related hemorrhage or pneumothorax or central line-associated bacteremia), along with transfusion reactions to plasma such as TRALI. There is also a risk of viral transmission, although this along with allergenic potential may be reduced by the use of plasma processed with solvent detergents [20].
   - When the availability of PLEX is delayed, the administration of FFP may transiently raise the circulating ADAMTS13 levels and ameliorate some symptoms of TTP. It is not a substitute for PLEX!

2. Transfusion of platelets is controversial due to possible exacerbation of disease and worsening of microvascular thrombi. Some studies have demonstrated no difference in the frequency of death or serious neurologic outcomes in TTP patients receiving platelet transfusions [19], while other retrospective analyses have found an association between platelet transfusion in TTP and higher rates of arterial thrombosis and mortality [20, 21]. It is likely available data are confounded by the more frequent use of platelet transfusions in patients with more unstable clinical status, and in a severely thrombocytopenic TTP patient with life-threatening hemorrhage, the use of platelet transfusions is likely justified to provide a workable substrate for normal hemostasis.

3. Clinicians may seek to utilize heparin infusions for TTP patients with signs of myocardial infarction or cardiac ischemia from microthrombi; however the likelihood of intended clinical effect is questionable. Heparin binds antithrombin III and inhibits thrombosis by inactivation of Factor X and inhibition of thrombin, preventing the cross-linking of fibrin. The microthrombi produced by TTP do not form via this pathway and do not contain significant amounts of fibrin.

4. Caplacizumab (Cablivi®): This humanized llama immunoglobulin fragment binds to vWF and prevents it from binding to platelets, thereby blocking the characteristic platelet plug formation. A recent study compared PLEX plus caplacizumab vs. PLEX plus placebo. It showed that patients receiving caplacizumab had a 74% decrease in the composite endpoint of death, recurrence of TTP during the study period or thromboembolic event. As expected, a drug that interferes with the vWF-platelet interaction would have mucocutaneous bleeding as a side effect. Most of the bleeding was mild to moderate, but 11% had severe bleeding events. None of the treatment arm patients died as a result of bleeding [22].

Case Conclusion

The patient underwent plasmapheresis, but during the process, she suffered a run of ventricular tachycardia. Another bolus of amiodarone was given with no change. 2 grams of magnesium sulfate was administered. Just prior to attempts at cardioversion, the patient went into ventricular fibrillation. Despite multiple shocks, including dual-sequential defibrillation and the administration of antiarrhythmics, spontaneous circulation could not be restored. The patient's rhythm deteriorated to asystole and resuscitative efforts were terminated.

Discussion

As an emergency physician, I've often heard the utility of the routine CBC questioned in an era of value-focused health care and institutional expectations of a rationale for all testing. A review of the evidence shows, however, that TTP can present with some of the most vague and exceedingly common complaints in the emergency department (headache, nonspecific abdominal pain, etc.). Establishing this diagnosis will require high clinical suspicion and a comprehensive approach to excluding other possible diagnoses, and in this case, the routine CBC may provide a crucial prompt for further evaluation. Remember…thrombocytopenia and MAHA with schistocyte on peripheral smear +/− neurologic and renal abnormalities are key in suspecting TTP. We will go as far as to say that every emergency physician should be able to recognize two things on a peripheral smear (yes, we said "emergency physician and looking at a peripheral smear…by yourself" in the same sentence)!! These are schistocytes and blasts (*see chapter on Blast Crisis*).

The emergency physician can play a crucial role in expediting appropriate treatment of TTP via expedient placement of a central catheter for plasma exchange. While the procedure is similar to the placement of a standard central line, practitioners should familiarize themselves with the kit available at their institution, due to the large-bore catheter and the need for two-stage dilation. Complications of plasma exchange are often related to catheter placement; therefore sterile technique and ultrasound guidance should be prioritized to minimize adverse outcomes.

Patients with acquired TTP are at risk for recurrence, particularly in the first year of illness. The recurrence may present with milder symptoms but should not be taken or treated lightly! My first patient with TTP presented with a recurrent episode with the only symptom being the return of a mild petechial rash on his thighs. In consultation with hematology, the patient received urgent plasma exchange with catheter placement and initiation of treatment prior to his leaving the emergency department. He ultimately survived.

Pattern Recognition

- Thrombocytopenia and anemia on CBC
- Normal coagulation studies (PTT, INR)
- Microangiopathic hemolytic anemia (schistocytes on peripheral smear)
- End-organ dysfunction (neurologic symptoms, MI, renal injury)
- Frequently recurrent within the first year of the initial episode

Disclosure Statement Joshua Faucher: No disclosures.

Colin Kaide: Callibra, Inc.-Discharge 123 medical software company. Medical Advisory Board Portola Pharmaceuticals. I have no relationship with a commercial company that has a direct financial interest in subject matter or materials discussed in article or with a company making a competing product.

References

1. Kappler S, Ronan-Bentle S, Graham A. Thrombotic Microangiopathies (TTP, HUS, HELLP). Hematol Oncol Clin North Am. 2017;31:1081–103.
2. Reese JA, Muthurajah DS, Hovinga JAK, Vesely SK, Terrell DR, George JN. Children and adults with thrombotic thrombocytopenic purpura associated with severe, acquired Adamts13

deficiency: comparison of incidence, demographic and clinical features. Pediatr Blood Cancer. 2013;60:1676–82.

3. Terrell DR, Vesely SK, Hovinga JAK, Lämmle B, George JN. Different disparities of gender and race among the thrombotic thrombocytopenic purpura and hemolytic-uremic syndromes. Am J Hematol. 2010;85:844–7.

4. Koyfman A, Brém E, Chiang VW. Thrombotic thrombocytopenic purpura. Pediatr Emerg Care. 2011;27:1085–8.

5. George JN. The thrombotic thrombocytopenic purpura and hemolytic uremic syndromes: evaluation, management, and long-term outcomes experience of the Oklahoma TTP-HUS registry, 1989–2007. Kidney Int. 2009; https://doi.org/10.1038/ki.2008.622.

6. Tsai H-M. Mechanisms of microvascular thrombosis in thrombotic thrombocytopenic purpura. Kidney Int. 2009; https://doi.org/10.1038/ki.2008.610.

7. Furlan M, Robles R, Galbusera M, et al. von Willebrand factor–cleaving protease in thrombotic thrombocytopenic purpura and the hemolytic–uremic syndrome. N Engl J Med. 1998;339:1578–84.

8. Nokes T, George JN, Vesely SK, Awab A. Pulmonary involvement in patients with thrombotic thrombocytopenic purpura. Eur J Haematol. 2013;92:156–63.

9. Sadler JE. Pathophysiology of thrombotic thrombocytopenic purpura. Blood. 2017;130(10):1181–8. https://doi.org/10.1182/blood-2017-04-636431.

10. Zakarija A, Kwaan HC, Moake JL, et al. Ticlopidine- and clopidogrel-associated thrombotic thrombocytopenic purpura (TTP): review of clinical, laboratory, epidemiological, and pharmacovigilance findings (1989–2008). Kidney Int. 2009; https://doi.org/10.1038/ki.2008.613.

11. Amorosi EL, Ultmann JE. Thrombotic thrombocytopenic purpura. Medicine. 1966;45:139–60.

12. Page EE, Hovinga JAK, Terrell DR, Vesely SK, George JN. Thrombotic thrombocytopenic purpura: diagnostic criteria, clinical features, and long-term outcomes from 1995 through 2015. Blood Adv. 2017;1:590–600.

13. George JN. Measuring ADAMTS13 activity in patients with suspected thrombotic thrombocytopenic purpura: when, how, and why? Transfusion. 2015;55:11–3.

14. Bendapudi PK, Hurwitz S, Fry A, et al. Derivation and external validation of the PLASMIC score for rapid assessment of adults with thrombotic microangiopathies: a cohort study. Lancet Haematol. 2017;4(4):e157.

15. Li A, Khalighi PR, Wu Q, Garcia DA. External validation of the PLASMIC score: a clinical prediction tool for thrombotic thrombocytopenic purpura diagnosis and treatment. J Thromb Haemost. 2017;16(1):164–9. https://doi.org/10.1111/jth.13882.

16. Rock GA, Shumak KH, Buskard NA, Blanchette VS, Kelton JG, Nair RC, Spasoff RA. Comparison of plasma exchange with plasma infusion in the treatment of thrombotic thrombocytopenic purpura. N Engl J Med. 1991;325:393–7.

17. Michael M, Elliott EJ, Craig JC, Ridley G, Hodson EM. Interventions for hemolytic uremic syndrome and thrombotic thrombocytopenic purpura: a systematic review of randomized controlled trials. Am J Kidney Dis. 2009;53:259–72.

18. Scully M, Mcdonald V, Cavenagh J, Hunt BJ, Longair I, Cohen H, Machin SJ. A phase 2 study of the safety and efficacy of rituximab with plasma exchange in acute acquired thrombotic thrombocytopenic purpura. Blood. 2011;118:1746–53.

19. McClain RS, Terrell DR, Vesely SK, George JN. Plasma exchange complications in patients treated for thrombotic thrombocytopenia purpura-hemolytic uremic syndrome. 2011 to 2014. Transfusion. 2014;54:3257–9.

20. Scully M. Trends in the diagnosis and management of TTP: European perspective. Transfus Apher Sci. 2014;51:11–4.

21. Swisher KK, Terrell DR, Vesely SK, Hovinga JAK, Lämmle B, George JN. Clinical outcomes after platelet transfusions in patients with thrombotic thrombocytopenic purpura. Transfusion. 2009;49:873–87.

22. Scully M, Cataland SR, Peyvandi F, et al. Caplacizumab treatment for acquired thrombotic thrombocytopenic purpura. N Engl J Med. 2019; [e-pub].; https://doi.org/10.1056/NEJMoa1806311.

Tumor Lysis Syndrome: *Cancer Toxic Dump*

Michelle Nassal and Colin G. Kaide

Case

Pertinent History

This patient is a 65 year-old-male with a past medical history (PMH) of diabetes mellitus (DM), coronary artery disease (CAD) s/p left anterior descending artery (LAD) stent who was recently diagnosed with diffuse large B-cell lymphoma (DLBCL), the most common variety of Non-Hodgkin's Lymphoma (NHL) He presented with generalized fatigue, muscle cramps, nausea, difficulty urinating, and palpitations. He initiated R-CHOP* chemotherapy 3 days ago. Since then, he has had nausea, generalized fatigue and muscle cramping. Today he also noticed difficulty urinating and sensations of "his heart flip-flopping." He denies any chest pain, shortness of breath or syncope. He denies any fevers or chills, cough or changes in bowel habits. *Rituximab, cyclophosphamide, hydroxydanorubicin, Oncovin (vincristine) and prednisone.

Pertinent Physical Exam

Except as noted below, the findings of the complete physical exam are within normal limits.

M. Nassal · C. G. Kaide (✉)
Department of Emergency Medicine, Wexner Medical Center at The Ohio State University, Columbus, OH, USA
e-mail: michelle.nassal@osumc.edu; Colin.kaide@osumc.edu

© Springer Nature Switzerland AG 2020
C. G. Kaide, C. E. San Miguel (eds.), *Case Studies in Emergency Medicine*,
https://doi.org/10.1007/978-3-030-22445-5_59

- Temperature: 100.6 °F/38.1 °C, Blood Pressure: 135/65, Heart Rate: 105, Respiratory Rate: 18, Peripheral capillary oxygen saturation (SpO2): 99% on room air.
- *General*: Alert, ill-appearing, oriented times 3
- *HEENT*: mucous membranes dry, positive Chvostek's sign, conjunctivae are pale
- *Cardiovascular*: tachycardic

Past Medical History Non-Hodgkin's Lymphoma with 10 cm mediastinal mass and positive inguinal lymph nodes, DM not on insulin, CAD s/p LAD stent 2 years prior

Social History social alcohol use, denies illicit drugs and smoking

Family History CAD father, DM mother

Pertinent Test Results

EKG Sinus Tachycardia, with peaked T-waves, no ST elevations or depressions

Lab results			
Test	Results	Units	Normal range
WBC	4.3	K/uL	3.8–11.0 10^3 / mm^3
Hgb	8.9	g/dL	(Male) 14–18 g/dL (female) 11–16 g/dL
Platelets	35	K/uL	140–450 K /uL
BUN	23	mg/dL	6–23 mg/dL
Creatinine	2.4	mg/dL	0.6–1.5 mg/dL
Potassium	7.4	mEq/L	3.5–5.5 mEq/L
Chloride	105	mEq/L	96–112 mEq/L
Bicarbonate	21	mEq/L	21–34 mEq/L
Glucose	145	mg/dL	65–99 mg/dL
Calcium	6.5	mg/dL	8.6–10.5 mg/dL
Troponin	<0.01	ng/ml	< 0.04
Uric acid	12.1	mg/dL	3.5–7.7 mg/dL
Phosphate	6.2	mg/dL	2.2–4.6 mg/dL

Emergency Department Management

Based on the patient's History and Physical exam findings, concern for electrolyte imbalance due to Tumor Lysis Syndrome (TLS) is suspected. With patient history of CAD and palpitations, cardiac work up was also ordered. Electrolytes, EKG, and Complete Blood Count were ordered. EKG was found to have peaked T-waves concerning for hyperkalemia. Hyperkalemia treatment was initiated including calcium gluconate and bicarbonate.

Labs returned confirming hyperkalemia and revealing also hypocalcemia and acute kidney injury (AKI) with elevated creatinine. Patient was given insulin and D5 0.9% Normal saline boluses to treat hyperkalemia and AKI. Further labs including phosphate and uric acid were ordered. The oncology team was consulted for inpatient admission and management.

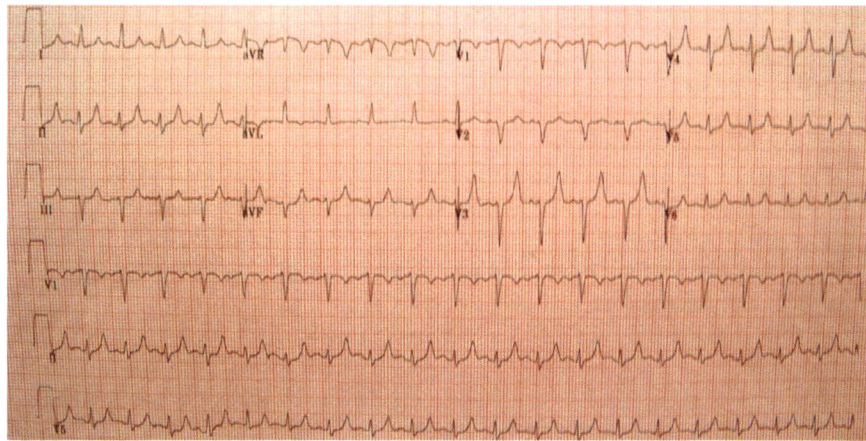

Fig. 59.1 Electrocardiogram (EKG) With Peaked T Waves (Published with kind permission of © Colin G. Kaide 2019. All Rights Reserved)

Updates on ED Course

After 2 L boluses were given, repeat electrolytes revealed potassium levels to be 6.4 mmol/L. Patient also had continued physical exam findings supportive of symptomatic hypocalcemia.

Learning Points

Priming Questions

1. When to suspect tumor lysis syndrome? Risk factors and the time period in which one should expect tumor lysis.
2. How is tumor lysis syndrome diagnosed? Compare laboratory versus clinical Tumor lysis Syndrome criteria.
3. Current clinical management recommendations of basic tumor lysis syndrome versus more severe tumor lysis syndrome.

Introduction/Background

1. Tumor Lysis syndrome is a metabolic emergency resulting from mass expulsion of potassium, purine nucleotides and phosphate upon tumor lysis. Majority of presentations are following treatment initiation; however, rare cases of spontaneous tumor lysis syndrome have also been reported [1].
2. Electrolyte imbalances from tumor lysis syndrome can be observed as early as 6 h after treatment to 72 h after treatment [2, 3]. Patients with higher probability of developing tumor lysis syndrome frequently have hematologic malignancies

rather than solid tumors, specifically lymphoproliferative cancers with high chemotherapy sensitivity.

- Patient Factors that increase likelihood of tumor lysis syndrome
  - Advanced age
  - Dehydration status
  - Increased baseline creatinine level
- Tumor-related factors that increase likelihood of tumor lysis syndrome
  - Mediastinal mass
  - Increased sensitivity to chemotherapy
  - Larger cancer mass
- Chemotherapy-related factors that increase the likelihood of tumor lysis syndrome
  - In children, aggressive versus slow introduction chemotherapy increased likelihood of chemotherapy.
  - Polychemotherapy has also been associated with increased likelihood

Physiology/Pathophysiology

Chemotherapy induced lysis of tumor cells results in release of large amounts of potassium, purine nucleotides, and phosphate. These metabolic derangements can result in benign symptoms such as muscle cramping to more severe consequences such as seizures or even sudden cardiac death. The following sections review the metabolic effects of tumor lysis. Summary of pathophysiology is shown in Fig. 59.3 below.

1. Hyperkalemia: Hyperkalemia affects neuromuscular and cardiac tissue most significantly resulting in muscle cramps, fatigue, paresthesias, cardiac dysfunction, arrhythmias, and potential for sudden cardiac death [4]. This makes hyperkalemia the most severe consequence of tumor lysis syndrome (Fig. 59.2).
   - ECG findings
     - Peaked T-waves→widened QRS→flattened P waves→ventricular tachycardia/ventricular fibrillation/asystole
2. Hyperuricemia: Large amounts of purine nucleic acids are broken down into uric acid. (See Fig. 59.1).
   - Hyperuricemia develops 48–72 h after treatment initiation. [5]
   - Large uric acid levels results in formation and deposition of urate crystals in renal tubules, resulting in acute kidney injury or more severely renal failure [6, 7]. Acute Kidney Injury (AKI) is the most common clinical manifestation of tumor lysis syndrome [8].
3. Hyperphosphatemia: Malignant cells have large quantities of phosphate, which spills into serum with cell lysis.
   - Hyperphosphatemia can occur 24–48 h after chemotherapy [9, 10].
   - Hyperphosphatemia can result in nausea, vomiting, diarrhea, lethargy, and seizures [5, 9, 11].

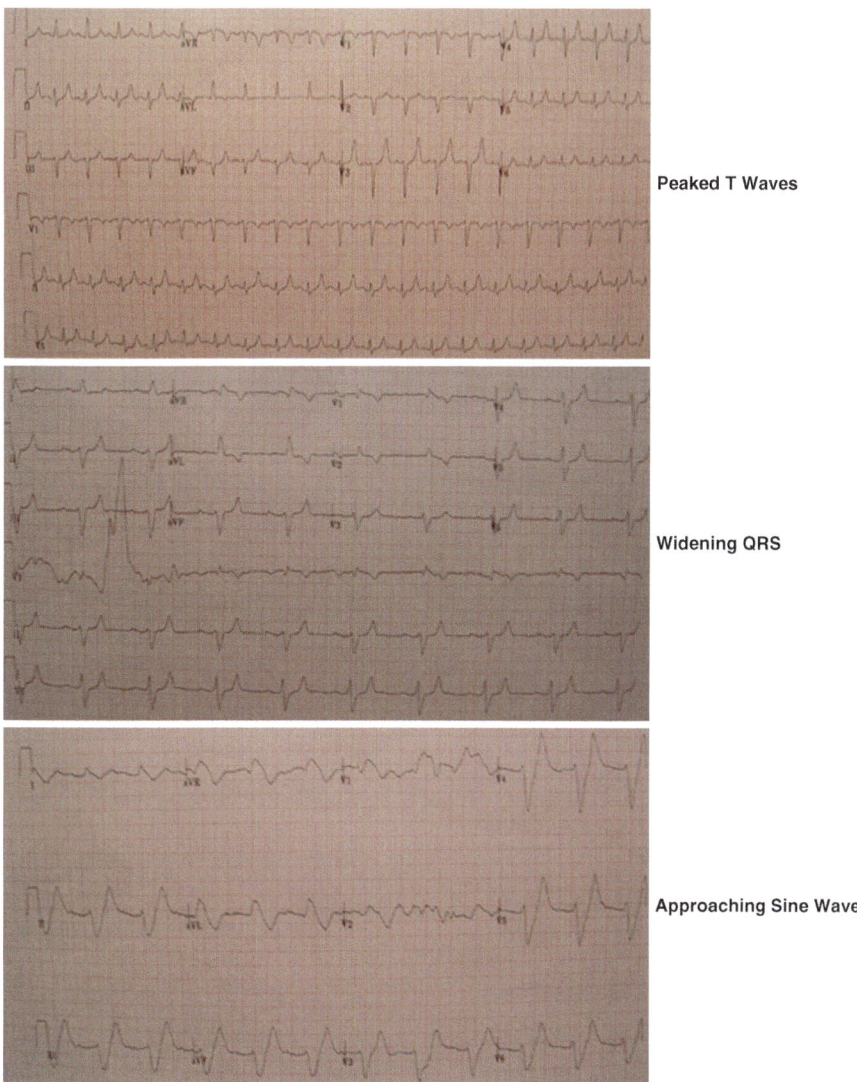

Peaked T Waves

Widening QRS

Approaching Sine Wave

Fig. 59.2 Progression of EKG Changes With Hyperkalemia (Published with kind permission of © Colin G. Kaide 2019. All Rights Reserved)

4. Hypocalcemia: Hypocalcemia is not directly from tumor cell lysis, rather from hyperphosphatemia. Excessive amounts of phosphate binds to serum calcium resulting in hypocalcemia.
   • Calcium phosphate crystals precipitate in renal tubules further contributing to acute kidney injury (AKI) [5].
   • Hypocalcemia can result in muscle cramps, paresthesias, tetany, altered mental status, hypotension, cardiac dysrhythmias or ECG changes and seizures [5, 12].

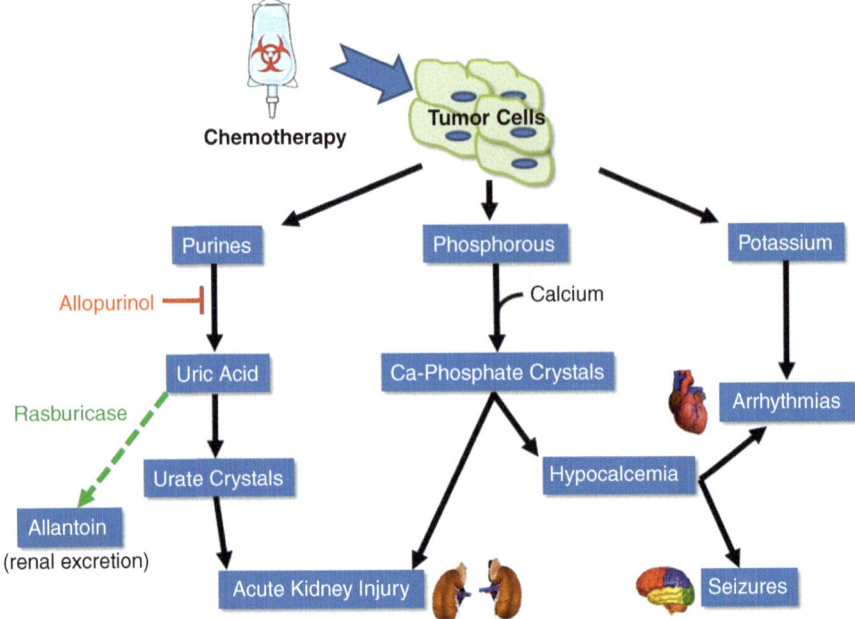

Fig. 59.3 Pathophysiology of Tumor Lysis Syndrome (Image courtesy of Colin Kaide, MD and Michelle Nassal, MD

Making the Diagnosis

Differential Diagnosis
- Chemotherapy side-effects
- Tumor lysis syndrome
- Invasive metastatic disease specifically to bone
- Isolated electrolyte abnormalities,
- Hypercalcemia of malignancy
- Infection

1. TLS can present as asymptomatic lab abnormalities or with severe clinical manifestations such as renal failure, sudden cardiac death or seizures.
2. Cairo-Bishop classification is the most widely accepted definition of TLS.
   - Laboratory TLS: Two or more of the following metabolic abnormalities within 3 days prior to or 7 days post-chemotherapy.
     - Potassium ≥6 meq/L or 25% increase from baseline
     - Uric acid ≥8 mg/dL or 25% increase from baseline
     - Phosphate ≥4.5 mg/dL or 25% increase from baseline
     - Calcium ≤7 mg/dL or 25% decrease from baseline

- Clinical TLS: Laboratory TLS criteria and one or more of following clinical consequences
  - Creatinine ≥1.5 times upper limit of normal (ULN)
  - Cardiac dysrhythmia
  - Seizure
- Howard et al. 2011 has further modified the Cairo-Bishop classification by adding the following qualifications [13].
  - Any two of the prior metabolic abnormalities over a 24-hour time-period. This has allowed for inclusion of patients who present with only one lab abnormality but develop more metabolic abnormalities during their evaluation.
  - Clinical TLS to include any level of symptomatic hypocalcemia.
3. Basic work-up for TLS should minimally include
   - Basic metabolic panel
   - Calcium
   - Phosphorous
   - Uric acid
   - Urinalysis-also evaluate crystals
   - EKG

Treating the Patient

1. Patients with established TLS; patients should be admitted to the ICU in order to have electrolytes evaluated every 4–6 h and for correction of any abnormalities that arise. They should also have continuous cardiac monitoring.
2. Hydration is the first measure to treat TLS. This allows for dilution of potassium, uric acid and phosphorous. Second, this also allows for increased renal blood flow improving acute kidney injury.
   - Current hydration goals: Minimally 2–3 L of isotonic fluid (mixture ¼ normal saline and 5% dextrose) daily for adults. Children <10 kg = 200 ml/kg/d [14].
   - Goal urine output 80–100 ml/h in adults and 4–6 ml/kg/h in children <10 kg
   - Patients with congestive heart failure or end-stage renal disease should be treated more cautiously with frequent remonitoring of fluid status.
3. With hyperkalemia potentially being the fatal consequence of TLS, hyperkalemia should be treated aggressively and early when suspected.
   - Immediate cardiomyocyte electrical stability can be provided by calcium gluconate [15].
   - Insulin with glucose and albuterol can work to shift potassium intracellularly.
   - Sodium bicarbonate and loop diuretics can help distal tubule secretion of potassium [15]. However, direct alkalization of urine is no longer a recommended treatment for TLS, as it may precipitate calcium phosphate and metabolic acidosis [16].

4. Hyperuricemia is treated by either preventing the formation of uric acid or encouraging the degradation of uric acid.
   • Allopurinol prevents formation of uric acid by inhibiting xanthine oxidase see Fig. 59.1. A newer agent, febuxostat, is also a competitive inhibitor of xanthine oxidase that is better tolerated by patients with renal dysfunction. These medications are helpful when given as a preventative agent 1–2 days prior induction of chemotherapy as they block the formation of uric acid; however, these agents do not treat the hyperuricemia in TLS [10, 14, 17].
   • In TLS patients, rasburicase has been proven effective in reducing uric acid levels within hours [18, 19]. Rasburicase is a synthetic urate oxidase enzyme not found in humans that breaks down uric acid into allantoin, which is more soluble and excreted in urine. Per the 2008 TLS expert panel, recommended dosing is 0.2 mg/kg daily for TLS treatment [14].
5. Hyperphosphatemia and Hypocalcemia are treated concomitantly.
   • Oral phosphate binders such as aluminum hydroxide (30 mL every 6 h) will reduce gut absorption of phosphate.
   • Correction of hyperphosphatemia should correct hypocalcemia. Caution should be taken when giving calcium alone to correct hypocalcemia as this may precipitate additional calcium phosphate crystals [13].
6. Acute Renal Failure may result from urate and calcium phosphate crystals. Although this is less common than acute kidney injury, dialysis has been considered a possibility early in the course of treatment to prevent severe kidney injury.
   • Indications for nephrology consult and potential dialysis include [13, 14].
     – Severe oliguria.
     – Persistent hyperkalemia after hyperkalemia interventions.
     – Hyperphosphatemia-induced symptomatic hypocalcemia.
     – Volume overload.

Case Conclusion

Nephrology was consulted for potential dialysis as patient remained hyperkalemic after interventions were performed. Phosphorus and uric acid were elevated. The patient was given aluminum hydroxide. The urinalysis showed crystals. Continuous hydration was maintained. He was admitted to the ICU with q4H–q6H electrolyte evaluation.

Discussion

Tumor lysis syndrome is a life-threatening oncologic emergency. It should be suspected in any patient presenting with the electrolyte abnormalities mentioned above and acute kidney injury. TLS should be highly suspected in patients with known cancer, especially hematologic malignancies. Because of electrolyte abnormalities, stability can be tenuous and frequent electrolyte monitoring is required. These patients are often admitted to higher levels of care, usually the intensive care unit (ICU).

Pattern Recognition

Tumor Lysis Syndrome
- *Hyper*kalemia
- *Hyper*uricemia
- *Hyper*phosphatemia with reflexive *hypo*calcemia
- Renal involvement: Acute kidney injury to acute kidney failure

Disclosure Statement Michelle Nassal: I have no relationship with a commercial company that has a direct financial interest in subject matter or materials discussed in article or with a company making a competing product

Colin Kaide: Callibra, Inc-Discharge 123 medical software company. Medical Advisory Board Portola Pharmaceuticals. I have no relationship with a commercial company that has a direct financial interest in subject matter or materials discussed in article or with a company making a competing product.

References

1. Liu JH, Zhou F, Zhang XI. Spontaneous fatal tumor lysis syndrome in a patient with t-cell lymphoblastic lymphoma/leukemia: successful treatment with continuous renal replacement therapy and increasing-dose gradually chemotherapy. J Clin Case Rep. 2014;4:361–3.
2. Yarpuzlu AA. A review of clinical and laboratory findings and treatment of tumor lysis syndrome. Clinica chimica acta; Int J Clin Chem. 2003;333:13–8.
3. Flombaum CD. Metabolic emergencies in the cancer patient. Semin Oncol. 2000;27:322–34.
4. McCullough PA, Beaver TM, Bennett-Guerrero E, Emmett M, Fonarow GC, Goyal A, Herzog CA, Kosiborod M, Palmer BF. Acute and chronic cardiovascular effects of hyperkalemia: new insights into prevention and clinical management. Rev Cardiovasc Med. 2014;15:11–23.
5. Davidson MB, Thakkar S, Hix JK, Bhandarkar ND, Wong A, Schreiber MJ. Pathophysiology, clinical consequences, and treatment of tumor lysis syndrome. Am J Med. 2004;116:546–54.
6. Shimada M, Johnson RJ, May WS Jr, Lingegowda V, Sood P, Nakagawa T, Van QC, Dass B, Ejaz AA. A novel role for uric acid in acute kidney injury associated with tumour lysis syndrome. Nephrol, Dialysis, Transplant: Off Publ Eur Dialysis Transpl Assoc – European Renal Association. 2009;24:2960–4.
7. Atchison DK, Humes HD. A case of tumor lysis syndrome and acute renal failure associated with elotuzumab treatment in multiple myeloma. Clin Nephrol Case Stud. 2017;5:78–81.
8. Lameire N, Vanholder R, Van Biesen W, Benoit D. Acute kidney injury in critically ill cancer patients: an update. Crit Care. 2016;20:209.
9. Cairo MS, Bishop M. Tumour lysis syndrome: new therapeutic strategies and classification. Br J Haematol. 2004;127:3–11.
10. Bclay Y, Yirdaw K, Enawgaw B. Tumor lysis syndrome in patients with hematological malignancies. J Oncol. 2017;2017:9684909.
11. Qunibi WY. Consequences of hyperphosphatemia in patients with end-stage renal disease (esrd). Kidney Int Suppl. 2004;90:S8–S12.
12. Thomas TC, Smith JM, White PC, Adhikari S. Transient neonatal hypocalcemia: presentation and outcomes. Pediatrics. 2012;129:e1461–7.
13. Howard SC, Jones DP, Pui CH. The tumor lysis syndrome. N Engl J Med. 2011;364:1844–54.
14. Coiffier B, Altman A, Pui CH, Younes A, Cairo MS. Guidelines for the management of pediatric and adult tumor lysis syndrome: an evidence-based review. J Clin Oncol. 2008;26:2767–78.
15. Weisberg LS. Management of severe hyperkalemia. Crit Care Med. 2008;36:3246–51.

16. Wilson FP, Berns JS. Onco-nephrology: tumor lysis syndrome. Clin J Am Soc Nephrol: CJASN. 2012;7:1730–9.
17. Wagner J, Arora S. Oncologic metabolic emergencies. Hematol Oncol Clin North Am. 2017;31:941–57.
18. Jeha S, Kantarjian H, Irwin D, Shen V, Shenoy S, Blaney S, Camitta B, Pui CH. Efficacy and safety of rasburicase, a recombinant urate oxidase (elitek), in the management of malignancy-associated hyperuricemia in pediatric and adult patients: final results of a multicenter compassionate use trial. Leukemia. 2005;19:34–8.
19. Trifilio S, Gordon L, Singhal S, Tallman M, Evens A, Rashid K, Fishman M, Masino K, Pi J, Mehta J. Reduced-dose rasburicase (recombinant xanthine oxidase) in adult cancer patients with hyperuricemia. Bone Marrow Transplant. 2006;37:997–1001.

Typhlitis: *A Real Pain in the Gut!*

60

Kimberly Bambach and Michael Purcell

Case

A 60-year-old female with a history of acute myelogenous leukemia (AML) presents to the emergency department with abdominal pain for the past 2 days. She is currently undergoing induction chemotherapy with cytarabine and daunorubicin with her last treatment being 10 days ago. She describes the pain as dull, constant, severe, and progressively worsening over the past 2 days. Her pain is localized to the right lower quadrant without radiation or obvious exacerbating or relieving factors. She also notes abdominal distension and profuse watery diarrhea with some bright red blood. She endorses subjective fever and chills at home.

Past medical history (PMH) Acute myeloid leukemia (AML)

Past surgical history (PSH) No prior surgical history.

Pertinent Physical Exam

Except as noted below, the findings of the complete physical exam are within normal limits.

- Vital Signs: BP 95/56, HR 110, RR 18, Temp 102 °F.
- General: Appears uncomfortable, holding her abdomen in bed.

K. Bambach (✉) · M. Purcell
Department of Emergency Medicine, Wexner Medical Center at The Ohio State University, Columbus, OH, USA
e-mail: Kimberly.Bambach@osumc.edu; Michael.Purcell@osumc.edu

© Springer Nature Switzerland AG 2020
C. G. Kaide, C. E. San Miguel (eds.), *Case Studies in Emergency Medicine*,
https://doi.org/10.1007/978-3-030-22445-5_60

- Abdomen: Normoactive bowel sounds, soft, mildly distended, and exquisitely tender to palpation in the RLQ, no guarding or rebound tenderness, no masses or organomegaly.

Pertinent Diagnostic Testing

CBC, chem 10, hepatic function panel, lipase, lactate, type and cross, urinalysis (UA) + culture, C. diff stool assay, 2x blood cultures, and a CT abdomen and pelvis with oral and IV contrast were ordered. Significant findings are below.

Test	Result	Units	Normal range
WBC	2.0	K/uL	3.8–11.0 10^3/mm^3
18% neutrophils, 1% bands, ANC 380			
Hgb	7.5	g/dL	Male: 14–18 g/dL
			Female: 11–16 g/dL
Lactate	4.0	mmol/L	< 2.0 mmol/L

ED Management

The differential diagnosis included acute appendicitis, infectious colitis, ischemic colitis, perforated viscus, and typhlitis.

Fluid resuscitation and empiric broad-spectrum antibiotics to cover enteric bacteria and *Pseudomonas aeruginosa* were immediately initiated.

The CBC was notable for WBC count of 2000 cells/mm^3 with 18% neutrophils, 1% bands, and an absolute neutrophil count (ANC) of 380 cells/mm^3. The patient was placed on neutropenic precautions. The lactate was 4.0 mm/L, and the CT demonstrated dilation and wall thickening of the cecum with adjacent mesenteric fat stranding.

Learning Points

Priming Questions
1. What patient population is classically associated with typhlitis?
2. How do you determine if a patient is neutropenic?
3. What is the pathophysiology of typhlitis?
4. What are possible complications of typhlitis?
5. What are the important steps in managing neutropenic fever and typhlitis?

Introduction/Background

1. Typhlitis, also known as neutropenic enterocolitis, is an acute inflammatory disorder of the bowels, usually affecting the cecum and ascending colon. The word "typhlitis" comes from the word "typhlon," the Greek equivalent of the Latin term "cecum." Typhlitis is an oncologic emergency and classically occurs in patients who are neutropenic after receiving cytotoxic chemotherapy for treatment of hematologic malignancy [1]. However, typhlitis may also occur in the setting of solid organ malignancy or other states of profound immunosuppression.
2. Patients classically present with right lower quadrant abdominal pain due to involvement of the cecum and fever.

Physiology/Pathophysiology

1. The pathophysiology of typhlitis is incompletely understood, and thought to be multifactorial: [1–3]

Pathophysiology of Typhlitis

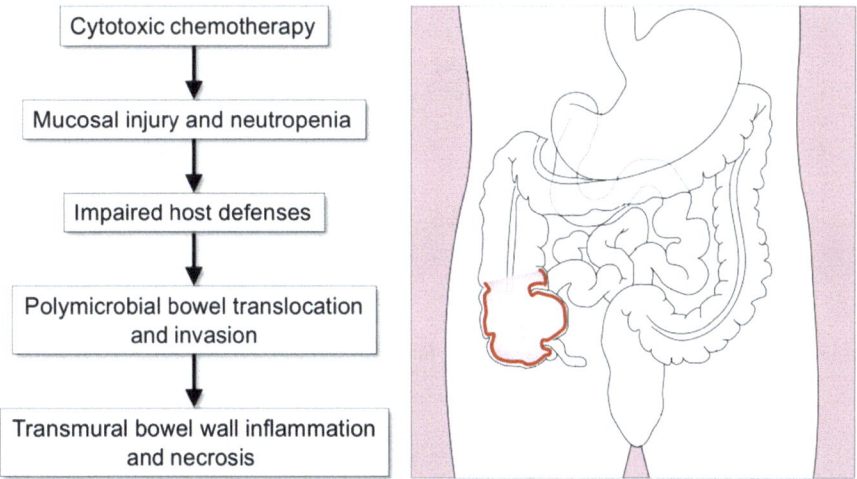

Image Courtesy of Wikimedia. William Crochot (https://commons.wikimedia.org/wiki/File: Stomach_colon_rectum_diagram-en.svg), Stomach colon rectum diagram-en

2. Patients are most vulnerable to infection at approximately 5–10 days after chemotherapy or when absolute neutrophil count reaches nadir [4]. Since different

agents will confer a different WBC nadir, it can be useful to note the patient's specific chemotherapy regimen.
3. The associated inflammation has a predilection for the cecum but can involve any segment of the bowels. Based on autopsy reports, inflammation often extends to the right colon and terminal ileum [5].

Making the Diagnosis

Differential Diagnosis
- Acute appendicitis.
- Pseudomembranous colitis (*Clostridium difficile* colitis).
- Other causes of infectious colitis.
- Ischemic colitis.
- Diverticulitis.
- Inflammatory bowel disease.

1. Considerations on history and physical include:
   - Is the patient immunocompromised?
   - When did the patient last receive chemotherapy, and with which agent?
   - Does the patient have a fever or report a history of fever at home?
   - Is there a history of appendectomy? *Typhlitis may mimic appendicitis.*
   - Are there any peritoneal signs on exam that would be concerning for bowel perforation?
   - Is hematochezia present?
   - Is the patient neutropenic with ANC <500 cells/mm^3 or <1000 cells/mm^3 with predicted decline to <500 cells/mm^3 in 48 hours? [6]

Absolute Neutrophil Count (ANC) Calculation
ANC = (% neutrophils + % Bands) × WBC Count (cells/μL)
Example: WBC = 2000 (cells/μL), neutrophils = 10%, bands = 2%
ANC = (10% + 2%) × 2000 (cells/μL) = 240 (cells/μL)

2. CT is the imaging modality of choice to make the diagnosis, with IV and oral contrast when possible. Findings most often include dilation of the cecum, wall thickening of the cecum, adjacent mesenteric fat stranding, and pericolic fluid [7].

Typhlitis on CT Demonstrating Gas in the Bowel Wall

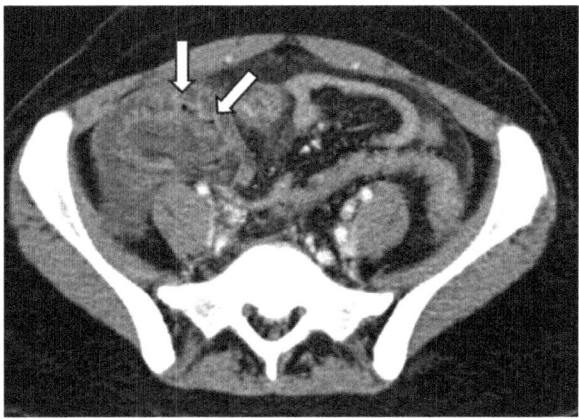

Open Access Image from Machado N (2010) Fig. 2. Neutropenic enterocolitis: A continuing medical and surgical challenge. North American Journal of Medical Sciences 2(7): 293–300. https://www.ncbi.nlm.nih.gov/pmc/articles/PMC3341635/bin/NAJMS-2-293-g002.jpg

- Plain films are useful for determining if free air is present under the diaphragm, but they are neither sensitive nor specific for typhlitis.
- Ultrasound may be a useful imaging modality to diagnose typhlitis, particularly in the pediatric setting. In pediatric typhlitis, bowel wall thickening on ultrasound may correlate with illness duration [8]. Findings include thickened, hypoechoic bowel wall, decreased peristalsis, and pericolic fluid [7, 8].
3. Typhlitis has a high mortality rate of 50% or higher, with death most commonly from sepsis [9]. Complications include sepsis, bowel perforation, and lower GI bleeding [1].

Treating the Patient

1. Treat the patient for presumed sepsis, including early fluid resuscitation and early administration of broad-spectrum antibiotics. *Obtaining results of diagnostic tests should not delay administration of broad-spectrum antibiotics in a patient presenting with signs of sepsis* [4].
   - Infections are often polymicrobial. Therefore, coverage should include gram-negative enteric organisms, *Pseudomonas*, and anaerobes [1].
   - As always, consult your local antibiogram for resistance patterns.
   - Possible regimens include: [10]
     - Piperacillin/tazobactam
     - Cefepime + Metronidazole
     - Ceftazidime + Metronidazole

- Reserve carbapenem antibiotics, such as Ertapenem, for pan allergic patients, or patients with known resistance.
- Typhlitis can occur due to fungal infection, but antifungals are not typically initiated in the ED empirically. Antifungals may be added to the treatment regimen in the setting of protracted fever >72 hours despite antibiotic therapy [5].
- Although not typically initiated in the ED, granulocyte colony-stimulating factor (G-CSF) is a potential therapeutic option to aid in recovery of the patient's neutrophil count. However, use of G-CSF is controversial due to lack of evidence-based benefit and potential to cause harm by further compromising the integrity of the bowel wall [1].
2. Supportive care
   • Bowel rest, nasogastric (NG) tube for decompression, and treatment of pain and nausea are all indicated [1].
3. Treat lower GI bleeding if present.
   • Type and cross, fluid resuscitation, and blood transfusion as clinically indicated.
4. Involve General Surgery if the patient has peritoneal signs or bowel perforation on imaging.

Case Conclusion

The patient was admitted to the intensive care unit and treated with fluid resuscitation, broad-spectrum antibiotics, and supportive care. The patient recovered with medical treatment as above and did not require surgical intervention.

Discussion

Typhlitis is an oncologic emergency and should be considered in patients presenting with neutropenia and abdominal pain or neutropenic fever. Patients may present along a spectrum of disease, from profound sepsis to subtle discomfort with minimal abdominal tenderness without peritoneal signs on exam [4]. This case demonstrates how subtle exam findings in the immunocompromised patient can mask life-threatening pathology. Typhlitis is not exclusive to patients with cancer. Of note, there are case reports of typhlitis occurring in other immunocompromised states such as advanced HIV [11, 12]. The high mortality of this disease process underscores the need for emergency physicians to keep typhlitis on the differential for abdominal pain in immunocompromised patients and to anticipate the associated complications. It is also important to bear in mind that typhlitis may mimic more common diagnoses such as appendicitis and *C. difficile* colitis.

Pattern Recognition

Typhlitis
- History of malignancy and recent chemotherapy.
- Neutropenia.
- Abdominal pain, particularly RLQ.
- Bowel wall thickening and necrosis.

Disclosure Statement The authors of this chapter report no significant disclosures.

References

1. Nesher L, Rolston KVI. Neutropenic Enterocolitis, a growing concern in the Era of widespread use of aggressive chemotherapy. Clin Infect Dis. 2012;56:711–7.
2. Bow EJ, Meddings JB. Intestinal mucosal dysfunction and infection during remission-induction therapy for acute myeloid leukaemia. Leukemia. 2006;20:2087–92.
3. Rolston KVI, Bodey GP, Safdar A. Polymicrobial infection in patients with cancer: an underappreciated and underreported entity. Clin Infect Dis. 2007;45:228–33.
4. Mickley M, et al. Oncologic and hematologic emergencies in children. In: Tintinalli's emergency medicine: a comprehensive study guide. McGraw-Hill, Columbus, Ohio, USA. 2016.
5. Katz JA, Mahoney DH, Fernbach DJ, Wagner ML, Gresik MV. Typhlitis. An 18-year experience and postmortem review. Cancer. 1990;65:1041–7.
6. Lewis MA, Hendrickson AW, Moynihan TJ. Oncologic emergencies: pathophysiology, presentation, diagnosis, and treatment. CA Cancer J Clin. 2011; https://doi.org/10.3322/caac.20124.
7. Block J, et al. Chapter 7: Atraumatic conditions of the abdomen. In: The atlas of emergency radiology. McGraw-Hill, Columbus, Ohio, USA. 2013.
8. Mccarville MB, Adelman CS, Li C, Xiong X, Furman WL, Razzouk BI, Pui C-H, Sandlund JT. Typhlitis in childhood cancer. Cancer. 2005;104:380–7.
9. Gorschluter M, Mey U, Strehl J, Ziske C, Schepke M, Schmidt-Wolf IGH, Sauerbruch T, Glasmacher A. Neutropenic enterocolitis in adults: systematic analysis of evidence quality. Eur J Haematol. 2005;75:1–13.
10. McAninch S, Clinton C. Gastrointestinal emergencies. In: CURRENT diagnosis & treatment: emergency medicine. McGraw-Hill, Columbus, Ohio, USA. 2017.
11. Till M. Typhlitis in patients with HIV-1 infection. Ann Intern Med. 1992;116:998.
12. Jumper C. Typhlitis and HIV. Ann Intern Med. 1992;117:698.

Radiology Case 12

61

James Flannery and Joshua K. Aalberg

Indication for Exam *66 y/o m presents after being found down outside of his house. On examination, he has right-sided hemiplegia and global aphasia.*

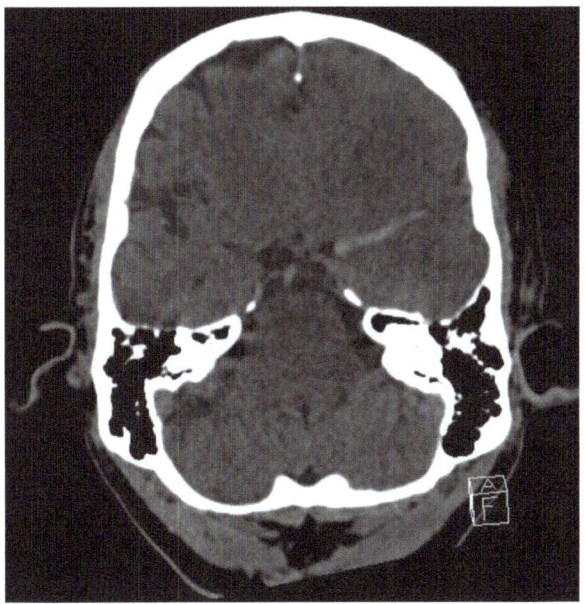

J. Flannery · J. K. Aalberg (✉)
Department of Emergency Medicine, Wexner Medical Center at The Ohio State University, Columbus, OH, USA
e-mail: James.flannery@osumc.edu; joshua.aalberg@osumc.edu

© Springer Nature Switzerland AG 2020
C. G. Kaide, C. E. San Miguel (eds.), *Case Studies in Emergency Medicine*,
https://doi.org/10.1007/978-3-030-22445-5_61

Radiologic Findings Hyperdense vessel sign – acute thrombus in the left middle cerebral artery.

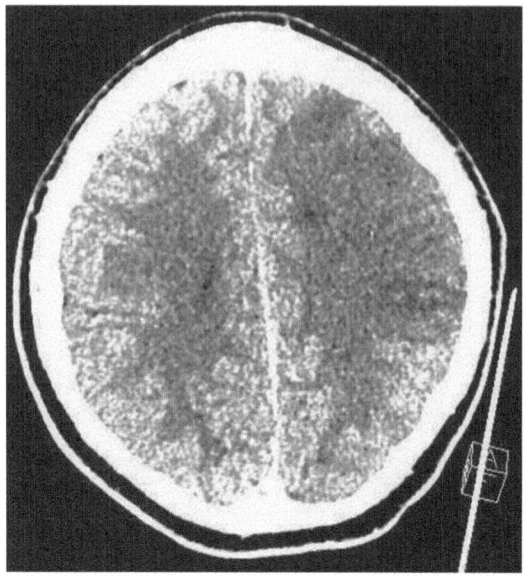

Radiologic Findings Loss of the gray–white differentiation of the left cerebral hemisphere.

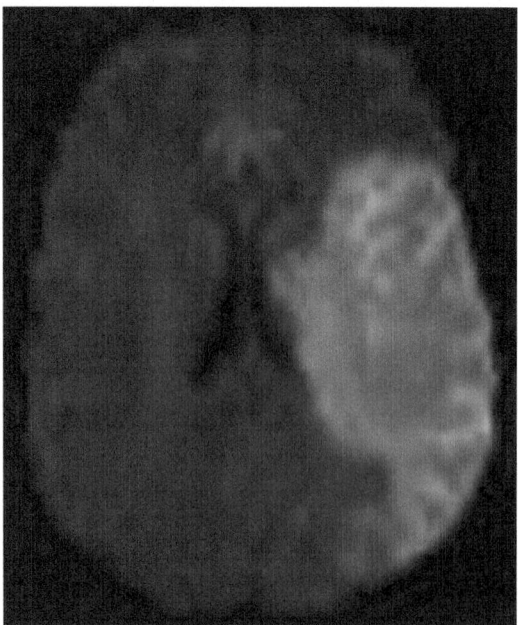

Radiologic Findings Restricted diffusion – Hyperintense Diffusion Weighted Imaging (DWI) signal (bright) in the Left Middle Cerebral Artery (MCA) distribution.

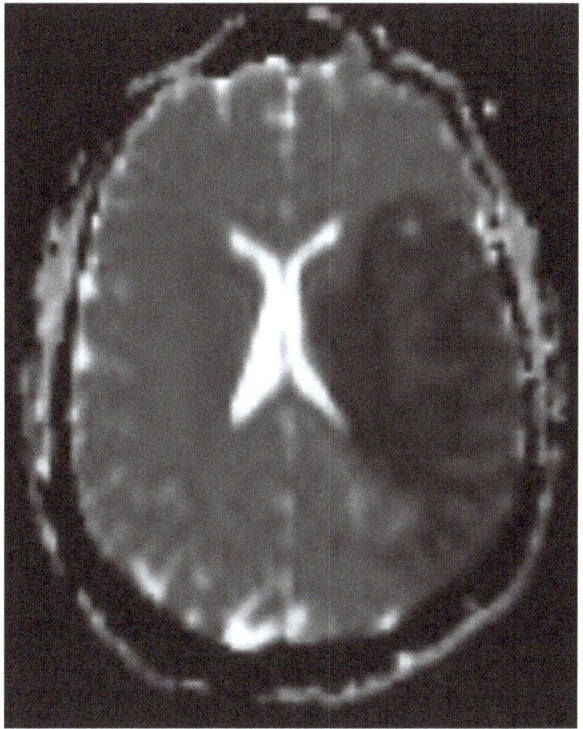

Radiologic Findings Restricted diffusion must correlate with hypointense signal (dark) on the Apparent Diffusion Coefficient (ADC) sequence.

Diagnosis Left Middle Cerebral Artery Ischemic Stroke.

Learning Points

Priming Questions
- What imaging findings signify "acute" stroke?
- What features are important on the initial noncontrasted head CT?
- What features would change the management of acute ischemic stroke?

Introduction/Background

Acute stroke can be defined by interruption of blood flow to the brain. Ischemic strokes constitute 87% of strokes. Acute strokes are the second most common cause of death worldwide and leading cause of morbidity in the United States [1].

Pathophysiology/Mechanism

Ischemia of brain tissue is usually secondary to either a thrombus or embolus in a cerebral artery. There is a wide range of stroke symptoms depending on the vessels involved but the classical symptoms are typically related to the MCA distribution. This includes contralateral weakness, contralateral numbness, contralateral facial droop, and slurred speech.

Making the Diagnosis

- One of the earliest signs of acute ischemic stroke on noncontrasted head CT is the dense vessel sign, which will be hyperdense relative to the contralateral side and represents acute thrombus. This is typically present at the proximal portion of the vessel and can be seen within 90 minutes [2]. A later sign of acute ischemia is loss of the gray–white differentiation of the effective territory which can become apparent in the first 3 hours [4]. Using comparison to the contralateral, normal hemisphere is a powerful tool in both findings. These findings are very highly specific but not very sensitive [2–4].
- If the noncontrasted head CT is negative or equivocal for acute stroke, a brain MRI can be utilized for higher sensitivity evaluation. Hyperintense DWI signal correlating with hypointense ADC signal is indicative of ischemic stroke in the acute phase. Restricted diffusion in the setting of stroke means simply that water cannot escape brain cells and cytotoxic edema ensues. Restricted diffusion can be seen as early as 30 minutes of the event [6] and sensitivity is >90% [6–8]. Hypointense ADC signal will normalize over the course of days to weeks and is useful to age the infarct [7, 8].

Treating the Patient

Two main treatment arms exist for acute ischemic stroke: intravenous thrombolytic agents and mechanical thrombectomy.

- Tissue plasminogen activator (tPA, alteplase) is a thrombolytic agent and is recommended within the first 4.5 hours of symptom onset [5].
  - There are numerous contraindications to tPA therapy, including intracranial hemorrhage, coagulopathy, iatrogenic-elevated international normalized ratio (INR), and severe hypertension. Institutionally, these are typically delineated in a tPA checklist.

- – Excluding intracranial hemorrhage is imperative during the initial workup, and indeed this is the main function of the initial noncontrast head CT for suspected stroke patients.
  - • If the noncontrasted head CT does not demonstrate intracranial bleeding, or another explanation for the patient's symptoms, they are presumed to be suffering an ischemic stroke and if there are no contraindications, they can be consented for tPA treatment.
- • Mechanical thrombectomy is a relatively recent development in stroke care and is only currently available at limited specialized facilities.
  - – Criteria generally include occlusion of the internal cerebral artery or proximal cerebral arteries, a so-called large vessel occlusion (LVO).
  - – Thrombectomy can generally be considered up to 16 hours since the onset of symptoms, though in specific cases this treatment therapy is an option up to 24 hours after the onset of symptoms [5].
  - – Receiving systemic tPA is not a contraindication to thrombectomy; therefore, it is generally recommended to continue to offer this therapy, if the patient qualifies as above, unless the patient will be immediately undergoing thrombectomy.

Discussion

- • Given the time-dependent treatment options in ischemic stroke, prompt CT evaluation is essential.
  - – CT is used to rule out intracranial hemorrhage as a cause for symptoms.
    - ○ Acute intracranial hemorrhage will be hyperdense outside the expected course of a vessel and typically demonstrates mass effect.
  - – Linear hyperdensity along the expected course of the cerebral vessel indicates an acute ischemic stroke.
  - – Asymmetric cerebral findings may further indicate acute stroke, including loss of the grey–white differentiation.
- • Ischemic stroke in the acute setting (6–72 hours) is most sensitively diagnosed by restricted diffusion on MRI (Hyperdense on DWI sequence AND hypodense on ADC sequence):
  - – Sensitivity to detect acute ischemic stroke is >90%.
  - – Imaging characteristics of restricted diffusion can persist for 7–10 days, and ADC sequence will slowly normalize (aka become less dark).
  - – MRI useful for distinguishing other etiology for stroke-like symptoms.
- • Management of the acute ischemic stroke is complex based on the patient's history and onset of symptoms. In general terms:
  - – Intravenous thrombolytic agent such as tPA can be administered within the first 4.5 hours of symptom onset.
  - – Mechanical thrombectomy is reserved for a large vessel occlusion, but in certain circumstances can be offered up to 24 hours after symptom onset.

Disclosure Statement   The authors of this chapter report no significant disclosures.

References

1. Yang Q, Tong X, Schieb L, Vaughan A, Gillespie C, Wiltz JL, King S, Odom E, Merritt R, Hong Y, George M. Vital signs: recent trends in stroke death rates — United States, 2000–2015. MMWR Morb Mortal Wkly Rep. 2017;66(35):933–9. https://doi.org/10.15585/mmwr.mm6635e1.
2. Tomandl BF, et al. Comprehensive imaging of ischemic stroke with multisection CT. Radiographics. 2003;23(3):565–92.
3. Leys D, Pruvo JP, Godefroy O, Rondepierre P, Leclerc X. Prevalence and significance of hyperdense middle cerebral artery in acute stroke. Stroke. 1992;23:317–24.
4. Beauchamp NJ Jr, Barker PB, Wang PY, vanZijl PC. Imaging of acute cerebral ischemia. Radiology. 1999;212:307–24.
5. Powers WJ, Rabinstein AA, Ackerson T, Adeoye OM, Bambakidis NC, Becker K, Biller J, Brown M, Demaerschalk BM, Hoh B, Jauch EC, Kidwell CS, Leslie-Mazwi TM, Ovbiagele B, Scott PA, Sheth KN, Southerland AM, Summers DV, Tirschwell DL, American Heart Association Stroke Council. 2018 Guidelines for the early management of patients with acute ischemic stroke: a guideline for healthcare professionals from the American Heart Association/American Stroke Association. Stroke. 2018;49:e46–e110.
6. Srinivasan A, Goyal M, Al Azri F, et al. State-of-the-art imaging of acute stroke. Radiographics. 2006;26(suppl 1):S75–95.
7. Schwamm LH, Koroshetz WJ, Sorensen AG, et al. Time course of lesion development in patients with acute stroke: serial diffusion- and hemodynamic-weighted magnetic resonance imaging. Stroke. 1998;29:2268–76.
8. Okorie CK, et al. Role of diffusion-weighted imaging in acute stroke management using low-field magnetic resonance imaging in resource-limited settings. West Afr J Radiol. 2015;22(2):61–6.

The Unvaccinated Febrile Child: *No Shot, Too Hot!*

Elaise Hill and Jennifer Mitzman

Case

Pertinent History

The patient is a 22-month-old female who presented to the emergency department (ED) with her mother following two days of fever of up to 103 °F (39.4 °C) orally at home. Her mother reported that she seemed more tired and has been eating less, but had continued to drink well at home. She had not had any upper respiratory tract infection symptoms, vomiting, diarrhea, abdominal pain, or rash. They reported that they just returned home from a trip to Disneyland last week. The patient's mother was concerned because her child is always healthy and has never been sick despite being unvaccinated.

Pertinent Physical Exam
- BP 98/40, Pulse 155, Temp 103.4 °F (39.7 °C), RR 32, SpO2 99%.

Except as noted below, the findings of the complete physical exam are within normal limits.

- General: Alert, awake, comfortably held by parent, crying on physician approach.
- Head, Eyes, Ears, Nose and Throat (HEENT): Nares without discharge, tympanic membranes clear, clear and moist oropharynx, and neck supple.

E. Hill
Nationwide Children's Hospital, Columbus, OH, USA
e-mail: elaise.hill@nationwidechildrens.org

J. Mitzman (✉)
Nationwide Children's Hospital, Columbus, OH, USA

Department of Emergency Medicine, Wexner Medical Center at The Ohio State University, Columbus, OH, USA

© Springer Nature Switzerland AG 2020
C. G. Kaide, C. E. San Miguel (eds.), *Case Studies in Emergency Medicine*,
https://doi.org/10.1007/978-3-030-22445-5_62

- Pulmonary: Tachypnea with good aeration, no wheeze, rales, or rhonchi.
- Cardiac: Tachycardia without murmur, warm extremities, and capillary refill <2 seconds.
- Abdominal: Nontender, no mass, and no hepatosplenomegaly.
- Skin: No rashes.

Pertinent Diagnostic Testing

Test	Result	Units	Normal range
Urinalysis – Leukesterase	Positive	–	Negative
Urinalysis – Nitrites	Positive	–	Negative
Urinalysis – White Blood Cells	Positive	–	Negative

Plan Antipyretics (10 mg/kg of ibuprofen), oral cephalexin dose, and urine culture sent.

Updates on ED Course The child tolerated ibuprofen, oral antibiotics, and a popsicle. After one hour, vitals were rechecked and had normalized. The patient was sent home with next day pediatrician follow-up, and return precautions were discussed with the family.

Learning Points: Serious Bacterial Infections

Priming Questions
1. In the unvaccinated child, how likely is a serious bacterial infection?
2. What is the epidemiology of serious bacterial infection in children?
3. What are the appropriate tests that should be performed in the Emergency? Department and what is the appropriate follow up?

Introduction/Background

1. Fever is one of the most common reasons a child will present to the pediatric emergency department (ED) accounting for approximately 20% of all ED visits [1–3]. It is often a cause of parental worry and fear [4, 5].
2. The etiology of fever in children is often difficult to determine and may be the only sign in infants and young children of serious bacterial infection [6]. In the well-appearing child, it is often challenging to determine the appropriate screening for safe discharge from the ED [3].
3. There are substantiated guidelines for the ED workup of infants less than 3 months of age with fever. However, guidelines for children 3–36 months have yet to change dramatically after the widespread vaccination against

Haemophilus influenza b (*Hib*) and *Streptococcus penumoniae* (*Sp*). These vaccines have resulted in a significant decrease in rates of serious bacterial infections (SBI) and occult infection [7, 8].

Physiology/Pathophysiology/Epidemiology

1. For the majority of well-appearing children presenting with fever without a source, the etiology for their symptoms will be a minor viral illness [9, 10]. Prior to vaccination development, *Hib* and *Sp* were both common causes of SBI in young children [11].
   - Since the introduction of the *Hib* vaccine in 1987, rates of invasive disease have fallen by 99% [12–14].
   - Since the introduction of the *Sp* vaccine in 2000, rates of invasive disease have fallen 75% [12–14].
   - Rates of occult bacteremia in the well-appearing child with fever without a source have decreased from as high as 10% to less than 0.5% for children aged 3–36 months. This reduction is also seen in undervaccinated children [3, 15].
2. In the last 20 years, the epidemiology and cause of childhood SBI had changed. Urinary tract infection (UTI) is now the most common cause of SBI in children, including children without a source. [3, 16, 17] Whereas *Sp* used to be the predominant pathogen of infant bacteremia, *E.coli* now predominates [3, 14]. Now, 96% of all SBIs are attributable to pneumonia and UTI, with bacteremia only accounting for 0.14% [18].
3. The vaccination strategies against *Hib* and *Sp* have had a dramatic positive effect on the unvaccinated and under-vaccinated. In fact, the largest effect of *Sp* vaccination has been on those who were not vaccinated [19, 20].

Making the Diagnosis

The decision to test, treat, or admit the ill-appearing child or child with focal disease is often easier than managing the well-appearing child without a source. This dilemma is further complicated if the patient is under-vaccinated.

1. Updated clinical guidelines from the American College of Emergency Physicians (ACEP) in 2016 provide a Level C recommendation that emergency physicians should consider urinary testing in the well-appearing child less than 2 years of age with fever. However, the guidelines do not comment on previous recommendations of empiric antibiotic use from a pre- *Hib* and *Sp* vaccination era. The current National Institute for Health and Care Excellence (NICE) guidelines from the United Kingdom (UK) recommend very little testing in an otherwise healthy febrile child younger than 5 years [3, 9, 21–26].
2. Urine: For fever without a source in girls under 24 months, screening for urinary tract infection with urinalysis and urine culture is recommended [27]. The

current guidelines of American Academy of Pediatrics recommend assessing a patient's risk of UTI prior to urinalysis and culture.

3. Blood work: New research has gone into predicting SBI through blood testing. However, with current epidemiology, screening white blood cell count and absolute neutrophil count has not proved effective in ruling in or out SBI, nor have inflammatory markers such as procalcitonin and C reactive protein [17, 18, 21, 28]. Screening complete blood count and blood culture are no longer cost-effective in well-appearing children now that occult bacteremia rates are less than 0.5%. [29] With current low pathogenic bacteremia rates, screening blood cultures prove to have contamination rates as high as 70% [14, 15, 18].

4. Chest Radiograph: The 2016 ACEP clinical guidelines make a level B recommendation, that "physicians should consider obtaining a chest radiograph for those with cough, hypoxia, rales, high fever ($\geq 39°C$), fever duration greater than 48 hours, or tachycardia and tachypnea out of proportion to fever" [3]. However, if the clinical picture includes wheezing and otherwise is consistent with bronchiolitis, there is a level C recommendation against obtaining a chest radiograph [3].

5. Clinical insight: Guidelines provide guidance; however, physician acumen is important in the workup of a febrile child. Studies have shown that a gut feeling that a child may be sicker than meets the eye may avoid missed SBI [30, 31].

Treating the Patient

1. Appropriate antibiotics are recommended for any child with a known source of bacterial infection [3, 21, 27].

2. The empiric use of antibiotics is *not* recommended in otherwise healthy children older than 3 months with fever. The use of empiric antibiotics for fever without a source leads to frequent antibiotic treatment for viral infection [10].

3. Despite some controversy, empiric use of antibiotics for febrile illness was also discouraged prior to regular vaccination against *Hib* and *Sp* and would therefore not be recommended for children who are under-vaccinated [32].

4. All guidelines for children who are discharged from the ED recommend close pediatrician follow-up. Reassuringly, compared with those children who had their SBI diagnosed in the ED, children who were diagnosed with an SBI at a subsequent healthcare encounter (after discharge from the ED) had no increased morbidity [33, 34].

Case Conclusion

The child was seen at her primary care physician's office the next day. The child no longer had fever and had been tolerating oral medication without difficulty. The urine culture returned positive for >100,000 CFU of *E. coli*. The patient was continued on a course of antibiotics without sequelae.

Case Discussion

- Vaccination rates have led to decreased prevalence of SBI even in patients who have not themselves received the vaccines. While tempting to think about unusual illnesses in the unvaccinated or under-vaccinated child, the reality is that common things are common and the overwhelming majority of fevers in this population are caused by minor viral illnesses.
- It is recommended to follow the guidelines for urinalysis, as this is the most common bacterial source. Blood work, indicated in the ill-appearing child, is not indicated or effective as a screening tool in the well-appearing child. Antibiotics were indicated in this patient because a bacterial source was identified. They should not be utilized in the absence of a source, even if the patient is unvaccinated or undervaccinated.
- In the United States, the workup of a febrile, well-appearing child without a clear source is the same, regardless of vaccination status.

Disclosure Statement   The authors of this chapter report no significant disclosures.

References

1. Sands R, Shanmugavadivel D, Stephenson T, Wood D. Medical problems presenting to paediatric emergency departments: 10 years on. Emerg Med J. 2012;29(5):379–82.
2. Alpern ER, Stanley RM, Gorelick MH, Donaldson A, Knight S, Teach SJ, et al. Epidemiology of a pediatric emergency medicine research network: the PECARN Core Data Project. Pediatr Emerg Care. 2006;22(10):689–99.
3. Mace SE, Gemme SR, Valente JH, Eskin B, Bakes K, Brecher D, et al. Clinical policy for well-appearing infants and children younger than 2 years of age presenting to the emergency department with fever. Ann Emerg Med. 2016;67(5):625–39.e13.
4. Poirier MP, Collins EP, McGuire E. Fever phobia: a survey of caregivers of children seen in a pediatric emergency department. Clin Pediatr (Phila). 2010;49(6):530–4.
5. Armon K, Stephenson T, Gabriel V, MacFaul R, Eccleston P, Werneke U, et al. Determining the common medical presenting problems to an accident and emergency department. Arch Dis Child. 2001;84(5):390–2.
6. Watson RS, Carcillo JA, Linde-Zwirble WT, Clermont G, Lidicker J, Angus DC. The epidemiology of severe sepsis in children in the United States. Am J Respir Crit Care Med. 2003;167(5):695–701.
7. Huppler AR, Eickhoff JC, Wald ER. Performance of low-risk criteria in the evaluation of young infants with fever: review of the literature. Pediatrics. 2010;125(2):228–33.
8. Irwin AD, Wickenden J, Le Doare K, Ladhani S, Sharland M. Supporting decisions to increase the safe discharge of children with febrile illness from the emergency department: a systematic review and meta-analysis. Arch Dis Child. 2016;101(3):259–66.
9. Jhaveri R, Byington CL, Klein JO, Shapiro ED. Management of the non-toxic-appearing acutely febrile child: a 21st century approach. J Pediatr. 2011;159(2):181–5.
10. Colvin JM, Muenzer JT, Jaffe DM, Smason A, Deych E, Shannon WD, et al. Detection of viruses in young children with fever without an apparent source. Pediatrics. 2012;130(6):e1455–62.
11. Martin NG, Sadarangani M, Pollard AJ, Goldacre MJ. Hospital admission rates for meningitis and septicaemia caused by Haemophilus influenzae, Neisseria meningitidis, and Streptococcus

pneumoniae in children in England over five decades: a population-based observational study. Lancet Infect Dis. 2014;14(5):397–405.

12. Hamilton JL, John SP. Evaluation of fever in infants and young children. Am Fam Physician. 2013;87(4):254–60.

13. Yildirim I, Shea KM, Pelton SI. Pneumococcal disease in the era of pneumococcal conjugate vaccine. Infect Dis Clin N Am. 2015;29(4):679–97.

14. Herz AM, Greenhow TL, Alcantara J, Hansen J, Baxter RP, Black SB, et al. Changing epidemiology of outpatient bacteremia in 3- to 36-month-old children after the introduction of the heptavalent-conjugated pneumococcal vaccine. Pediatr Infect Dis J. 2006;25(4):293–300.

15. Bressan S, Berlese P, Mion T, Masiero S, Cavallaro A, Da Dalt L. Bacteremia in feverish children presenting to the emergency department: a retrospective study and literature review. Acta Paediatr. 2012;101(3):271–7.

16. Craig JC, Williams GJ, Jones M, Codarini M, Macaskill P, Hayen A, et al. The accuracy of clinical symptoms and signs for the diagnosis of serious bacterial infection in young febrile children: prospective cohort study of 15 781 febrile illnesses. BMJ. 2010;340:c1594.

17. Manzano S, Bailey B, Gervaix A, Cousineau J, Delvin E, Girodias JB. Markers for bacterial infection in children with fever without source. Arch Dis Child. 2011;96(5):440–6.

18. Rudinsky SL, Carstairs KL, Reardon JM, Simon LV, Riffenburgh RH, Tanen DA. Serious bacterial infections in febrile infants in the post-pneumococcal conjugate vaccine era. Acad Emerg Med. 2009;16(7):585–90.

19. Centers for Disease Control and Prevention (CDC). Direct and indirect effects of routine vaccination of children with 7-valent pneumococcal conjugate vaccine on incidence of invasive pneumococcal disease – United States, 1998–2003. MMWR Morb Mortal Wkly Rep. 2005;54(36):893–7.

20. Yildirim I, Hanage WP, Lipsitch M, Shea KM, Stevenson A, Finkelstein J, et al. Serotype specific invasive capacity and persistent reduction in invasive pneumococcal disease. Vaccine. 2010;29(2):283–8.

21. Davis T. NICE guideline: feverish illness in children--assessment and initial management in children younger than 5 years. Arch Dis Child Educ Pract Ed. 2013;98(6):232–5.

22. American College of Emergency Physicians Clinical Policies Committee, American College of Emergency Physicians Clinical Policies Subcommittee on Pediatric Fever. Clinical policy for children younger than three years presenting to the emergency department with fever. Ann Emerg Med. 2003;42(4):530–45.

23. Brook I. Unexplained fever in young children: how to manage severe bacterial infection. BMJ. 2003;327(7423):1094–7.

24. Baraff LJ, Bass JW, Fleisher GR, Klein JO, McCracken GH Jr, Powell KR, et al. Practice guideline for the management of infants and children 0 to 36 months of age with fever without source Agency for Health Care Policy and Research. Ann Emerg Med. 1993;22(7):1198–210.

25. Baraff LJ. Editorial: clinical policy for children younger than three years presenting to the emergency department with fever. Ann Emerg Med. United States. 2003;42:546–9.

26. Barbi E, Marzuillo P, Neri E, Naviglio S, Krauss BS. Fever in children: pearls and pitfalls. Children (Basel). 2017;4(9).

27. Subcommittee On Urinary Tract I. Reaffirmation of AAP clinical practice guideline: the diagnosis and management of the initial urinary tract infection in febrile infants and young children 2–24 months of age. Pediatrics 2016;138(6).

28. Van den Bruel A, Thompson MJ, Haj-Hassan T, Stevens R, Moll H, Lakhanpaul M, et al. Diagnostic value of laboratory tests in identifying serious infections in febrile children: systematic review. BMJ. 2011;342:d3082.

29. Lee GM, Fleisher GR, Harper MB. Management of febrile children in the age of the conjugate pneumococcal vaccine: a cost-effectiveness analysis. Pediatrics. 2001;108(4):835–44.

30. Van den Bruel A, Thompson M, Buntinx F, Mant D. Clinicians' gut feeling about serious infections in children: observational study. BMJ. 2012;345:e6144.

31. Van den Bruel A, Haj-Hassan T, Thompson M, Buntinx F, Mant D. Diagnostic value of clinical features at presentation to identify serious infection in children in developed countries: a systematic review. Lancet. 2010;375(9717):834–45.
32. Jaffe DM, Tanz RR, Davis AT, Henretig F, Fleisher G. Antibiotic administration to treat possible occult bacteremia in febrile children. N Engl J Med. 1987;317(19):1175–80.
33. Vaillancourt S, Guttmann A, Li Q, Chan IY, Vermeulen MJ, Schull MJ. Repeated emergency department visits among children admitted with meningitis or septicemia: a population-based study. Ann Emerg Med. 2015;65(6):625–32.e3.
34. Green SM, Nigrovic LE, Krauss BS. Sick kids look sick. Ann Emerg Med. 2015;65(6):633–5.

Electrical Storm of the Heart: *A Shocking Experience!*

63

Patrick Sylvester and Christopher E. San Miguel

Case

Palpitations, Syncope, Recurrent VT

Pertinent History

A 47-year-old female is brought in to the emergency department by EMS. The paramedics report that the patient was found unresponsive at a high school basketball game where she was a spectator. Witnesses did not report any seizure-like activity. She awoke without any post-event confusion. Her blood glucose was 113. During transport, the cardiac monitor showed frequent runs of nonsustained ventricular tachycardia (VT). As she arrives, she is connected to your monitor and has a run of polymorphic VT for approximately 30 seconds during which time she reports feeling "light-headed" with palpations, shortness of breath (SOB), and diffuse chest discomfort. The patient is alert, oriented, and able to provide some additional history. She does not recall any prodromal symptoms prior to the event. She recalls that for the past three days she has been feeling extremely fatigued and has had episodes of palpitations with shortness of breath. Thinking back further, she has noted increased lower extremity edema over the past 1–2 weeks and was recently started on furosemide for "lower extremity edema."

Pertinent Physical Exam

- BP 97/62. HR 104, Temp 98.9F, RR 22. SpO2 94% on 4 L NC.

Except as noted below, the findings of the complete physical exam are within normal limits.

P. Sylvester · C. E. San Miguel (✉)
Department of Emergency Medicine, Wexner Medical Center at The Ohio State University, Columbus, OH, USA
e-mail: christopher.sanmiguel@osumc.edu

© Springer Nature Switzerland AG 2020
C. G. Kaide, C. E. San Miguel (eds.), *Case Studies in Emergency Medicine*, https://doi.org/10.1007/978-3-030-22445-5_63

- General: Somewhat pale, diaphoretic. Alert and oriented.
- Cardiovascular: Jugular venous distension (JVD) appreciated to the level of the thyroid cartilage while sitting upright. Regular rate and rhythm during exam. +S3. Pitting edema of lower extremities to upper tibias. Lower extremities cool to touch.
- Pulmonary: No apparent respiratory distress, trachea midline, posterior auscultation with crackles up to the mid-thorax bilaterally.
- Abdomen: Soft, nondistended, nontender to palpation.

Past Medical History (PMH)
Hypertension, Hyperlipidemia, Type II DM, Chronic Kidney Disease Stage III.

Social History (SH)
Former smoker (~ 10 pack-years), occasional ETOH use, denies illicit substance use.

Family History (FH)
Family history notable for "enlarged heart" in her brother and father, with early cardiac death of her father at age 50. Her brother has "some kind of pacemaker."

Pertinent Test Results

Test	Result	Units	Normal range
WBC	11.3 ↑	K/uL	$3.8–11.0\ 10^3/\ mm^3$
Hgb	8.4 ↓	g/dL	Male: 14–18 g/dL
			Female: 11–16 g/dL
Platelets	400	K/uL	140–450 K/uL
Potassium	3.4 ↓	mEq/L	3.5–5.5 mEq/L
Magnesium	1.6	mg/dL	1.6–2.6 mg/dL
Creatinine	2.1 ↑	mg/dL	0.6–1.5 mg/dL
Lactate	3.1 ↑	mmol/L	< 2.0 mmol/L
Troponin	1.3 ↑	ng/Ml	< 0.11 ng/mL
BNP	12580 ↑	pg/ml	<100 pg/ml

EKG Sinus rhythm with frequent PVCs, left axis deviation, nonspecific T-wave inversions. QTc read as 457.

Chest X-ray (CXR) Cardiomegaly, bilateral airspace disease consistent with pneumonia vs pulmonary edema. Small bilateral pleural effusions.

ED Management

There was concern for syncope secondary to primary dysrhythmia (VT/ventricular fibrillation (VF)) with new decompensated heart failure. Acute coronary syndrome was considered, and the patient was given 324 ASA, with serial troponins ordered. The admission order was placed to the cardiology service.

Updates on ED Course

Update 1 (1910)   While awaiting triage to the inpatient service, the patient is noted to have a period of sustained monomorphic VT (see EKG below). On reassessment, the patient is diaphoretic, and confused. Her blood pressure is noted to be 86/50. The crash cart is brought into the room, the patient is sedated with 10 mg of etomidate, and is successfully cardioverted with 100J (synchronized) to sinus rhythm.

- Repeat EKG remains stable from prior.
- The case was discussed with cardiology who recommended a 150 mg amiodarone bolus followed by a drip, but declined catheterization lab activation.
- 40 mg PO potassium was ordered as well as 4g IV magnesium.

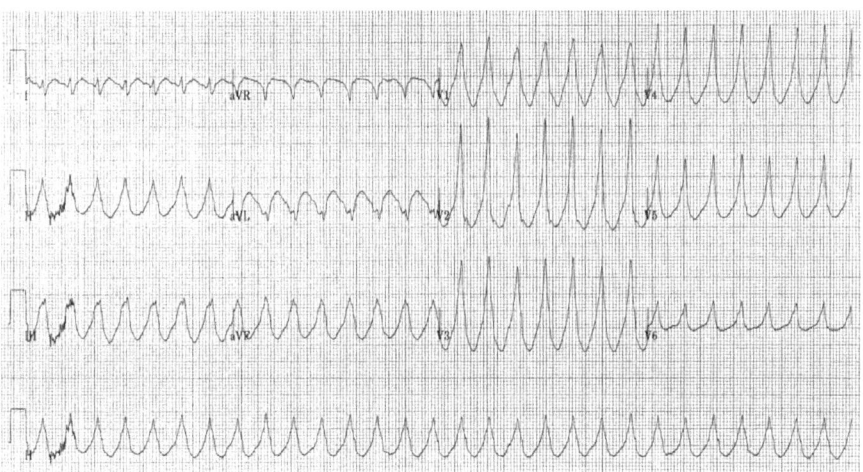

https://en.wikipedia.org/wiki/Ventricular_tachycardia#/media/File:Electrocardiogram_of_
Ventricular_Tachycardia.png

Update 2 (1950)   Shortly after completion of the amiodarone bolus, the patient again has another run of sustained VT requiring additional synchronized cardioversion, again at 100J which successfully restores sinus rhythm. However, frequent runs of non-sustained VT are noted.

- A loading dose of lidocaine 1 mg/kg was ordered.
- Due to declining mentation, the patient was intubated for airway protection.

Update 3 (2011) As nursing begins to prime a pump of propofol for post-intubation sedation, the patient is noted again to be in a wide-complex tachyarrhythmia. The patient then lost pulses. Code blue was called and chest compressions were started.

- Initial rhythm was consistent with coarse ventricular fibrillation (VF), defibrillation was attempted at 360 J unsuccessfully. The patient was given 1 mg epinephrine IV, and compressions were resumed.
- At the next rhythm check, the patient reamined in VF, and defibrillation was unsuccessful at 360J. The patient was given 300 mg amiodarone IVP, and compressions were resumed.
- The patient remained in VF at subsequent 2 pulse/rhythm checks.
- A second external defibrillator was brought to the resuscitation room, and a second set of pads were placed in the anterior-posterior (A-P) orientation on the patient's chest. At the next rhythm check with persistent VF, both external defibrillators were fired simultaneously at 360 J. No immediate change was noted to the rhythm.
- Dual-sequence defibrillation was repeated at the next rhythm check with apparent conversion to sinus tachycardia, achieving return of spontaneous circulation (ROSC).
- Postarrest EKG showed inferior ST depressions, cardiology was called, and the catheterization lab was activated.
- Left heart catheterization showed mild luminal irregularities and an ejection fraction (EF) <15% by ventriculogram. Therefore, an intra-aortic balloon pump was placed.
- The patient was admitted to the Coronary Care Unity for further management and propranolol 40 mg q6 was added to her medication regimen.

Learning Points: Electrical Storm

Priming Questions
1. Describe some of the common mechanisms by which ventricular dysrhythmias originate.
2. What criteria are used to diagnose electrical storm in patients with and without an implantable cardioverter defibrillator (ICD)?
3. Outside of anti-arrhythmic medications, what pharmacologic and non-pharmacologic therapies exists for treatment of electrical storm?

Introduction/Background

1. For emergency physicians, the diagnosis, treatment, and management of unstable ventricular dysrhythmias are rather simple. These patients are dead or dying. They fall quite neatly into the ACLS algorithms which are firmly engrained in our resuscitative minds. However, those patients who are "stable-ish" are at risk

for devolving into electrical anarchy and may continue to require repeated therapies (electrical or pharmacologic) for their symptomatic ventricular dysrhythmias. This can be a challenging patient population to manage.

2. Electrical storm is the proper term for a syndrome characterized by persistent or refractory ventricular dysrhythmias. Most commonly, this is ventricular tachycardia; hence, this entity is most frequently encountered and described as "VT storm."

   - Review of multiple retrospective studies suggests that monomorphic VT accounts for 86–97% of electrical storms, with VF accounting for 1–21%. There are varying incidence of mixed VT/VF and polymorphic VT [1].

3. The incidence of this syndrome is unclear. However, since the widespread implementation of ICDs, there has been perhaps a greater identification of patients with recurrent ventricular dysrhythmias as recorded on interrogation of these devices as well as the therapies that are then delivered as a result. Admittedly, these are patients with known cardiac disease; therefore, the application of this data to the general public is unclear.

   - For patients with ICDs placed for primary prevention (i.e., ejection fraction (EF) <35% despite revascularization and guideline-directed medical therapy), the incidence of electrical storm has been reported to be anywhere from 1.5 to 6.1%/year.
   - Not surprisingly, when you look at patients who had ICDs placed for secondary prevention of ventricular dysrhythmias, the incidence of electrical storm increases to upwards of 8%/year [2].

Physiology/Pathophysiology

1. With regard to the pathogenesis of a particular ventricular dysrhythmia, there are three basic mechanisms by which such a rhythm is generated. This includes the following [3]:

   - Abnormal automaticity: Often seen in the acute phase of myocardial ischemia due to changes in membrane potential, it results in the spontaneous depolarization of ventricular myocytes or Purkinje fibers.
   - Triggered activity/afterdepolarizations: This occurs when another depolarization takes place at an inappropriate time during the cycle of a myocytes action potential, often seen when the action potential duration is abnormally long (e.g., prolonged QT)
   - Re-entry: Most commonly seen in structural heart diseases, with either functional re-entry circuits or anatomic circuits (e.g., scar/fibrosis).

2. With this in mind, the most common primary precipitants of electrical storm can be thought of as those conditions that create or exacerbate one of these mechanisms [4].

   - Myocardial ischemia – frequently polymorphic VT/VF.
   - Drug toxicity.
   - Electrolyte abnormalities.
   - New/Decompensated heart failure – frequently monomorphic VT.

Making the Diagnosis

Differential Diagnosis
- Supra-ventricular tachycardia (SVT) with aberrancy.
- Pacemaker mediated tachycardia.
- ICD malfunction/lead fracture.

1. In one sense, this is a very easy diagnosis to make. Electrical storm is defined as three or more episodes of sustained VT, VF, or appropriate shocks from an implantable defibrillator within 24 hours [5].
   - VT is considered sustained if is lasts for at least 30 seconds, requires intervention to terminate, or if it causes hemodynamic compromise.
   - For patients with an ICD, the question that needs to be answered is whether they are receiving appropriate shocks, meaning the device is terminating lethal arrhythmias, or inappropriate shocks, which can be the result of oversensing, improper settings, or device failure among other things.
     - Keeping the patient on continual cardiac monitoring will allow for review of telemetry should the patient receive additional shocks while in the ED.
     - The key to answering this question most often lies in interrogating the device. Not only does it supply information on the patient's previous rhythms, it also performs diagnostics that can identify device failure. Advanced interpretation of the report should generally be performed in collaboration with a cardiologist familiar with ICDs.
     - If device interrogation is not an option, a magnet can be placed on the device. This inhibits the defibrillator function while maintaining pacemaker capabilities. The patient can then be kept on telemetry to evaluate for any new arrhythmic events. External defibrillator pads should be placed on the patient in the event that they were receiving appropriate shocks and they have another arrhythmia. If this is found to be the case, the magnet can be removed, and the device should resume defibrillator function [5].
   - Perhaps the most difficult distinction to make is whether the patient is experiencing VT or SVT with aberrancy. Both cause wide complex tachycardias and both have a wide range of clinical presentation, from asymptomatic to hemodynamic collapse [5].
     - If there is hemodynamic compromise, the debate becomes a bit of an academic one, at least in terms of initial management, as both arrhythmias would in that case warrant emergent synchronized cardioversion.
     - For patients who are relatively stable, this determination does in fact have significant impact on the next best steps in management.
     - The first step is to look at the patient's old EKG. If you are lucky, it will show a bundle branch block pattern that matches the morphology seen on

their current EKG. If this is the case, then the patient is likely experiencing an SVT with aberrancy. Similarly, a previous diagnosis or EKG features of Wolff-Parkinson-White syndrome (short PR, delta wave, and broad QRS) also increases the likelihood that this is SVT and not VT.

- Patient factors which are more likely to indicate VT are age > 35 years (positive predictive value of 85%), previous heart disease, and family history of sudden cardiac death [6].
- Looking at the current EKG, there are numerous individual features which increase the likelihood of VT. Of note, most are highly specific, but not sensitive. Therefore, it is possible to have a patient in VT without any of the typical features seen on EKG. Lifeinthefastlane.com has a great post on this exact topic with example EKGs that we have mostly summarized for this section. If you see any of the following, the patient is likely in VT:
  ○ Extreme axis deviation with a positive QRS in aVR and a negative QRS in I and aVF.
  ○ QRS complexes broader than 160 ms.
  ○ Capture beat – a narrow complex QRS beat among the wide complex QRS beats.
  ○ Josephson sign – a notch just before the S wave's nadir.
  ○ Lack of an RS complex in precordial leads – either all positive monophasic r waves or all negative monophasic s waves in V1–V6 [6]
- For advanced EKG interpreters, there do exist EKG interpretation algorithms that help distinguish the difference between SVT and VT. These include the Brugada and Vereckei Algorithms. Details of each are bit beyond our discussion here.
- A key point of emphasis is that if you are unsure of whether you are treating VT or SVT, treat it like VT! With the exception of beta-blockers, all the below treatments for VT are safe for use in SVT with a wide-complex. Some are even effective at treating SVT. Beta-blockers are also acceptable in SVT with aberrancy (wide-complex) as long as it is secondary to a bundle branch block. They are dangerous only in the setting of specific conduction pathways secondary to Wolff-Parkinson-White syndrome causing an irregular wide complex tachycardia. On the other hand, giving adenosine and/calcium blockers (first-line treatment for SVT) to a patient in VT can precipitate sudden cardiac death [5].

2. After emergent stabilization, part of your workup should be directed at identifying reversible causes of the arrhythmia. This includes electrolyte abnormalities (potassium, calcium, and magnesium are particularly important), cardiac ischemia, acute infection, and thyroid dysfunction. A review of the patient's medication list is also warranted to identify any drugs which may be causing prolonged QT.

Treating the Patient

1. When it comes to the ventricular dysrhythmias (VT/VF), the most straightforward patient to care for is the one who presents with cardiac arrest. To be clear, this is not to say that this resuscitation is going to be simple, or that patient is going to have a good outcome. Rather, these patients are universally recognized as critically ill immediately upon assessment, and providers of nearly all levels of training (as well as many laypersons) have at least some understanding of the initial steps in management. Several large-scale efforts are to thank for this, including:
   - Public awareness campaigns by the American Heart Association regarding bystander CPR.
   - Automated external defibrillators (AEDs) in public locations.
   - Widespread education (generally required) of hospital staff in Advanced Cardiac Life Support (the specifics of which will not be reviewed here).
2. The general management of the patient with electrical storm involves the classic ED mantra of "IV, O_2, and monitor." The latter, in this case, is of significant importance.
   - Indeed, for someone with symptomatic or hemodynamically significant ventricular dysrhythmias, a cardiac monitor is not sufficient. The patient should be connected to the pads of the defibrillator which should be in the room and be ready to deliver appropriate therapies.
     – In terms of pad placement, the traditional two methods include the anterior-lateral position, and the anterior-posterior position. There is no robust set of data to recommend one or other; however, many factors likely play a role into the success of one over the other including patient body habitus, need for ongoing CPR, etc.
   - For a patient as sick as the one described in our vignette, it goes without saying that activation of proper staff and resources is important. This is a patient who should be placed in an acute resuscitation area/trauma bay/etc. (not a hallway bed). Appropriate nursing, respiratory therapy, and ancillary staff should be available with clearly designated roles.
3. As one can imagine, anti-arrhythmic medications have a large role in the management of electrical storm. While there are many options to consider (along with an intimidating variety of various mechanisms, dosages, and side effects), there are a select few agents that the emergency physician should be comfortable reaching for and using.
   - If you were stuck on an island with only one anti-arrhythmic medication, amiodarone seems like the ideal choice [7]. Although listed as a Class III anti-arrhythmic based on primary mechanism, it has properties that overlap with all four classes.
     – To review, the code dose of amiodarone is 300 mg IVP, followed by a repeat 150 mg dose during pulseless VT/VF.
     – For a stable ventricular dysrhythmia, the typical starting point is a 150 mg bolus over 10 minutes, followed by a 1 mg/min drip for 6 hours, followed by a step-down to 0.5 mg/min for the following 18 hours.

○ Of note, the practice of doing a bolus dose, followed by tapered drip is designed primarily for the purposes of getting close to a 1g load over 24 hours. If clinical conditions mandate more urgent control of a ventricular dysrhythmias, it is appropriate to redose the 150 mg bolus dose q10 minutes as indicated (with a maximum dose of around 2g in the first 24 hours) [8].

– Amiodarone has a whole slew of side effects that are outside the scope of this discussion (and frankly outside the scope of emergency medicine in general). These are typically encountered with chronic use of this medication.

• As a second-line anti-arrhythmic medication, one should consider the use of lidocaine (which thankfully is also stocked in code carts). This is a class IB anti-arrhythmic. It is thought to have a predilection for blockade of ischemic myocardium and is thought to be effective in preventing re-entrant ventricular dysrhythmias [9].

– The dosing for this starts with a 1–1.5 mg/kg bolus, followed by repeated doses of 0.5–0.75 mg/k every 5–10 minutes as needed up to a total of 3 mg/kg. If there is a positive effect, an infusion can be continued at a rate of 1–4 mg/min. Serum lidocaine levels can and should be followed for monitoring of toxicity [6].

– While lidocaine historically was a very popular anti-arrhythmic (even being used prophylactically after myocardial ischemia for a time), it has slowly fallen out of favor due to a lack of data supporting improved outcomes with its use. While that can be said for many (or all) of the anti-arrhythmic drugs in the setting of cardiac arrest, at least in the setting of electrical storm, there is head to head data supporting the use of amiodarone over lidocaine. For that reason, lidocaine is considered a second-line agent after amiodarone [10].

4. Beyond the anti-arrhythmic, there are a couple of important pharmacologic therapies, which should be considered and initiated in the throes of electrical storm.

• Electrolyte abnormalities such as hypokalemia and hypomagnesemia should be corrected rapidly, with minimum goals of K>4 and Mg >2.

– Rather than waiting for labs, empiric treatment, particularly with magnesium and calcium seems to be a high-reward/low-risk intervention, particularly if there is any concern for underlying prolonged Qt or presentation in Torsades.

– Note that the code dose for magnesium is 2g IVP over minutes – significantly faster than the 4g hung over 4 hours that typically defaults when ordered.

• While it probably is not the first agent that comes to mind, as a class, the beta-blockers have a significant role in the management of electrical storm, as it pertains to limiting the catecholamine surge that can propagate these dysrhythmias.

– The IV beta-blockers such as metoprolol and esmolol are often used initially due to their short duration of action, with the thought that their effect on hemodynamics can be carefully titrated and stopped in the setting of profound hypotension.

- However, the beta-blocker that has the best data supporting its use in electrical storm is propranolol. Given at a dose of 40 mg q6 hours via PO/enteral access, a recent study showed that this reduced the rate of ICD discharges in electrical storm by 90% at 24 hours, compared to 53% in a group who received metoprolol [11].
- Sedation is critical to the management of patients in electrical storm, most pertinently in situations in which there are ongoing attempts at cardioversion. With that said, sedation may also play a role in limiting sympathetic output and thus can be a treatment modality in and of itself.
  - While a variety of agents could be chosen, propofol is well regarded as an ideal agent both for conscious sedation and for ongoing sedation (i.e., in the case of sedation for mechanical ventilation). Studies have suggested its superiority over other agents, and there has been much discussion as to whether propofol may have intrinsic sympatholytic activity [12].
5. Nonpharmacologic therapies
   - Cardioversion should be considered at the earliest sign of clinical instability, and defibrillation should be performed immediately on detection of ventricular fibrillation or loss of pulses.
     - To review, synchronized cardioversion should be utilized in patients with a pulse, whereas unsynchronized cardioversion/defibrillation is performed in the setting of cardiac arrest.
     - For energy selection, current ACLS guidelines recommend starting at 100 joules for stable VT, and 120–200 joules for VF or pulseless VT.
   - Anti-tachycardia pacing (ATP) (aka overdrive pacing) could be considered, although it is uncommonly performed in the emergency department. This is most pertinent in ventricular tachycardia and involves pacing at a rate higher than the VT for a few beats, with the thought being that this brief period can overcome re-entrant activity and prevent progression to VF.
     - Most commonly, this is seen occurring in patients with advanced ICDs that contain this feature. These devices often attempt ATP as a means of minimizing the frequency of defibrillation therapies delivered for VT.
     - In a patient without an ICD, this can be performed temporarily via external pacing. Case series have shown the efficacy of this, notably with the requirement of fairly high amperage necessary to obtain this (~150 mA). Of note, this may not be available in all standard defibrillator/pacer control units as some manufacturers set an upper limit of pacing (e.g., 120 BPM) which may not be high enough to overcome the rate of ongoing VT [13].
   - As mentioned elsewhere, one should have a high degree of suspicion for myocardial ischemia as a trigger for VT/VF. EKG analysis should be performed and discussed with cardiology for consideration of left heart catheterization and potential percutaneous coronary intervention (PCI), especially if an ST-segment elevation myocardial infarction (STEMI) is identified [14].
   - Depending on one's resources, or personal skills with regional blocks, consideration could be made for the use of a stellate ganglion block during cases of electrical storm.

- The stellate ganglion is a collection of sympathetic fibers from the lower cervical and upper thoracic spinal cord, which lies under the sternocleidomastoid around the level of the cricoid cartilage. While more frequently done as an outpatient procedure in the setting of complex regional pain disorders, the injection of local anesthetic in the region of this ganglion may result in decreased sympathetic outflow to the heart.
  - One study showed improved outcomes with regard to mortality when compared to traditional anti-arrhythmic therapy [15].
    - ○ Of note, however, the group receiving the block also was primarily treated with beta blockade at a rate different than the anti-arrhythmic group, so the isolated effect of the stellate ganglion block is less clear.
- Although not performed within the emergency department, ablation can be a definitive means of treating recurrent ventricular dysrhythmias. These are generally more successful in ischemic cardiomyopathies, where there is a large burden of scar acting as a source for re-entry; however, techniques for a wide variety of etiologies have been described in electrophysiology literature using less invasive percutaneous methods [16]. In very rare refractory cases, epicardial ablation may be needed using a surgical approach [17].
- In cases where additional time is needed to allow some of the above therapies to take effect or to get a patient to percutaneous coronary intervention (PCI) or electrophysiology (EP) ablation, mechanical support may be initiated as a temporizing measure.
  - An intra-aortic balloon pump (IABP) is a fairly common device within interventional cardiology, which can be utilized peri-procedurally for high-risk PCI or on its own in patients with recurrent VT/VF. This device relies on a system of counter-pulsation in which a percutaneously inserted aortic balloon is inflated during diastole and collapsed during systole. The effect is a decrease in systolic BP, and an increase in diastolic BP with an overall increase in mean arterial pressure (MAP). For patients with recurrent VT/VF, this provides a number of benefits – increasing coronary perfusion pressure (particularly useful if ischemia is the underlying etiology) and by reducing afterload and increasing cardiac output which may assist if decompensated heart failure is the underlying etiology [18].
  - Along the same lines, extra-corporeal life support (ECLS or ECMO) can provide hemodynamic support for patients with recurrent VT/VF, most often as a bridge to procedure, more durable mechanical support (i.e., LVAD) or transplantation. Veno-arterial ECMO can be used for this purpose via peripheral (femoral artery/vein) or central access and can assist (or even totally replace) the patient's entire cardiac output [19].
    - ○ Food for thought: On full mechanical support, patients can be fully conscious and perfused with sustained VT/VF which would ordinarily be nonperfusing.
6. Coming back to the coding patient with VT or VF, treatment that fails to achieve ROSC with the ACLS algorithm can be particularly frustrating, as there is the feeling that more should be done for these potentially reversible dysrhythmias.

Recently, there has been a lot of buzz about additional therapies/procedures that one can try as a "Hail Mary."

- One of the most interesting developments has been the use of so-called "Double Sequential External Defibrillation" or DSED. This involves connecting two sets of pads connected to two external defibrillators – one set in an anterior-posterior orientation, and the other being in the standard right upper-left lower configuration. When it is time for defibrillation, both devices are charged and the shock is delivered by pushing the buttons at the same time (most frequently with one provider coordinating the delivery) [20].
  - The principle behind this tactic is that for those patients with refractory dysrhythmias, they may require a greater vector of depolarization to reset the ongoing electrical chaos.
  - While studies have shown that there appears to be an increased rate of successful cardioversion and ROSC, there has not been any significant benefit with regard to neurologic outcome or mortality. Indeed, the most recent meta-analysis concluded that the usefulness of this technique was unclear and that more robust studies were needed [21].
  - It is also worth noting that this technique may cause damage to the defibrillator and could also potentially void the manufacturer's warranty [22]. We would encourage you to discuss this technique with your biomedical engineering departments before implementing it into your practice.
- There have been several studies that have investigated the role of high-dose esmolol in refractory VT/VF which also seems promising [23]. While the idea of giving a beta-blocker in a grossly hemodynamically unstable patient might give you pause, one should stop and consider what is happening several rounds deep into the standard ACLS algorithm. Specifically, with several rounds of high-dose epinephrine in, it may be possible that the benefit obtained from a vasopressor standpoint is at odds with the persistent adrenergic tone propagating the underlying ventricular dysrhythmia.
  - Like DSED, there does appear to be a promising effect on conversion/ROSC (up to 3x more likely in some retrospective studies); however, there has been no prospective study comparing the use of high dose esmolol to current standard practices, and even the current retrospective studies have very limited sample sizes.
  - Dosages and delivery methods (bolus vs infusion) may vary, and there is no consensus as to how and when this should be attempted. However the most recent study which showed benefit gave a 500 mcg/kg bolus followed by a 0-100 mcg/kg/minute infusion.
7. The disposition for patients with electrical storm should be fairly clear early in the patient's ED course. Early consideration for the patient's disposition should be considered. At minimum, patients with stable and infrequent runs of VT should be placed in a telemetry bed/cardiac service. Clearly, patients with hemodynamic instability associated with their ventricular dysrhythmias will require ICU/CCU admission.

- Early consultation with on-call cardiologist (including interventional cardiology/EP subspecialties if available) should be done to help facilitate admission vs transfer.

Case Conclusion

The patient was carefully diuresed, with careful monitoring of electrolytes. No further sustained VT/VF events were noted. The patient was subsequently started on guideline-directed medical therapy for new diagnosis of heart failure. The IABP was weaned and subsequently removed. The patient underwent cardiac MRI which showed a severely dilated left ventricle (LV) and a pattern of fibrosis consistent with nonischemic cardiomyopathy. Given her family history, the patient was referred to cardiac genetics for workup of a familial cardiomyopathy. EP was consulted and did not recommend any ablative strategies but did place an ICD for secondary prevention prior to discharge.

Discussion

1. Electrical storm is defined as three episodes of sustained VT, Vfib, or appropriate shocks from an implantable defibrillator within 24 hours.
2. Use old EKGs, defibrillator interrogation, and careful examination of the current EKG to help determine if the patient is in VT or SVT with aberrancy. When in doubt, treat as VT!
3. If the patient is hemodynamically unstable with any tachydysrhythmia, they need to ride the lightning (aka be cardioverted).
4. In stable VT, the initial drugs of choice are amiodarone and propranolol. Consider intubation and sedation for those more symptomatic patients with repeated episodes of dysrhythmia. Correct electrolytes and evaluate for reversible causes.
5. In refractory VT causing cardiac arrest, "Hail Mary" maneuvers such as DSED and high-dose esmolol are gaining more attention, but there is a lack of robust research to support their use.

Pattern Recognition

Electrical Storm
- Repeated episodes of syncope, palpitations, or defibrillator firing.
- Family history of sudden cardiac death.
- Personal history of cardiac disease.

Disclosure Statement   The authors of this chapter report no significant disclosures.

References

1. Sagone A. Electrical storm: incidence, prognosis and therapy. J Atr Fibrillation. 2015;8(4):1150.
2. Israel CW, Barold SS. Electrical storm in patients with an implanted defibrillator: a matter of definition. Ann Noninvasive Electrocardiol. 2007;12(4):375–82.
3. Al-khatib SM, Stevenson WG, Ackerman MJ, et al. AHA/ACC/HRS Guideline for Management of Patients With Ventricular Arrhythmias and the Prevention of Sudden Cardiac Death: A Report of the American College of Cardiology/American Heart Association Task Force on Clinical Practice Guidelines and the Heart Rhythm Society. J Am Coll Cardiol. 2017:2017.
4. Ueno A, Kobayashi Y, Murata H, et al. The short-term prognosis of the patients with ventricular tachycardia and fibrillation: from the registry data of Tokyo CCU Network for 3 years. The proceedings of the 37th scientific meeting of Tokyo CCU Network. ICU and CCU. 2018 (In press).
5. Eifling M, Razavi M, Massumi A. The evaluation and management of electrical storm. Tex Heart Inst J. 2011;38:111–21.
6. Burns B. VT versus SVT LITFL Medical Blog ECG library basics. In: Life in the fast lane. https://litfl.com/vt-versus-svt-ecg-library/; 2019. Accessed 4 Mar 2019.
7. Dorian P, Cass D, Schwartz B, Cooper R, Gelaznikas R, Barr A. Amiodarone as compared with lidocaine for shock-resistant ventricular fibrillation. N Engl J Med. 2002;346(12):884–90.
8. Muser D, Santangeli P, Liang JJ. Management of ventricular tachycardia storm in patients with structural heart disease. World J Cardiol. 2017;9(6):521–30.
9. Panchal AR, Berg KM, Kudenchuk PJ, et al. 2018 American Heart Association Focused Update on Advanced Cardiovascular Life Support Use of Antiarrhythmic Drugs During and Immediately After Cardiac Arrest: An Update to the American Heart Association Guidelines for Cardiopulmonary Resuscitation and Emergency Cardiovascular Care. Circulation. 2018;138(23):e740–9.
10. Dorian P, Cass D, Schwartz B, Cooper R, Gelaznikas R, Barr A. Amiodarone as compared with lidocaine for shock-resistant ventricular fibrillation. N Engl J Med. 2002;346(12):884–90.
11. Chatzidou S, Kontogiannis C, Tsilimigras DI, et al. Propranolol versus metoprolol for treatment of electrical storm in patients with implantable cardioverter-defibrillator. J Am Coll Cardiol. 2018;71(17):1897–906.
12. Burjorjee JE, Milne B. Propofol for electrical storm; a case report of cardioversion and suppression of ventricular tachycardia by propofol. Can J Anaesth. 2002;49(9):973–7.
13. Grubb BP, Temesy-Armos P, Hahn H, Elliott L. The use of external, noninvasive pacing for the termination of ventricular tachycardia in the emergency department setting. Ann Emerg Med. 1992;21(2):174–6.
14. Kobayashi Y. How to manage various arrhythmias and sudden cardiac death in the cardiovascular intensive care. J Intensive Care. 2018;6:23.
15. Nademanee K, Taylor R, Bailey WE, Rieders DE, Kosar EM. Treating electrical storm: sympathetic blockade versus advanced cardiac life support-guided therapy. Circulation. 2000;102(7):742–7.
16. Liang JJ, Santangeli P, Callans DJ. Long-term outcomes of ventricular tachycardia ablation in different types of structural heart disease. Arrhythmia Electrophysiol Rev. 2015;4(3):177–83.
17. Anter E, Hutchinson MD, Deo R, et al. Surgical ablation of refractory ventricular tachycardia in patients with nonischemic cardiomyopathy. Circ Arrhythm Electrophysiol. 2011;4(4):494–500.
18. Zhang ZP, Su X, Yan H, et al. Reversal of electrical storm after intraaortic balloon pump counterpulsation in a patient with acute myocardial infarction. Am J Emerg Med. 2015;33(5):734. e1–3.

19. Uribarri A, Bravo L, Jimenez-candil J, Martin-moreiras J, Villacorta E, Sanchez PL. Percutaneous extracorporeal membrane oxygenation in electrical storm: five case reports addressing efficacy, transferring allowance or radiofrequency ablation support. Eur Heart J Acute Cardiovasc Care. 2017:2048872617730036.
20. Cortez E, Krebs W, Davis J, Keseg DP, Panchal AR. Use of double sequential external defibrillation for refractory ventricular fibrillation during out-of-hospital cardiac arrest. Resuscitation. 2016;108:82–6.
21. Delorenzo A, Nehme Z, Yates J, Bernard S, Smith K. Double sequential external defibrillation for refractory ventricular fibrillation out-of-hospital cardiac arrest: a systematic review and meta-analysis. Resuscitation. 2019;135:124–9.
22. D Gerstein NS, Mclean AR, Stecker EC, Schulman PM. External defibrillator damage associated with attempted synchronized dual-dose cardioversion. Ann Emerg Med. 2018;71:109–12.
23. Lee YH, Lee KJ, Min YH, et al. Refractory ventricular fibrillation treated with esmolol. Resuscitation. 2016;107:150–5.

Vertigo: *"You Spin Me Right Round Baby Right Round"*

64

Bradley M. End and Colin G. Kaide

Case

Pertinent History

This patient is a 45-year-old male physician who was doing some paperwork in his office when he developed sudden, severe debilitating vertigo. He was found on the office floor by a colleague. He was complaining of a severe spinning sensation. He was actively vomiting at the time. He cannot recall anything that might have provoked the event. He appeared very stoic and had trouble answering questions. He was completely unable to ambulate or sit in an upright position. He denied headache, chest pain, numbness, tingling or overt weakness.

Physical Exam

- Vitals: T 98.5 °F/36.9 °C, BP 160/98, P 110, RR 16.
- General: Alert and oriented × 3, male in severe distress.
- Head: Atraumatic.

B. M. End
Department of Emergency Medicine, Robert C. Byrd Health Sciences Center, West Virginia University, Morgantown, WV, USA

C. G. Kaide (✉)
Department of Emergency Medicine, Wexner Medical Center at The Ohio State University, Columbus, OH, USA
e-mail: Colin.kaide@osumc.edu

© Springer Nature Switzerland AG 2020
C. G. Kaide, C. E. San Miguel (eds.), *Case Studies in Emergency Medicine*,
https://doi.org/10.1007/978-3-030-22445-5_64

- Ears: within normal limits.
- Eyes: Pupils equal, round and reactive to light, direction-changing nystagmus noted on exam.
- Neck: Nontender, trachea midline; thyroid is normal.
- Lungs: Bilaterally clear to auscultation.
- Heart: S1/S2 increased rate with regular rhythm. No murmurs.
- Abdomen: Soft, non-tender/non-distended, bowel   sounds present, no mass or bruit.
- Skin: Warm and dry with no rashes.
- Neuro: Cranial nerve exam.
  - III, IV, VI (eye movements) – Significant direction-changing nystagmus.
  - V (facial sensory) – Normal
  - VII (facial motor) – Normal
  - VIII (auditory) – Normal
  - XI (glossopharyngeal) – Symmetrical palate movement.
  - X (vagus) – Normal
  - XI (accessory) – Normal
  - XII (hypoglossal) – Tongue protrudes to midline.
- Speech: Mild slurring of speech.
- Reflexes: 2+ bilaterally.
- Sensory: Grossly intact.
- Motor: Upper extremity strength is 5/5 bilaterally; Lower extremity strength is 5/5.
- Pronator drift: Unable to perform.
- Tandem gait: Unable to stand.
- Romberg: Inability to maintain balance even with eyes open.
- Finger to nose/heel to shin: Left-sided abnormality compared to the left.
- Rapid alternating movements: Abnormal coordination.
- Nystagmus: Nystagmus is horizontal and bidirectional.

Past Medical History
None

Social History
- Alcohol: Social use
- Tobacco: None
- Drugs of abuse: Denies

Family History
Coronary artery disease

Pertinent Test Results

CT Scans and MRI

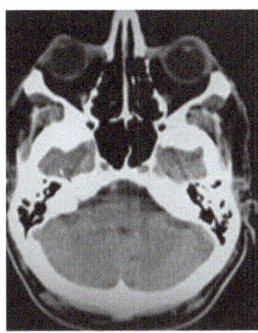 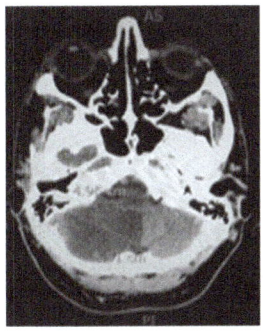 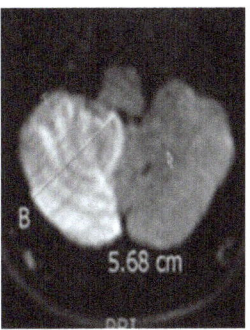

Initial CT at time 2 h post onset   Repeat CT 24 hours later   Initial MRI at 2.5 hpost onset

Images courtesy of Colin Kaide, MD and Michael Dick, MD

ED Management

The patient was brought to the ED from his office on an ED cart. He had persistent vomiting and profound vertigo with nystagmus. He was given Ativan, Phenergan, and Zofran with little relief of symptoms. He had a CT scan that was normal. He was sedated and taken for immediate MRI/MRA. The MRI showed and acute right cerebellar infarct and the MRA showed a vertebral artery dissection on the right side. He was given repeat doses of medication for nausea and vertigo but they were not particularly effective. He was transferred to the main campus hospital to be admitted to the neurology service.

Learning Points

Priming Questions
1. What are the most common etiologies of vertigo in patients presenting to the Emergency Department?
2. What provocative testing and imaging are required for patients presenting with vertigo?
3. What is the Head Impulse, Nystagmus, and Test of Skew (HINTS) exam and how can it contribute to the evaluation of vertigo in the ED?

Introduction/Background

1. Dizziness and vertigo account for about four million Emergency Department (ED) visits annually in the United States [1].
   - Between 160,000 and 240,000 (4–6%) are caused by cerebrovascular disease [1].
   - Approximately, one quarter of vertebrobasilar stroke patients had at least one transient neurologic symptom within 3 months prior to stroke [2].
   - In one small sample, 42% (21/50) had attacks with an isolated nonfocal symptom that was not considered typical transient ischemic attack (TIA)-like, and neuroimaging confirmed acute infarction in four of them. *Vertigo was the most common of these non-focal symptoms* [2].
2. Elderly patients and "dizziness."
   - Most common ED complaint in patients over 75 years old; up to 20% report symptoms significant enough to interfere with activities of daily living [2].
   - Chronic: Average five visits without resolution.
3. The first step is to differentiate the complaint of "dizziness." Since dizziness can mean anything the patient wants it to mean, it must be more precisely described to categorize it as one of the following:
   - Light-headedness: The feeling of passing out. Common phrases used to describe this feeling include:
     - "Lightheadedness."
     - "Going to pass out."
     - "Swimmy-headed."
     - "Stood up too fast."
   - True balance problems: Often described as falling to one side or not being able to coordinate movements. This can be a true ataxia representing posterior fossa disease.
   - Vertigo: The sensation of perceived motion, typically spinning but may also be described as swaying, tumbling, or tilting [3–5].
   - Nonspecific vague complaints. You will never figure this out! Ensure it is not something dangerous and send them back to their family doctor.

Physiology/Pathophysiology

A complete review of the vestibular organs and vestibulo-ocular interface is beyond the scope of this chapter. Know that the vestibular organ consists of three semi-circular canals and two otolith structures located in the inner ear that detect angular and linear acceleration, respectively. The movement of fluid (endolymph) contained within these structures activates or inhibits hair cells which in turn convey information to the cerebral cortex. These organs interface with the visual system and play a significant role in balance [6].

In turn, dysfunction of the central component of the system occurs in the vestibular structures in the brainstem or cerebellum. It is usually caused by an interruption in blood flow to those areas.

The key to evaluation of the patient with vertiginous symptoms is to differentiate the source of the symptoms as either central or peripheral.

1. Characteristics of PERIPHERAL Vertigo [7].
   - Acute onset, intense spinning, swaying with nausea, vomiting, diaphoresis aggravated by change in position.
   - Fatigable, unidirectional nystagmus inhibited by fixing on an object.
   - Otic symptoms sometimes present (pain, tinnitus, occasionally decreased hearing).
   - No central focal examination findings.
2. Characteristics of CENTRAL Vertigo:
   - Gradual onset (but can be sudden with acute loss of blood flow), less intense with mild peripheral symptoms.
   - Nonfatigable, direction-changing nystagmus, uninhibited by eye fixation.
   - Vertical nystagmus (almost always central – may be seen in anterior canal benign paroxysmal positional vertigo (BPPV)) [8].
   - Focal cerebellar or brain stem findings such as dysmetria, dysdiadochokinesia, and gait ataxia [9].

Nystagmus

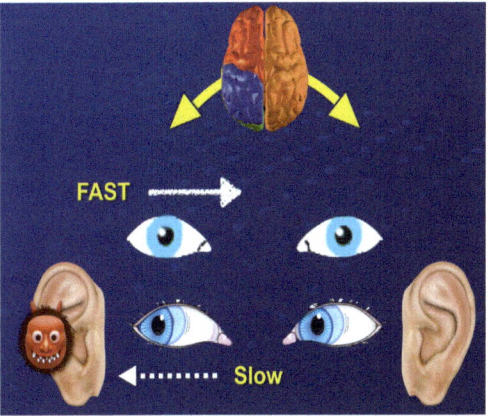

The direction of the nystagmus is described by the fast component, which generally moves away from the side of the lesion. The fast component of the nystagmus is a cortically-mediated correction of the deviated direction of gaze. When in doubt about the direction of the nystagmus, use your smart phone camera in the slow-motion setting. It is easy to tell when the image is slowed.

Making the Diagnosis

Differential Diagnosis
- Benign Paroxysmal Positional Vertigo (BPPV).
- Meniere's Disease.
- Vestibular Neuronitis.
- Labyrinthitis.
- Cerebrovascular Accident (CVA).
- Transient Ischemic Attack (TIA).
- Vertebrobasilar Insufficiency (VBI).
- Intracranial Mass.
- Intracranial Hemorrhage.

1. Determine if this vertigo is amenable to this algorithmic approach. The types of patients in whom the algorithm works are those with acute vestibular syndrome (AVS). Patients with light-headedness or the feeling of fainting when standing can be excluded immediately from this algorithm.
   - Determine that the patient has an acute vestibular syndrome.
     - This is an acute, persistent vertigo lasting for at least 24 hours to several weeks with associated nausea or vomiting, head motion intolerance, gait unsteadiness, and nystagmus. It accounts for 10–20% of ED "dizziness" presentations. It is typically peripheral in 80% of cases and central in ~20% [10]. These patients *will* have symptoms while they are being seen in the ED.
   - There are types of vertigo that you can immediately remove from this workup paradigm.
     - The first is the patient with TIA-like symptoms. A sudden, acute, self-limited, intense vertigo that began spontaneously and is clearly not provoked or alleviated by movement or rest. It usually lasts for minutes and is resolved by the time the patient is seen in the ED. This is potentially a vertebrobasillar TIA or may be related to vertebrobasilar insufficiency [6]. They should get a TIA workup to include the cervical and intracerebral vasculature with an MRA or CT angiogram (CTA), along with a brain MRI and cardiac echo [11].
     - The second type is vertigo with any hard neurologic finding, excluding isolated nystagmus. *These patients should be presumed to have central vertigo until proven otherwise.* They fall out of the algorithm and get and MRI, neuro consult, etc.
     - The third type is the patient who has had symptoms for months, especially vague nonspecific ones. You will never figure this out!
2. When you have decided that the patient has AVS, the next step depends on the provoking factors. If the patient has symptoms that are specifically *and only* provoked in special positions, such as when the head is realigned with respect to gravity (this means head positions such as when the patient rolls over in bed or looks down or looks up toward the ceiling), it is called positional vertigo

[12]. Vertigo that is mostly present and transiently made somewhat worse by looking side-to-side or going from a sitting to standing position *is not* "positional vertigo," but rather "spontaneous vertigo." If the vertigo is positional… it is often from crystal disease. The next step in this setting is to "provoke the crystals." If it is clearly spontaneous vertigo/nystagmus…proceed to the HINTS exam.

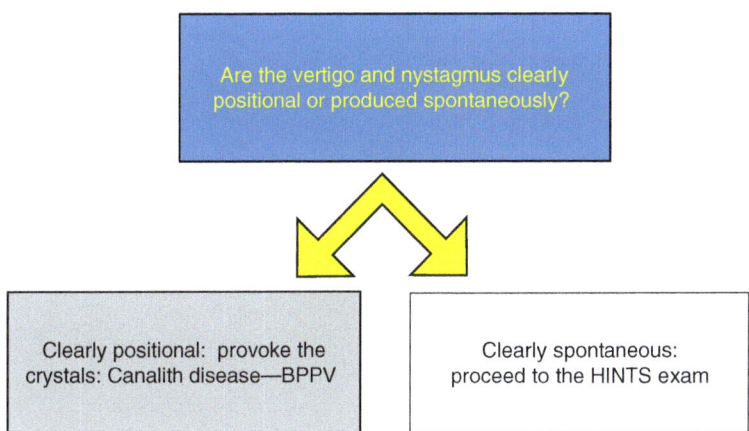

- *Provoking the Crystals:* The Dix-Hallpike and the Pagnini-McClure Maneuvers test for canalithiasis in the posterior and horizontal semicircular canals respectively. The best way to learn how to do these tests is to watch a *YouTube* video of them being performed. This will be easy to find!
    - A positive test implies "Benign Paroxysmal Positional Vertigo (BPPV)."
    - BPPV incidence increases with age and is more common in women. Despite its designation as "benign," note that up to 30% of elderly patients with BPPV will sustain multiple falls over the course of a single year which may contribute to morbidity and mortality [12, 13].
    - If either of these tests is positive, then the diagnosis of Benign Positional Paroxysmal Vertigo can be assigned. The Modified Epley Maneuver should be performed in a positive Dix-Hallpike test. If the Roll Test is positive, a barbeque roll maneuver should be performed
- **HINTS Exam** [1, 14]: The HINTS exam is an acronym for Head Impulse, Nystagmus, and Test of Skew. HINTS is based on differentiating central from peripheral causes of vertigo, not etiology per se, making it well suited to the ED diagnostic environment that values prompt disposition decisions over exact etiologic diagnoses. As expected, HINTS performs best in predicting "a" central cause (as opposed to specifically predicting stroke or gauging the presence of a structural lesion by MRI).

Dix-Hallpike Maneuver: Tests for otoliths in the posterior semi-circular canal
Steps:
1. Sit the patient on the bed.
2. Extend the neck and turn to one side.
3. Place patient supine rapidly (head hangs over the edge of the bed).
4. Keep patient in this position for 30 seconds, if no nystagmus occurs.
5. Return patient to upright position and observe for 30 seconds for nystagmus.
6. Repeat with the head turned to the other side.

Positive Test If:
- Horizontal/rotary (torsional) nystagmus to the stimulated side.
- Lasts 15–45 seconds.
- Latency of 2–15 seconds.
- Fatigues easily, meaning repeat Dix-hallpike tests show significantly fewer symptoms.
- Nystagmus may reverse on sitting.

Pagnini-McClure Maneuver (Roll Test) [5]: Tests for otoliths in the horizontal semi-circular canal

Steps: Similar in execution to the Dix-Hallpike,
1. Lie the patient supine with the head placed flat in a supine position not over-hanging the bed.
2. The head is then quickly rotated approximately 90° to the right and then returned to baseline and rotated 90° to the left
3. Ensure the head is left in place for at least 30 seconds or until symptoms resolve.

Positive Test If:
- Test is positive as above with the Dix-Hallpike, except the nystagmus is horizontal and not torsional.

– HINTS to Diagnose Stroke in the Acute Vestibular Syndrome. This study also proves that finding one of three dangerous, subtle oculomotor signs is more sensitive than the combined presence of all other traditional neurological signs for identifying stroke or other central problem as a cause of AVS [14].
  o HIT suggests a peripheral vertigo.
  o Horizontal nystagmus that changes direction in eccentric gaze.
  o Skew deviation.

- Using HINTS vs. ABCD2: HINTS would yield 98% fewer missed strokes at 87% lower cost. ABCD2 score was designed to help predict the risk of cerebrovascular accident (CVA) in patients presenting with a TIA. Each value is assigned points depending on the presence or degree of abnormality and this score is used to predict the risk of developing a stroke at different intervals postpresentation [1].
  - **A**ge ≥ 60 years.
  - **B**lood Pressure with either the systolic ≥140 or the diastolic ≥90.
  - **C**linical features.
  - **D**uration of symptoms.
  - History of **D**iabetes.
- The HINTS exam does have a significant learning curve. It takes a while to be able to recognize when it suggests central or peripheral vertigo. It is very important for anyone who wants to use this exam clinically to exclude a central cause of vertigo to watch the exam many times and perform it with someone who is good at it! It helps a lot to video the patient's eyes during the exam using the slow-motion feature of your device. It is much easier to see corrective saccades or the direction of the nystagmus in slow motion.

3. When the HINTS exam points to a central cause, imaging with MRI of the head and MRA (or CTA) of the head and neck is indicated. When the HINTS exam clearly indicates a peripheral cause (see caution above), the patient can be treated symptomatically [1, 14]. In some cases, this will require medications and in others, it will require a particle repositioning procedure such as the Epley maneuver.

HINTS Exam
Head Impulse Test:
- Examiner tells patient to look forward and keep this or her eyes focused on the examiner's nose. The head is quickly turned to one side, then back to the middle. This is repeated in the opposite direction. In a patient with a PERIPHERAL vertigo, there will be a corrective saccade in which the eye has to seemingly jump to keep up with the rapid head turn. This will occur when the head is turned toward the side with the pathology. CENTRAL vertigo does not have a corrective saccade. Normal patients with absolutely no pathology at all will also NOT have a corrective saccade. Positive HIT equals the presence of corrective saccade.
- Implication of a Positive HI Test (In a patient with spontaneous nystagmus):
  - Positive HI test = presence of corrective saccade. Strongly implies a peripheral cause!
  - Central vertigo DOES NOT have a corrective saccade.

Nystagmus in Vertigo
- **In Peripheral Vertigo:** The direction of the nystagmus (fast component) stays the same and increases in intensity when the patient looks in the direction of the fast phase. So…when looking forward, if the fast beat is to the left:
  - *Looking to the L, the fast beat moves faster to the L.*
  - *Looking to the R, the fast beat still moves to the L.*
- **In Central Vertigo:** Vertical or rotational nystagmus reliably predicts an underlying central pathology…*BUT* patients with central vertigo more often have horizontal-beating nystagmus. In central vertigo, the direction of the horizontal nystagmus changes when the direction of gaze.
  - *The fast phase beats in one direction when looking to the right, and the opposite direction when looking to the left (or on returning to the midline).*

Skew Deviation
- Eyes should remain aligned and keep their original point of fixation when one is covered. Skew is a repositioning of an eye back to the correct point of fixation upon uncovering. Have the patient look at your nose. Cover then uncover the left eye then do the same on the right. Each eye should remain fixed on the position it was in prior to being covered—It should not drift and have to "correct" itself back to the original point of fixation. Skew deviation is strongly linked to the presence of brainstem lesions, most often ischemic strokes in the lateral medulla or pons.

HINTS to INFARCT

H
I 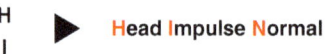 **Head Impulse Normal**

N 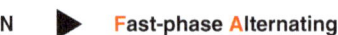 **Fast-phase Alternating**

T
S 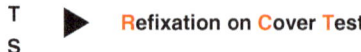 **Refixation on Cover Test**

If any one of these is positive in a patient with spontaneous nystagmus, consider this as a central vertigo.
False negative MRIs happen in HINTS positive patients in the first 24–48 hours after symptom onset.

An Algorithm for Characterizing Vertigo

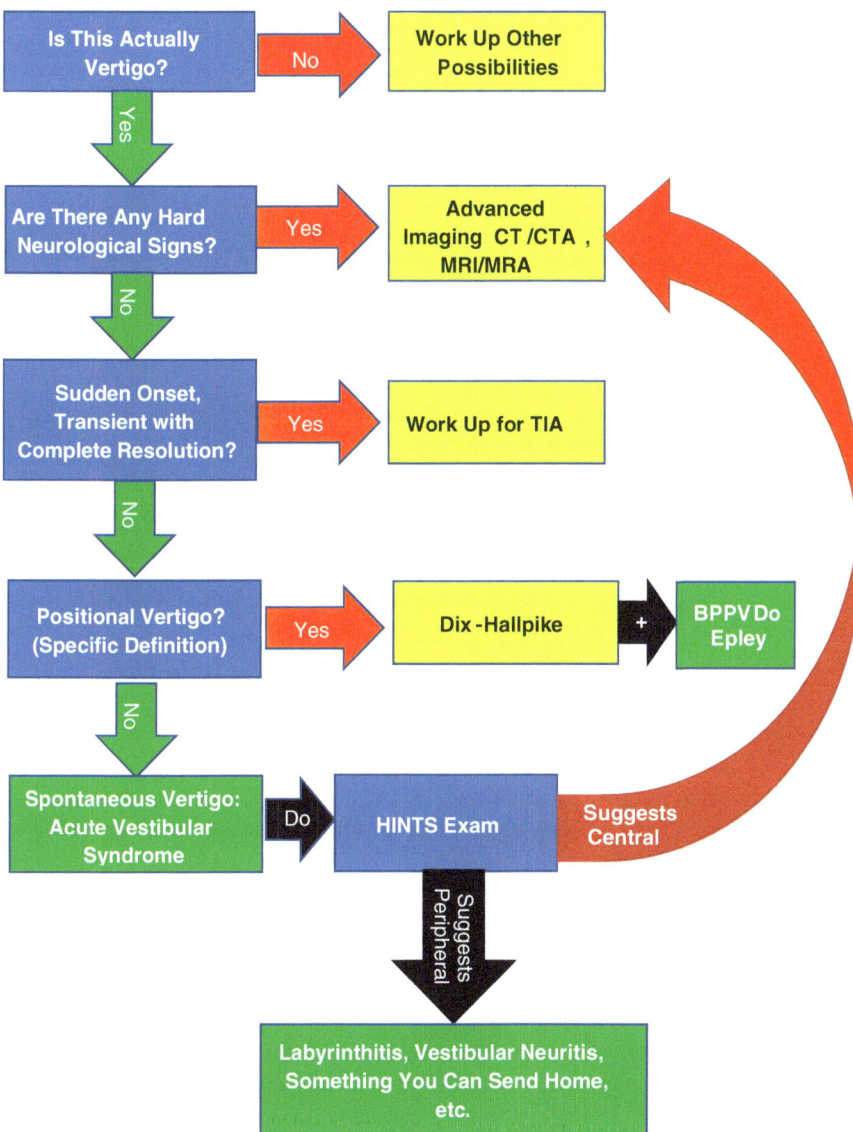

Published with kind permission of © Colin G. Kaide 2019. All Rights Reserved

Treating the Patient [15]

1. Regardless of whether the cause is presumed to be central or peripheral, symptomatic treatment is appropriate.
2. Different classes of medications can be used to help with symptoms. These include the following.

- Antihistamines: These have their anti-vertigo effect primarily because of their anticholinergic properties.
    - Meclizine (Antivert®): 25–50 mg PO q6h PRN.
    - Diphenhydramine (Benadryl®): 25–50 mg PO q6h PRN.
    - Dimenhydrinate (Dramamine®): 50–100 mg PO/IM/IV q4–6h PRN. Max 400 mg PO qd; Max 600 mg IM/IV qd.
    - Betahistadine: 24–36 mg/qd divided in 2–3 doses (14).
- Benzodiazepines
    - Diazepam (Valium®): 5–10 mg PO/IV q6h PRN.
    - Lorazepam (Ativan®): 1–2 mg PO/IV/IM q8h PRN.
- Anticholinergics
    - Atropine: 1 mg in 500–1000 mL NS, IV over 30–-60 minutes.
    - Hyoscyamine (Levsin®): 0.125–0.25 mg PO/SL q4h PRN.
    - Scopolamine: 0.4–0.8 mg PO q8h PRN.
3. Epley Maneuver: This is appropriate for patients with BPPV. It will not have any effect on non-BPPV causes of vertigo.
    - When doing an Epley maneuver, make sure to keep the patient in each of the positions until all symptoms of vertigo resolve or at least 30 seconds.
    - Repeating the maneuver increases success.
    - You can initiate the maneuver as soon as you see a positive Dix-Hallpike, using that as the first position of the Epley Maneuver.
        - Recurrence rate of approximately 36%.
        - Epley maneuver outcomes equivalent to Semont and Gans maneuvers, all superior to Brandt-Darhoff exercises [16]. Mastoid oscillation during the maneuver or "augmented" maneuvers do not routinely improve success rates [17].
        - Of note, postural restrictions following these maneuvers has not been shown to improve efficacy [18].
4. For the patient with a CVA or other central cause, referral to a stroke center is appropriate.

Case Conclusion

After admission to the neurology service for a brief period, the symptoms gradually began to improve. The patient was transferred to a rehab facility where extensive physical therapy and cognitive testing was performed. After a briefer than expected time in rehab, the patient made a full recovery and went back to practicing medicine, fully healed.

Discussion

Patients may present with nonspecific symptoms. While vertigo is defined as the perception of movement in the absence of a stimulus, patients may have difficulty conveying symptoms and so inappropriate descriptors may still be due to an underlying vertiginous cause.

Leave the ability to fully comprehend the vestibular organ, its neural interfaces and feedback mechanisms and the endless differential list to the neuro-otologists. Your job in the Emergency Department is to reliably differentiate between peripheral and central causes of vertigo.

Always consider a posterior TIA or VBI in patients with intense symptoms that have remitted by the time they reach the ED. Do not ignore subtle neurologic deficits. Ensure that you see all patients walk prior to ruling out a central etiology.

Perform the Dix-Hallpike maneuver or roll test to see if vertigo is positional and reproducible. If these tests are positive, attempt to abate symptoms using the Epley maneuver or barbeque roll, respectively.

All vertigo symptoms are made worse by head movement. Most studies regarding the use of the HINTS exam were performed by neurologists and often in the office setting. If your exam is equivocal or you are uncertain in the face of multiple risk factors, consider consultation or imaging to exclude central causes.

Physician, Heal Thyself—*An Emergency Physician's Perspective on Being the Patient*
Michael R. Dick, MD

I am an emergency physician, and the medical director of The Ohio State University Emergency Department—East Campus. A few years ago, I was in my office, just off the clinical area of the ED working on the physician schedule. I had one last hole to fill, when out of the blue, I experienced the sudden onset of vertigo…and I mean sudden; like I had been hit in the head with a baseball bat! I had never had vertigo before. My first response was to grab my desk. By holding on as tight as I could, maybe I could stop the constant sensation of movement. Instead, the vertigo just became worse. Maybe, I though, if I were to lie down, and hold perfectly still, it would stop. This must be garden variety vertigo, right? BPPV, Labyrinthitis maybe? It never occurred that it could be anything other than that. I slid to the floor and stretched my arms out, palms down, in an attempt to keep the floor – or me – from moving. Fortunately, one of my attending partners, Brandy, happened by and realized that is was not typical for me to be lying flat on my office floor. "Are you OK?" she asked. The effort that it took to answer was the first hint that maybe I wasn't. Brandy grabbed another attending to help me from behind the desk. I couldn't stand, let alone walk. That was odd! They helped me onto an ED cart. That is when the marathon of vomiting began. Even then, everything felt strangely calm, I barely noticed the stream of people in an out of the room. I don't remember the CT. I vaguely remember another attending partner, Kurt, telling me that I had a stroke. It didn't register. I said, "Ok," and kept my eyes closed. I still wonder at the sense of calm. Was it the medication? Edema? (it is odd to have a ventriculostomy tray by your bed day after day), remodeling? Fatigue? I have a slight recollection of the MRI/MRA that confirmed a right vertebral artery dissection and right cerebellar stroke. When they took me for a TEE, I remember thinking, "Well that will be great with this constant puking." The wonders of Midazolam-like it never happened! The only position that made things tolerable, was lying on my right side, eyes closed, holding on to the bed railing as tightly as possible. Prior to this, I had always slept on my left side. To this day, I now sleep on my right side.

After several days, the physical therapists began their visits. Over time, I progressed from a broad-based waddle to eventually walking close to normal. Ultimately, I was transferred from the floor to our rehab hospital. I hated rehab. I felt totally out of control. I was being tested to see if my cognitive function had been affected. Was I fit to practice medicine? Oddly, this was the first time I was worried. Fortunately, things progressed very quickly and my rehab stay was short. My stroke occurred in August, and in October, I was able to run a full marathon as I had planned. What caused the dissection? The night before, two of my kids and I went to the driving range and hit golf balls. The repeated twisting of the neck? I have no connective tissue disease or any other risk factors. I will never know for sure.

What are the take home points? Vertigo is miserable…absolutely miserable! Do whatever you can help the patient get some relief. H2 blockers and PPIs do make emesis less acidic and easier to tolerate. The sense of detachment that you often see with stroke victims is something inherent in the brain insult. If they don't seem concerned, they just don't understand what is happening. I don't believe that I had any true decision-making capacity during the acute phase of this event. Beware of sudden onset severe vertigo without any of the classic findings of a benign entity. Listen to your gut. Dig deeper if something doesn't seem right. Yes, we all hate to see the chief complaint of dizziness, but it can be a sign of real pathology.

Pattern Recognition

Vertigo
- The sensation of movement, must differentiate from presyncope.
- Intense short-lived, nonreproducible vertigo or vertigo + neuro deficit is TIA/CVA until proven otherwise.
- In AVS, perform provocative maneuvers and the HIINTS exam to attempt to differentiate between central and peripheral causes of vertigo.

Disclosure Statement Bradley End: No disclosures.

Colin Kaide: Callibra, Inc.-Discharge 123 medical software company. Medical Advisory Board Portola Pharmaceuticals. I have no relationship with a commercial company that has a direct financial interest in subject matter or materials discussed in article or with a company making a competing product.

References

1. Newman-Toker DE, Kerber KA, Hsieh YH, et al. HINTS outperforms ABCD2 to screen for stroke in acute continuous vertigo and dizziness. Acad Emerg Med. 2013;20(10):986–96.
2. Saber-Tehrani AS, Coughlan D, Hsieh YH, et al. Rising annual costs of dizziness presentations to US emergency departments. Acad Emerg Med. 2013;20:689–96.
3. Furman JM, Barton JS. Evaluation of the patient with vertigo. In: Aminoff MJ, Deschler DG, Hockberger RS, Wilterdink JL, editors. UpToDate; 2015. Retrieved May 8 2018 from https://www.uptodate.com/contents/evaluation-of-the-patient-with-vertigo.
4. Goldman B. Vertigo. In: Tintinalli JE, Stapczynski J, Ma O, Yealy DM, Meckler GD, Cline DM, editors. Tintinalli's emergency medicine: a comprehensive study guide. 8th ed. New York: McGraw-Hill; 2016.
5. Lustig LR, Schindler JS. Ear, nose, & throat disorders. In: Papadakis MA, SJ MP, Rabow MW, editors. Current medical diagnosis & treatment. New York: McGraw-Hill; 2017.
6. Baloh RW, Jen JC. Hearing and equilibrium. In: Goldman-Cecil medicine, vol. 428. Philadelphia: Elsevier/Saunders; 2016. p. 2593–2601.e2.
7. Ferri FF. Vertigo. In: Ferri's clinical advisor. Philadelphia: Elsevier; 2018. p. P1756–62.
8. Barton JS. Benign paroxysmal positional vertigo. In: Aminoff MJ, Deschler DG, Brazis PW, Wilterdink JL, editors. UpToDate; 2018. Retrieved May 8 2018.
9. Chang AK. Dizziness and vertigo. In: Rosen's emergency medicine: concepts and clinical practice. Philadelphia: Elsevier; 2018. p. 145–152.e1.
10. Furman JM. Pathophysiology, etiology, and differential diagnosis of vertigo. In: Aminoff MJ, Deschler DG, Wilterdink JL, editors. UpToDate; 2017. Retrieved May 8 2018 from https://www.uptodate.com/contents/pathopysiology-etiology-and-differential-diagnosis-of-vertigo.
11. Angtuaco EJ, Wippold FJ II, Cornelius RS, Aiken AH, Berger KL, Broderick DF, Brown DC, Bykowski J, Douglas AC, Germano IM, Kesser BW, Kessler MM, McConnell CT Jr, Mechtler LL, Smirniotopoulos JG, Vogelbaum MA. Expert panel on neurologic imaging. In: ACR Appropriateness Criteria® hearing loss and/or vertigo. [online publication]. Reston: American College of Radiology (ACR); 2013. 14 p.
12. Kim JS, Zee DS. Benign paroxysmal positional vertigo. N Engl J Med. 2014;370(12):1138.
13. Wang Y, Liu J, Cui Z, Yan L, Si J. Analysis of risk factors in patients with peripheral vertigo or central vertigo. Neurologist. 2018;23:75–8. https://doi.org/10.1097/NRL.0000000000000179.
14. Kattah JC, Talkad AV, Wang DZ, et al. HINTS to diagnose stroke in the acute vestibular syndrome: three-step bedside oculomotor examination more sensitive than early MRI diffusion-weighted imaging. Stroke. 2009;40:3504–10.
15. Furman JM, Barton JS. Treatment of vertigo. In: Aminoff MJ, Deschler DG, Wilterdink JL, editors. UpToDate. Wolters Kluwer; 2015.
16. Hilton MP, Pinder DK. The Epley (canalith repositioning) manoeuvre for benign paroxysmal positional vertigo. Cochrane Database Syst Rev. 2014;(12):Art. No.: CD003162. https://doi.org/10.1002/14651858.CD003162.pub3.
17. Hunt WT, Zimmermann EF, Hilton MP. Modifications of the Epley (canalith repositioning) manoeuvre for posterior canal benign paroxysmal positional vertigo (BPPV). Cochrane Database Syst Rev. 2012;(4):Art. No.: CD008675. https://doi.org/10.1002/14651858.CD008675.pub2.
18. Cromwell C, et al. The necessity for post-maneuver restrictions in the treatment of benign paroxysmal positional vertigo: an updated meta-analysis of the literature. Otol Neurotol. 2018;39:671–9.

Volatile Alcohol Ingestion: *A Good Ole Boy Drinking Ethylene Gly, Singin This'll Be How I Get AKI*

65

Matthew Schwab and Christopher E. San Miguel

Case

Pertinent History

The patient is a 45-year-old male with a history of alcohol abuse and depression who was brought in by Emergency Medical Services (EMS) after an intentional ingestion of an unknown substance.

Per EMS, the patient appeared significantly intoxicated at the scene. The patient had been consuming what they assumed was alcohol throughout the day per family and was mumbling that his drink tasted "so bitter." He was combative for EMS causing him to be sedated and ultimately intubated en route to the hospital. Of note, the paramedics reported difficulty with the intubation secondary to a large amount of emesis.

Pertinent Physical Exam

Except as noted below, the findings of the complete physical exam are within normal limits.

M. Schwab · C. E. San Miguel (✉)
Department of Emergency Medicine, Wexner Medical Center at The Ohio State University, Columbus, OH, USA
e-mail: matthew.schwab@osumc.edu; christopher.sanmiguel@osumc.edu

© Springer Nature Switzerland AG 2020
C. G. Kaide, C. E. San Miguel (eds.), *Case Studies in Emergency Medicine*,
https://doi.org/10.1007/978-3-030-22445-5_65

- BP 136/77, Pulse 122, Temperature 97.9 °F (36.6 °C), Resp. Rate 18, SpO$_2$ 96.00%.
- Constitutional: He appears well-developed and well-nourished. Intubated with vomitus around the mouth.
- HENT: Normocephalic and atraumatic.
- Eyes: Conjunctivae are normal. Pupils are equal, round, and reactive to light. No scleral icterus.
- Cardiovascular: Tachycardia, regular.
- Pulmonary/chest: Intubated, clear bilaterally.
- Abdomen: Soft. Bowel sounds are normal. He exhibits no distension.
- Neuro: Intubated and paralyzed.

Pertinent Test Results

Test	Result	Units	Normal range
WBC	26 ↑	K/µL	3.8–11.0 10^3/mm^3
Hgb	15.1 ↑	g/dL	Male: 14–18 g/dL
			Female: 11–16 g/dL
Platelets	379	K/µL	140–450 K/µL
Sodium	142	mEq/L	135–148 mEq/L
Potassium	5.6 ↑	mEq/L	3.5–5.5 mEq/L
Chloride	109	mEq/L	96–112 mEq/L
Bicarbonate	9 ↓	mEq/L	21–34 mEq/L
BUN	15	mg/dL	6–23 mg/dL
Creatinine	1.54 ↑	mg/dL	0.6–1.5 mg/dL
Glucose	208 ↑	mg/dL	65–99 mg/dL
pH (venous)	6.92 ↓	–	7.320–7.420
Lactate	3.8 ↑	mmol/L	<2.0 mmol/L
Alcohol	0	mg/dL	<10 mg/dL
Measured osmoles	348 ↑	mOsm/kg	285–295 mOsm/kg
UA – Other	Muddy brown casts, Ca-oxalate crystals	–	–

Chest X-ray: Dense opacity at the left base may represent atelectasis and/or air-space disease. Small adjacent left pleural effusion noted.

ED Course and Medical Decision-Making

Based on the history of ingestion and the patient's family's concern for self-harm, the above lab-work, as well as a volatile alcohol panel, was sent on the patient. While awaiting results of the alcohol panel, the clinicians calculated an increased osmolar and anion gaps (see below), leading them to conclude that the patient was currently poisoned with a toxic alcohol. He was therefore started on fomepizole and bicarb. However, the patient continued to display a refractory acidosis, and nephrology was consulted for immediate dialysis. This was initiated in the ED and the patient was admitted to the ICU for further care.

Learning Points

Priming Questions

1. When would you suspect toxic alcohol ingestion in someone with altered mental status if there is no clear history of ingestion?
2. What are the various treatment options for toxic alcohol ingestion and what are their indications?
3. How does ethylene glycol compare to methanol and isopropyl alcohol regarding presentation and management?

Introduction/Background

1. The term toxic alcohol is a bit ambiguous and could technically refer to any alcohol, as even ethanol causes inebriation and has end-organ effects. For our purposes, we will be discussing the most commonly ingested, nonrecreational alcohols: ethylene glycol, methanol, and isopropyl alcohol [1].
2. Ethylene glycol is found in antifreeze and engine coolant. It naturally has a very sweet odor and flavor which historically has thought to account at least in part for its accidental ingestion. Ethylene glycol's metabolite, oxalic acid, bind with calcium to form calcium oxalate monohydrate crystals in the renal tubules, causing acute tubular necrosis and renal failure [1].
3. Methanol (or wood alcohol) is found in cologne and windshield washer fluid. In addition to ingestion, methanol poisonings can also occur via inhalation and transdermal exposure [1, 2]. Methanol's metabolite, formate, is a mitochrondrial toxin that for unclear reasons only has significant effects on retinal cells and cells of the basal ganglia [1].
4. Isopropyl Alcohol is the most frequently ingested toxic alcohol, likely due to it being easily obtained, inexpensive, and confused with ethanol due to having the word "alcohol" in its name. It is found in rubbing alcohol and hand sanitizer. While ingestion causes intoxication, there is little in the way of significant end-organ damage [1].
5. A high clinical suspicion is needed to identify a toxic alcohol exposure when the patient is unable to give a clear history as in the case above. An intoxicated patient without clear history of ethanol use or smell of ethanol should raise suspicion. Other "red flag" initial findings include vision changes (methanol), gastric irritation, acetone smell (isopropyl), calcium oxalate crystals in urine, and fluorescent urine (ethylene glycol) [1].
6. All alcohols contribute to the oncotic pressure of a solution; therefore, all alcohols will cause an osmolar gap. Only methanol and ethylene glycol have metabolites which act as acids and cause an anion gap acidosis. Isopropyl alcohol is metabolized to acetone and therefore causes the classically described ketosis without acidosis [1].
7. In treating ethylene glycol and methanol poisonings, the mainstay of treatment involves halting the production of toxic metabolites and/or facilitating the excretion of toxic metabolites. Treatment of ethanol and isopropyl alcohol ingestions on the other hand is largely composed of supportive care.

Physiology/Pathophysiology

1. When thinking about alcohol metabolism, there are two main enzymes to keep in mind: alcohol dehydrogenase and aldehyde dehydrogenase. The alcohol component itself causes intoxication; however, it is toxic metabolites which cause the most significant pathology in toxic alcohol ingestions.
   - Under "normal" drinking circumstances, alcohol dehydrogenase converts ethanol to acetaldehyde. Acetaldehyde is then converted to acetate by aldehyde dehydrogenase. Acetate is a rather benign compound which is then further broken down and eventually repurposed and/or excreted.
   - Following the same sequence methanol is metabolized to formaldehyde and then formic acid [3].
     - Formic acid is then converted to formate, a mitochrondrial toxin that is believed to cause most of the end-organ damage in methanol toxicity. For unclear reasons, its significant effects appear to be localized to retinal cells and cells of the basal ganglia. These effects tend to be permanent [1].

   Drunk as a Skunk and Red as a Beet! [4]
   Some people of East Asian descent have a variant of the alcohol dehydrogenase enzyme which is significantly more efficient at converting alcohol to acetaldehyde leading to increased acetaldehyde concentrations. Also, aldehyde dehydrogenase has two isoenzymes. Caucasians have both isoenzymes. Up to 50% of East Asians lack one form of aldehyde dehydrogenase. This increased efficiency of alcohol dehydrogenase and decreased efficiency of aldehyde dehydrogenase results in increased acetaldehyde concentrations. Elevated acetaldehyde levels cause many downstream effects, but the most evident is histamine release. This leads to a condition called "Asian Flush" which is erythema of the face neck and shoulders and occasionally the whole body. Most interestingly, elevated acetaldehyde levels are linked to higher risk of esophageal cancer, and thought to be the main cause of increased rates of esophageal cancer seen in Japan.

     - Acute kidney injury (AKI) and pancreatitis have also been described in methanol toxicity, though this too is not fully understood [1].
   - Ethylene glycol metabolism has several additional steps (as shown below) but starts with these two enzymes.

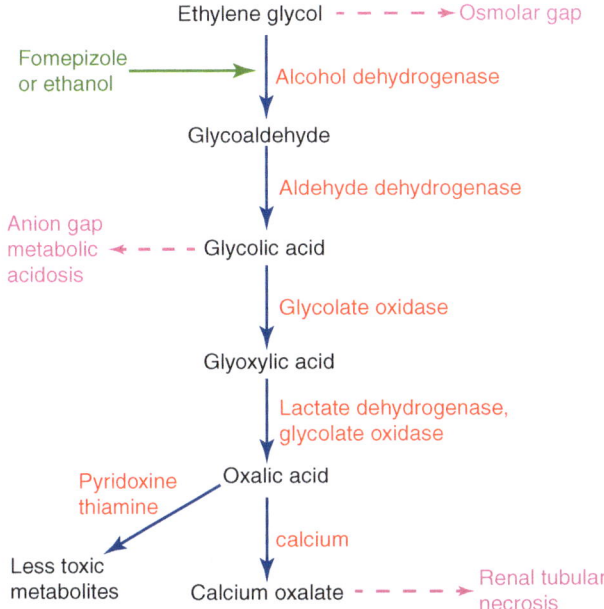

Metabolic pathway of Ethylene Glycol [1, 3] (Diagram courtesy of Matthew Schwab, MD)

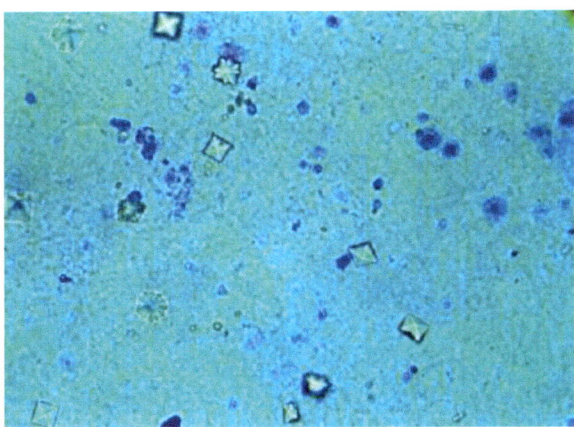

Calcium Oxalate Crystals—aka "Envelope Crystals". NASA/JSC (https://commons.wikimedia. org/wiki/File:Calcium_oxalate_crystals_in_urine.jpg), "Calcium oxalate crystals in urine", marked as public domain, more details on Wikimedia Commons: https://commons.wikimedia.org/ wiki/Template:PD-US

– As you can see in the diagram, the final metabolite of ethylene glycol, oxalic acid interacts with calcium to form calcium oxalate monohydrate crystals, which precipitate in the renal tubules. This causes acute tubular necrosis (ATN) and results in AKI. As seen above, the calcium oxalate

monohydrate crystals can be seen in the urine. Take caution though as this is a late finding, and has nontoxicological causes. Indeed, calcium oxalate crystals are the components of most kidney stones [3].
– In extreme poisonings, this process can use up enough calcium to cause a systemic deficiency, which can result in a prolonged QT interval.
– Other toxic metabolites of ethylene glycol cause:
    o Oxidative phosphorylation and cellular respiration.
    o Glucose and serotonin metabolism.
    o Protein synthesis.
    o DNA replication.
    o Ribosomal RNA formation.
• Isopropyl alcohol has the least complex metabolism as it is converted only by alcohol dehydrogenase to acetone. Acetone is then eliminated in urine and through respiration.

2. Anion Gap: Serum has a net neutral charge. Since there are molecules with negative charges (anions) and molecules with positive charges (cations), the concentration of each much balance out to result in a neutral charge. This is the basic principal behind the anion gap. We take the positive ions and subtract the negative ions. In an artificial setting where we were actually measuring all positive and negative ions, the difference would be zero. In patients, however, we do not actually measure all the ions, just the major contributors.
• The most classic formula is $Na^+ - (Cl^- + HCO_3^-)$. Some people add K^+ to the positive ion side of the equation. We know that there are several anions that we are not measuring and that during normal physiology there are roughly 10 mEq/L that are unaccounted for in our formula. Thus, we expect for the difference between positive and negative measured ions to be about 10, though <12 is our lab's reference range. If the difference is elevated above 12, we know that there is an excess amount of an unmeasured anion in the solution.
    – For our patient the anion gap is calculated:

$$Na - (Cl + HCO_3) = 142 - (109 + 9) = 24 \text{ mEq/L}$$

• In the case of toxic alcohol ingestion, the unmeasured anion is either formic acid (if the parent alcohol is methanol) or glycolic acid (if the parent alcohol is ethylene glycol). Ethanol and isopropyl alcohol do not have acidic metabolites that would cause an anion gap acidosis.
• Of course, in the undifferentiated patient, there are several other potential causes of this anion gap acidosis [1].

Anion Gap Acidosis differential diagnosis

• **C**   Cyanide
• **A**   Alcoholic Ketoacidosis
• **T**   Toluene (in solvents and glues)

- **M** Methanol
- **U** Uremia
- **D** DKA
- **P*** Paracetamol (acetaminophen), Phenformin (substitute metformin since phenformin is not available anymore).
- **I** Isoniazid, Iron, Ibuprofen (in massive doses)
- **L** Lactic acidosis
- **E** Ethylene Glycol
- **S** Salicylate

Volatile alcohols to consider in an osmolar gap include:

- **M** Methanol (aka wood alcohol)
- **E** Ethanol
- **D** Diuretics (osmotic diuretics like glycerol)
- **I** Isopropyl alcohol (aka rubbing alcohol)
- **E** Ethylene Glycol (EtGly)

3. Osmolar Gap: In the serum, large molecules are unable to freely cross membranes out of solution and instead contribute to an oncotic pressure. Similar to anion gap, we know which compounds have the greatest contribution to the serum's osmolality, and we use the concentrations of these compounds to calculate the osmolality. We then compare our calculated osmolality to the measured osmolality which is conducted in the medical laboratory. Again, we know that we are not accounting for all the compounds and thus we expect there to be some difference between the measured osmoles and our calculated osmoles.
   - A normal osmolar gap is <10. When the difference exceeds 10, we know that there is an additional unaccounted-for compound contributing to the osmolar force. **All alcohols contribute to the osmolar force and therefore cause an osmolar gap**. Thus, this is a measurement of the circulating parent alcohol in the serum. As toxic alcohols are often co-ingested with ethanol, it can be helpful to account for the ethanol in our calculation to see if there remains an unexplained gap.
   - The formula for osmolar gap is Measured Osmoles – (2 × Na + Glc/18 + BUN/2.8 + ETOh/4.6)
     - For our patient, the osmolar gap is calculated:

$$348 - \left(2 \times 142 + 208/18 + 15/2.8 + 0/4.6\right) = 47$$

   - An osmolar gap >10 is generally considered a reason to search for an unmeasured volatile alcohol, and a markedly elevated gap (>50) is virtually diagnostic for a toxic alcohol. Conversely, a "normal" gap cannot exclude toxic alcohol poisoning as the range of normal extends from −14 to +10 osmols depending on the individual [1]. So, if an individual's normal osmolar gap is −14, their osmolar gap during an acute ingestion of a toxic alcohol could be 9. This would be considered a "normal" but it is in reality quite a change from their baseline gap and could represent a dangerous ingestion. Furthermore, if the patient seeks medical care at a time remote from the original ingestion, they could certainly continue to have symptoms from the toxic metabolites but have no parent compound remaining to cause an osmolar gap [1].

4. Ethylene glycol is a "glycol molecule" and is essentially a sugar compound resulting in a sweet, palatable flavor. Many but not all ethylene glycol-containing radiator fluid products have a chemical additive called denatonium benzoate (under trade name Bitrex®) [5]. It is the most bitter chemical compound known to man and is added to create a "taste deterrent" to prevent ingestion of the substance by humans, cats, and dogs.

Bitrex®, Better or Just Bitter? [5–8]

The addition of a bittering agent to ethylene glycol containing products, typically denatonium benzoate (commonly known as Bitrex), is currently required by law in seventeen states in hopes of reducing accidental and intentional ingestions. However, studies aimed at evaluating the effectiveness of this strategy have failed to demonstrate a decrease in the number or severity of ethylene glycol ingestions, both intentional and in pediatric patients. Therefore, while there are no significant disadvantages to adding compounds such as Bitrex to ethylene glycol, this strategy cannot take the place of other ingestion prevention strategies such as child-proof containers and public health education.

Making the Diagnosis

Differential Diagnosis
- Alcohol Intoxication
- Other toxic alcohol ingestion
- Hypoglycemia
- Intracranial Hemorrhage
- Infection with Delirium

1. The most common physical exam finding with ingestion of any of these substances is clinical intoxication. Without a history of ingestion, it can be a very difficult diagnosis to make, as clinically it can be indistinguishable from ethanol intoxication.

2. Intoxication with ethylene glycol produces three major stages of toxic effects [2].

	Onset of effects	System affected	Signs and symptoms
1	30 minutes to 12 hours	Central Nervous System	Similar to EtOH: Inebriation, euphoria, ataxia, slurred speech, drowsiness, irritation, restlessness, and disorientation.
		Gastrointestinal	Nausea and vomiting
		Systemic	Increased osmolar gap
2	12–24 hours	Cardiovascular	Hypertension, tachycardia, and shock.
		Pulmonary	Tachypnea, Acute Respiratory Distress Syndrome (ARDS), pulmonary edema, and pneumonitis.
		Systemic	Metabolic acidosis with anion gap, possible tetany from hypocalcemia. As EtGly is metabolized, osmolar gap decreases.
3	24–72 hours	Renal	Flank pain, ATN with renal failure.
		Systemic	Normalizing anion and osmolar gaps.

3. Many ethylene glycol-containing radiator fluid products have fluorescein added in order to facilitate finding a leak of fluid from the radiator. It fluoresces under black light (Wood's Lamp). If you suspect ethylene glycol toxicity, you can place the patient's urine under a blacklight and examine for fluorescence. However, it may be very difficult to distinguish the fluorescing from fluorescein from the normal color of urine (which appears to fluoresce on its own). The plastic urine containers also look like they glow under black light. DO NOT use this method to "rule out" ethylene glycol poisoning [2].

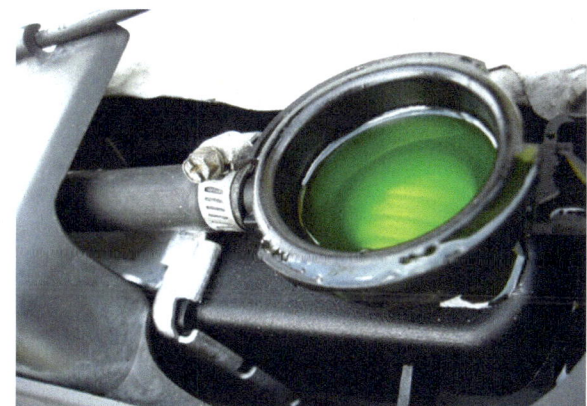

Ethylene Glycol in Radiator Fluid with Fluorescein Added. EvelynGiggles (https://commons.wikimedia.org/wiki/File:Antifreeze_in_the_radiator.jpg), "Antifreeze in the radiator", https://creativecommons.org/licenses/by/2.0/legalcod

4. The diagnosis is made definitively by finding an elevated level of ethylene glycol. Prior to the level coming back, the possibility of a volatile alcohol ingestion should be suspected if the patient has symptoms of intoxication and a metabolic acidosis (in the case of ethylene glycol or methanol) or the profound odor of acetone (isopropyl alcohol).

   • Clinically, without a history of ingestion, investigation of an otherwise unexplained anion gap metabolic acidosis is the first step in making this diagnosis.

   • Obtaining a measured osmoles lab test and calculating an osmolar gap can be a helpful step, if volatile alcohol levels are not quickly available at your facility. An elevated osmolar gap suggests a volatile alcohol and the concomitant metabolic acidosis suggests either methanol or ethylene glycol ingestion.

      – The challenge in making this diagnosis is that the surrogate labs change based on the time since ingestion. As discussed above, the parent alcohol accounts for the osmolar gap while metabolites cause the anion gap metabolic acidosis. So, in the hyperacute ingestion, there will be a significant osmolar gap, but there may be no anion gap metabolic acidosis. However, late after ingestion, there may be no osmolar gap, but a significant anion gap metabolic acidosis.

      – Since ethanol has a higher affinity for alcohol dehydrogenase than any of the volatile alcohols, if there is a co-ingestion with ethanol and a volatile alcohol, the time from ingestion to metabolism is significantly extended.

Reciprocal relationship of anion gap an osmolar gap over time. Osmolar gap decreases as levels of toxic metabolites increase [1, 2]. (Figure courtesy of Matthew Schwab, MD)

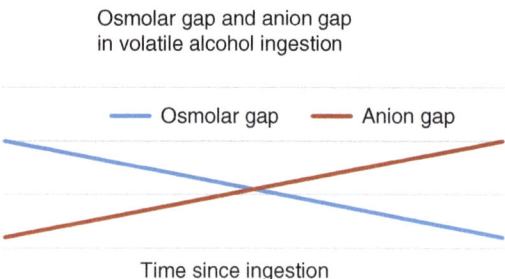

Osmolar gap and anion gap in volatile alcohol ingestion

── Osmolar gap   ── Anion gap

Time since ingestion

Treating the Patient

1. Isopropyl ingestion is essentially treated the same as ethanol ingestion. The hallmarks of treatment are supportive care, ensuring resolution of inebriation, and evaluation for other pathology. As with ethanol, only extreme cases require care beyond fluids and anti-emetics. Hemodialysis is an option for assisting with the clearance of the parent alcohol.

2. Ethylene glycol and methanol ingestions follow essentially the same treatment path and are aimed at preventing the metabolism of the alcohol to its toxic metabolites, eliminating the parent compound, and treating the symptoms of the intoxication.

   • Preventing Metabolism of the Alcohol to its Toxic Metabolites
     – Competitive Inhibition – By competitively inhibiting alcohol dehydrogenase, the parent alcohol remains unmetabolized in circulation. Although this will cause intoxication, it prevents the end-organ damage and acidosis caused by the toxic metabolites.
     – 4-methylpyrazole (fomepizole or Antizole®): This is a pure alcohol dehydrogenase competitive inhibitor. The dose is a loading dose of 15 mg/kg infused intravenously over 30 minutes, followed by doses of 10 mg/kg every 12 hours for four doses, then 15 mg/kg every 12 hours until ethylene glycol levels are below 20 mg/dL [3]. The addition of ethanol to fomepizole is not necessary.
     – Ethanol: Because alcohol dehydrogenase has a higher affinity for ethanol than for ethylene glycol and methanol, the administration of ethanol will competitively inhibit the metabolism of the parent alcohol to its toxic metabolites. The goal of ethanol therapy is to maintain the blood ethanol level between 100 and 150 mg/dL to saturate the body's full complement of alcohol dehydrogenase [3]. Ethanol can be difficult to use in these ingestions and fomepizole is extremely effective and easier to administer, making ethanol much less frequently used.
   • Eliminating the Parent Compound
     – Initiation of competitive inhibition therapy prolongs the time required for the body to reach nontoxic levels of the alcohol since the alcohol is no longer metabolized via its typical pathway. Ethylene glycol is readily excreted by the kidneys provided renal function is intact. Methanol is primarily removed through respiration. However, half-lives can be as high as 71 hours and 16 hours for methanol and ethylene glycol respectively [1]. Additionally, competitive inhibition does not protect the body from the toxic metabolites already formed prior to initiation of treatment which is critical if there has been a prolonged time between ingestion and presentation to the ED. For these reasons, hemodialysis may be necessary in addition to fomepizole therapy.
     – Hemodialysis can be used to remove ethylene glycol, methanol, and to ameliorate the acidosis. Indications for dialysis include the presence of any of the following situations [2]:
       ○ Metabolic acidosis (pH < 7.3), regardless of drug level.
       ○ Elevated serum levels of ethylene glycol or methanol more than 50 mg/dL (8.1 mmol/L), unless arterial pH is above 7.3. Dialysis is rarely necessary for isopropyl ingestion, but a level >500 mg/dL is an indication.
       ○ Evidence of end-organ damage (renal failure or vision changes).

- If the patient is stable, without meeting any of the above criteria, you may consider admitting them on fomepizole and awaiting for the body to eliminate the parent compound.
- Cofactor Therapy
  - o Thiamine and pyridoxine act as metabolic cofactors in the metabolism of ethylene glycol. They promote the transformation of glyoxylic acid to less toxic metabolites and may decrease the formation of oxalate [1]. The degree of usefulness of this therapy is not clear, but it won't hurt! Current recommendations from the Centers of Disease Control and Prevention (CDC) suggest 100 mg IV daily in the form of a single dose, especially if the patient has a history of alcohol abuse and there is a concern for malnutrition.
- Supportive Care
  - Airway, Breathing, and Circulation
    - o These may require active management particularly in the setting of severe acidemia.
  - Sodium Bicarbonate
    - o This can be titrated and used to control the pH; it should be considered in patients who are significantly acidotic.
3. Most patients who are treated aggressively and early do very well.

Case Conclusion

Our patient's volatile alcohol panel ultimately revealed an ethylene glycol level of 144 mg/dL. The patient underwent several more rounds of hemodialysis in the intensive care unit. His renal function returned to baseline, and he was able to be extubated within 48 hours and transferred out of the ICU. Psychiatry was consulted to begin treatment for substance abuse, depression, and suicidality.

Discussion

1. Toxic alcohol ingestion can be difficult to catch without a history of exposure. It should be considered in any intoxicated or altered patient, especially if they do not smell of ethanol. Other causes of altered mental status should also be considered including infection, trauma, polysubstance abuse, and other metabolic abnormalities.
2. Do not forget to think about volatile alcohol ingestion in the setting of an unexplained anion gap metabolic acidosis.
3. An increased osmolar gap and negative or insufficient ethanol level to explain the gap can be used to diagnosis toxic alcohol ingestion when a volatile alcohol panel is not readily available.
4. If an ingestion of methanol or ethylene glycol is suspected, treatment with fomepizole should be initiated prior to confirmatory testing to prevent the buildup of toxic metabolites and resulting end-organ damage. If confirmed or highly suspected, the patient may require hemodialysis in addition to fomepizole.

Toxic alcohols [1, 2]	Ethylene glycol	Methanol	Isopropyl alcohol
Source	Radiator fluid/engine coolant, antifreeze.	Wood alcohol, sterno, windshield washer fluid, cologne.	Rubbing alcohol, hand sanitizer.
Physical exam	Intoxication; fluorescent urine under wood's lamp.	Intoxication, vison changes and blindness (snow storm effect), Parkinsonian symptoms (rare)	Intoxication/CNS depression, sweet odor (from ketones), abdominal pain
Lab findings	Osmolar and anion gap acidosis; calcium oxalate crystals in urine causing ATN (also deposit in lung and heart causing organ damage), hypocalcemia, lactate gap (discrepancy between Point of Care (POC) analyzer and lab test), prolonged QT.	Osmolar and anion gap acidosis, basal ganglia hemorrhage (in severe cases).	Osmolar gap without acidosis, ketosis, acetonemia.
Metabolites	Glycolic acid (causes acidosis), oxalic acid (causes toxic effects).	Formic acid.	Acetone
Systemic effects	ATN from oxylic acid crystals; glycoxylate produces myocardial depression, prolonged QT.	Basal ganglia hemorrhage.	Respiratory depression, mucosal irritant.
Onset of clinical and laboratory features (hours after ingestion	Without coingested ethanol: 12–24 hours With coingested ethanol: 48–72 hours	Without coingested ethanol: 6–24 hours. With coingested ethanol: 72–96 hours.	Without coingested ethanol: 2–4 hours. With coingested ethanol: n/a.
Treatment	Fomepizole, ethanol, hemodialysis.	Fomepizole, ethanol, hemodialysis.	Supportive care (metabolite not toxic).

Pattern Recognition

- Intoxication
- Osmolar gap (especially if ethanol is accounted for in the equation)
- Possible anion gap (methanol, ethylene glycol)
- Calcium oxalate crystals in the the urine (ethylene glycol)

References

1. Wiener SW. Toxic alcohols. In: Nelson LS, Howland M, Lewin NA, Smith SW, Goldfrank LR, Hoffman RS, editors. Goldfrank's toxicologic emergencies. 11th ed. New York: McGraw-Hill; 2019.
2. Kraut JA, Mullins ME. Toxic alcohols. N Engl J Med. 2018;378:270–80.
3. Mcmartin K, Jacobsen D, Hovda KE. Antidotes for poisoning by alcohols that form toxic metabolites. Br J Clin Pharmacol. 2016;81:505–15.
4. Brooks PJ, Enoch M-A, Goldman D, Li T-K, Yokoyama A. The alcohol flushing response: an unrecognized risk factor for esophageal cancer from alcohol consumption. PLoS Med. 2009;6:e50. https://doi.org/10.1371/journal.pmed.1000050.
5. Schwartz L. Poison prevention and education. In: Hoffman RS, Howland M, Lewin NA, Nelson LS, Goldfrank LR, editors. Goldfrank's toxicologic emergencies. 10th ed. New York: McGraw-Hill; 2015.
6. Jobson MA, Hogan SL, Maxwell CS, Hu Y, Hladik GA, Falk RJ, Beuhler MC, Pendergraft WF. Clinical features of reported ethylene glycol exposures in the United States. PLoS One. 2015;10:e0143044. https://doi.org/10.1371/journal.pone.0143044.
7. White NC, Litovitz T, Benson BE, Horowitz BZ, Marr-Lyon L, White MK. The impact of bittering agents on pediatric ingestions of antifreeze. Clin Pediatr. 2009;48:913–21.
8. White NC, Litovitz T, White MK, Watson WA, Benson BE, Horowitz BA, Marr-Lyon L. The impact of bittering agents on suicidal ingestions of antifreeze. Clin Toxicol (Phila). 2008;46(6):507–14.

Joshua K. Aalberg

Indication for Exam A 24 year-old female presents after a fall on an outstretched hand. On exam, she has pain at the elbow, most prominently at the lateral aspect and with motion.

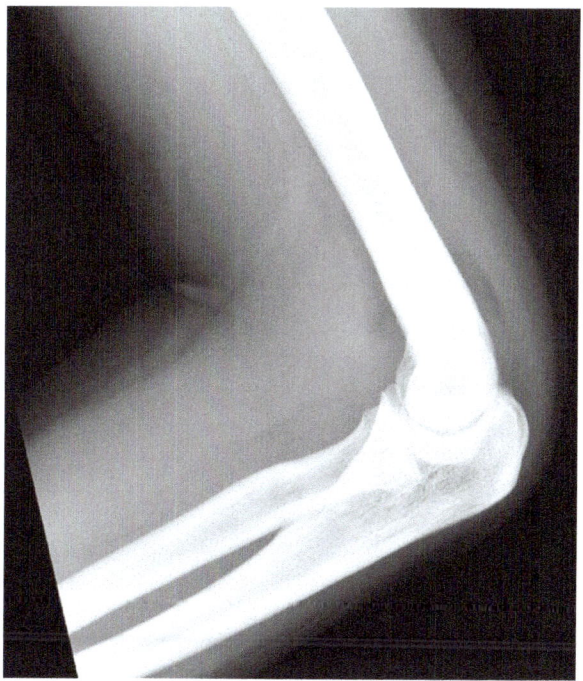

J. K. Aalberg (✉)
Department of Emergency Medicine, Wexner Medical Center at The Ohio State University,
Columbus, OH, USA
e-mail: joshua.aalberg@osumc.edu

© Springer Nature Switzerland AG 2020
C. G. Kaide, C. E. San Miguel (eds.), *Case Studies in Emergency Medicine*,
https://doi.org/10.1007/978-3-030-22445-5_66

Radiological Findings Joint effusion with displacement of the anterior and posterior fat pads.

Diagnosis Radial Head Fracture

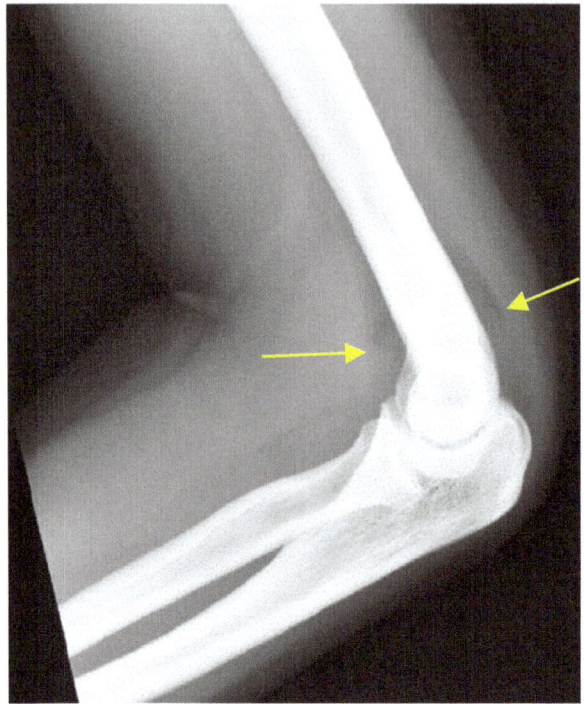

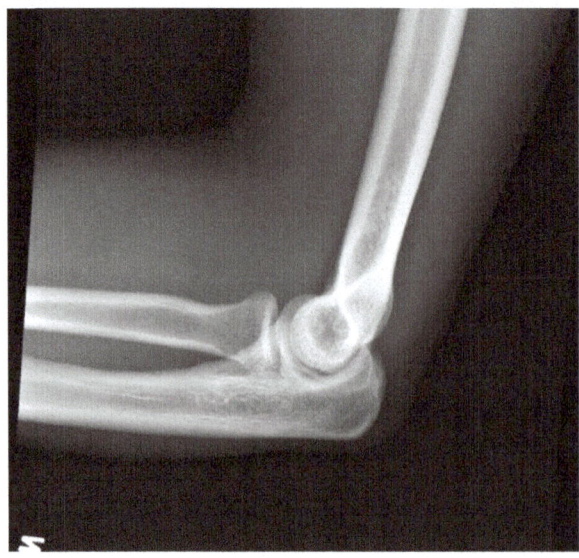

Normal elbow X-ray for comparison

Learning Points

Priming Questions
- What are the secondary signs that help identify radial head fractures on X-ray?
- What are other commonly associated fractures/injuries?
- What features of the fracture can necessitate surgical management?

Introduction/Background

A radial head fracture is a common injury that accounts for approximately of one-third of adult elbow fractures [1].

Pathophysiology/Mechanism

These fractures are typically caused by indirect trauma; most commonly an axial load causing the radial head to impact on the humeral capitellum, such as seen in a fall on an outstretched hand (FOOSH) type injury. Fractures from direct trauma to the radial head can occur but are rare.

Injuries commonly associated with radial head fractures include:

- Essex-Lopresti lesion: tear of the interosseous membrane and disruption of distal radioulnar joint.
- "Terrible triad of elbow" which includes elbow dislocation, coronoid fracture, and radial head fracture.
- Capitellar fracture.
- Ligamentous (medial collateral) injuries.
- Joint dislocation.
- Wrist injuries.

Making the Diagnosis

- Linear lucency/lucencies in the radial head are certainly diagnostic of fracture, however, these may not always be visible when a fracture is present. Presence of a joint effusion (+ fat pad sign) visualized on the lateral view in the setting of trauma suggests an occult radial head fracture is present.
- If necessary, addition of a radiocapitellar x-ray view may be helpful, although visualization of a discrete fracture line is not necessary in the presence of a joint effusion. Additionally, noncontrast CT could be obtained for more complete detection and/or characterization, though this is not typically necessary.

Treating the Patient

Radial head fractures are typically graded with the Mason Classification [1, 2]:

- Type I: Displacement <2 mm (noncomminuted).
- Type II: Displacement >2 mm (noncomminuted).
- Type III: Comminuted fractures involving entire radial head.
- Type IV: Comminuted fracture with dislocation of the elbow joint.

In general, Type I fractures can be treated conservatively with short-term immobilization in a sling while Type II+ can require surgical management [1]. The vast majority of radial head fractures are Type I.

Discussion

- Knowledge of imaging findings of a joint effusion aka a positive fat pad sign on plain film radiography is a powerful tool in identification of radial head fractures when a discrete fracture line is not visualized. If a joint effusion is present, the injury can be treated as a nondisplaced fracture even if a discrete fracture line is not visualized. Presence of joint effusion is assessed on the lateral view and is manifested by either one or both of these findings:
  - Visualization of posterior fat pad which is always abnormal.
  - Convex anterior margin of anterior fat pad (sail sign). Although the anterior fat pad can be visualized in a normal patient, the anterior margin should always be straight or concave.
- Surgical consultation is typically indicated only if fracture displacement is >2 mm, there is a mechanical block limiting the range of motion of the joint, and/or comminution is present [1].

Disclosure Statement The authors of this chapter report no significant disclosures.

References

1. Dr Sachintha Hapugoda and R Bronson et al. Radial head fractures. Radiopaedia. Accessed 26 June 2018. https://radiopaedia.org/articles/radial-head-fractures.
2. Sheps DM, Kiefer KR, Boorman RS, Donaghy J, Lalani A, Walker R, Hildebrand KA. The interobserver reliability of classification systems for radial head fractures: the Hotchkiss modification of the Mason classification and the AO classification systems. Can J Surg. 2009;52:277–82.

Wolff-Parkinson-White: *Who's Afraid of the Big Bad Wolff?*

67

Serena Hua and Andrew King

Case 1

Pertinent History

A 32-year-old male presented to the emergency department complaining of a "racing heart beat." He explained that earlier in the morning, while eating breakfast, he felt his heart pounding and beating very fast. He expressed that he felt somewhat light-headed when walking. He denied any associated symptoms such as fever, chest pain or pressure, cough, or recent alcohol use. He drank a cup of coffee this morning which is a normal for him to do.

No Relevant Past Medical or Surgical History

Social History Married with one child. He is a nonsmoker and denies illicit drug use. He admitted to occasional alcohol use.

Family History There was no family history of sudden cardiac death.

S. Hua (✉) · A. King
Department of Emergency Medicine, Wexner Medical Center at The Ohio State University, Columbus, OH, USA
e-mail: serena.hua@osumc.edu; andrew.king3@osumc.edu

© Springer Nature Switzerland AG 2020
C. G. Kaide, C. E. San Miguel (eds.), *Case Studies in Emergency Medicine*,
https://doi.org/10.1007/978-3-030-22445-5_67

Pertinent Physical Examination

Except as noted below, the findings of a complete physical exam are within normal limits.

- Vitals: 98.7F/37C; HR, 203; BP, 115/62; RR, 18.
- General: Alert, thin, and pale male sitting on the cot in minimal distress.
- Cardiovascular: Tachycardic, regular rhythm, 2+ peripheral pulses, warm and well perfused.

Pertinent Test Results

Laboratory studies were unremarkable.

ED Management

The patient was connected to a continuous 12-lead ECG machine. Carotid massage and Valsalva maneuvers were attempted without termination of his rhythm; 12 mg of adenosine was administered via rapid push method and the rhythm subsequently terminated. The following ECG was obtained prior to adenosine.

Patient's EKG Before Adenosine

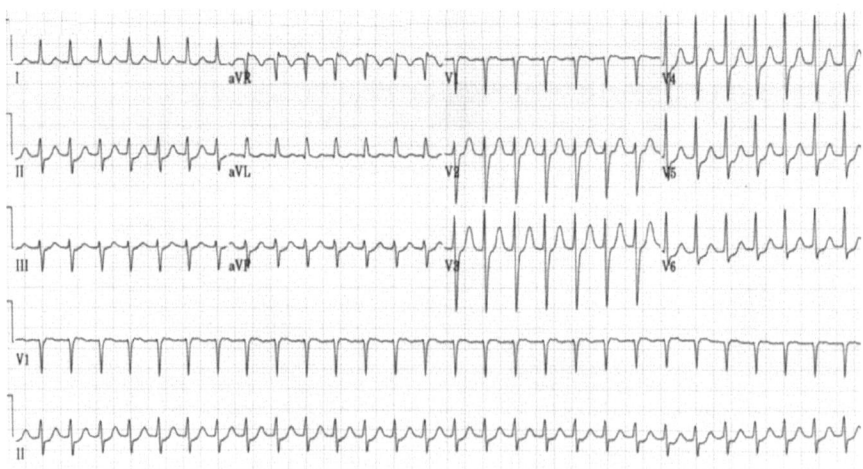

EKG courtesy of Colin Kaide, MD

Patient's EKG After Adenosine

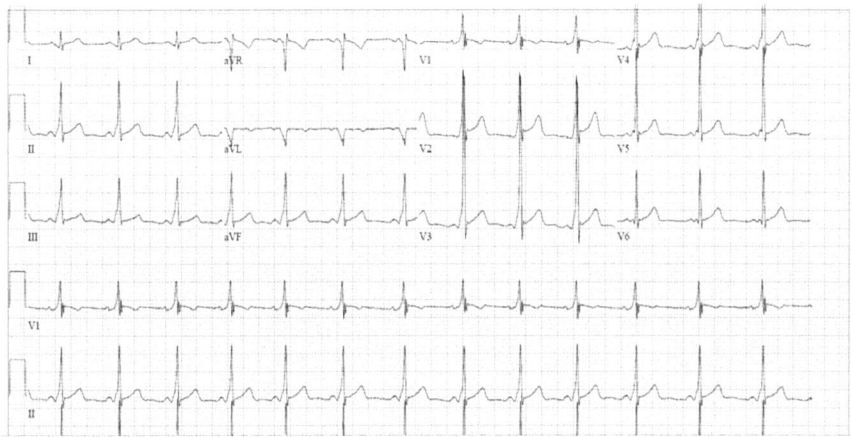

EKG courtesy of Colin Kaide, MD

Case 2

Pertinent History

A 40-year-old female was brought to the emergency department by EMS after she had an episode of syncope while at work. She expressed that she had been feeling unwell throughout the day and felt especially out of breath. She had associated nausea without vomiting or fevers. She worked at a warehouse and had been carrying some boxes when she suddenly became lightheaded and collapsed to the floor. Per bystanders, she was unconscious for only a few seconds. Upon awakening, she was immediately alert and oriented. Coworkers did not witness tonic-clonic activity. Upon EMS arrival, the patient's blood glucose was 124. EMS reported that the ECG obtained showed an irregularly irregular wide-complex rhythm.

No Relevant Past Medical or Surgical History

Social History Employed at a warehouse. She smokes marijuana and cigarettes daily, while using alcohol socially. She denied other drug use.

Relevant Family History The patient's father had an unknown heart condition and suffered from a sudden cardiac death.

Pertinent Physical Examination

Except as noted below, the findings of a complete physical exam are within normal limits.
- Vitals: 99.1, BP 102/50; HR, 210; RR, 18; O_2, 97%.
- General: An alert, age-appropriate female sitting up in the cot, who appears somewhat diaphoretic.
- HEENT: Dry mucous membranes.
- Cardiovascular: Tachycardic, irregularly irregular rhythm, thready pulses.
- Extremities: Clammy extremities and skin.

Pertinent Labs

Laboratory studies, including thyroid studies and HCG, were unremarkable.

Patient's EKG

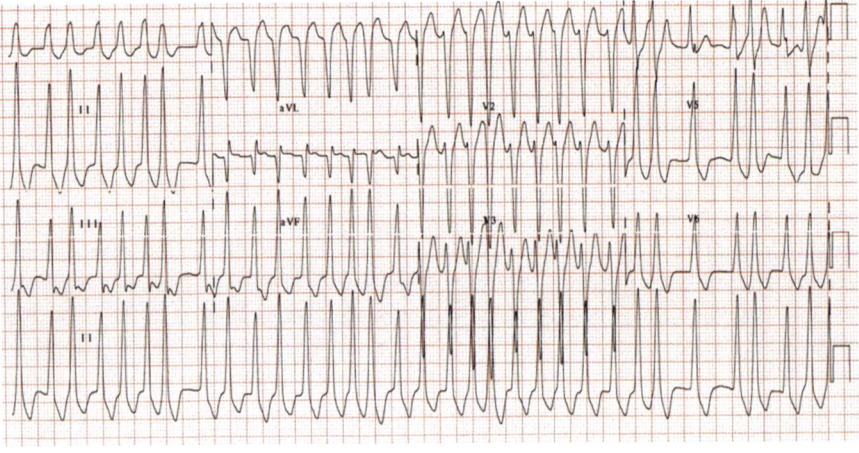

EKG courtesy of Andrew King, MD

ED Management

The patient was placed on a cardiac monitor and intravenous access was obtained. The ECG was read as atrial fibrillation with rapid ventricular response (RVR) and was given diltiazem 15 mg intravenously in attempt to improve the ventricular rate; however, over the next few minutes, the patient appeared more diaphoretic, pale, and drowsy. Repeat vitals showed a BP 70/42 with a HR 261. Given her decompensation, synchronized cardioversion was performed which terminated the rhythm. A repeat ECG showed findings that were concerning for underlying WPW.

Learning Points

Priming Questions

1. What is the pathophysiology for WPW and what are the characteristic EKG findings?
2. What is the best approach to management of a symptomatic WPW patient?
3. What agents should be avoided in WPW patients presenting with irregular wide complex tachycardia?

Introduction/Background

1. The Wolff-Parkinson-White (WPW) pattern was first described by Drs. Wolff, Parkinson, and White in 1930 from 11 case reports of patients identified to have short PR intervals and bundle branch block who resultantly developed supraventricular tachycardia and atrial fibrillation [1, 2].
2. WPW is a form of ventricular pre-excitation in which an accessory pathway exists between the atria and the ventricles. These pathways allow for conduction of impulses between the atria and ventricle to occur *in addition to* the normal conduction through the atrioventricular (AV) node and the His-Purkinje pathway.
3. The pattern occurs in about 0.13–0.25% of the general population, whereas the syndrome, the development of a tachyarrhythmia leading to symptoms, occurs in 0.07–1.8% of those with the pattern. Most people with WPW are asymptomatic with no associated arrhythmias [3, 4]. Sudden cardiac death is rare, with a rate of 0.00125–0.0015 per patient-year [5] with rates being slightly higher in children [6].

Physiology/Pathophysiology

1. Normal conduction between the atria and ventricles occurs through the AV node and then proceeds rapidly down the His-Purkinje system to cause ventricular contraction. When accessory pathways exist, some of these signals will transmit down these pathways to reach the ventricle.
   - A shortened PR interval is created because unlike the AV node which slows electrical signals, the accessory pathway allows for signals to pass quickly.
   - Once these accessory signals reach the ventricles, they travel much slower than those signals which propagate through the His-Purkinje system. In WPW, there are signals going down both the AV node/His-Purkinje system and the accessory pathway. This leads to the characteristic delta wave, or slurred upstroke of the QRS, on ECG [7].

Accessory Pathway

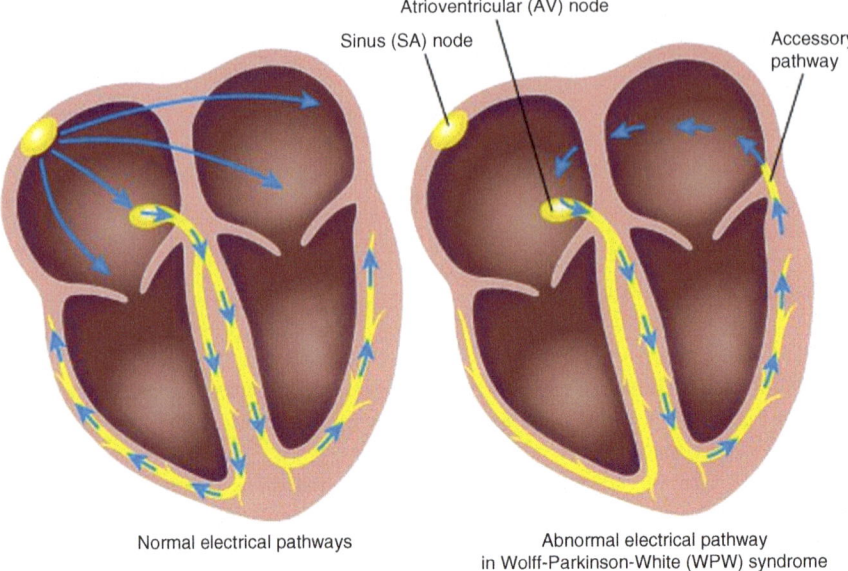

Normal electrical pathways

Abnormal electrical pathway
in Wolff-Parkinson-White (WPW) syndrome

Tom Lück (https://commons.wikimedia.org/wiki/File:WPW.jpeg), "WPW", https://creativecommons.org/licenses/by/3.0/legalcode

2. Not all WPW accessory pathways are created alike [8].
   - 60–75% of accessory pathways can conduct bidirectionally.
   - 17–35% can only conduct retrograde (ventricle to atria) and therefore have no delta wave (concealed pathway).
   - 13% of patients with WPW have multiple accessory pathways.
3. Not all WPW patients are the same: [3–5, 9]
   - Some patients will simply have the WPW pattern on resting ECG and never develop symptoms.
   - Some will have a concealed pathway (retrograde-only accessory pathway) with no delta wave but can still develop tachyarrhythmias.
   - A smaller subset will become symptomatic with supraventricular tachycardia such as atrioventricular re-entrant tachycardia or atrial fibrillation, which can result in sudden cardiac death.

Making the Diagnosis

Differential Diagnosis
- Atrioventricular nodal reentry tachycardia (AVNRT)
- Multifocal atrial tachycardia
- Sinus tachycardia
- Ventricular tachycardia
- Atrial fibrillation with bundle branch block
- Frequent premature atrial contractions (PACs) or premature ventricular contractions (PVCs)

WPW Pattern

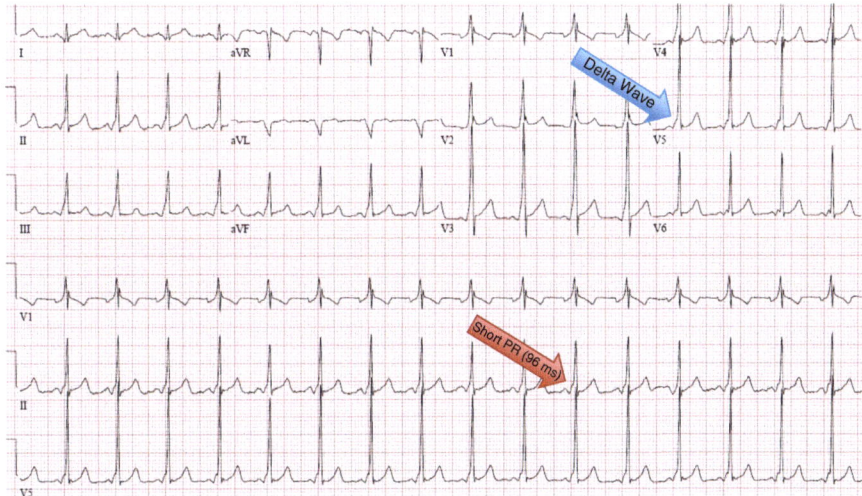

- Short PR interval <0.12s or <3 small boxes.

- Normal P wave.

- Delta wave: slurred upstroke of QRS.

- Can see QRS prolongation >0.11s

Delta Wave

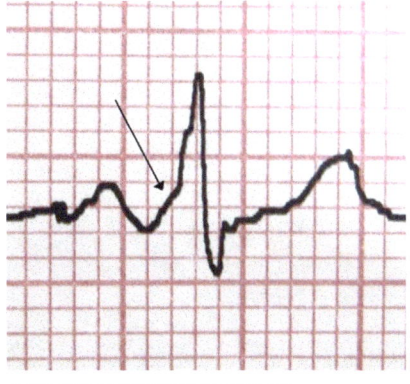

James Heilman, MD wikimedia commons

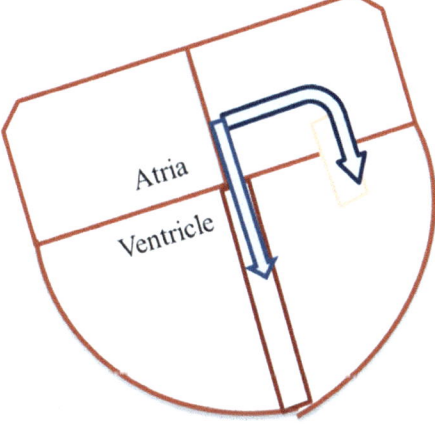

EKG courtesy of Colin Kaide, MD

WPW Syndrome: WPW Pattern + Arrhythmia

Atrioventricular nodal re-entrant tachycardia (AVNRT)

1. The Orthodromic Circuit (down AV node and up the accessory pathway (AP) - occurs in up to 95% of WPW patients [10].
   - There is usually a narrow QRS (<120 ms) unless there is also a pre-existing bundle branch block.

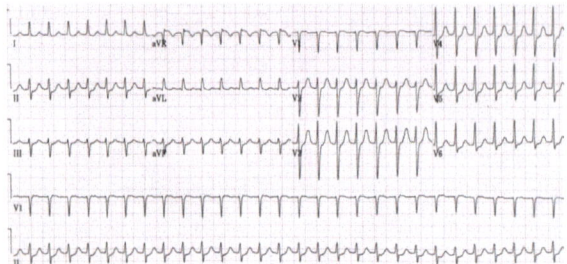 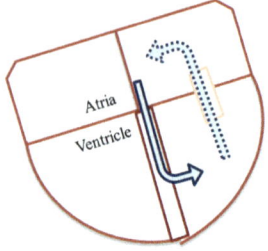

2. The Antidromic Circuit (down AP and up AV) - occurs in about 10% of WPW patients [10].
   - There is usually a wide QRS (>120 ms).

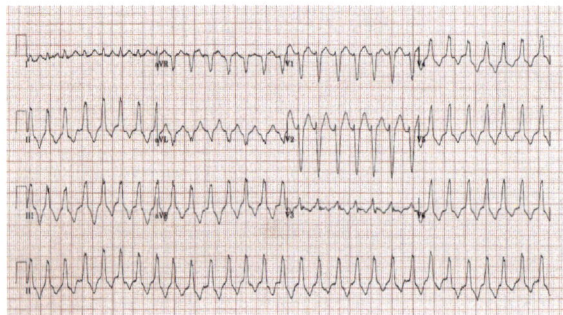 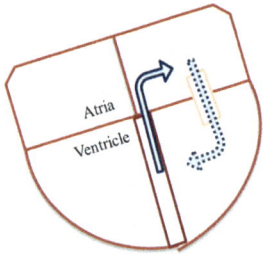

3. Atrial fibrillation with WPW.
   - This is a fast, irregularly irregular wide-complex rhythm. Atrial impulses are rapidly firing down both the normal conduction pathway as well as from the accessory pathway.
   - QRS complexes can vary in morphology and can change in axis.

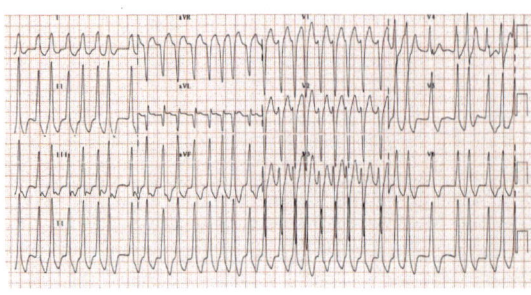 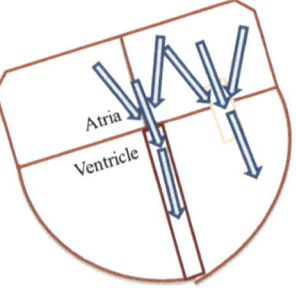

- What can happen when you treat the above with AV nodal blockers?... ventricular fibrillation!
  - Blocking the AV node encourages faster conduction thorough the accessory pathways which can degenerate to ventricular fibrillation. Ventricular fibrillation tends to occur in patients who have a history of SVT or atrial fibrillation and have multiple accessory pathways [11].

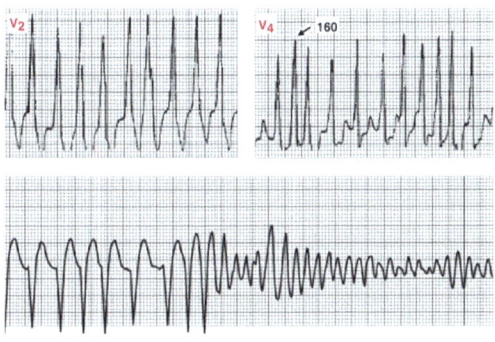
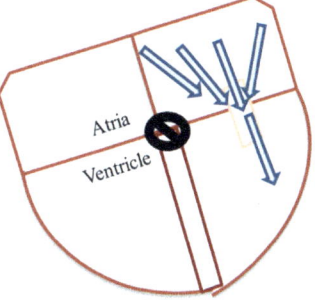

Treating the Patient [12]

Attend to your patient's Airway, Breathing, and Circulation (ABCs)...but then...

1. For an *asymptomatic* patient in normal sinus rhythm...most of them will not develop any arrhythmias associated with WPW. One study of 212 patients with asymptomatic WPW found that 20% eventually develop AVNRT or atrial fibrillation upon follow-up at 60 months [13]. It is therefore reasonable to refer to a cardiologist who can discuss the potential option of cardiac ablation.
2. For a *symptomatic* patient with a tachyarrhythmia: Ask yourself...are they hemodynamically stable?
   - NO: Shock! Synchronized cardioversion.
   - YES: Consider the different types of SVT.
     - Orthodromic (typically narrow QRS complex) - block the AV node to disrupt the circuit.
       o Vagal maneuvers- carotid sinus massage or valsalva [14].
       o Adenosine.
       o Verapamil.
       o Procainamide.
       o Shock if unsuccessful with chemical cardioversion.
     - Antidromic (Wide QRS) – It can be difficult to differentiate antidromic SVT vs VT. Guidelines are unclear.
       o If you know your patient has underlying WPW and is stable, then use procainamide.
       o It is reasonable in unclear cases to treat the patient as you would for stable VT, or one could or ere on the side of caution and use

procainamide in case your patient does have WPW... avoid beta blockers and calcium channel blockers which can lead to VF in WPW patients.
  ○ Shock.
– Atrial fibrillation with WPW (Wide, irregular, polymorphic QRS) – *no AV nodal blockers*, which could promote conduction through the accessory pathway. Instead, use a drug that would slow conduction down both pathways.
  ○ Procainamide
  ○ Shock!
  ○ NO adenosine, amiodarone, B-blockers, calcium channel blockers!
Take away: If in doubt or wide complex, give Procainamide or shock!
All symptomatic patients should be referred for cardiac ablation.

The Adenosine Challenge 1996…Only the Strong Survive! EKG of a Patient Given Adenosine with WPW and Atrial Fibrillation*

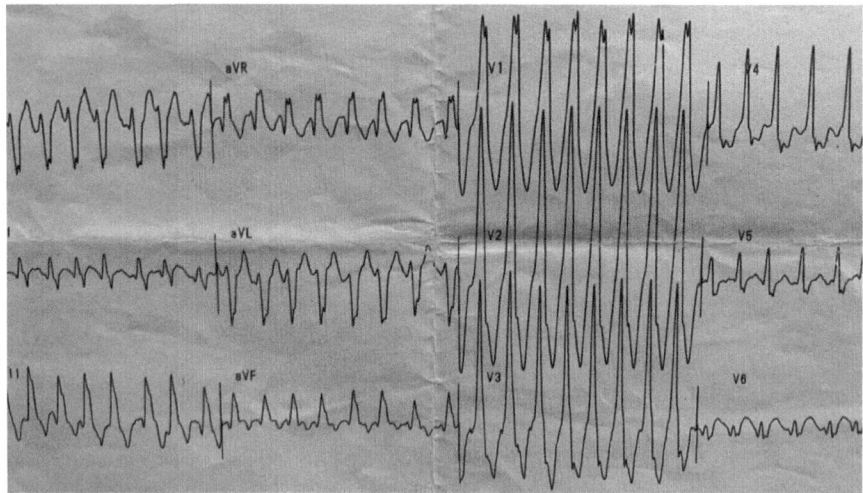

Rhythm Strip Pre-Adenosine

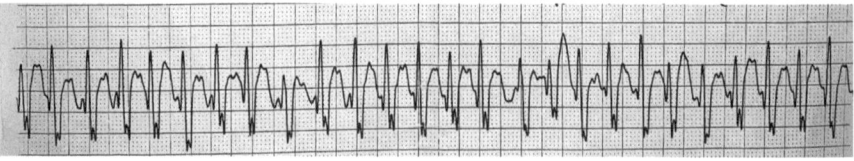

Rhythm Strip After Adenosine (for 10 seconds)

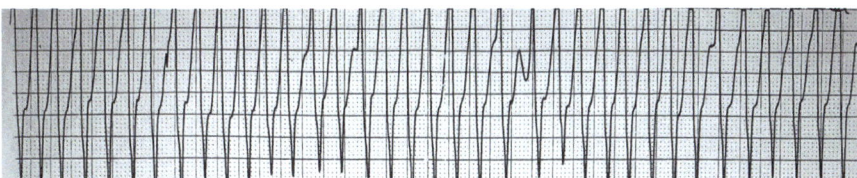

*Misinterpreted as being simple SVT with aberrancy. After the heart rate went through the roof and the moonlighting resident nearly lost bladder control, the adenosine wore off and the HR went back to 200. Electricity followed! Images Courtesy of Colin Kaide, MD

> **What About Amiodarone? Is Amiodarone Safe in WPW?** [15, 16]
> Originally, ACLS guidelines in 2005 and 2008 recommended "expert consultation" or amiodarone for WPW patient in atrial fibrillation. However, there have been some studies and case reports that support not using amiodarone, as it seems to be associated with conversion to ventricular fibrillation, owing to its AV nodal blocking properties. Consider erring on the side of caution for now and avoid amiodarone until we have more conclusive data.

Case Conclusion

The patient in case 1 was discharged from the ED after a period of observation with close cardiology follow-up. Decision was made for cardiac ablation of the accessory pathway.

The patient in case 2 was admitted to the cardiology service where an EP study performed an ablation on the accessory pathways. She was discharged in stable condition.

Case Discussion

Consider WPW when encountering any patient with tachycardia. Evaluate if the QRS is wide or narrow, which can help determine the appropriate treatment. Remember that the characteristic delta wave, shortened PR interval, and widened QRS usually do not appear on ECG of a patient who is having AVNRT or atrial fibrillation!

Re-entrant tachycardia is the most common arrhythmia seen in WPW patients – up to 80%.

While you treat rapid, narrow complex tachycardias (orthodromic AVNRT) with AV nodal blockers, avoid them in wide complex tachycardia which could be antidromic AVNRT or more dangerously, AF related to WPW!

Any wide-complex, irregularly irregular rhythm should be assumed to be related to WPW. Electricity is the drug of choice if unstable. Procainamide is #2.

Pattern Recognition

WPW
- PR < 0.12 with a normal P wave.
- Wide QRS > 0.11.
- Delta Wave.
- Secondary ST-T wave changes.
- Up to 30% of patients with WPW will develop atrial fibrillation.

Disclosure Statement The authors of this chapter report no significant disclosures.

References

1. Boyer NH. The Wolff-Parkinson-white syndrome. N Engl J Med. 1946;234:111–4. https://doi.org/10.1056/NEJM194601242340402.
2. Scheinman MM. The history of the Wolff–Parkinson–white syndrome. Rambam Maimonides Med J. 2012;3(3):e0019. https://doi.org/10.5041/RMMJ.10083.
3. Krahn AD, Manfreda J, Tate RB, Mathewson FA, Cuddy TE. The natural history of electrocardiographic preexcitation in men. The Manitoba Follow-up Study. Ann Intern Med. 1992;116(6):456–60.
4. Kim SS, Knight BP. Long term risk of Wolff-Parkinson-White pattern and syndrome. Trends Cardiovasc Med. 2017;27(4):260–8, ISSN 1050-1738. https://doi.org/10.1016/j.tcm.2016.12.001T.
5. Munger M, Packer DL, Hammill SC, Feldman BJ, Bailey KR, Ballard DJ, Holmes DR, Gersh BJ. A population study of the natural history of Wolff-Parkinson-White syndrome in Olmsted County, Minnesota, 1953–1989. Circulation. 1993;87:866–73, originally published March 1, 1993
6. Obeyesekere MN, Leong-Sit P, Massel D, Manlucu J, Modi S, Krahn AD, Skanes AC, Yee R, Gula LJ, Klein GJ. Risk of arrhythmia and sudden death in patients with asymptomatic preexcitation: a meta-analysis. Circulation. 2012;125(19):2308–15. https://doi.org/10.1161/CIRCULATIONAHA.111.055350. Epub 2012 Apr 24.
7. Bhatia A, Jasbir Sra J, Akhtar M. Preexcitation syndromes. Curr Probl Cardiol. 2016;41(3):99–137, ISSN 0146-2806. https://doi.org/10.1016/j.cpcardiol.2015.11.002.
8. Zachariah JP, Walsh EP, Triedman JK, Berul CI, Cecchin F, Alexander ME, Bevilacqua LM. Multiple accessory pathways in the young: the impact of structural heart disease. Am Heart J. 2013;165(1):87–92. https://doi.org/10.1016/j.ahj.2012.10.025. Epub 2012 Nov 20.
9. Santinelli V, Radinovic A, Manguso F, Vicedomini G, Gulletta S, Paglino G, et al. The natural history of asymptomatic ventricular pre-excitation a long-term prospective follow-up study of 184 asymptomatic children. J Am Coll Cardiol. 2009;53(3):275–80.

10. Josephson ME. Preexcitation syndromes. In: Clinical cardiac electrophysiology, 4th. Philadelphia: Lippincot Williams & Wilkins; 2008. p. 339.
11. Klein GJ, Bashore TM, Sellers TD, Pritchett EL, Smith WM, Gallagher JJ. Ventricular fibrillation in the Wolff-Parkinson-white syndrome. N Engl J Med. 1979;301:1080–5.
12. Page RL, Joglar JA, Caldwell MA, Calkins H, Conti JB, Deal BJ, Estes NA 3rd, Field ME, Goldberger ZD, Hammill SC, Indik JH, Lindsay BD, Olshansky B, Russo AM, Shen WK, Tracy CM, Al-Khatib SM. Evidence Review Committee Chair. 2015 ACC/AHA/HRS guideline for the Management of Adult Patients with supraventricular tachycardia: a report of the American College of Cardiology/American Heart Association task force on clinical practice guidelines and the Heart Rhythm Society. Circulation. 2016;133(14):e506. Epub 2015 Sep 23.
13. Pappone C, Santinelli V, Rosanio S, Vicedomini G, Nardi S, Pappone A, Tortoriello V, Manguso F, Mazzone P, Gulletta S, Oreto G, Alfieri O. Usefulness of invasive electrophysiologic testing to stratify the risk of arrhythmic events in asymptomatic patients with Wolff-Parkinson-White pattern: results from a large prospective long-term follow-up study. J Am Coll Cardiol. 2003;41(2):239–44.
14. Mehta D, Wafa S, Ward DE, Camm AJ. Relative efficacy of various physical manoeuvres in the termination of junctional tachycardia. Lancet. 1988;1(8596):1181–5.
15. Tijunelis MA, Herbert ME. Myth: intravenous amiodarone is safe in patients with atrial fibrillation and Wolff-Parkinson-White syndrome in the emergency department. CJEM. 2005 Jul;7(4):262–5.
16. Simonian SM, Lotfipour S, Wall C, Langdorf MI. Challenging the superiority of amiodarone for rate control in Wolff-Parkinson-White and atrial fibrillation. Intern Emerg Med. 2010;5(5):421–6.

Correction to: Peripartum Cardiomyopathy. *"Babies Are Breaking My Heart"!*

Meenal Sharkey and Natasha Boydstun

Correction to:
C. G. Kaide, C. E. San Miguel (eds.), *Case Studies in Emergency Medicine*
https://doi.org/10.1007/978-3-030-22445-5_50

Dr. Natasha Boydstun's name had been misspelt throughout in the original version of the book. This has now been corrected.

The updated online version of this chapter can be found at
https://doi.org/10.1007/978-3-030-22445-5_50

Index

© Springer Nature Switzerland AG 2020
C. G. Kaide, C. E. San Miguel (eds.), *Case Studies in Emergency Medicine*,
https://doi.org/10.1007/978-3-030-22445-5

The manufacturer's authorised representative in the EU is Springer
Nature Customer Service Centre GmbH, Europaplatz 3, 69115 Heidelberg,
Germany. If you have any concerns regarding our products, please
contact ProductSafety@springernature.com

Printed and bound by CPI Group (UK) Ltd, Croydon, CR0 4YY
29/04/2026
02099451-0014